Advances in Retrovirology

Advances in Retrovirology

Edited by Adeline Foley

hayle
medical

New York

Hayle Medical,
750 Third Avenue, 9th Floor,
New York, NY 10017, USA

Visit us on the World Wide Web at:
www.haylemedical.com

This book contains information obtained from authentic and highly regarded sources. Copyright for all individual chapters remain with the respective authors as indicated. All chapters are published with permission under the Creative Commons Attribution License or equivalent. A wide variety of references are listed. Permission and sources are indicated; for detailed attributions, please refer to the permissions page and list of contributors. Reasonable efforts have been made to publish reliable data and information, but the authors, editors and publisher cannot assume any responsibility for the validity of all materials or the consequences of their use.

ISBN: 978-1-63241-796-1

Trademark Notice: Registered trademark of products or corporate names are used only for explanation and identification without intent to infringe.

Cataloging-in-Publication Data

Advances in retrovirology / edited by Adeline Foley.
   p. cm.
Includes bibliographical references and index.
ISBN 978-1-63241-796-1
1. Retroviruses. 2. Virology. 3. Virus diseases. 4. Medical virology.
5. Medical microbiology. I. Foley, Adeline.
QR414.5 .A38 2019
616.019--dc23

Table of Contents

Preface...VII

Chapter 1   Modulation of the functional association between the HIV-1 intasome
             and the nucleosome by histone amino-terminal tails 1
             Mohamed S. Benleulmi, Julien Matysiak, Xavier Robert, Csaba Miskey,
             Eric Mauro, Delphine Lapaillerie, Paul Lesbats, Stéphane Chaignepain,
             Daniel R. Henriquez, Christina Calmels, Oyindamola Oladosu,
             Eloïse Thierry, Oscar Leon, Marc Lavigne, Marie-Line Andreola,
             Olivier Delelis, Zoltán Ivics, Marc Ruff, Patrice Gouet and
             Vincent Parissi

Chapter 2   Importance of Fc-mediated functions of anti-HIV-1 broadly neutralizing
             antibodies...17
             Matthew S. Parsons, Amy W. Chung and Stephen J. Kent

Chapter 3   Predominant envelope variable loop 2-specific and gp120-specific
             antibody-dependent cellular cytotoxicity antibody responses in acutely
             SIV-infected African green monkeys 29
             Quang N. Nguyen, David R. Martinez, Jonathon E.Himes,
             R. Whitney Edwards, Qifeng Han, Amit Kumar, Riley Mangan,
             Nathan I. Nicely, Guanhua Xie, Nathan Vandergrift, Xiaoying Shen,
             Justin Pollara and Sallie R. Permar

Chapter 4   HIV latency reversing agents act through Tat post translational modifications............43
             Georges Khoury, Talia M. Mota, Shuang Li, Carolin Tumpach,
             Michelle Y. Lee, Jonathan Jacobson, Leigh Harty, Jenny L. Anderson,
             Sharon R. Lewin and Damian F. J. Purcell

Chapter 5   CD8$^+$ T cells specific for conserved, cross-reactive Gag epitopes with strong
             ability to suppress HIV-1 replication 60
             Hayato Murakoshi, Chengcheng Zou, Nozomi Kuse, Tomohiro Akahoshi,
             Takayuki Chikata, Hiroyuki Gatanaga, Shinichi Oka, Tomáš Hanke and
             Masafumi Takiguchi

Chapter 6   Rapid HIV disease progression following superinfection
             in an HLA-B*27:05/ B*57:01-positive transmission recipient 74
             Jacqui Brener, Astrid Gall, Jacob Hurst, Rebecca Batorsky,
             Nora Lavandier, Fabian Chen, Anne Edwards, Chrissy Bolton,
             Reena Dsouza, Todd Allen, Oliver G. Pybus, Paul Kellam,
             Philippa C. Matthews and Philip J. R. Goulder

Chapter 7   Engineering multi-specific antibodies against HIV-1 87
             Neal N. Padte, Jian Yu, Yaoxing Huang and David D. Ho

Chapter 8   **Reticuloendotheliosis virus and avian leukosis virus subgroup J synergistically increase the accumulation of exosomal miRNAs** 103
Defang Zhou, Jingwen Xue, Shuhai He, Xusheng Du, Jing Zhou, Chengui Li, Libo Huang, Venugopal Nair, Yongxiu Yao and Ziqiang Cheng

Chapter 9   **Selective resistance profiles emerging in patient-derived clinical isolates with cabotegravir, bictegravir, dolutegravir and elvitegravir** 113
Maureen Oliveira, Ruxandra-Ilinca Ibanescu, Kaitlin Anstett, Thibault Mésplède, Jean-Pierre Routy, Marjorie A. Robbins and Bluma G. Brenner

Chapter 10   **Pre-exposure prophylaxis (PrEP) in an era of stalled HIV prevention: Can it change the game?** 127
Robyn Eakle, Francois Venter and Helen Rees

Chapter 11   **The HIV-1 accessory proteins Nef and Vpu downregulate total and cell surface CD28 in CD4$^+$ T cells** 137
Emily N. Pawlak, Brennan S. Dirk, Rajesh Abraham Jacob, Aaron L. Johnson and Jimmy D. Dikeakos

Chapter 12   **Promoter expression of HERV-K (HML-2) provirus-derived sequences is related to LTR sequence variation and polymorphic transcription factor binding sites** 159
Meagan Montesion, Zachary H. Williams, Ravi P. Subramanian, Charlotte Kuperwasser and John M. Coffin

Chapter 13   **A CRISPR screen for factors regulating SAMHD1 degradation identifies IFITMs as potent inhibitors of lentiviral particle delivery** 175
Ferdinand Roesch, Molly OhAinle and Michael Emerman

Chapter 14   **Measuring integrated HIV DNA ex vivo and in vitro provides insights about how reservoirs are formed and maintained** 191
Marilia Rita Pinzone and Una O'Doherty

Chapter 15   **Myricetin antagonizes semen-derived enhancer of viral infection (SEVI) formation and influences its infection-enhancing activity** 203
Ruxia Ren, Shuwen Yin, Baolong Lai, Lingzhen Ma, Jiayong Wen, Xuanxuan Zhang, Fangyuan Lai, Shuwen Liu and Lin Li

Chapter 16   **Assessment of the gorilla gut virome in association with natural simian immunodeficiency virus infection** 227
Mirela D'arc, Carolina Furtado, Juliana D. Siqueira, Héctor N. Seuánez, Ahidjo Ayouba, Martine Peeters and Marcelo A. Soares

Permissions

List of Contributors

Index

Preface

The type of RNA virus, which inserts a copy of its genome into the DNA of a host cell that it invades, and changes the genome of that cell, is known as a retrovirus. Such type of viruses are classified as single-stranded positive-sense RNA viruses. The study of retroviruses is called retrovirology. On entering the host cell's cytoplasm, the retroviruses use their own reverse transcriptase enzyme to produce DNA from their RNA genome, which is the reverse or retro of the usual pattern. Then the new DNA incorporates into the host cell genome with the help of an integrase enzyme. Some retroviruses such as Rous sarcoma virus and mouse mammary tumor virus can trigger tumor growth. Some others can cause infections like HIV. This book aims to shed light on some of the unexplored aspects of retrovirology and the recent researches in this field. It traces the progress of this field and highlights some of its key concepts and applications. It will help the readers in keeping pace with the rapid changes in this field.

The researches compiled throughout the book are authentic and of high quality, combining several disciplines and from very diverse regions from around the world. Drawing on the contributions of many researchers from diverse countries, the book's objective is to provide the readers with the latest achievements in the area of research. This book will surely be a source of knowledge to all interested and researching the field.

In the end, I would like to express my deep sense of gratitude to all the authors for meeting the set deadlines in completing and submitting their research chapters. I would also like to thank the publisher for the support offered to us throughout the course of the book. Finally, I extend my sincere thanks to my family for being a constant source of inspiration and encouragement.

Editor

Preface

The type of RNA virus, which inserts a copy of its genome into the DNA of a host cell that it invades, and changes the genome of that cell, is known as a retrovirus. Such type of viruses are classified as single-stranded positive-sense RNA viruses. The study of retroviruses is called retrovirology. On entering the host cell's cytoplasm, the retroviruses use their own reverse transcriptase enzyme to produce DNA from their RNA genome, which is the reverse or retro of the usual pattern. Then the new DNA incorporates into the host cell genome with the help of an integrase enzyme. Some retroviruses such as Rous sarcoma virus and mouse mammary tumor virus can trigger tumor growth. Some others can cause infections like HIV. This book aims to shed light on some of the unexplored aspects of retrovirology and the recent researches in this field. It traces the progress of this field and highlights some of its key concepts and applications. It will help the readers in keeping pace with the rapid changes in this field.

The researches compiled throughout the book are authentic and of high quality, combining several disciplines and from very diverse regions from around the world. Drawing on the contributions of many researchers from diverse countries, the book's objective is to provide the readers with the latest achievements in the area of research. This book will surely be a source of knowledge to all interested and researching the field.

In the end, I would like to express my deep sense of gratitude to all the authors for meeting the set deadlines in completing and submitting their research chapters. I would also like to thank the publisher for the support offered to us throughout the course of the book. Finally, I extend my sincere thanks to my family for being a constant source of inspiration and encouragement.

Editor

Modulation of the functional association between the HIV-1 intasome and the nucleosome by histone amino-terminal tails

Mohamed S. Benleulmi[1,10†], Julien Matysiak[1,10†], Xavier Robert[2†], Csaba Miskey[3†], Eric Mauro[1,10], Delphine Lapaillerie[1,10,11], Paul Lesbats[1,10], Stéphane Chaignepain[4], Daniel R. Henriquez[5], Christina Calmels[1,10,11], Oyindamola Oladosu[6], Eloïse Thierry[7], Oscar Leon[5], Marc Lavigne[8,9,11], Marie-Line Andreola[1,10,11], Olivier Delelis[7,11], Zoltán Ivics[3], Marc Ruff[6,11], Patrice Gouet[2,11] and Vincent Parissi[1,10,11*]

Abstract

Background: Stable insertion of the retroviral DNA genome into host chromatin requires the functional association between the intasome (integrase·viral DNA complex) and the nucleosome. The data from the literature suggest that direct protein–protein contacts between integrase and histones may be involved in anchoring the intasome to the nucleosome. Since histone tails are candidates for interactions with the incoming intasomes we have investigated whether they could participate in modulating the nucleosomal integration process.

Results: We show here that histone tails are required for an optimal association between HIV-1 integrase (IN) and the nucleosome for efficient integration. We also demonstrate direct interactions between IN and the amino-terminal tail of human histone H4 in vitro. Structure/function studies enabled us to identify amino acids in the carboxy-terminal domain of IN that are important for this interaction. Analysis of the nucleosome-binding properties of catalytically active mutated INs confirmed that their ability to engage the nucleosome for integration in vitro was affected. Pseudovirus particles bearing mutations that affect the IN/H4 association also showed impaired replication capacity due to altered integration and re-targeting of their insertion sites toward dynamic regions of the chromatin with lower nucleosome occupancy.

Conclusions: Collectively, our data support a functional association between HIV-1 IN and histone tails that promotes anchoring of the intasome to nucleosomes and optimal integration into chromatin.

Keywords: Retroviral integration, HIV-1, Integrase, Chromatine, Nucleosome, Histone tails

Background

Retroviral integrases (INs) are key enzymes that catalyze the insertion of viral DNA into infected cells genome (for a recent review see [1]). Integration occurs in strongly preferred regions of the genome that depend on the virus. Although the IN is a major viral determinant in the integration site selection [2], cellular targeting factors such as BET or LEDGF/p75 proteins, which bind specific histone marks, also contribute to this process by interacting with the IN·viral DNA complex (i.e., the intasome) in these specific chromatin regions (reviewed in [3]). Additional parameters, such as the nuclear import pathway, the nuclear architecture and the interaction of cellular factors like CPSF6 with other viral components, also affect retroviral integration selectivity [4]. Thus, integration site selection is a multi-step process that first involves a global targeting of the intasome toward

*Correspondence: vincent.parissi@u-bordeaux.fr
†Mohamed S. Benleulmi, Julien Matysiak, Xavier Robert and Csaba Miskey have contributed equally to this work
[1] Fundamental Microbiology and Pathogenicity Laboratory, UMR 5234 CNRS-University of Bordeaux, SFR TransBioMed, 146 rue Léo Saignat, Bordeaux Cedex, France
Full list of author information is available at the end of the article

a suitable chromatin region via the association between IN and cellular factors, followed by local insertion step requiring IN-nucleosome interaction.

This final association between IN and its nucleosomal target substrate is a process governed by the intasome and nucleosomal DNA constraints and regulated by nucleosome density and remodeling activities [5–8]. Indeed, the data from the literature also indicate that while HIV-1 integration occurs at the surface of the nucleosomes, their compaction into dense chromatin limits efficient integration [6, 8]. We have previously shown that chromatin remodeling processes overcome this integration inhibition and favor HIV-1 integration [8]. Furthermore, we have recently reported that local nucleosome dissociation by the FACT histone chaperon generates chromatin structures favoring HIV-1 integration both in vitro and in cells [9]. Taken together these data suggest that additional contacts between the HIV-1 intasome and the nucleosome, which may be prevented during compaction and made accessible during chromatin remodeling, could be required for efficient integration. This hypothesis is supported by the cryoEM structure of the PFV intasome in complex with a mononucleosome showing direct interactions between IN protomers and histones [10]. Moreover, integration assays performed on DNA mini-circles (MCs) mimicking the nucleosomal DNA structure in the absence of histones also suggested that both this structure and additional IN/histone interactions can act in synergy during nucleosomal integration [11]. Consequently, due to the lack of information regarding the mechanisms of nucleosome capture by the HIV-1 intasome, we investigated the potential role of IN/histone interactions in regulating HIV-1 integration.

Using various biochemical and cellular approaches, we show that histone tails are required for efficient HIV-1 IN binding to nucleosomes and optimal integration. We also report that IN binds preferentially to the amino-terminal peptide tail of histone H4 (H4) in vitro and this binding is required for efficient functional interaction between the intasome and the nucleosome. Mutations affecting the IN/histone tail interaction also affect the integration step in cells. Consequently, our data lead us to conclude that the direct interaction between HIV-1 IN and histone tails may facilitate the tethering of the retroviral intasome to the nucleosomes for efficient integration into the host genome.

Results
Amino-terminal histone tails modulate the interaction between HIV-1 IN and the nucleosome in vitro
To determine whether the presence of histone tails was required for the association between HIV-1 IN and the nucleosome, we performed in vitro pull-down experiments using recombinant purified IN and either native human mononucleosomes (MNs) or tailless MNs (TL MNs) assembled on the previously described 147-bp W601 Widom sequence [12] biotinylated on its 5′ end (see the MN assembly analysis in Additional file 1: Figure S1). As shown in Fig. 1, IN exhibited different affinities for native MNs and TL MNs. Indeed, increasing salt concentrations decreased the association between IN and TL MNs more efficiently than the association between IN and native MNs (Fig. 1a, b). Similar results were obtained with the IN·LEDGF/p75 complex, indicating that this functional complex also required the presence of native tails for optimal association with the nucleosome (Fig. 1c). To better determine the contribution of each histone tail in the IN/MN binding, we next performed pull-down experiments with MNs assembled using octamers lacking the tails of either H4, H3, H2A or H2B. As shown in Fig. 1d, e, the efficiency of IN binding to the H4TL MNs was approximately 50–60% less efficient than for the native and other MN variants. Interestingly, the deletion of all the histone tails had a larger impact on IN/MN binding than deletion of the H4 tail only. This may indicate that several histone tails could participate together in the binding process, the histone H4 tail appearing the most important protein determinant of this binding. To further determine the impact of histone tails on active IN/viral DNA intasomes, we next performed functional integration assays using the different MN variants.

Amino-terminal histone tails modulate the integration into nucleosomes catalyzed by HIV-1 IN in vitro
The impact of histone tails on integration activity was then evaluated in in vitro integration assays. For this purpose, the quantitative assay schematized in Fig. 2a was set up using MNs immobilized on streptavidin beads, recombinant IN and a viral DNA donor carrying the 40/42 final base pairs of the HIV-1 U5 sequence (see the "Methods" section for the description of the donor DNA). Optimized reaction conditions set up in the presence of PEG and DMSO (see materials and methods section) were first used to allow analysis of IN activity in the absence of LEDGF. The quantification of the radioactivity that remained on the beads after the reaction, washing and deproteinization, allowed us to quantify the integration efficiency. Control experiments first showed that viral DNA integrated more efficiently into MNs than into naked DNA (Fig. 2b). This result confirmed very early data reporting that MNs are the preferred substrate for HIV-1 integration [13, 14] and validated our system. Integration kinetics experiments showed that viral DNA integrated less efficiently into TL MNs than into native MNs (Fig. 2c). Speed and efficiency of integration were also

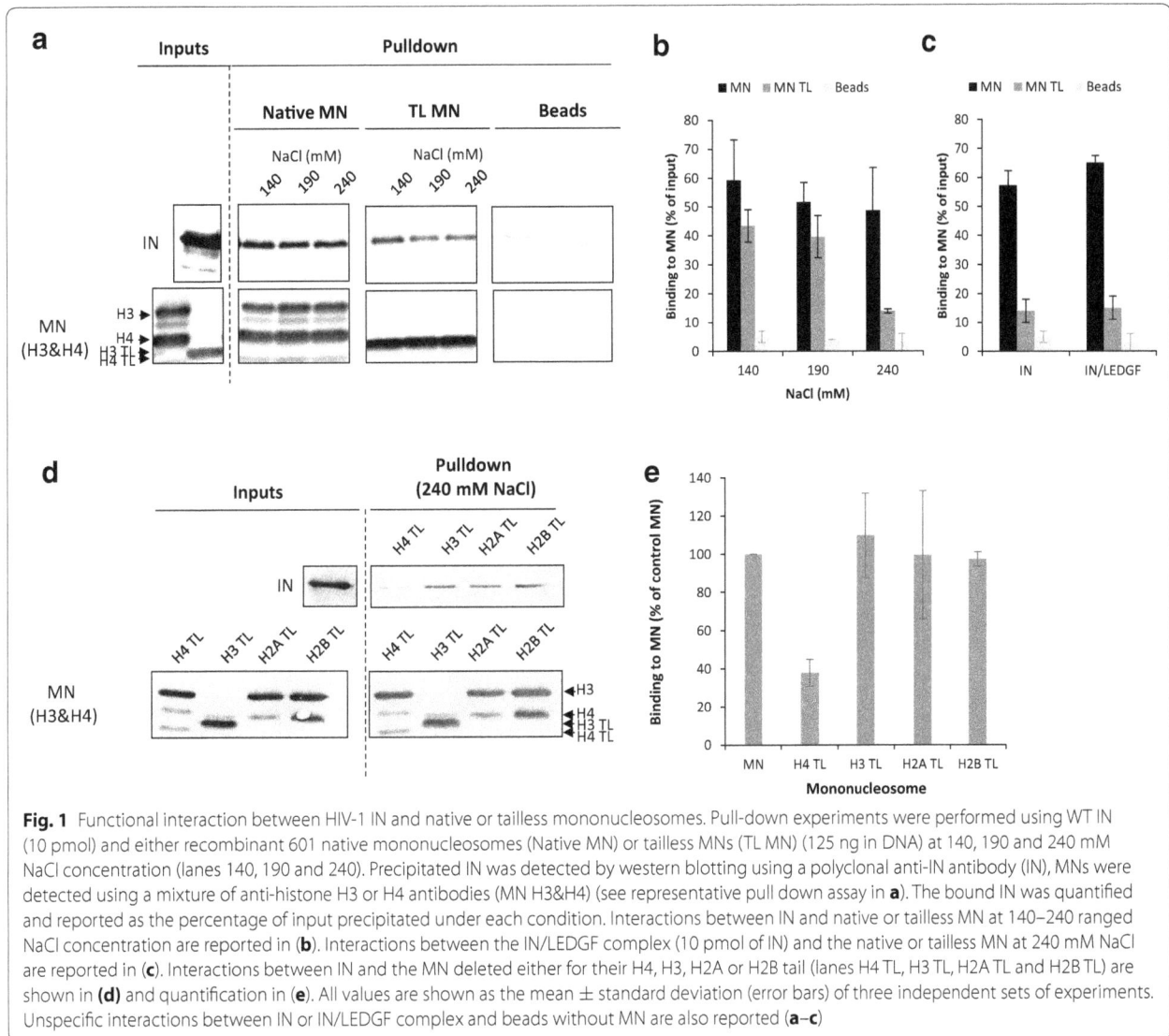

Fig. 1 Functional interaction between HIV-1 IN and native or tailless mononucleosomes. Pull-down experiments were performed using WT IN (10 pmol) and either recombinant 601 native mononucleosomes (Native MN) or tailless MNs (TL MN) (125 ng in DNA) at 140, 190 and 240 mM NaCl concentration (lanes 140, 190 and 240). Precipitated IN was detected by western blotting using a polyclonal anti-IN antibody (IN), MNs were detected using a mixture of anti-histone H3 or H4 antibodies (MN H3&H4) (see representative pull down assay in **a**). The bound IN was quantified and reported as the percentage of input precipitated under each condition. Interactions between IN and native or tailless MN at 140–240 ranged NaCl concentration are reported in (**b**). Interactions between the IN/LEDGF complex (10 pmol of IN) and the native or tailless MN at 240 mM NaCl are reported in (**c**). Interactions between IN and the MN deleted either for their H4, H3, H2A or H2B tail (lanes H4 TL, H3 TL, H2A TL and H2B TL) are shown in (**d**) and quantification in (**e**). All values are shown as the mean ± standard deviation (error bars) of three independent sets of experiments. Unspecific interactions between IN or IN/LEDGF complex and beads without MN are also reported (**a–c**)

decreased when H4TL MNs were used, but to a lesser extent. Notably, integration efficiency was found to be lower when using TL MNs than when using H4TL MNs, suggesting that several histone tails could act in concert for optimal integration as suggested by the binding data. Deletion of the H3 tail slightly increased the integration efficiency, while deletion of the tails of other histone variants had no significant effect on the global integration efficiency. The presence of LEDGF/p75 did not alter the effect of histone tail deletion on integration under these conditions (Fig. 2d) and even when non-optimized reactions allowing a maximal LEDGF/p75 stimulatory effect were used (i.e. without PEG and DMSO, Additional file 1: Figure S2).

Taken together, these data indicate that native amino-terminal histone tails are required for optimal IN binding to MNs and efficient integration in vitro. Binding

experiments between IN and histone tails were next performed to further investigate whether this integration modulation could be due to such direct interactions.

Interaction between HIV-1 IN and histone amino-terminal peptide tails

Possible direct interactions between HIV-1 IN and histone tails were analyzed using a far dot blot approach with recombinant IN and peptides derived from the H3, H4, H2A and H2B amino-terminal tail (see peptide sequences in Additional file 1: Figure S3). As reported in Fig. 3a and quantification in b, interaction was significantly detected only in the presence of the histone H4 tail. Similar results were obtained with the purified IN·LEDGF/p75 complex, indicating that the LEDGF/p75 cofactor did not affect IN binding to the peptide (Fig. 3c). Additional analyzes showed that the IN/H4 tail

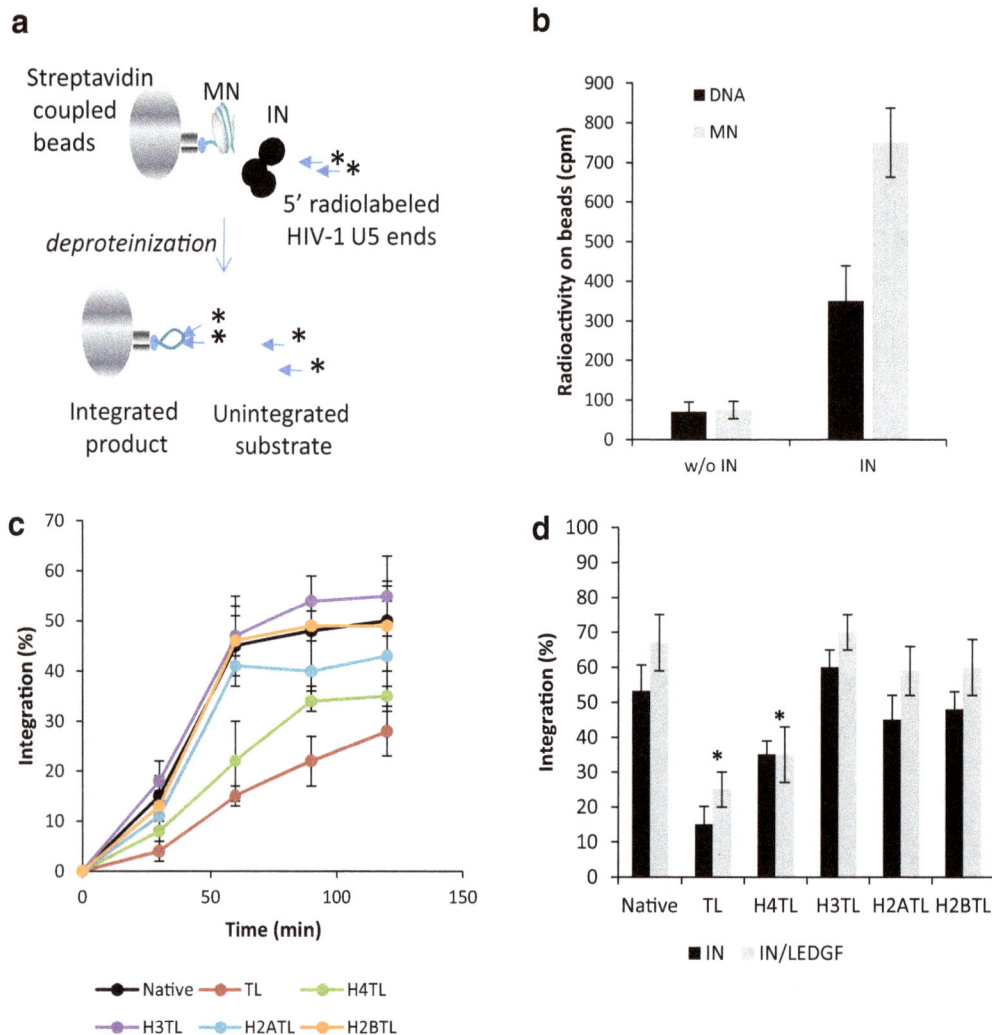

Fig. 2 In vitro Integration onto mononucleosomes. Either the 5′ biotinylated naked 601 DNA fragment or the native MNs (50 ng in DNA) were coupled to streptavidin beads and incubated with HIV-1 WT IN (400 nM) under integration conditions reported in the "Methods" section (**a**). After 0–2 h incubations the samples were deprotenized and washed after beads magnetization, then radioactivity was measured on both the pellet and supernatant. Quantification of the radioactivity remaining on beads after reaction performed with naked 601 DNA or MN and with or without IN is reported (**b**). The percentage of integrated product over time for each MN construct was reported in (**c**). Comparison of data obtained with IN alone and IN/LEDGF complex is reported in (**d**). All values are shown as the mean ± standard deviation (error bars) of three to four independent sets of experiments. The p values were calculated by Student's t-test and are shown as *p < 0.05 to represent the probability of obtaining significant differences compared with the data obtained with the native MNs control

interaction could be negatively or positively modulated by amino acid modifications as methylation of K20 or K20 or K16 acetylation (Additional file 1: Figure S4).

The far dot blot approach was then adapted to compare different IN truncation mutants in order to identify the IN domains involved in the interaction to H4 tail. Under these conditions, the engineered IN 50–288 amino acid construct lacking the amino-terminal domain (ΔNTD) and the isolated 220–288 amino acid CTD domain construct (CTD) show similar binding properties when compared to the wild-type (WT) enzyme (Fig. 3d). By contrast, the association with the histone H4 tail was

almost completely abolished for the 1-212 amino acid construct lacking the carboxy-terminal domain (ΔCTD). These results show that the CTD domain is responsible for the interaction between IN and histone tail. In order to study the role of this interaction in the integration process we further searched for specific amino-acids mutations that could affect the IN binding to the tail.

Identification of IN mutations affecting the binding to histone H4 tail

We first adopted an in silico blind docking simulation approach starting from a fragment spanning residues

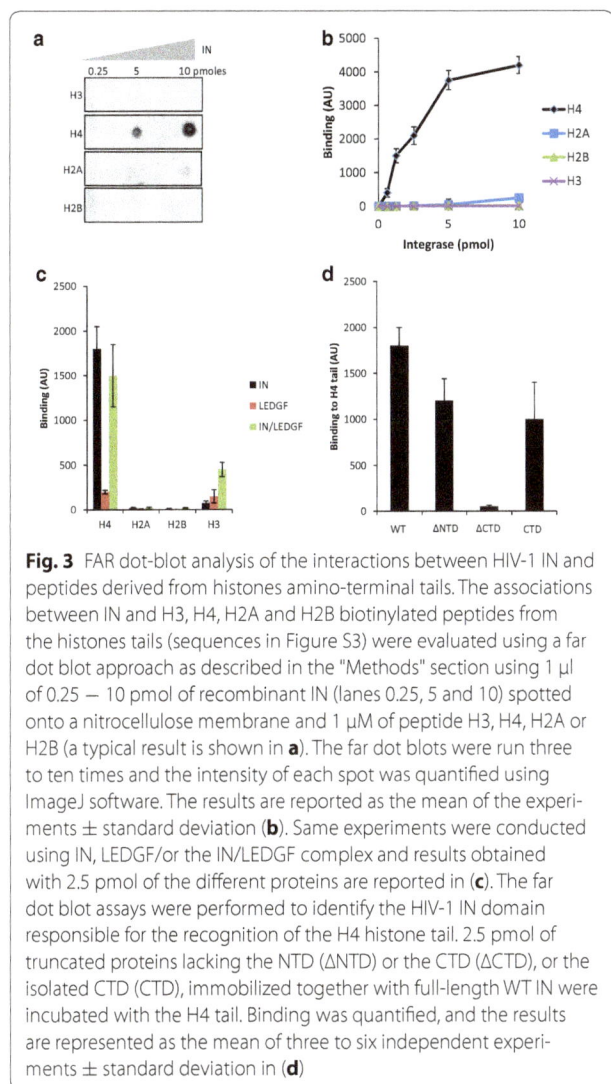

Fig. 3 FAR dot-blot analysis of the interactions between HIV-1 IN and peptides derived from histones amino-terminal tails. The associations between IN and H3, H4, H2A and H2B biotinylated peptides from the histones tails (sequences in Figure S3) were evaluated using a far dot blot approach as described in the "Methods" section using 1 µl of 0.25 − 10 pmol of recombinant IN (lanes 0.25, 5 and 10) spotted onto a nitrocellulose membrane and 1 µM of peptide H3, H4, H2A or H2B (a typical result is shown in **a**). The far dot blots were run three to ten times and the intensity of each spot was quantified using ImageJ software. The results are reported as the mean of the experiments ± standard deviation (**b**). Same experiments were conducted using IN, LEDGF/or the IN/LEDGF complex and results obtained with 2.5 pmol of the different proteins are reported in (**c**). The far dot blot assays were performed to identify the HIV-1 IN domain responsible for the recognition of the H4 histone tail. 2.5 pmol of truncated proteins lacking the NTD (ΔNTD) or the CTD (ΔCTD), or the isolated CTD (CTD), immobilized together with full-length WT IN were incubated with the H4 tail. Binding was quantified, and the results are represented as the mean of three to six independent experiments ± standard deviation in (**d**)

210–270 from the 2.8 Å resolution HIV-1 IN CCD-CTD structure [15] and a pentapeptide mimicking the 18–22 residues from the H4K20me1-modified histone ($H_{18}RK_{me}VL$), which corresponds to the best IN binder in the previous analyzes (see Additional file 1: Figure S4). In the first set of experiments, the AutoDock and AutoDockVina programs were used in parallel to determine a potential binding region based on a blind docking analysis of the entire surface of the receptor, namely, the IN CTD fragment, which was treated as rigid. Following a cluster analysis of all docked conformations computed by AutoDock, a potential binding site emerged in the HIV-1 IN CTD encompassing a V-shaped groove area delineated by loops 228–235 and 253–257 (one connecting strands β1 and β2 and the other connecting β3 and β4, respectively) (Fig. 4a). The resulting docking solution is compatible with the 3.9 Å resolution cryoEM structure of

the HIV-1 strand transfer complex (STC) intasome [16], in which the V-shaped CTD grooves are accessible in all the assembled IN protomers.

To determine the IN residues that may be involved in the CTD-H4 tail interaction, we focused on this latter region, where several amino acid side-chains surrounding the V-shaped groove of the receptor were treated as flexible (namely, Y227, D229, S230, R231, D232, L234, W235, K236, D253, N254, S255, D256, K258 and K264). RMSD cluster analysis of 1000 independent docking solutions using the AutoDock program allowed 56 distinct conformational groups to be defined. Considering the binding energies one solution stood out in particular, where the peptide was engaged in a total of 7 intermolecular hydrogen bonds (with the side-chains of D229, R231, S255, D256, and K258 and the backbone of L234 in the HIV-1 CTD) and 15 hydrophobic contacts (with the side-chains of Y227, D229, D232, K236, D256, K258 and V260 and the backbones of D229, S255 and D256). In this model, the peptide adopted an elongated shape at the surface of the IN CTD, with the H4K20me1 side-chain pointing down into the V-shaped groove, and formed 9 of the 16 predicted hydrophobic contacts (involving Y227, D229, K236, K258 and V260 HIV-1 CTD amino-acids residues) as well as one hydrogen bond (with D229) (Fig. 4a). Slight side-chain movements were observed to accommodate the pentapeptide, with the exception of R231 IN residue, whose side-chain flipped to form a hydrogen bond with H18 from histone 4 tail. This model was used to design a site-directed mutagenesis approach. The CTD domain has been shown to be involved in multiple functions during the viral life cycle, including interactions with reverse transcriptase and target DNA [17–19]. This made it difficult to generate CTD mutants that only affected histone binding. We focused on amino acids Y227, D229, R231, W235, K236 and D253, which were expected (1) to be located in the V-shaped groove of the IN CTD and (2) to be involved directly or indirectly in modulating the interaction. Alanine, glycine or histidine substitutions were introduced at the chosen positions to test peptide binding. The D232G substitution was also included because it represents a natural polymorphism in HIV-1 IN.

All mutants were purified, and their overall functional structures were examined in in vitro concerted integration assay. As shown in Additional file 1: Figure S5, the Y227A and W235A mutations severely affected integration (90–70% loss of activity). The K236A and D229G mutations also influenced IN catalysis, but to a lesser extent (20–40% loss). By contrast, the D232G, R231G/A/H and D253H proteins were fully active. A far dot blot assay was the used to determine the ability of the mutants to bind to and recognize the histone H4 tail. The

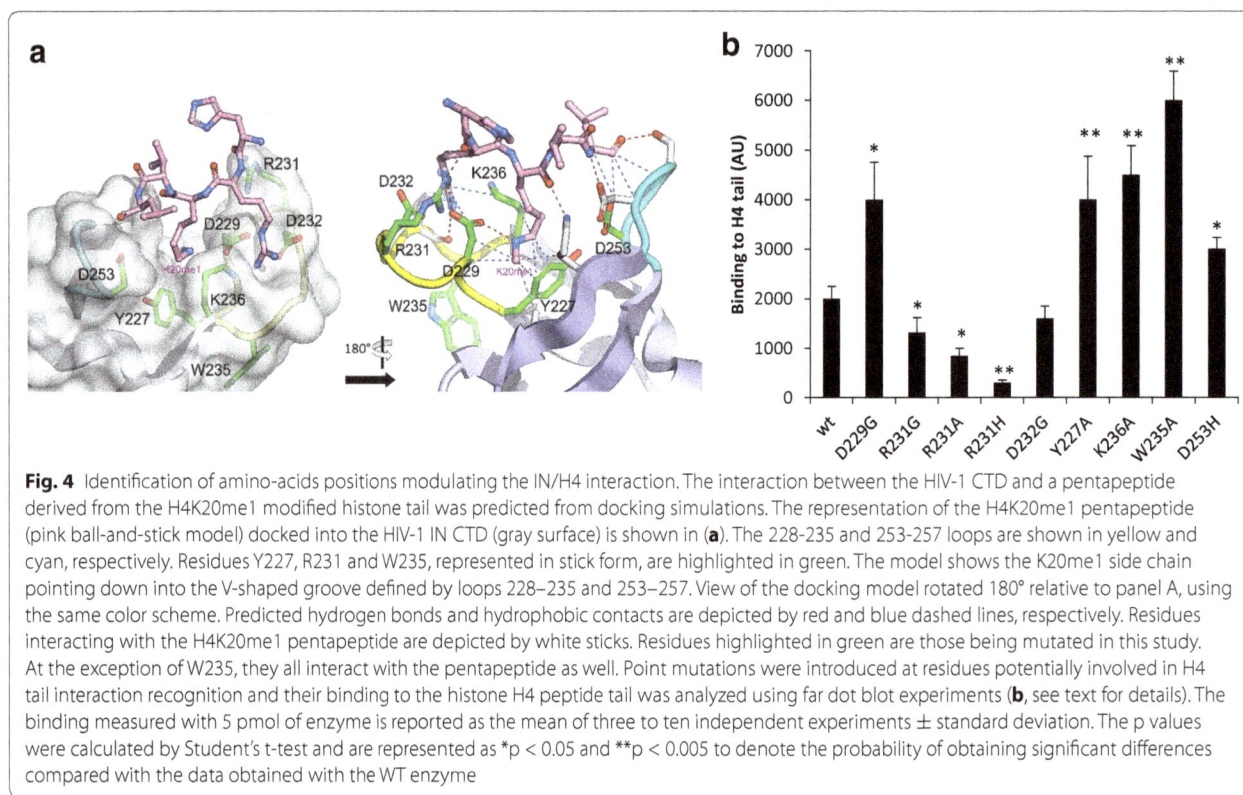

Fig. 4 Identification of amino-acids positions modulating the IN/H4 interaction. The interaction between the HIV-1 CTD and a pentapeptide derived from the H4K20me1 modified histone tail was predicted from docking simulations. The representation of the H4K20me1 pentapeptide (pink ball-and-stick model) docked into the HIV-1 IN CTD (gray surface) is shown in (**a**). The 228-235 and 253-257 loops are shown in yellow and cyan, respectively. Residues Y227, R231 and W235, represented in stick form, are highlighted in green. The model shows the K20me1 side chain pointing down into the V-shaped groove defined by loops 228–235 and 253–257. View of the docking model rotated 180° relative to panel A, using the same color scheme. Predicted hydrogen bonds and hydrophobic contacts are depicted by red and blue dashed lines, respectively. Residues interacting with the H4K20me1 pentapeptide are depicted by white sticks. Residues highlighted in green are those being mutated in this study. At the exception of W235, they all interact with the pentapeptide as well. Point mutations were introduced at residues potentially involved in H4 tail interaction recognition and their binding to the histone H4 peptide tail was analyzed using far dot blot experiments (**b**, see text for details). The binding measured with 5 pmol of enzyme is reported as the mean of three to ten independent experiments ± standard deviation. The p values were calculated by Student's t-test and are represented as *p < 0.05 and **p < 0.005 to denote the probability of obtaining significant differences compared with the data obtained with the WT enzyme

R231G/A/H mutants showed a decrease in their overall binding to the H4 amino-terminal tail (30, 44 and 77%, respectively; Fig. 4b). Additionally, the binding properties of the D232G mutant were virtually unaffected, whereas D229G showed a global increase in H4 tail affinity. Conversely, the Y227A, W235A, K236A and D253H mutants displayed a significant increase in affinity for the histone H4 tail.

In summary, most of the designed mutations, except the natural D232G variant, significantly affected the IN binding to the H4 tail suggesting that the corresponding amino-acids position modulate the IN/H4 interaction directly or indirectly. The identified mutants were then used to further investigate the role of the IN/H4 interaction in the association with nucleosomes.

Effect of mutations affecting IN binding to H4 on the functional interaction with nucleosomes in vitro

To avoid any biases in the analysis of the MN-binding properties of the mutated INs due to the alteration of IN-DNA interaction, we first evaluated their DNA-binding properties by pull-down experiments using the naked W601 fragment. The Y227A, W235A and K236A mutants each showed decreased affinity for DNA (Additional file 1: Figure S6), which correlates well with their relative levels of in vitro integration activity. Consequently, we

excluded these enzymes from the MN interaction studies, and the mutants that showed unaffected DNA-binding capability were further analyzed for their capacity to associate with MNs.

As shown in Fig. 5a (see detailed analysis in Additional file 1: S6), the R231A/H mutants showed a significant decrease in MN binding affinity, which parallels their reduced affinity for the histone tail. The R231G mutant also had a decreased affinity for MN, but to a lesser extent, as a significant decrease in IN/MN binding was detected only at NaCl concentrations above 190 mM. By contrast, the D229G and D253H mutants, which showed an increased affinity for the H4 histone tail, also showed increased binding to MNs. The MN-binding capabilities of the natural D232G variant were not significantly affected. We next tested the effect of the mutations on the catalysis of integration into nucleosomes.

In vitro integration assays were performed using the recombinant W601 MNs used in the pull-down experiments (Fig. 5b). Control experiments performed with the unassembled W601 DNA fragment confirmed that the ability of the mutants to catalyze integration into naked DNA was not affected. In contrast, the R231G/A/H IN mutants exhibited a 25–60% decrease in efficiency of integration into MNs, and the D253H mutant was 20–40% more active than the WT enzyme. This result finely correlates with the capability of the

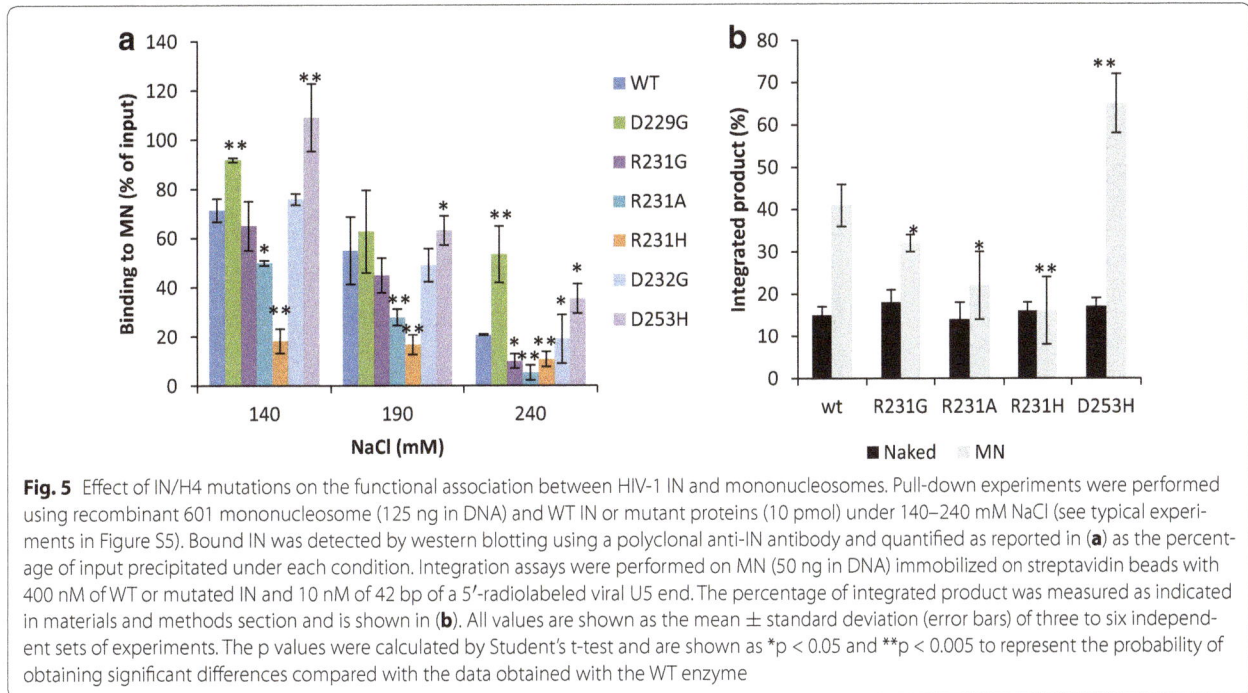

Fig. 5 Effect of IN/H4 mutations on the functional association between HIV-1 IN and mononucleosomes. Pull-down experiments were performed using recombinant 601 mononucleosome (125 ng in DNA) and WT IN or mutant proteins (10 pmol) under 140–240 mM NaCl (see typical experiments in Figure S5). Bound IN was detected by western blotting using a polyclonal anti-IN antibody and quantified as reported in (**a**) as the percentage of input precipitated under each condition. Integration assays were performed on MN (50 ng in DNA) immobilized on streptavidin beads with 400 nM of WT or mutated IN and 10 nM of 42 bp of a 5'-radiolabeled viral U5 end. The percentage of integrated product was measured as indicated in materials and methods section and is shown in (**b**). All values are shown as the mean ± standard deviation (error bars) of three to six independent sets of experiments. The p values were calculated by Student's t-test and are shown as *p < 0.05 and **p < 0.005 to represent the probability of obtaining significant differences compared with the data obtained with the WT enzyme

different INs to bind the H4 tail/MNs and fully supports our hypothesis that the binding to the tail is required for optimal integration into MNs in vitro. Therefore, we next investigated the impact of this IN/H4 interaction in a viral context.

Effect of IN/H4 mutations on viral infectivity and integration efficiency

Retroviral vectors carrying the selected R231G/A/H and D253H IN mutations, which modified the IN/H4 interaction without affecting the intrinsic IN catalytic properties, were produced, and their early replication steps were examined. The infectivity of the mutants was compared to that of WT vectors using a single-round infection assay performed in 293T cells. As shown in Fig. 6a, the infectivity of the R231G/A/H viruses was reduced by 20, 40 and 60% when compared with the WT virus, respectively. By contrast, the D253H mutation showed a 40–60% increase in viral infectivity.

The replication stages affected by the mutations were further characterized by comparing the viral DNA population size of the mutants to that of the known catalytically inactive D116A integrase (class I mutant, Fig. 6b). Under these conditions, viral cDNA production was found to be unaffected in all the viruses, indicating that there was no significant defect in the reverse transcription step, in contrast to the results observed with RT inhibition (AZT treatment). By contrast, the amount of integrated viral DNA detected for the R231G/A/H mutants was reduced by approximately 25, 60 and 80%,

respectively, with a characteristic accumulation of 2-LTR circles over time, which is indicative of normal nuclear import of the pre-integration complex. However, the D253H mutant showed a 20–40% increase in the amount of integrated DNA compared with the WT levels. This increase was associated with a decrease in the quantity of 2-LTR circles, indicating that the integration step was more efficient for this mutant, as confirmed by time-course analyses.

According to the biochemical data, one explanation for these replication phenotypes was a change in the functional association between the mutants intasomes and the chromatine/nucleosomes. To further investigate this hypothesis we next analyzed the chromatin structures surrounding the integration loci.

Effect of IN/H4 mutations on genomic integration sites selection

K562 cells were chosen because chromatin features, including histone modifications and nucleosome positions, are well annotated in this cell line. When K562 cells were transduced with lentiviruses carrying the D253H, R231G, R231A and R231H IN versions, we detected a decrease in transduction efficiency of approximately 20, 30 and 60% for the R231G/A/H mutants, respectively, and an increase in efficiency of approximately 40% for the D253H mutant compared with the WT enzyme (Fig. 7a and DNA population analyzes in Additional file 1: Figure S7). Three days post-transduction, the isolated genomic

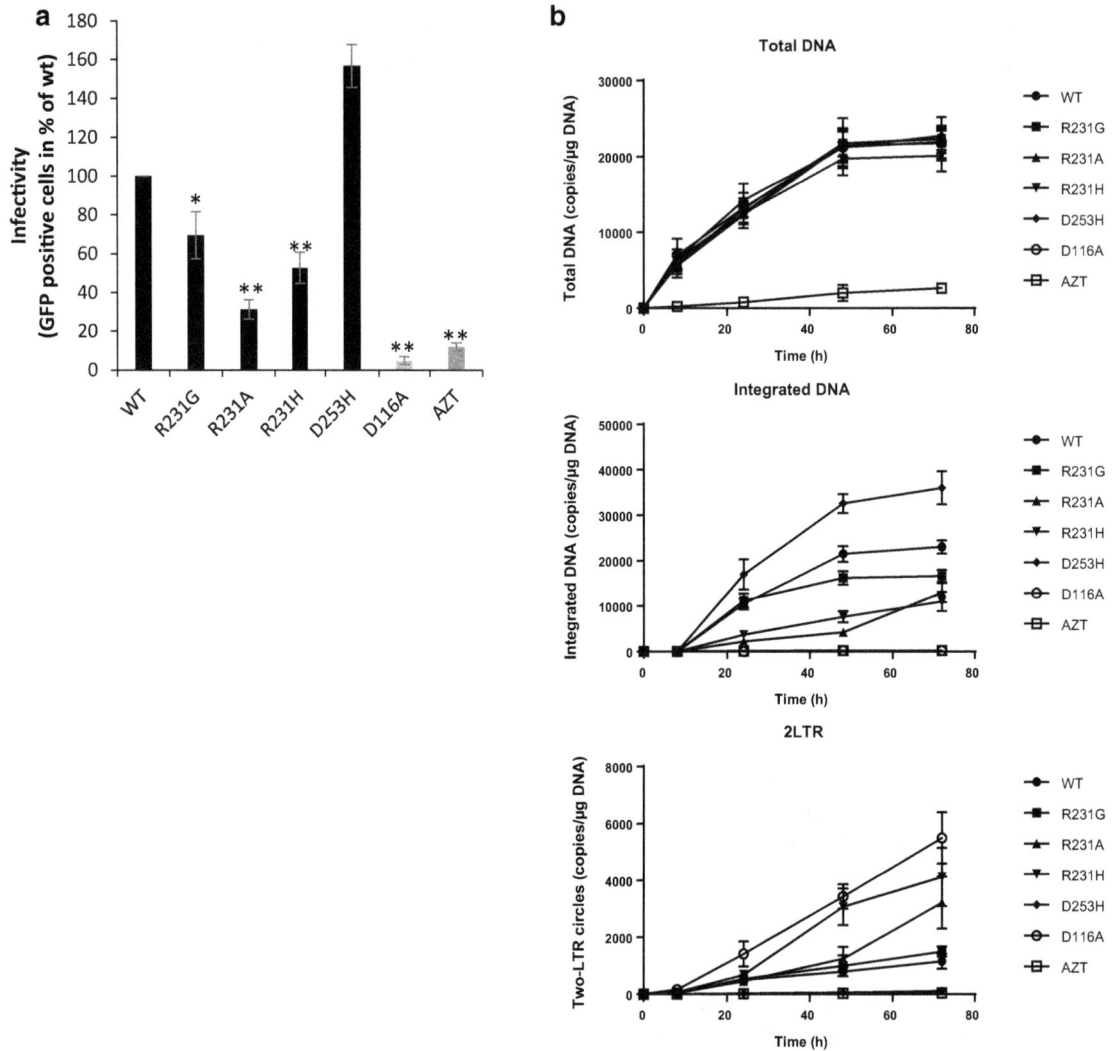

Fig. 6 Effects of mutations affecting the IN/H4 interaction during early steps of viral replication. HEK-293T cells were transduced with VSV-G pseudotyped lentiviruses encoding either WT IN or the R231A/H/G or D253H IN mutants or the catalytically inactive class I D116A mutant with or without AZT 1 µM. Viral replication was quantified based on eGFP fluorescence measured by FACS 48 h post-transduction. The data shown in (**a**) are expressed as the percentage of eGFP-positive cells at a MOI of 1. The replication steps affected by the mutations were determined by measuring the amounts of the different viral DNA species produced using qPCR. Levels of total viral DNA, integrated DNA and 2-LTR circles shown respectively in (**b**) were monitored between 0 and 72 h post-transduction to check for potential defects at the steps of reverse transcription, integration and nuclear import of the preintegration complex, respectively. The data are represented as the mean of at least three independent experiments ± standard deviation. The p-values were calculated by Student's t-test and are shown as *p < 0.05 and **p < 0.005 to represent the probability of obtaining significant differences compared with the WT data

DNA samples of the transduced cells were subjected to integration sites library preparation and high-throughput sequencing.

Between 4638 and 13,931 independent integration sites were obtained and analyzed. In agreement with previous findings [20, 21], analyses using genome-wide histone modification data obtained from ChIP-seq experiments performed on the chromatin of K562 cells showed that the WT insertion sites were underrepresented in heterochromatin (H3K27me3-enriched regions) and highly associated with histone marks characteristic of active transcription and open chromatin, including H3K36me3 (Additional file 1: Figure S8). We detected no significant differences in the distribution of the integration sites of the WT and the mutant INs in chromatin segments with various histone marks. By contrast, the insertion sites of the R231G/A/H mutants were more frequently localized in intragenic regions than those of the WT and D253H vectors (p value = 2.53E−4, 3.68E−11 and 1.68E−10,

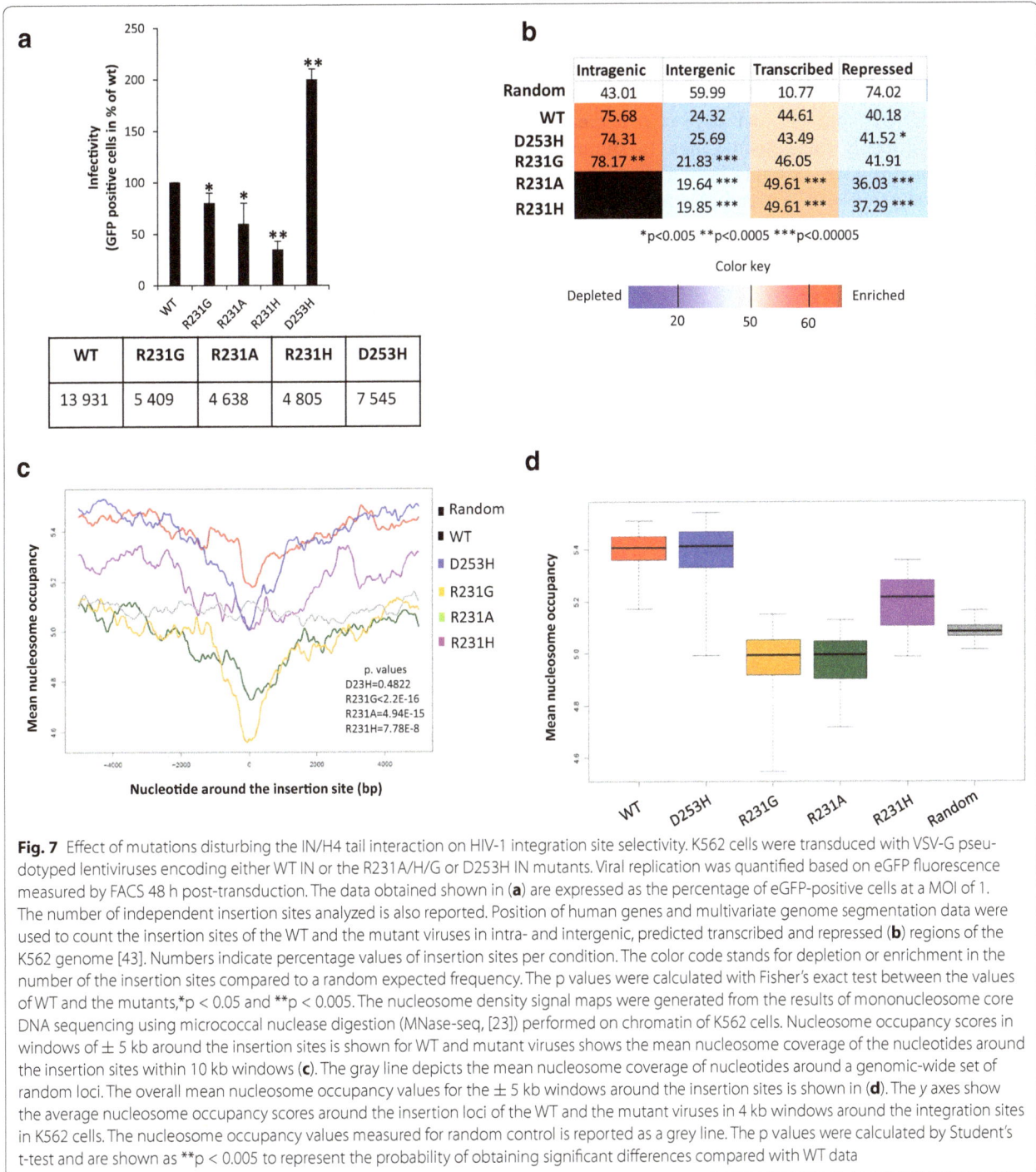

Fig. 7 Effect of mutations disturbing the IN/H4 tail interaction on HIV-1 integration site selectivity. K562 cells were transduced with VSV-G pseudotyped lentiviruses encoding either WT IN or the R231A/H/G or D253H IN mutants. Viral replication was quantified based on eGFP fluorescence measured by FACS 48 h post-transduction. The data obtained shown in (**a**) are expressed as the percentage of eGFP-positive cells at a MOI of 1. The number of independent insertion sites analyzed is also reported. Position of human genes and multivariate genome segmentation data were used to count the insertion sites of the WT and the mutant viruses in intra- and intergenic, predicted transcribed and repressed (**b**) regions of the K562 genome [43]. Numbers indicate percentage values of insertion sites per condition. The color code stands for depletion or enrichment in the number of the insertion sites compared to a random expected frequency. The p values were calculated with Fisher's exact test between the values of WT and the mutants,*p < 0.05 and **p < 0.005. The nucleosome density signal maps were generated from the results of mononucleosome core DNA sequencing using micrococcal nuclease digestion (MNase-seq, [23]) performed on chromatin of K562 cells. Nucleosome occupancy scores in windows of ± 5 kb around the insertion sites is shown for WT and mutant viruses shows the mean nucleosome coverage of the nucleotides around the insertion sites within 10 kb windows (**c**). The gray line depicts the mean nucleosome coverage of nucleotides around a genomic-wide set of random loci. The overall mean nucleosome occupancy values for the ± 5 kb windows around the insertion sites is shown in (**d**). The y axes show the average nucleosome occupancy scores around the insertion loci of the WT and the mutant viruses in 4 kb windows around the integration sites in K562 cells. The nucleosome occupancy values measured for random control is reported as a grey line. The p values were calculated by Student's t-test and are shown as **p < 0.005 to represent the probability of obtaining significant differences compared with WT data

respectively), and the R231 mutants integrated less frequently in intergenic territories (p value = 1.15E−5, 3.3E−13 and 1.6E−12 for R231G, R231A and R231H, respectively; Fig. 7b). Additionally, the R231A/H integrase substitutions resulted in a significant increase of approximately 5% in the representations of the

integrants in transcribed regions compared with those of the WT and D253H versions (p value = 3.91E−9 and 1.67E−8, respectively). Concordantly, integration sites of the R231A/H mutants were less frequently found in repressed genomic territories (p value = 1.72E−20 and 3.51E−15, respectively). In these analyses, the R231G mutant presented an intermediate state, as its preference for intragenic regions and transcribed genes was also affected, but to a lesser extent. Interestingly, the D253H mutant exhibited a trend opposite to that of the R231G/A/H mutants and showed a decreased preference for highly transcribed genes. In summary, we found that the R231 mutants have a stronger bias toward actively transcribed chromatin segments than the WT virus. Since the level of transcription is positively correlated with chromatin accessibility [22], we next studied the nucleosome content of the chromatin neighboring the insertion sites.

The nucleosome occupancy of the chromatin around the insertion loci was analyzed using the results of mononucleosome core DNA sequencing (MNase-seq [23]) performed on chromatin from K562 cells [22]. Similar to previous results [6, 8], measuring nucleosome occupancy in windows of $\pm$ 5 kb around the insertion sites showed that insertions of the WT vectors occurred in nucleosome-rich chromatin and that this preference declined toward the immediate insertion locus (Fig. 7c). We also found a lower mean nucleosome occupancy in the chromatin region around the R231G/A/R IN insertions sites with regards to the chromatin region surrounding the WT insertions (Wilcoxon test, $p_{R231G} < 2.2E-16$, $p_{R231A} = 4.94E-15$, $p_{R231H} = 7.78E-8$; Fig. 7c, d). These results suggest that the above vectors carrying IN/H4-disrupting mutations are less biased toward nucleosome-rich target DNA.

Since recent data suggest that residues in the HIV-1 CTD are involved in target DNA binding and recognition [7, 16, 24], we analyzed the nucleotide composition of the integration sites of the mutants. No major changes in the known weak consensus sequence of target site nucleotides typical of the WT IN were detected (Additional file 1: Figure S9). These findings, together with the results of the integration catalysis and DNA binding assays in vitro, argue against the possibility that the altered IN/target DNA interaction is responsible for the changes in the insertion site patterns of the mutants.

Altogether, our findings suggest that mutations disrupting the IN/H4 interaction may decrease the ability of the mutated INto bind and functionally integrate within nucleosomes. This would explain the shift of insertion patterns toward more accessible, dynamic and nucleosome-sparse chromatin regions.

Discussion

Using multiple complementary approaches, we demonstrated that the presence of histone tails is required for efficient HIV-1 integration into nucleosomes. Additionally, we report here that HIV-1 IN binds histone amino-terminal tails, with a significant preference for the H4 tail. This interaction was shown to be required for efficient interaction with nucleosomes and optimal integration in vitro. Docking calculations, mutagenesis studies and binding analyses enabled us to identify several amino acid positions in the CTD of HIV-1 IN, more precisely in its V-groove, that modulate the interaction between IN and the histone tail. Analysis of the nucleosome-binding properties of the selected mutants and their capability to integrate into nucleosomes showed strong correlations between their ability to bind to the H4 tail and to nucleosomes and their ability to catalyze efficient integration into nucleosomes.

Functional analyses showed that mutations preventing the IN/H4 association also reduced viral infectivity and partly impaired the integration process. A simplest explanation for this phenotype is a deficiency in the interaction between IN and a cellular cofactor. Because all of the mutated enzymes in this study were able to interact with LEDGF/p75 (data not shown), we propose that the loss of the interaction between IN and the histone tails, leading to a loss of interaction with the nucleosome, was directly responsible for the observed integration deficiency. Importantly, the LEDGF/p75 IN cofactor did not affect IN/H4 binding or its effect on MN association and integration. This indicates that the IN/LEDGF and IN/H4 interactions may occur simultaneously, which further suggests the physiological role of this histone interaction. This is also supported by the cellular data indicating that mutations preventing the IN/H4 interaction redirect integration into genes and more dynamic regions of the chromatin. Recent studies have also reported mutations in the CTD that redirect integration. Notably, the R231G polymorphism showed more pronounced integration into GeneSeq genes but in less gene-dense and transcribed regions of the host chromatin [24]. While the redirection of this mutant into genes appears to be consistent with our data, the difference in the preference for less transcribed regions could result from differences between our and the published experimental conditions.

Interestingly, the phenotype reported in our work is reminiscent of that observed for PFV IN, which was recently reported to bind to nucleosomes via the direct interaction of IN with histones, namely, the H2A/H2B dimer surface [10]. Indeed, in both cases, PFV and HIV-1 mutants exhibiting impaired binding to MNs also showed impaired integration and an increased preference for transcribed genes and lower nucleosome occupancy regions ([10] and this work, see Fig. 7). Consequently, these data support the hypothesis that the direct binding of retroviral INto human histones contributes to optimal integration. Retroviral intasomes may have developed various histone-binding mechanisms involving different intasome organizations.

Although several amino acid positions that modulate the HIV-1 IN/H4 interaction, including Y227, D229, R231, K236 and D253, have been identified, the putative histone-binding site has yet to be fully mapped using structural approaches. Indeed, although the mutations introduced in these positions clearly affect the association between IN and histone H4, we cannot conclude at this stage whether these positions are indirectly or directly involved in the interaction. Furthermore, the CTD has also been reported to bind target DNA [7] 33) and reverse transcriptase [17–19], making it difficult to discriminate between these pleiotropic functions and histone binding. Interestingly, the analysis of the cryoEM structure of the HIV-1 STC intasome [16] indicated that the histone tail binding site is accessible in the CTDs of all assembled IN protomers (Additional file 1: Figure S10). The CTDs of the two inner protomers contact the host DNA and are the best candidates for histone tail binding. This observation remains to be verified for the two synaptic CTDs of the lentiviral maedi-visna virus (MMV) STC intasome, whose hexadecameric 4.9 Å resolution cryoEM structure reflects a plausible higher macromolecular assembly for HIV-1 IN [25]. Additionally, these recent structural data also indicate that lentiviral integration is mediated by supramolecular complexes involving a hexadecamer of IN [16, 25]. Thus, these structures show that (1) a CTD within the catalytic protomers can interact with both target DNA and the H4 tail and (2) although some CTDs of the intasome are clearly engaged with target DNA, other CTDs from other non-catalytic protomers may be available for additional protein–protein contacts. For similar reasons, it remains difficult to discriminate between the effect of R231 mutations on target DNA binding, as previously reported [7, 24], and on histone binding as reported here. However, the effect of R231 mutations on nucleotide preferences within the target site has been shown to be considerably lower than that reported for analogous PFV mutations ([16] and our own data (Additional file 1: Figure S6)). This phenotype is better explained by the recently reported structure showing a weaker interaction between the R231 HIV-1 IN residue and target DNA compared with the homologous R229 residue of PFV IN [10, 16]. This is also confirmed by the results of our integration assays and DNA binding experiments reported in Additional file 1: Figures S5 and S6 showing that the catalytic properties of these R231 mutants are not significantly affected. Furthermore, using DNA MCs mimicking the nucleosomal DNA curvature in the absence of histones, we recently showed that mutations in the CTD residues involved in target DNA binding and recognition do not significantly affect their preference for specific DNA curvatures found at the

surface of the nucleosome [11]. These data suggest that the change in target nucleosomal DNA selectivity previously observed in vivo [24] likely does not solely result from a loss of target DNA structure recognition but also results from a possible additional interaction with other histone-like components, as reported in our work.

Our data provide also an explanation for the inhibition of HIV-1 integration in dense chromatin templates as previously reported [6, 8]. Indeed, in these polynucleosome templates, the H4 tail is known to interact with neighboring nucleosomes, and access to the tail can be modulated by several processes, such as local chromatin remodeling [26–28]. Interestingly, the integration-refractory property of dense chromatin can be overcome by such remodeling activity (6, 8). These data suggest that local nucleosome remodeling could be required for efficient integration by allowing additional protein/protein interactions between the incoming intasome and the nucleosome, such as the interactions between IN and histones reported herein. Moreover, we have recently shown that local remodeling by the FACT histone chaperone complex allows HIV-1 integration into poly-nucleosomes by generating partially dissociated nucleosomes which fully supports this hypothesis [9]. One direct effect of the chromatin remodeling by FACT would be thus to make accessible the H4 tails for interaction with the incoming intasomes.

Interestingly, the higher impact observed on in vitro integration when using tail less nucleosomes in comparison to H4 TL constructs suggests that several tails may act in synergy to modulate HIV-1 integration. Further structural determination of the intasome/nucleosome contacts by crystallography or cryo-electron microscopy, will be required to fully depict the role of each histone tails as well as histone core in the integration modulation in the context of the functional intasome/nucleosome complex.

Conclusion

The HIV-1 IN/H4 interaction reported in our work constitutes a new host/pathogen interaction important for the functional association between the incoming intasomes and the targeted nucleosome. Additional cellular processes and additional cellular protein factors, such as the recently discovered CPSF6 protein [39], participate also in regulating this multi-factorial mechanism. Consequently, optimal retroviral integration would result from an equilibrium being reached among efficient chromatin targeting, nucleosome anchoring and recognition of local DNA features. In this complex process, the interaction between IN and the H4 histone tail reported here could be an additional important determinant and, thus, constitute a potential novel therapeutic target.

Methods

Proteins, peptides and antibodies

Wild type (WT), mutated full-length and His-tagged truncated HIV-1 INs were purified as previously reported [6, 29]. GST-tagged HIV-1 IN CTD (220–288 amino-acids) was expressed in *Escherichia coli* BL21 cells (DE3) [29]. LEDGF/p75 and IN·LEDGF complex were purified as following the previously reported protocol [30, 31]. Polyclonal anti-HIV-1 IN antibodies were purchased from Bioproducts MD (Middletown, MD, USA). Antibodies directed against histones H3 (ab70550) and H4 (pAb61521 clone MABI 0400) were purchased from Abcam and Active Motif (Carlsbad, CA, USA) respectively. Recombinant mononucleosome assembled on 601 sequence biotinylated in 5′ and the naked corresponding sequence were purchased from TEBU-Bio or were home-made using typical salt dialysis protocole described in [6, 8]. We used either native human histone octamers or tailless octamers purified in the Protein Expression and Purification Facility (PEPF) from the Department of Biochemistry and Molecular Biology, Colorado State University. The quality of the assembly was checked on gel shift in 0.8% agarose gel and protein content analysis on SDS-PAGE (see Additional file 1: Figure S1). Biotinylated peptides were purchased from Eurogentech (Angers, France).

In vitro integration assays

Concerted integration assays were performed as previously reported [6] using recombinant purified IN or IN·LEDGF/p75 complex (200 nM in IN monomers). IN/viral DNA complex were preassembled using previously optimized conditions [6, 32] and 10 ng of donor DNA containing the U5 viral ends (see description of the different donors in Additional file 1: Figure S11). Preassembled complexes were then incubated with 50 ng of pBSK-derived p481 plasmid DNA in 20 mM HEPES pH7, 15% DMSO, 8% PEG, 10 mM MgCl2, 20 µM ZnCl2, 100 mM NaCl, 10 mM DTT final concentration.

After the reaction, the resultant integration products were deproteinized by Proteinase K treatment and phenol/chloroform/isoamyl alcohol (25/24/1 v/v/v) treatment before loading onto a 1% agarose gel. The gel was then dried and submitted to autoradiography. The bands corresponding to free substrate (S), donor/donor, linear FSI (FSI) and circular HSI + FSI (HSI + FSI) products were quantified. The circular FSI products were specifically quantified by cloning them into bacteria and determining the numbers of ampicillin-, kanamycin- and tetracycline-resistant clones as percentages of the integration reaction control, which was performed using the WT enzyme. Integration assays using recombinant 601 mononucleosomes or naked 601 DNA fragments were performed using the same procedure, except that a shorter viral DNA fragment corresponding to the 42 final base pairs of the HIV-1 U5 viral ends was used (see sequence in Additional file 1: Figure S11) and the concentration of IN was increased to 400 nM. Either 250 ng of MN or 125 ng of acceptor DNA were used. Acceptor substrates were immobilized on streptavidin-coupled beads before reaction and the reaction products were deproteinized as described above and the integration was quantified by counting the remaining radioactivity bound to magnetized beads.

Docking calculations

In all docking experiments, the fragment corresponding to residues A210-A270 from the HIV-1 IN catalytic core and the CTD crystal structure (PDB entry 1EX4) [15] was used as a protein receptor. For the ligand, we used the crystal structure of the H4K20me1 pentapeptide from the human MSL3 chromodomain complex (PDB entry 3OA6) [33]. The receptor and ligand structures were prepared for docking with AutoDockTools 1.5.6 [34]. Polar hydrogen atoms were added, non-polar hydrogens were merged, and Gasteiger partial atomic charges were computed. All possible rotatable bonds were subsequently assigned for the H4K20me1 ligand molecule. In the first set of experiments, a blind docking was performed on the entire surface of the receptor, which was treated as rigid, using the programs AutoDock 4.2.6 [34] and AutoDockVina 1.1.2 [35]. The combined docking results from these two methods enabled us to determine a unique consensus binding area. Second, experiments focusing on this area were conducted to predict the residues that may be involved in the binding of the ligand. To this end, a set of 14 residue side-chains surrounding the predicted binding area was treated as flexible. AutoGrid was used to produce grid maps that were properly centered to encompass the area of interest, with a grid box size of $76 \times 84 \times 98$ points and a grid spacing value of 0.264 Å. AutoDock performed a total of 1000 independent runs with step sizes of 0.2 Å for translations and 5 Å for torsions. The Lamarckian Genetic Algorithm was used with a population size of 150 individuals, the maximum number of energy evaluations set to 10,000,000, the maximum number of generations set to 27,000, the maximum number of top individuals that automatically survived set to 1, and mutation and crossover rates of 0.02 and 0.8, respectively. The final cluster analysis of all docked conformations was achieved with a cluster tolerance of 3.5Å. Finally, the top-ranked docking solutions were analyzed with AutoDockTools.

Pull-down experiments

Recombinant purified WT, mutant HIV-1 INs or IN·LEDGF/p75 complex (10 pmol of IN monomers) were incubated with either native recombinant W601 mono-nucleosomes, tailless MNs (250 ng, i.e., 125 ng DNA), or the naked 601 DNA sequence (125 ng) in 10 µl interaction buffer (50 mM HEPES, pH7.5; 1 µg/ml BSA; 1 mM DTT; 0.1% Tween 20;10% glycerol; and 50–240 mM NaCl) for 20 min on ice and then for 30 min at room temperature. A 12.5 µl aliquot of DynabeadsMyOne Streptavidin T1 (Invitrogen, ref. 65601) was then added to a total volume of 300 µl interaction buffer and incubated at room temperature for 1 h under rotation. The beads were washed three times with 300 µl interaction buffer, and the precipitated products were resuspended in 10 µl of Laemmli buffer, after which they were separated on a 12% gel via SDS-PAGE. Interacting proteins were detected by western blot analysis using anti-HIV-1 IN and anti-histone antibodies. Nucleosomal DNA was detected using a 1% agarose gel stained with SYBR® Safe. 140–240 mM NaCl conditions were chosen for analyzes since salt concentrations lower than 140 mM led to unspecific binding of HIV-1 INto the beads masking its interaction with nucleosomes.

FAR dot blot experiments

One µl of HIV-1 IN solution (1–10 pmol) was spotted onto a nitrocellulose membrane and dried for 1 h at room temperature. The membrane was then saturated for 3 h at room temperature with 5 ml of 1% BSA in PBS. After two washes, the membrane was incubated with 1 µM of the requisite peptide in 4 ml of PBS for 1 h at 37 °C. After two washes with PBS, the membrane was incubated with ExtrAvidin coupled to horseradish peroxidase (Sigma ref. E2886 1/4000) in 4 ml of 0.3% BSA in PBS for 1 h at room temperature. The interactions were detected by ECL using a LAS4000 device. The far dot blots were run three to ten times and the intensity of each spot was quantified using ImageJ software.

Transduction of human cells with lentiviral vectors

HEK-293T (Human Embryonic Kidney 293 cells, laboratory cell line) were transduced as previously described [36]. An optimized multiplicity of infection (MOI) of 1 was used, which resulted in 25–35% of the cells containing one copy of proviral DNA as determined before. Fluorescence was quantified 48 h post-transduction by counting 10,000 cells on a FACSCalibur flow cytometer (Becton–Dickinson, San Jose, CA, USA). HIV-1 DNA species were quantified at 24, 48 and 72 h post-transduction as previously described [37]. The total and integrated HIV-1 DNA levels were determined as copy numbers per 10^6 cells. Integrated cDNA and 2-LTR circles were expressed as a percentage of the total viral DNA.

Integration site library preparation

To remove any non-integrated viral DNA (and one-, or two-LTR circles) per condition, 5 µg genomic DNA (gDNA) samples isolated from K562 (human immortalized myelogenous leukemia cell line purchased from ATCC company) 72 h post-transfection were subjected to 0.6% agarose gel electrophoresis and high-molecular gDNA was isolated from the gel using the Zymoclean™ Large Fragment DNA Recovery Kit, (Zymo Research). The eluents were sonicated to an average of 600 bp-long fragments in screw-cap cuvettes with the Covaris M220 ultrasonicator with the following settings: peak power: 50.0, duty factor: 20, cycle/burst: 200, duration: 28 s. After bead purification the DNA was end-repaired and 5′-phosphorylated with the NEBNext End Repair Module (New England Biolabs, (NEB)). The DNA was prepared for ligation with NEBNextdA-Tailing Module, (NEB) and eluted after bead purification in 10 µl water. Ligation with double-stranded linkers (see Additional file 1: Figure S10) was performed in 15 µl for 15 min at room temperature using the Blunt/TA Ligase Master Mix (NEB). After purification with 0.8 volumes of AMPure XP beads (Beckman Coulter), the ligated DNA was eluted in 20 µl of 10 mM Tris/HCl, pH 8.0 and the whole DNA solution was used for multiple PCR reactions to amplify the virus-gDNA junctions with the primers SIN-HIV1 and linker primer using NEBNext High-Fidelity 2× PCR Master Mix (NEB) with the following cycling conditions: 98 °C 30 s; 20 cycles of: 98 °C 10 s, 68 °C 30 s, 72 °C 30 s; 10 cycles of: 98 °C 10 s, ramp to 63 °C 1 °C/s 30 s, 72 °C 30 s; 72 °C 3 min. The PCR products were isolated using 1 volume of AMPure XP beads (Beckman Coulter), eluted in 20 µl of 10 mM Tris/HCl, pH 8.0 and 2 µl of the eluents served as template for 5 parallel PCR reactions with the primers: SIN-HIV-BC-N-Ill and PE-nest ind-N (where N stands for the sequences of Illumina TrueSeq indexes, or their corresponding reverse complement sequences) using the following cycling conditions: 98 °C 30 s; 20 cycles of: 98 °C 10 s, 67 °C 30 s, 72 °C 30 s; 72 °C 3 min. The 200–500 bp size range of the indexed libraries were agarose gel-isolated and mixed equimolarly for 100 base, single-end Illumina sequencing on a HiSeq 2000 instrument using 40% PhiX DNA spike-in at Genewiz, USA.

Analysis of sequencing data

The raw reads starting with condition-specific indexes were grouped and filtered for the presence of the virus-specific nested primer followed by LTR sequences at the tip of the LTR. The rest of the reads were quality-trimmed as soon as 2 out of 5 bases had quality scores less than a Phred score of 20. We used *bowtie* [38] with the TAPDANCE tool [39] to map the reads to the hg19 human genome assembly in cycles with decreasing read length of 60, 55, 50, 45, 40, 35 allowing 3, 3, 3, 2, 1, 0 mismatches, respectively, with the following bowtie parameters in the mapping cycles: [$-quiet$ $-a$ $-v$ $<$ $nu.$ $mismatches$ $allowed$ $>$ $-m$ 1 $-suppress$ $5,6,7$ $-f$]. Any insertion site was considered valid if there were at least 5 independent reads supporting it. All read pre-processing and follow-up analyses were done in R (R Development Core Team (2008). R: A language and environment for statistical computing. R Foundation for Statistical Computing, Vienna, Austria. ISBN 3-900051-07-0, URL http://www.R-project.org).

Analysis of insertion sites in chromatin features

Nucleosome occupancy signal datasets for K562 cells were obtained from ENCODE [22]. Genomic coordinates with an associated nucleosome occupancy density signal value greater than zero were used to calculate occupancy matrixes and to plot nucleosome densities with the *genomation* R package [40]. BEDTools [41] and *genomation* were used to analyze the representation of ISs in histone mark distributions [42] and in chromatin state segment datasets making use of a consensus merge of the segmentations produced by the ChromHMM and Segway software [43]. We applied the Wilcoxon test on the row-sums of the score matrixes generated from nucleosome occupancy datasets to check for any statistical difference between the conditions. Fisher's exact test was used to calculate statistical significance between the representations of ISs of the WT and the integrase mutant viruses within methylated histone ChIP-seq peaks.

Additional files

Additional file 1: Figure S1. Structure of the native and tailless mononucleosomes used in the work. The globular structure of the nucleosomes was analyzed by loading 250 ng of native or tailless MN on 0.8% native agarose gel run 4 h at 50 V and 4 °C then stained with SYBR®Safe 20 min. Assembled MNs migrate between 600 and 700 bp and the naked 601 DNA fragment at 147 bp. **Figure S2.** A. Effect of LEDGF/p75 on HIV-1 integration in vitro. Integration assay was performed as done in Fig. 2 using naked 601 DNA coupled to magnetic beads and increasing concentration of LEDGF in the presence or absence of PEG and DMSO. B. Integration activity catalyzed by IN and IN/LEDGF complex on native or tail less nucleosomes in the absence of PEG and DMSO. Integration assay was performed as done in Fig. 2 using native or tail less nucleosomes coupled to magnetic beads and either IN or IN/LEDGF complex. All values are shown as the mean ± standard deviation (error bars) of three independent sets of experiments. The p values were calculated by Student's t test and are shown as *p < 0.05 to represent the probability of obtaining significant differences compared with the data obtained with the native MNs control. **Figure S3.** Sequence of the peptide tails used in the work. **Figure S4.** FAR dot-blot analysis of the interactions between HIV-1 IN and peptides derived from histone 4 amino-terminal tails. The associations between IN and unmodified H4, or modified H4 peptides were evaluated using a far dot blot approach as described in the "Methods" section using 1 µl of 2.5 pmol of recombinant IN spotted onto a nitrocellulose membrane and 1 µM of peptides. The far dot blots were run three to ten times and the intensity of each spot was quantified using ImageJ software. The results are reported as the mean of the experiments ± standard deviation. **Figure S5.** In vitro integration activities of wild type and mutant integrases. A concerted integration assay was performed using 200 nM of different enzymes which were purified using a similar procedure, in addition to 10 ng of donor DNA and 50 ng of pBSK-derived p481 plasmid DNA. The reaction products were loaded onto 1% agarose gels and a representative set of experiments is shown in (A). The positions and structures of the donor substrate and the different half-site (HSI), full-site (FSI) and donor/donor integration (d/d) products are shown. Quantification of the total integration is shown in (B) as a percentage of WT activity. The circular FSI products were quantified by cloning them into bacteria and are shown in (C) as the numbers of ampicillin-, kanamycin- and tetracycline-resistant clones as percentages of the integration reaction control performed using the WT enzyme. All values are shown as the mean ± standard deviation (error bars) of at least three independent sets of experiments. The p-values were calculated by Student's t-test and are shown as *p < 0.05 and **p < 0.005 to represent the probability of obtaining significant differences compared with WT data set at 100%. **Figure S6.** HIV-1 IN and mononucleosome pull-down experiment. Naked 147 bp 601 DNA sequence or MN assembled on this fragment were used (structure of the naked and assembled 601 DNA is reported in the gel shift experiment shown in **Figure S1.** WT IN was efficiently pulled down using a biotinylated naked 601 DNA fragment (left panel) or 601 mononucleosomes assembled on the same DNA (right panel) immobilized on streptavidin beads using 140–240 mM of NaCl (A). Experiments were performed using different mutated enzymes. Each pull-down was run three to six times and the intensity of each band was quantified using ImageJ software. The results obtained with naked DNA are reported as the mean of the experiments ± standard deviation in (B). The p values were calculated by Student's t-test and are shown as *p < 0.05 and **p < 0.005 to represent the probability of obtaining significant differences compared with the WT data in each condition. **Figure S7.** Time course analysis of the early steps of replication of wild type and mutants viral vectors in K562 cells. K562 cells were transduced with VSV-G pseudotyped lentiviruses encoding either WT IN or the R231A/H/G or D253H IN mutants. The replication steps affected by the mutations were determined by measuring the amounts of the different viral DNA species produced using qPCR. Levels of total viral DNA, integrated DNA and 2-LTR were monitored between 0 and 72 h post-transduction to check for potential defects at the steps of reverse transcription, integration and nuclear import of the preintegration complex. The data are represented as the mean of at least three independent experiments ± standard deviation. The p-values were calculated by Student's t-test and are shown as *p < 0.05 and **p < 0.005 to represent the probability of obtaining significant differences compared with the WT data. **Figure S8.** Effect of mutations affecting the IN/H4 tail interaction on HIV-1 integration site selectivity. Integration sites of the WT and the mutant viruses were annotated in signal peaks of ChIP-seq experiments for genome-wide histone modifications in K562 cells. Numbers indicate percentage values of insertion sites per condition. The p values were calculated with Fisher's exact test between the values of WT and the mutants,*p < 0.05 and **p < 0.005. **Figure S9.** Consensus sequences directly neighboring insertion sites of pseudoviral vectors carrying IN/H4 mutations. The target DNA consensus diagrams were generated with the *seqLogo* package in R. The triangles show the insertion sites. The relative height of individual bases at each position is proportional to the frequency of the base at that position. **Figure S10.** Superimposition of the HIV-1 IN CTD-H4K20me1 docking model with the structure of the tetrameric HIV-1 strand transfer complex intasome (PDB entry 5U1C). The model is presented in magenta cartoon representation with the docked H4K20me1 pentapeptide highlighted in green. The CTDs of the two inner protomers contacting the host DNA (colored in gold) are depicted in salmon and cyan. The grey cartoon corresponds to the rest of the HIV-1 strand transfer complex structure. **Figure S11.** Sequence of the viral DNA donors used in concerted integration assays. For concerted integration on MNs the two HIV1_U5 (+) and HIV1_U5 (-) (A) were hybridized and the resulting 42/40 bp hybrid was radiolabeled in 5′ with T4 DNA kinase. For concerted integration on naked DNA plasmid we used the 246 bp DNA fragment shown in (B) generated by PCR on a pUC19 supF. After purification the fragment was radiolabeled in 5′ with T4 DNA kinase. Sequence of oligonucleotides used for integration selectivity analyses (C).

Additional file 2. List of insertion sites of all the tested conditions. Raw sequencing reads are available upon request.

Authors' contributions
MSB, JM, EM, DL, PL, DRH ant VP performed the in vitro assays. CC purified the full length and truncated HIV-1 IN.1 ET and OD perform the viral DNA quantification. OO and MR performed the thermophoresis experiments and purified the HIV-1 IN CTD. XR and PG performed the docking calculation. CM and ZI performed the integration selectivity analyzes. MSB, XR, CM, PL, SC, OL, ML, MLA, OD, ZI, MR, PG and VP analyzed and discussed the data. MSM, XR, MR, OD, PG and VP wrote the manuscript. All authors read and approved the final manuscript.

Author details
[1] Fundamental Microbiology and Pathogenicity Laboratory, UMR 5234 CNRS-University of Bordeaux, SFR TransBioMed, 146 rue Léo Saignat, Bordeaux Cedex, France. [2] MMSB-Institute of the Biology and Chemistry of Proteins, UMR 5086 CNRS-Lyon 1 University, Lyon, France. [3] Division of Medical Biotechnology, Paul Ehrlich Institute, Langen, Germany. [4] UMR CNRS 5248 CBMN (Chimie Biologie des Membranes et Nanoobjets), Université de Bordeaux, 33076 Bordeaux, France. [5] Virology Program, ICBM, Faculty of Medicine, University of Chile, Santiago of Chile, Chile. [6] Département de Biologie Structurale Intégrative, UDS, U596 INSERM, UMR7104 CNRS, IGBMC (Institut de Génétique et de Biologie Moléculaire et Cellulaire), Illkirch, France. [7] LBPA, UMR8113, CNRS, ENS-Cachan, 94235 Cachan, France. [8] Dpt de Virologie, UMR 3569, CNRS, Institut Pasteur, Paris, France. [9] Institut Cochin-Inserm U1016-CNRS UMR8104-Université Paris Descartes, Paris, France. [10] International Associated Laboratory (LIA) of Microbiology and Immunology, CNRS, University de Bordeaux/Heinrich Pette Institute-Leibniz Institute for Experimental Virology, Bordeaux, France. [11] Viral DNA Integration and Chromatin Dynamics Network (DyNAVir), Bordeaux, France.

Acknowledgements
The authors are deeply grateful to Dr. Simon Litvak for fruitful discussions. The manuscript was edited by NPG Language Editing and Prof Ray Cooke.

Competing interests
The authors declare that they have no competing interests.

Funding
This work was supported by the French National Research Agency [ANR, RETROSelect program]; the French National Research Agency against AIDS (ANRS, AO 2016-2, ECTZ18624); SIDACTION (AO-27-1 10465, 16-1-AEQ-10465); the French Infrastructure for Integrated Structural Biology (FRISBI) [ANR-10-INSB-05-01]; Instruct, a part of the European Strategy Forum on Research Infrastructures (ESFRI); the Centre National de la Recherche Scientifique (CNRS); the University Victor Segalen Bordeaux 2; and the ECOS-CONICYT C12B03 program.

References
1. Lesbats P, Engelman AN, Cherepanov P. Retroviral DNA integration. Chem Rev. 2016;116(20):12730–57.
2. Lewinski MK, Yamashita M, Emerman M, Ciuffi A, Marshall H, Crawford G, et al. Retroviral DNA integration: viral and cellular determinants of target-site selection. PLoS Pathog. 2006;2:e60.
3. Kvaratskhelia M, Sharma A, Larue RC, Serrao E, Engelman A. Molecular mechanisms of retroviral integration site selection. Nucleic Acids Res. 2014;42(16):10209–25.
4. Sowd GA, Serrao E, Wang H, Fadel HJ, Poeschla EM, et al. A critical role for alternative polyadenylation factor CPSF6 in targeting HIV-1 integration to transcriptionally active chromatin. Proc Natl Acad Sci USA. 2016;113:E1054–63.
5. Naughtin M, Haftek-Terreau Z, Xavier J, Meyer S, Silvain M, Jaszczyszyn Y, et al. DNA physical properties and nucleosome positions are major determinants of HIV-1 integrase selectivity. PLoS ONE. 2015;10:e0129427.
6. Benleulmi MS, Matysiak J, Henriquez DR, Vaillant C, Lesbats P, Calmels C, et al. Intasome architecture and chromatin density modulate retroviral integration into nucleosome. Retrovirology. 2015;12:13.
7. Serrao E, Krishnan L, Shun MC, Li X, Cherepanov P, Engelman A, et al. Integrase residues that determine nucleotide preferences at sites of HIV-1 integration: implications for the mechanism of target DNA binding. Nucleic Acids Res. 2014;42:5164–76.
8. Lesbats P, Botbol Y, Chevereau G, Vaillant C, Calmels C, Arneodo A, et al. Functional coupling between HIV-1 integrase and the SWI/SNF chromatin remodeling complex for efficient in vitro integration into stable nucleosomes. PLoS Pathog. 2011;7:e1001280.
9. Matysiak J, Lesbats P, Mauro E, Lapaillerie D, Dupuy J-W, Lopez AP, et al. Modulation of chromatin structure by the FACT histone chaperone complex regulates HIV-1 integration. Retrovirology. 2017;14(1):39.
10. Maskell DP, Renault L, Serrao E, Lesbats P, Matadeen R, Hare S, et al. Structural basis for retroviral integration into nucleosomes. Nature. 2015;523:366.
11. Pasi M, Mornico D, Volant S, Juchet A, Batisse J, Bouchier C, et al. DNA minicircles clarify the specific role of DNA structure on retroviral integration. Nucleic Acids Res. 2016;44:7830.
12. Lowary PT, Widom J. New DNA sequence rules for high affinity binding to histone octamer and sequence-directed nucleosome positioning. J Mol Biol. 1998;276:19–42.
13. Pryciak PM, Sil A, Varmus HE. Retroviral integration into minichromosomes in vitro. EMBO J. 1992;11:291–303.
14. Pryciak PM, Müller H-P, Varmus HE. Simian virus 40 minichromosomes as targets for retroviral integration in vivo. Proc Natl Acad Sci USA. 1992;89:9237–41.
15. Chen JC, Krucinski J, Miercke LJ, Finer-Moore JS, Tang AH, Leavitt AD, et al. Crystal structure of the HIV-1 integrase catalytic core and C-terminal domains: a model for viral DNA binding. Proc Natl Acad Sci USA. 2000;97:8233–8.
16. Passos DO, Li M, Yang R, Rebensburg SV, Ghirlando R, Jeon Y, et al. Cryo-EM structures and atomic model of the HIV-1 strand transfer complex intasome. Science. 2017;355:89–92.
17. Lu R, Ghory HZ, Engelman A. Genetic analyses of conserved residues in the carboxyl-terminal domain of human immunodeficiency virus type 1 integrase. J Virol. 2005;79:10356–68.
18. Lu R, Limón A, Ghory HZ, Engelman A. Genetic analyses of DNA-binding mutants in the catalytic core domain of human immunodeficiency virus type 1 integrase. J Virol. 2005;79:2493–505.
19. Tekeste SS, Wilkinson TA, Weiner EM, Xu X, Miller JT, Le Grice SFJ, et al. Interaction between reverse transcriptase and integrase is required for reverse transcription during HIV-1 replication. J Virol. 2015;89:12058–69.
20. Mitchell RS, Beitzel BF, Schroder AR, Shinn P, Chen H, Berry CC, et al. Retroviral DNA integration: ASLV, HIV, and MLV show distinct target site preferences. PLoS Biol. 2004;2:E234.
21. Wang GP, Ciuffi A, Leipzig J, Berry CC, Bushman FD. HIV integration site selection: analysis by massively parallel pyrosequencing reveals association with epigenetic modifications. Genome Res. 2007;17:1186–94.

22. Mieczkowski J, Cook A, Bowman SK, Mueller B, Alver BH, Kundu S, et al. MNase titration reveals differences between nucleosome occupancy and chromatin accessibility. Nat Commun. 2016;7:11485.

23. Valouev A, Johnson SM, Boyd SD, Smith CL, Fire AZ, Sidow A. Determinants of nucleosome organization in primary human cells. Nature. 2011;474:516–20.

24. Demeulemeester J, Vets S, Schrijvers R, Madlala P, De Maeyer M, De Rijck J, et al. HIV-1 integrase variants retarget viral integration and are associated with disease progression in a chronic infection cohort. Cell Host Microbe. 2014;16:651–62.

25. Ballandras-Colas A, Maskell DP, Serrao E, Locke J, Swuec P, Jónsson SR, et al. A supramolecular assembly mediates lentiviral DNA integration. Science. 2017;355:93–5.

26. Luger K, Mader AW, Richmond RK, Sargent DF, Richmond TJ. Crystal structure of the nucleosome core particle at 2.8 A resolution. Nature. 1997;389:251–60.

27. Dorigo B, Schalch T, Bystricky K, Richmond TJ. Chromatin fiber folding: requirement for the histone H4 N-terminal tail. J Mol Biol. 2003;327:85–96.

28. Song F, Chen P, Sun D, Wang M, Dong L, Liang D, et al. Cryo-EM study of the chromatin fiber reveals a double helix twisted by tetranucleosomal units. Science. 2014;344:376–80.

29. Busso D, Delagoutte-Busso B, Moras D. Construction of a set Gateway-based destination vectors for high-throughput cloning and expression screening in *Escherichia coli*. Anal Biochem. 2005;343:313–21.

30. Botbol Y, Raghavendra NK, Rahman S, Engelman A, Lavigne M. Chromatinized templates reveal the requirement for the LEDGF/p75 PWWP domain during HIV-1 integration in vitro. Nucleic Acids Res. 2008;36:1237–46.

31. Levy N, Eiler S, Pradeau-Aubreton K, Maillot B, Stricher F, Ruff M. Production of unstable proteins through the formation of stable core complexes. Nat Commun [Internet]. 2016 [cited 2017 Feb 16];7. https://www-ncbi-nlm-nih-gov.insb.bib.cnrs.fr/pmc/articles/PMC4800440/.

32. Lesbats P, Metifiot M, Calmels C, Baranova S, Nevinsky G, Andreola ML, et al. In vitro initial attachment of HIV-1 integrase to viral ends: control of the DNA specific interaction by the oligomerization state. Nucleic Acids Res. 2008;36:7043–58.

33. Kim D, Blus BJ, Chandra V, Huang P, Rastinejad F, Khorasanizadeh S. Corecognition of DNA and a methylated histone tail by the MSL3 chromodomain. Nat Struct Mol Biol. 2010;17:1027–9.

34. Morris GM, Huey R, Lindstrom W, Sanner MF, Belew RK, Goodsell DS, et al. AutoDock4 and AutoDockTools4: automated docking with selective receptor flexibility. J Comput Chem. 2009;30:2785–91.

35. Trott O, Olson AJ. AutoDock Vina: improving the speed and accuracy of docking with a new scoring function, efficient optimization, and multi-threading. J Comput Chem. 2010;31:455–61.

36. Cosnefroy O, Tocco A, Lesbats P, Thierry S, Calmels C, Wiktorowicz T, et al. Stimulation of the human RAD51 nucleofilament restricts HIV-1 integration in vitro and in infected cells. J Virol. 2012;86:513–26.

37. Munir S, Thierry S, Subra F, Deprez E, Delelis O. Quantitative analysis of the time-course of viral DNA forms during the HIV-1 life cycle. Retrovirology. 2013;10:87.

38. Langmead B, Trapnell C, Pop M, Salzberg SL. Ultrafast and memory-efficient alignment of short DNA sequences to the human genome. Genome Biol. 2009;10:R25.

39. Sarver AL, Erdman J, Starr T, Largaespada DA, Silverstein KAT. TAPDANCE: an automated tool to identify and annotate transposon insertion CISs and associations between CISs from next generation sequence data. BMC Bioinform. 2012;13:154.

40. Akalin A, Franke V, Vlahoviček K, Mason CE, Schübeler D. genomation: a toolkit to summarize, annotate and visualize genomic intervals. Bioinformatics. 2015;31:1127–9.

41. Quinlan AR, Hall IM. BEDTools: a flexible suite of utilities for comparing genomic features. Bioinformatics. 2010;26:841–2.

42. Ernst J, Kheradpour P, Mikkelsen TS, Shoresh N, Ward LD, Epstein CB, et al. Systematic analysis of chromatin state dynamics in nine human cell types. Nature. 2011;473:43–9.

43. Hoffman MM, Buske OJ, Wang J, Weng Z, Bilmes JA, Noble WS. Unsupervised pattern discovery in human chromatin structure through genomic segmentation. Nat Methods. 2012;9:473–6.

2

Importance of Fc-mediated functions of anti-HIV-1 broadly neutralizing antibodies

Matthew S. Parsons[1]*, Amy W. Chung[1] and Stephen J. Kent[1,2,3]*

Abstract

Anti-HIV-1 broadly neutralizing antibodies (BnAbs) exhibit an impressive capacity to protect against chimeric SIV-HIV (SHIV) challenges in macaques and potently reduce viremia in both SHIV-infected macaques and HIV-1-infected humans. There is a body of evidence suggesting Fc-mediated functions of anti-HIV-1 binding antibodies are important in protecting from infection and controlling viremia. The degree to which the efficacy of BnAbs is assisted by Fc-mediated functions is of great interest. Challenge experiments with the older generation BnAb b12 showed that mutating the Fc region to abrogate Fcγ receptor binding reduced protective efficacy in macaques. Similar data have been generated with newer BnAbs using murine models of HIV-1. In addition, the degree to which therapeutically administered BnAbs reduce viremia suggests that elimination of infected cells through Fc-mediated functions may contribute to their efficacy. Fc-mediated functions that eliminate infected cells may be particularly important for challenge systems involving cell-associated virus. Herein we review data regarding the importance of Fc-mediated functions of BnAbs in mediating protective immunity and control of viremia.

Keywords: HIV-1, ADCC, Broadly neutralizing antibodies

Introduction

An HIV-1 vaccine is urgently needed, and new technologies to control HIV-1 infection in the absence of lifelong antiretroviral drug therapy are being actively pursued. Many highly potent neutralizing antibodies that neutralize broad arrays of HIV-1 isolates, termed broadly neutralizing antibodies (BnAbs), have been isolated in recent years [1]. Passive transfer of these antibodies reliably protects macaques from exposure to cell free chimeric Simian-Human Immunodeficiency Virus (SHIV) and reduces viremia in SHIV-infected macaques and HIV-1-infected humans [2–12]. Passive transfer of the BnAb VRC01 is currently under evaluation for its potential to protect humans from HIV-1 (NCT02716675 and NCT02568215).

Coincident with this exciting work on BnAbs, there is a growing body of literature on the importance of Fc-mediated functions of HIV-1 antibodies. Fc-mediated functions of non-neutralizing antibodies appeared to be important in the modest protective efficacy of the RV144 HIV-1 vaccine regimen [13–15]. Fc-mediated functions of HIV-1 antibodies generally correlate with slow HIV-1 disease progression and can force viral escape [16–19].

More potent Fc-mediated functions of BnAbs should theoretically enhance their efficacy and there is some evidence that this is the case [20]. This might be particularly important when HIV-1 is transmitted in the context of infected cells, which may partially evade neutralization by BnAbs. This review summarizes data on the importance of Fc-mediated functions of BnAbs.

Diversity of Fc-mediated functionality of isolated BnAbs

The breadth of viral recognition and much of the antiviral potency of BnAbs is derived from the recognition of key viral epitopes by BnAb paratopes that prevent the infection of cellular targets through viral neutralization. Importantly, BnAbs have the potential to mediate a diverse array of additional non-neutralizing functions through ligation of the Fc portion of the antigen-bound antibody by components of the complement system or

*Correspondence: mattp@unimelb.edu.au; skent@unimelb.edu.au
[1] Department of Microbiology and Immunology, The University of Melbourne, at the Peter Doherty Institute for Infection and Immunity, Victoria, Australia
Full list of author information is available at the end of the article

effector cells expressing Fc receptors (FcR). Indeed, HIV-1-infected cells bound by BnAbs can be targeted by FcR-expressing effector cells, such as natural killer (NK) cells, for elimination by antibody-dependent cellular cytotoxicity (ADCC) [21–23]. As well as cytolysis of infected cells opsonized by BnAbs, effector cells recognizing BnAb-coated target cells can become stimulated to produce soluble factors, such as beta chemokines, that can inhibit viral spread. The combination of ADCC, neutralization and effector cell derived soluble inhibitors of viral spread has been termed antibody-dependent cell-mediated viral inhibition (ADCVI), and this response can be mediated by BnAbs [24, 25]. Additionally, FcR-expressing phagocytic effector cells, such as monocytes, can eliminate BnAb-coated virions through an antibody-dependent uptake process, termed antibody-dependent phagocytosis (ADP) [26]. Lastly, infected cells coated by BnAbs can be targeted for elimination by the process of antibody-dependent complement-mediated lysis (ADCML) [22]. It should be noted that further diversity in these processes is introduced by the differential responsiveness of effector cells at different stages of ontogeny and differentiation, as well as polymorphisms in FcR that adjust effector cell responsiveness to antibody-coated target cells. Lastly, diversity in Fc-dependent non-neutralizing functions is driven by the differential capacity of individual BnAbs to trigger these functions.

Much research into the Fc-dependent functions of BnAbs has focused on ADCC. Indeed, several independent studies have assessed the capacity of panels of antibodies (including BnAbs) to trigger NK cell-mediated ADCC of target cells infected with diverse viral isolates [21–23]. Although these studies have revealed that the observed ADCC is highly dependent on the antibody and virus combination studied, several general characteristics of ADCC have been elucidated. It has now been demonstrated that: (1) the degree of antibody binding to target cells correlates with the susceptibility of the target cell to ADCC [21–23]; (2) the ability of the antibody to neutralize a virus isolate associates with the capacity of the antibody to trigger ADCC of target cells infected with the same isolate [21, 23]; and (3) combinations of antibodies trigger potent ADCC [21, 22]. It should be noted that exceptions to these generalizations have been reported. In particular, it has been reported that the 2G12 and 2F5 BnAbs trigger poor ADCC despite binding to infected cells [23]. Although the reasons for the reduced ADCC function of these two BnAbs have not been determined, roles for NK cell accessibility to 2F5 and the Fab swapped variable region of 2G12 have been proposed [23]. Importantly, some investigators have observed ADCC by 2F5 recognizing infected target cells [27], and 2G12 in monomeric and dimeric formats has been reported to induce ADCC [28, 29]. This suggests that the ADCC capacity of some BnAbs is highly context dependent, and this is an area for future research.

In addition to ADCC, recent research has also demonstrated BnAbs to bind to FcRs involved in ADP and to have the capacity to trigger phagocytosis of viral particles. Factors influencing BnAb ADP were recently investigated by Tay et al. [26]. These investigators employed the CD4 binding site specific CH31 BnAb to determine the effect of antibody isotype and IgG subclass on phagocytic activity. Primary monocytes were employed as effector cells and demonstrated to uptake viral particles opsonized by IgG1, monomeric IgA1 and monomeric IgA2 versions of CH31. Interestingly, IgG1 was a more potent inducer of viral particle uptake than IgA1 or IgA2. Next, the relative capacities of IgG1 and IgG3 to trigger ADP of viral particles by primary monocytes were assessed. The IgG3 version of CH31 was a more potent inducer of ADP than IgG1. This phenomenon of more potent ADP by IgG3 was shown to not be a result of enhanced antigen binding, and enhanced ADP of IgG3 compared to IgG1 was demonstrated for two additional BnAbs (CH27 and CH28) and non-broadly neutralizing antibodies directed to different epitopes.

As well as FcR binding, several BnAbs have now been screened for their capacity to trigger lysis of infected cells in a complement-dependent manner [22]. Furthermore, mutants of a CD4 binding site BnAb, b12, have been generated to exhibit different patterns of complement binding [30]. Passive immunization of these b12 mutants in macaques prior to mucosal SHIV challenge revealed no role for complement in b12-conferred protection from infection [5]. It remains undetermined if this observation extends to BnAbs other than b12. The capacity of a panel of antibodies (including BnAbs) to trigger ADCML of HIV-1-infected target cells was recently investigated by Mujib et al. [22]. An array of ADCML capacities was noted within the antibody panel. Although not statistically significant, a trend was noted between the level of antibody binding to infected cells and the ADCML observed.

As well as the Fc-dependent functions of BnAbs reviewed above, it is important to highlight additional functional roles of the antibody Fc that might be of significance for BnAb-conferred protection from HIV-1. For instance, interaction of antibody Fc with the neonatal FcR (FcRn) is important for extending antibody half-life, as well as localizing and sustaining antibody to mucosal sites of HIV-1 exposure [31]. Lastly, an understudied Fc-FcR interaction is that between antibodies and the inhibitory FcγRIIb. Interaction of immune complexes formed by live-attenuated SIV vaccine-induced antibodies with FcγRIIb expressed in the epithelium associates with

Table 1 Role for Fc-dependent BnAb functions for protection from cell free virus in vivo

Aim of study	BnAb studied	Model	Outcome	References
Compare wild type b12 with b12 versions deficient for FcR binding and/or complement binding for protection of macaques from high-dose SHIV challenge	b12	Macaque high-dose SHIV	Elimination of the ability of b12 to engage FcR diminished the ability of the antibody to protect macaques from high-dose SHIV challenge	[5]
Compare low doses of wild type b12 and b12 deficient for FcR binding for protection of macaques from repeated low-dose SHIV challenge	b12	Macaque repeated low-dose SHIV	More challenges did not result in infection of animals infused with wild type b12, as compared to animals infused with b12 deficient in FcR binding	[35]
Assess if low doses of a non-fucosylated version of b12, with enhanced ADCC potential, are better than wild type b12 for protecting macaques from repeated low-dose SHIV challenge	b12	Macaque repeated low-dose SHIV	Non-fucosylated b12 did not provide enhanced protection from repeated low-dose SHIV challenge, as compared to wild type b12	[36]
Screen panel of BnAbs with enhanced of diminished FcR binding for ability to block viral entry in a murine model	BnAb panel	Murine HIV-1 entry	BnAbs with enhanced FcR binding demonstrated enhanced in vivo blocking of HIV-1 entry	[20]
Determine if modifying VRC01 to enhance binding to FcRn improves the ability of suboptimal doses of the BnAb to protect against SHIV challenge	VRC01	Macaque SHIV	Suboptimal doses of VRC01 with enhanced binding to FcRn protected more macaques from SHIV challenge than wild type VRC01	[31]

live-attenuated vaccine-conferred protection from infection [32]. It is thought that this interaction prevents/diminishes the recruitment of target cells for SIV infection to the site of exposure. The importance of FcγRIIb for BnAb conferred protection from mucosal viral challenges in macaques has not yet been investigated.

Role of Fc-dependent functions in efficacy of BnAbs against cell free virus in vivo

A collection of studies demonstrate that BnAbs administered passively or through gene transfer using adeno-associated viral vectors protect against in vivo challenge with cell free virus in animal models of HIV-1 infection [5–8, 10, 12, 20, 31, 33–36]. While these studies clearly highlight the prophylactic capacity of BnAbs, only a few of the reports incorporated experiments to assess the potential mechanisms of BnAb-conferred protection (Table 1) [5, 20, 31, 35, 36]. Such experiments are important to gauge if neutralization function is sufficient, or if BnAbs need to trigger additional non-neutralizing functions through their Fc portions to protect against HIV-1 exposure.

Hessell et al. initially evaluated the involvement of non-neutralizing Fc-dependent functions in BnAb conferred protection from in vivo cell free virus challenge [5]. For this purpose the authors utilized a previously developed panel of variants of the CD4 binding site BnAb, b12 [30]. These variants included the b12 wild type (b12 WT), a version mutated to diminish FcγR and complement binding (b12 LALA), and a version only exhibiting diminished complement binding (b12 KA). Each of these b12 variants, or human IgG1 isotype control, were passively

administered intravenously to rhesus macaques prior to vaginal challenge with high-dose cell free $SHIV_{SF162P3}$. While all four animals receiving the isotype control were infected following challenge, animals receiving b12 WT and b12 KA exhibited similar robust levels of protection from infection (i.e. 8/9 animals protected in each group). Animals receiving the b12 LALA were less likely to be protected from challenge than animals receiving the b12 WT or b12 KA antibodies (i.e. 5/9 animals protected). These results imply that neutralization is often sufficient for protection from cell free virus challenge, but protection is optimized if BnAbs can trigger additional non-neutralizing effector cell functions through effector cells expressing FcγRs.

Following their observation of lower efficacy of b12 LALA than b12 WT in protecting against high-dose cell free virus challenge, Hessell et al. evaluated the potential role of non-neutralizing functions of b12 for protection of macaques from repeated low-dose cell free $SHIV_{SF162P3}$ challenge [35]. Animals were injected once weekly with low doses of b12 WT or b12 LALA and challenged twice weekly with low-dose virus. Animals inoculated with either b12 WT or b12 LALA required more challenges prior to becoming infected than animals administered isotype control prior to challenge. Although both b12 WT and b12 LALA provided protection compared to isotype control, protection conferred by b12 LALA appeared suboptimal as compared to b12 WT. Indeed, nearly twice as many challenges did not result in infection for b12 WT animals than b12 LALA animals (i.e. 104 vs. 61). These observations largely reflected the relative patterns of protection conferred by b12 WT and b12 LALA following high-dose viral challenge [5].

The major implication of the two studies assessing the relative protective efficacy of b12 variants with different FcγR binding potential is that neutralization is often sufficient for protection from infection with cell free virus. It is possible that neutralization might fail to be sufficient for protection when too large of a number of cells are infected following challenge. In these situations non-neutralizing Fc-dependent functions of BnAbs could be required to purge infected cells through ADCC or eliminate the virions produced by infected cells by ADP. The potential contribution of ADCC to protection conferred by b12 was evaluated by Moldt et al., who compared the relative protection from repeated low-dose SHIV$_{SF162P3}$ challenge conferred by b12 WT to a non-fucosylated version of b12 (NFb12) [36]. Despite exhibiting higher binding to human and rhesus macaque FcγRIIIa and mediating higher ADCC of HIV-1-infected cells, the NFb12 antibody did not confer enhanced protection from cell free viral challenge as compared to b12 WT. These results might reflect the importance of Fc-dependent functions other than ADCC in the protection conferred by BnAbs.

Until recently much of the research into the role of non-neutralizing Fc-dependent functions for BnAb-conferred protection from in vivo cell free virus challenge was conducted using the b12 BnAb. Since the isolation of b12 numerous anti-HIV-1 BnAbs have been isolated and demonstrated to exhibit enhanced neutralization breadth and potency [1]. The role of Fc-dependent functions in the protective efficacy of some of these BnAbs has been evaluated in mouse models of HIV-1 entry [20]. Inhibition of HIV-1 entry can be assessed in luciferase reporter mice by infusing adenovirus encoding HIV-1 receptor and co-receptor (i.e. CD4 and CCR5), infusing anti-HIV-1 or control antibodies, challenging with HIV-1 pseudovirus and full-body imaging. Employing this system Bournozos et al. [20] demonstrated that BnAbs with murine IgG2a Fc, which confers preferential binding to activating FcγRs, were better able to inhibit HIV-1 entry than BnAbs expressing wild type murine IgG1 or an IgG1 variant with diminished binding to FcγR. Reliance on Fc-dependent functions for optimal in vivo efficacy was observed for a panel of antibodies, suggesting Fc-dependent functions are important independent of the viral epitope targeted by the antibody. That this observation reflected FcγR engagement by antibodies is suggested by the absence of differences in efficacy between antibody variants in mice lacking FcγR expression. Lastly, it is important to note that the authors modified their mouse model by engineering mice to express human FcγRs. This allowed an assessment of the role of Fc-dependent

functions for BnAbs expressing human Fc in preventing viral entry. Employing wild type BnAb, as well as versions engineered to exhibit deficient or enhanced FcγR binding, the authors observed evidence for a role for human Fc/FcγR interactions in inhibition of in vivo viral entry. Cumulatively, these observations are largely supportive of the role for Fc/FcγR interactions in BnAb-conferred protection observed in macaques. The results from the murine experiments suggest that the role for Fc-dependent anti-viral functions of BnAbs for optimal protection extends beyond the b12 BnAb and might be a generalizable phenomenon.

Lastly, it should be noted that in addition to triggering anti-viral effector functions, interactions between BnAbs and FcRs are important for sustaining antibody concentrations and antibody transport. Indeed, antibody binding to the FcRn is important for homeostasis and antibody transport to mucosal surfaces. As such, the VRC01 antibody was recently mutated to enhance binding to the FcRn [31]. The resulting VRC01-LS antibody exhibited increased in vitro transcytosis, a 2.5-fold longer in vivo serum half-life in rhesus macaques and a tendency to accumulate in macaque rectal tissues through FcRn binding. Lastly, suboptimal concentrations of VRC01-LS provided enhanced protection against rectal SHIV$_{BaLP4}$ challenge, as compared to VRC01 WT (i.e. 7/12 vs. 2/12 animals protected from infection). These results highlight that Fc/FcR interactions are an important determinant of BnAb-conferred protection, even if the interaction does not directly stimulate anti-viral functions.

Utility of BnAbs for control of cell–cell virus transmission in vitro

Much evidence highlights the potential utility of BnAbs for preventing HIV-1 infection. A potential caveat for utilizing BnAbs to prevent HIV-1 infection is the presence of cell-associated virus within infectious bodily fluids, such as semen [37]. Cell-associated virus has long been proposed as a mechanism of transmission of HIV-1—the so-called "Trojan Horse" hypothesis [38, 39]. In macaques, cell-associated SIV is highly efficient at initiating infection, more so than cell free virus [40]. In humans, there are limited data based on virus sequencing that cell-associated virus may initiate a proportion of HIV-1 infections [41].

A key component of the "Trojan horse" hypothesis is that cell-associated virus may evade anti-viral immunity [38, 39]. There has been much research into this possibility, particularly with regards to cell-associated virus evading BnAbs. While some publications have reported BnAbs to prevent in vitro cell-to-cell transmission of HIV-1, others have demonstrated a decreased efficacy of BnAbs against cell-associated virus compared to cell free virus [42–51]. These divergent results likely reflect the utilization of different in vitro experimental systems. Nevertheless, decreased efficacy a BnAbs against cell-associated virus has been reported in terms of both higher 50% inhibitory concentrations (IC_{50}) and incomplete neutralization [45]. Importantly, the ability of BnAbs to prevent cell-to-cell spread is dependent on the virus/antibody combination [47]. Furthermore, combinations of BnAbs may be more efficient than single antibodies [44].

BnAb control of cell-associated challenge in vivo

We recently developed a cell-associated $SHIV_{SF162P3}$ infection model in pigtail macaques [52]. The model was adapted from a previously published cell-associated SIV model that used splenocytes from infected macaque donors to initiate infection [53]. Passive transfer of the BnAb PGT121 protected 6/6 pigtail macaques from an intravenous cell free $SHIV_{SF162P3}$ challenge but only 3/6 macaques from an intravenous cell-associated $SHIV_{SF162P3}$ challenge. However, the lack of efficacy in two macaques challenged with the cell-associated $SHIV_{SF162P3}$ appeared due to low levels of BnAb administered. Interestingly, one macaque had no viremia until eight weeks post challenge with cell-associated $SHIV_{SF162P3}$. It appeared that the $SHIV_{SF162P3}$ lay dormant, possibly existing as cell-associated virus in tissues, and only emerged when the passively transferred BnAb waned to low levels. Whether this anecdote will represent a common mode of evading strategies to control HIV-1 with BnAbs is unknown. We recently suggested that, given the capacity of HIV-1 to remain latent under ART for decades, HIV-1 could remain suppressed by BnAbs for years until the antibodies (whether delivered passively or induced by vaccination) wane to sub therapeutic levels [54]. This has implications for the long-term follow up of BnAb based clinical trials.

The use of BnAbs for HIV-1 therapy and cure: role of Fc-dependent responses

Following the isolation of first generation BnAbs there was much interest in their potential for therapeutic utilization. In an early study in hu-PBL-SCID mice, Poignard et al. observed limited utility of first generation BnAbs in mice infected with HIV-1$_{JR-CSF}$ or HIV-1$_{SF162}$ [55]. Indeed, monotherapy with the CD4 binding site BnAb, b12, did not significantly decrease plasma viral loads in mice infected with either virus, as compared to control animals. Furthermore, several viral isolates derived from animals treated with b12 developed resistance to the

BnAb. Similarly, treatment of mice infected with HIV-1$_{JR-CSF}$ with a cocktail of BnAbs (i.e. b12, 2G12 and 2F5) achieved unsatisfactory results. Temporary decreases in viral load were noted, but were followed by viral rebound and escape from one or all three BnAbs.

Trials of first generation BnAbs as therapeutics in HIV-1-infected humans also revealed transient therapeutic benefits followed by viral escape from BnAb. Trkola et al. administered a BnAb cocktail (i.e. 2G12, 2F5 and 4E10) to eight individuals with chronic HIV-1 infection and six individuals with acute HIV-1 infection one day before cessation of ART [56]. Trial participants received 13 BnAb injections over 11 weeks. Two of eight chronically infected donors exhibited a delay in viral rebound, as compared to historical data of the same individuals undergoing a treatment interruption in the absence of BnAb therapy. The acutely infected BnAb-treated participants exhibited a significant time delay prior to viral rebound as compared to a control group of acutely infected individuals undergoing treatment interruption in the absence of BnAb treatment (median 8 weeks vs. 3.75 weeks). The therapeutic benefits of the BnAb cocktail appeared to be primarily driven by 2G12, as viral rebound was accompanied by resistance to 2G12 in 12/14 trial participants. Mehandru et al. reported similar results in another trial assessing the therapeutic potential of the BnAb cocktail of 2G12, 2F5 and 4E10 [57]. As observed by Trkola et al. [56], these investigators noted that BnAb therapy slowed viral rebound following treatment interruption, as compared to historical controls. Furthermore, loss of viral control was associated with resistance to 2G12.

Since these initial trials, numerous BnAbs, with increased potency and breadth compared to first generation BnAbs, have been isolated from HIV-1-infected individuals [1]. The isolation of next generation BnAbs has reinvigorated interest in utilizing BnAbs as therapeutics for HIV-1 infection. Assessment of the therapeutic potential of next generation BnAbs in humanized mouse models suggested monotherapy to be inefficient, transiently controlling viremia before the development of viral resistance to BnAbs [58]. Combination therapy with five BnAbs, however, controlled viremia and did not result in viral resistance to BnAbs. Another study demonstrated that single BnAbs were sufficient to control viremia in a proportion of humanized mice, if viral replication was first controlled by ART and BnAb administrations were initiated prior to cessation of ART [59]. Studies in non-human primates have revealed that both combination therapy and monotherapy with BnAbs can control SHIV replication, but monotherapy can lead to the development of viral escape mutants [2, 11]. Furthermore, therapeutic administration of BnAbs to macaques during acute SHIV infection might facilitate the development of autologous antiviral immunity, thus conferring prolonged control of viral replication [9].

In addition to animal studies, next generation BnAbs have also been screened as therapeutics in HIV-1-infected humans [3, 4, 60]. Monotherapy with 3BNC117 and 10-1074 results in transient control of viremia, and 3BNC117 can delay viral rebound following treatment interruption. As noted in animal studies, viral resistance to BnAbs can develop in humans undergoing monotherapy.

As well as data highlighting the capacity of BnAbs to control viremia, several studies using murine models, as well as modelling of data from a human clinical trial, suggest a role for FcγRs in the therapeutic benefits conferred by BnAbs. A role for BnAb interactions with FcγR for controlling viremia in infected animals was demonstrated by Bournazos et al. [20]. Humanized mice infected with HIV-1 were treated with a cocktail of BnAbs (i.e. 3BNC117, PG16 and 10-1074) modified either to not interact with FcγR (FcR^{null}) or to exhibit enhanced binding to activating FcγR. A quicker and sustained control of viremia was observed in animals treated with the antibody cocktail containing antibodies designed to more strongly interact with activating FcγR. Halper-Stromberg et al. demonstrated that treatment of HIV-1-infected humanized mice with a BnAb cocktail (i.e. 10-1074, PG16 and 3BNC117) 4 days post infection reduced the establishment of a latent reservoir, as exhibited by a lack of viral rebound in a proportion of animals after waning of therapeutic BnAbs [61]. A rendition of this experiment using FcR^{null} versions of the BnAbs suggested a role for FcγR interactions in the observed interference with the establishment of a latent reservoir. Significantly more mice had rebounded viremia by 44 days post treatment with FcR^{null} versions of the BnAbs than those treated with wild type BnAbs capable of interacting with FcγR. Lastly, Lu et al. assessed the rate of viral load decline in HIV-1-infected humans treated with 3BNC117 [62]. Modelling suggested that the rate of decline in viremia was too rapid to be explained by neutralization of free virus alone. Indeed, the analysis suggested that non-neutralizing antibody effector functions, such as those involved in eliminating infected cells, were involved in the therapeutic benefits conferred by the antibody. Furthermore, the ability of BnAbs to eliminate human cells infected with the HIV-1$_{YU2}$ laboratory strain or isolates derived from HIV-1-infected patients was demonstrated in vivo in mice. The elimination of infected cells was demonstrated to be dependent on FcγR-mediated recognition of antibody, as infected cells were not eliminated by FcR^{null} BnAbs and in vivo blocking of FcγRs prevented the elimination of infected cells.

Diversity of Effector cells, FcγRs and antibody isotypes: potential influence on BnAb efficacy

While the BnAb paratope dictates neutralization breadth and potency, accumulating evidence indicates that Fc-dependent functions might be required for BnAbs to optimally protect from infection, suppress viral load and/or clear infected cells [5, 20, 61, 62]. These Fc-dependent functions might include ADCC, ADP, complement activation, effector cell release of cytokines, chemokines or enzymes, inhibition of transcytosis and mucus trapping. An antibody's Fc functional capacity can be modulated through multiple small biophysical differences of the Fc region [63], including the isotype (e.g., IgG, IgA, IgM, IgE, IgD), subclass (e.g., IgG1-4, IgA1, IgA2) [64], allotype [65, 66] and glycosylation of the Fc heavy chain [67, 68].

In humans, there are three distinct classes of Fcγ receptors: FcγRI, FcγRII (FcγRIIa, FcγRIIb, and FcγRIIc), and FcγRIII (FcγRIIIa and FcγRIIIb), which bind to different IgG subclasses with varying affinity, and can cause either activation or inhibition of the effector cell [64]. These FcγRs are expressed on a wide variety of innate immune cells including NK cells, monocytes, macrophages, dendritic cells, eosinophils, basophils and neutrophils. NK cells almost exclusively express the activating FcγRIIIa and are the effector cells most commonly associated with ADCC [69]. Macrophages, neutrophils, eosinophils, basophils and dendritic cells all express a more diverse range of FcγRs on their surfaces (both activating and inhibitory) and can mediate various effector functions, including ADCC, phagocytosis and trogocytosis (i.e., the exchange of cellular membrane fragments between effector and target cells) [70–72].

Human FcγRs are diverse. A range of FcγR polymorphisms have been identified, some of which have greater Fc binding affinity and are associated with enhanced Fc effector function capacity. For example, FcγRIIa has two common polymorphisms—H131 and R131. The FcγRIIa H131 polymorphism, which is commonly associated with enhanced ADP, is also related to HIV-1 disease progression status [73, 74]. The FcγRIIIa is also known to exhibit polymorphisms at position 158–V158 and F158. The high affinity FcγRIIIa V158 polymorphism, is associated with enhanced ADCC functionality and with better outcomes for cancer monoclonal therapeutics [75, 76]. Surprisingly, the FcγRIIIa V158 polymorphism might associate with HIV-1 disease progression [77] and associates with the risk of infection in recipients of the VAX004 vaccine [78].

While many factors can contribute to the Fc-dependent functions of antibodies, several studies have generated HIV-1-specific BnAbs with modified capacities to bind FcγRs and mediate Fc-dependent functions [5, 25, 36]. The aim of such studies is to gain an understanding of how to improve BnAb-conferred protection from infection. While abrogation of the Fc-dependent activity of BnAb b12 through introduction of the LALA mutation decreased the protective efficacy of the BnAb [5], a non-fucosylated version of b12, which exhibited an enhanced ability to bind to FcγRIIIa and trigger ADCC, did not confer any additional protection from repeated low-dose viral challenge [36]. These data suggest that engagement of FcγRIIIa and the triggering of ADCC activity are likely not essential to achieve in vivo BnAb-conferred protection from viral challenge. Alternatively, BnAbs that trigger a wide range of Fc-dependent functions or 'polyfunctional' Fc activity may be optimal. Indeed, several studies suggest that polyfunctional non-neutralizing Fc-dependent functions of HIV-1 binding antibodies can contribute to enhanced viral control and protection from infection [79–82]. Furthermore, the presence of antibodies with Fc polyfunctionality may contribute to the development of BnAbs. Richardson et al. recently observed that individuals that develop BnAbs have higher Fc polyfunctionality and increased subclass diversity [83].

It is important to note that studies have also assessed the effect of modifying the isotypes of BnAbs, especially to IgA, with varying results [84–88]. Isotype switching of 2F5 from IgG1 to IgA2 improved epitope affinity and improved inhibition of HIV-1 transcytosis [84]. In contrast, other studies have reported 2F5 IgA or 2F5 IgM variants to provide inferior protection against HIV-1 compared to 2F5 IgG [85, 86]. Indeed, 2F5 IgM failed to inhibit HIV-1 transcytosis [85], while 2F5 IgA failed to neutralize HIV-1 infection of PBMC [86]. In contrast, 2F5 IgG protected against HIV-1 infection in vitro and intravenous administration of 2F5 IgG protected macaques from intravaginal viral challenge [86]. Importantly, intravenous administration of 2F5 Fab exhibited no protection, emphasizing the importance of the Fc region of the 2F5 BnAb for protection. An additional study modified the V3 neutralizing antibody HGN194 from IgG1 to dimeric IgA1 and dimeric IgA2. The resulting antibodies exhibited similar neutralization potencies, but HGN194 dimeric IgA1 provided the best protection in vivo against intrarectal viral challenge. Protection was correlated with in vitro measurements of inhibition of viral transcytosis and virion capture [87]. Lastly, neutralizing CH31 IgG antibodies exhibited enhanced protection against intrarectal viral challenge in macaques compared to monomeric, dimeric or secretory IgA2 variants [88]. Clearly, these studies indicate that the isotype of BnAbs can contribute significantly to protection from mucosal viral challenge, but the contribution of isotype might be epitope specific and too few studies have been conducted to determine how the antibody isotype contributes mechanistically to protection. Similar to IgG, IgA can engage its Fcα receptor that is present on the surfaces of monocytes, macrophages and neutrophils to mediate phagocytosis, respiratory burst, and the release of various cytokines and inflammatory mediators [89]. The potential of Fc/FcR interactions between IgA and Fcα receptor is an area of research that has not yet been fully explored in terms of its potential for combatting HIV -1.

Potential importance of diverse human NK cell functionality on BnAb efficacy

In addition to polymorphisms in FcγRs, several additional variables might potentially impact the ability of effector cells to utilize BnAbs to mediate Fc-dependent functions. NK cells and the impact of the processes of education and differentiation on their functional potential best represent this.

Diversity in the capacity of NK cells to respond to stimuli is introduced through the process of NK cell education [90]. During the education process NK cells scan the self-environment for constitutively expressed ligands to their activating and inhibitory receptors. The receptors involved in this process include activating and inhibitory killer immunoglobulin-like receptors (KIR), which recognize classical major histocompatibility complex class I (MHC-I or HLA-I) molecules [91], and the inhibitory NKG2A receptor, which recognizes the non-classical HLA-E [92]. In general, education tunes the potential responsiveness of an NK cell in a manner that maintains self-tolerance, conferring functional capacity to cells expressing inhibitory receptors that recognize self-ligands [93–95] and reducing the functional capacity of cells expressing activating receptors that recognize self-ligands [96]. Several studies have now demonstrated that education determines the responsiveness of NK cells to direct stimulation with HLA-I-devoid target cells [93, 94], as well as FcγR-dependent stimulation of NK cells with antibody-coated target cells [93, 95].

The role of NK cell education in determining Fc-dependent NK cell functions via anti-HIV-1 antibodies has been investigated using HIV-1 envelope coated target cells and polyclonal antibodies derived from patients [97–100]. Most of these studies have evaluated the role of education in anti-HIV-1 Fc-dependent NK cell responses by focusing on single education-competent receptor/ligand combinations, such as KIR3DL1/HLA-Bw4 or KIR2DL1/HLA-C2. The highlighted studies have pointed to higher levels of antibody-dependent activation in NK cells educated through the studied receptor than in an autologous NK cell population containing both non-educated cells and cells educated through other inhibitory receptors. Isitman et al. compared anti-HIV-1 ADCC mediated by PBMC from individuals with NK cells educated through KIR3DL1/HLA-Bw4 and individuals with NK cells lacking education through KIR3DL1/HLA-Bw4 [101]. No differences in ADCC were noted between the two groups, leading the investigators to suggest that NK cell education may not be important for determining anti-HIV-1 ADCC capacity. Alternatively, it is possible that NK cells educated through inhibitory receptor/ligand combinations other than KIR3DL1/HLA-Bw4 conferred compensatory NK cell education in the individuals lacking this receptor/ligand combination. We recently attempted to evaluate the relative contributions of educated and non-educated NK cells within PBMC to anti-HIV-1 ADCC [99]. Briefly, PBMC were stained with fluorochrome-conjugated antibodies to identify cells expressing inhibitory receptors that would educate NK cells, given the donor's HLA-I profile. Stained cells were FACs sorted as a population enriched for educated NK cells (i.e. education$^+$ PBMC) and unstained cells were sorted as a population lacking educated NK cells (i.e. education$^-$ PBMC). Utilizing cell numbers reflecting the frequency of each population of cells within total PBMC, we evaluated the relative ability of each cell population to kill gp120-coated target cells in the presence of anti-HIV-1 antibodies. We observed robust ADCC mediated by total PBMC that was recaptured by the sorted education$^+$ PBMC. In contrast, the sorted education$^-$ PBMC mediated little-to-no ADCC, and were significantly less cytotoxic than either the whole PBMC or the education$^+$ PBMC population.

While our data imply that educated NK cells are the primary mediators of anti-HIV-1 ADCC within PBMC, it is important to note that these data were collected using gp120-coated target cells and with polyclonal antibody mixtures. Future experiments are needed to determine if education has a similar impact on the capacity of NK cells to utilize BnAbs to mediate anti-HIV-1 ADCC. Furthermore, it would be ideal to conduct these experiments with autologous HIV-1-infected target cells, which present viral envelope in physiological conformations and amounts. The implementation of autologous infected cells will also address the role of autologous HLA-I in inhibiting anti-HIV-1 ADCC, and how downregulation of HLA-I by HIV-1 nef influences the ability of self-HLA-I to inhibit anti-HIV-1 ADCC [102].

In addition to education, the relative responsiveness of an NK cell to antibody-dependent stimulation is determined by the stage of differentiation of the cell. NK cells differentiate in a defined pattern, proceeding from CD56^{bright} to CD56^{dim} before gaining expression of the CD57 differentiation marker [103]. Throughout this process NK cells gain expression of KIRs and FcγRIIIa and become more cytotoxic. Additionally, differentiated CD56^{dim}CD57$^+$ NK cells exhibit more robust responses through FcγRIIIa following stimulation with anti-receptor antibody or anti-viral antibody-coated target cells expressing HIV-1 antigens [100, 104].

Importantly, viral infections appear to influence the NK cell differentiation process. Indeed, individuals infected with human cytomegalovirus (HCMV) exhibit expansions of differentiated CD56^{dim}CD57$^+$ NK cells that also express the activating NKG2C receptor, which recognizes the non-classical HLA-E molecule [92, 105]. These NK cells exhibit robust function through FcγRIIIa [106]. Furthermore, these differentiated NK cells degranulate following ligation of NKG2C [105]. Interestingly, CD56^{dim}CD57$^+$NKG2C$^+$ NK cells have been noted to occur in HIV-1-infected individuals in a HCMV-dependent manner [107]. The frequency of these cells in HIV-1-infected donors, however, appears to be exaggerated compared to HCMV-infected HIV-1-uninfected donors. Further research is required to determine the anti-HIV-1 antibody-dependent functions of CD56^{dim}CD57$^+$NKG2C$^+$ NK cells. It will be interesting to determine if these cells can confer enhanced anti-viral benefits in individuals receiving BnAbs for the purposes of therapy or cure.

Lastly, the ability of NK cells to mediate Fc-dependent functions is influenced by virus-induced alterations on target cells. Much has been published on the ability of HIV-1 nef and vpu to downregulate CD4 on infected cells, prevent exposure of CD4-induced epitopes on viral envelope and facilitate the evasion of ADCC mediated by polyclonal patient-derived ADCC antibodies that predominantly recognize CD4-induced envelope epitopes [108, 109]. This phenomenon is less of a problem for BnAb-mediated ADCC, as BnAbs tend to recognize HIV-1 envelope in its native CD4-unbound trimeric state. In addition to downregulating CD4, HIV-1 nef can downregulate the expression of ligands for the activating NKG2D NK cell receptor, which can serve as a co-receptor for anti-HIV-1 ADCC [110–112]. Furthermore, HIV-1 vpu can downregulate cellular tetherin, which plays an essential role is concentrating virus at the cellular membrane. Downregulation of tetherin decreases the amount of viral antigen available on the surface of infected cells and is a means of evading anti-HIV-1 ADCC [113]. The potential for HIV-1 accessory proteins to influence ADCC readouts highlights the importance of carefully selecting viruses and assays that most closely portray the in vivo situation in which the antibody in question will be immersed [112, 114].

Conclusions

The weight of data supports the contention that Fc-mediated functions of BnAbs are important to their efficacy in preventing HIV-1 and controlling viremia. This contribution is likely to be even more important in the context of exposure to cell-associated virus, where virus may evade neutralization by BnAbs. Newer generation BnAbs have higher potency and are potential tools for preventing and controlling HIV-1 infection. Additional work characterizing the in vivo importance of Fc-mediated functions of newer generation BnAbs is needed.

Authors' contributions

All authors contributed to the writing of the manuscript. All authors approved the manuscript for final publication.

Author details

[1] Department of Microbiology and Immunology, The University of Melbourne, at the Peter Doherty Institute for Infection and Immunity, Victoria, Australia.
[2] ARC Centre of Excellence in Convergent Bio-Nano Science and Technology, The University of Melbourne, Victoria, Australia. [3] Melbourne Sexual Health Centre, Alfred Hospital, Monash University Central Clinical School, Victoria, Australia.

Competing interests

The authors declare that they have no competing interests.

Funding

Australian National Health and Medical Research Council Grant # 1052979.

References

1. McCoy LE, Burton DR. Identification and specificity of broadly neutralizing antibodies against HIV. Immunol Rev. 2017;275:11–20.
2. Barouch DH, Whitney JB, Moldt B, Klein F, Oliveira TY, Liu J, Stephenson KE, Chang HW, Shekhar K, Gupta S, et al. Therapeutic efficacy of potent neutralizing HIV-1-specific monoclonal antibodies in SHIV-infected rhesus monkeys. Nature. 2013;503:224–8.
3. Caskey M, Klein F, Lorenzi JC, Seaman MS, West AP Jr, Buckley N, Kremer G, Nogueira L, Braunschweig M, Scheid JF, et al. Viraemia suppressed in HIV-1-infected humans by broadly neutralizing antibody 3BNC117. Nature. 2015;522:487–91.
4. Caskey M, Schoofs T, Gruell H, Settler A, Karagounis T, Kreider EF, Murrell B, Pfeifer N, Nogueira L, Oliveira TY, et al. Antibody 10-1074 suppresses viremia in HIV-1-infected individuals. Nat Med. 2017;23:185–91.
5. Hessell AJ, Hangartner L, Hunter M, Havenith CE, Beurskens FJ, Bakker JM, Lanigan CM, Landucci G, Forthal DN, Parren PW, et al. Fc receptor but not complement binding is important in antibody protection against HIV. Nature. 2007;449:101–4.
6. Hessell AJ, Rakasz EG, Poignard P, Hangartner L, Landucci G, Forthal DN, Koff WC, Watkins DI, Burton DR. Broadly neutralizing human anti-HIV antibody 2G12 is effective in protection against mucosal SHIV challenge even at low serum neutralizing titers. PLoS Pathog. 2009;5:e1000433.
7. Moldt B, Rakasz EG, Schultz N, Chan-Hui PY, Swiderek K, Weisgrau KL, Piaskowski SM, Bergman Z, Watkins DI, Poignard P, Burton DR. Highly potent HIV-specific antibody neutralization in vitro translates into effective protection against mucosal SHIV challenge in vivo. Proc Natl Acad Sci U S A. 2012;109:18921–5.
8. Moog C, Dereuddre-Bosquet N, Teillaud JL, Biedma ME, Holl V, Van Ham G, Heyndrickx L, Van Dorsselaer A, Katinger D, Vcelar B, et al. Protective effect of vaginal application of neutralizing and nonneutralizing inhibitory antibodies against vaginal SHIV challenge in macaques. Mucosal Immunol. 2014;7:46–56.
9. Nishimura Y, Gautam R, Chun TW, Sadjadpour R, Foulds KE, Shingai M, Klein F, Gazumyan A, Golijanin J, Donaldson M, et al. Early antibody therapy can induce long-lasting immunity to SHIV. Nature. 2017;543:559–63.
10. Parren PW, Marx PA, Hessell AJ, Luckay A, Harouse J, Cheng-Mayer C, Moore JP, Burton DR. Antibody protects macaques against vaginal challenge with a pathogenic R5 simian/human immunodeficiency virus at serum levels giving complete neutralization in vitro. J Virol. 2001;75:8340–7.
11. Shingai M, Nishimura Y, Klein F, Mouquet H, Donau OK, Plishka R, Buckler-White A, Seaman M, Piatak M Jr, Lifson JD, et al. Antibody-mediated immunotherapy of macaques chronically infected with SHIV suppresses viraemia. Nature. 2013;503:277–80.
12. Veazey RS, Shattock RJ, Pope M, Kirijan JC, Jones J, Hu Q, Ketas T, Marx PA, Klasse PJ, Burton DR, Moore JP. Prevention of virus transmission to macaque monkeys by a vaginally applied monoclonal antibody to HIV-1 gp120. Nat Med. 2003;9:343–6.
13. Haynes BF, Gilbert PB, McElrath MJ, Zolla-Pazner S, Tomaras GD, Alam SM, Evans DT, Montefiori DC, Karnasuta C, Sutthent R, et al. Immune-correlates analysis of an HIV-1 vaccine efficacy trial. N Engl J Med. 2012;366:1275–86.
14. Rerks-Ngarm S, Pitisuttithum P, Nitayaphan S, Kaewkungwal J, Chiu J, Paris R, Premsri N, Namwat C, de Souza M, Adams E, et al. Vaccination with ALVAC and AIDSVAX to prevent HIV-1 infection in Thailand. N Engl J Med. 2009;361:2209–20.
15. Tomaras GD, Ferrari G, Shen X, Alam SM, Liao HX, Pollara J, Bonsignori M, Moody MA, Fong Y, Chen X, et al. Vaccine-induced plasma IgA specific for the C1 region of the HIV-1 envelope blocks binding and effector function of IgG. Proc Natl Acad Sci U S A. 2013;110:9019–24.
16. Chung AW, Isitman G, Navis M, Kramski M, Center RJ, Kent SJ, Stratov I. Immune escape from HIV-specific antibody-dependent cellular cytotoxicity (ADCC) pressure. Proc Natl Acad Sci U S A. 2011;108:7505–10.
17. Horwitz JA, Bar-On Y, Lu CL, Fera D, Lockhart AAK, Lorenzi JCC, Nogueira L, Golijanin J, Scheid JF, Seaman MS, et al. Non-neutralizing antibodies alter the course of HIV-1 infection in vivo. Cell. 2017;170:637–648.e10.
18. Lambotte O, Ferrari G, Moog C, Yates NL, Liao HX, Parks RJ, Hicks CB, Owzar K, Tomaras GD, Montefiori DC, et al. Heterogeneous neutralizing antibody and antibody-dependent cell cytotoxicity responses in HIV-1 elite controllers. AIDS. 2009;23:897–906.
19. Wren LH, Chung AW, Isitman G, Kelleher AD, Parsons MS, Amin J, Cooper DA, Asc investigators, Stratov I, Navis M, Kent SJ. Specific antibody-dependent cellular cytotoxicity responses associated with slow progression of HIV infection. Immunology. 2013;138:116–123
20. Bournazos S, Klein F, Pietzsch J, Seaman MS, Nussenzweig MC, Ravetch JV. Broadly neutralizing anti-HIV-1 antibodies require Fc effector functions for in vivo activity. Cell. 2014;158:1243–53.
21. Bruel T, Guivel-Benhassine F, Amraoui S, Malbec M, Richard L, Bourdic K, Donahue DA, Lorin V, Casartelli N, Noel N, et al. Elimination of HIV-1-infected cells by broadly neutralizing antibodies. Nat Commun. 2016;7:10844.
22. Mujib S, Liu J, Rahman A, Schwartz JA, Bonner P, Yue FY, Ostrowski MA. Comprehensive cross-clade characterization of antibody-mediated recognition, complement-mediated lysis, and cell-mediated cytotoxicity of HIV-1 envelope-specific antibodies toward eradication of the HIV-1 reservoir. J Virol. 2017;91:e00634–17.
23. von Bredow B, Arias JF, Heyer LN, Moldt B, Le K, Robinson JE, Zolla-Pazner S, Burton DR, Evans DT. Comparison of Antibody-dependent cell-mediated cytotoxicity and virus neutralization by HIV-1 Env-specific monoclonal antibodies. J Virol. 2016;90:6127–39.
24. Forthal DN, Landucci G, Daar ES. Antibody from patients with acute human immunodeficiency virus (HIV) infection inhibits primary strains

of HIV type 1 in the presence of natural-killer effector cells. J Virol. 2001;75:6953–61.

25. Moldt B, Schultz N, Dunlop DC, Alpert MD, Harvey JD, Evans DT, Poignard P, Hessell AJ, Burton DR. A panel of IgG1 b12 variants with selectively diminished or enhanced affinity for Fcgamma receptors to define the role of effector functions in protection against HIV. J Virol. 2011;85:10572–81.

26. Tay MZ, Liu P, Williams LD, McRaven MD, Sawant S, Gurley TC, Xu TT, Dennison SM, Liao HX, Chenine AL, et al. Antibody-mediated internalization of infectious HIV-1 virions differs among antibody isotypes and subclasses. PLoS Pathog. 2016;12:e1005817.

27. Tudor D, Bomsel M. The broadly neutralizing HIV-1 IgG 2F5 elicits gp41-specific antibody-dependent cell cytotoxicity in a FcgammaRI-dependent manner. AIDS. 2011;25:751–9.

28. Klein JS, Webster A, Gnanapragasam PN, Galimidi RP, Bjorkman PJ. A dimeric form of the HIV-1 antibody 2G12 elicits potent antibody-dependent cellular cytotoxicity. AIDS. 2010;24:1633–40.

29. Trkola A, Purtscher M, Muster T, Ballaun C, Buchacher A, Sullivan N, Srinivasan K, Sodroski J, Moore JP, Katinger H. Human monoclonal antibody 2G12 defines a distinctive neutralization epitope on the gp120 glycoprotein of human immunodeficiency virus type 1. J Virol. 1996;70:1100–8.

30. Hezareh M, Hessell AJ, Jensen RC, van de Winkel JG, Parren PW. Effector function activities of a panel of mutants of a broadly neutralizing antibody against human immunodeficiency virus type 1. J Virol. 2001;75:12161–8.

31. Ko SY, Pegu A, Rudicell RS, Yang ZY, Joyce MG, Chen X, Wang K, Bao S, Kraemer TD, Rath T, et al. Enhanced neonatal Fc receptor function improves protection against primate SHIV infection. Nature. 2014;514:642–5.

32. Smith AJ, Wietgrefe SW, Shang L, Reilly CS, Southern PJ, Perkey KE, Duan L, Kohler H, Muller S, Robinson J, et al. Live simian immunodeficiency virus vaccine correlate of protection: immune complex-inhibitory Fc receptor interactions that reduce target cell availability. J Immunol. 2014;193:3126–33.

33. Gardner MR, Kattenhorn LM, Kondur HR, von Schaewen M, Dorfman T, Chiang JJ, Haworth KG, Decker JM, Alpert MD, Bailey CC, et al. AAV-expressed eCD4-Ig provides durable protection from multiple SHIV challenges. Nature. 2015;519:87–91.

34. Saunders KO, Wang L, Joyce MG, Yang ZY, Balazs AB, Cheng C, Ko SY, Kong WP, Rudicell RS, Georgiev IS, et al. Broadly neutralizing human immunodeficiency virus type 1 antibody gene transfer protects nonhuman primates from mucosal simian-human immunodeficiency virus infection. J Virol. 2015;89:8334–45.

35. Hessell AJ, Poignard P, Hunter M, Hangartner L, Tehrani DM, Bleeker WK, Parren PW, Marx PA, Burton DR. Effective, low-titer antibody protection against low-dose repeated mucosal SHIV challenge in macaques. Nat Med. 2009;15:951–4.

36. Moldt B, Shibata-Koyama M, Rakasz EG, Schultz N, Kanda Y, Dunlop DC, Finstad SL, Jin C, Landucci G, Alpert MD, et al. A nonfucosylated variant of the anti-HIV-1 monoclonal antibody b12 has enhanced FcgammaRI-IIa-mediated antiviral activity in vitro but does not improve protection against mucosal SHIV challenge in macaques. J Virol. 2012;86:6189–96.

37. Ho DD, Schooley RT, Rota TR, Kaplan JC, Flynn T, Salahuddin SZ, Gonda MA, Hirsch MS. HTLV-III in the semen and blood of a healthy homosexual man. Science. 1984;226:451–3.

38. Anderson DJ, Politch JA, Nadolski AM, Blaskewicz CD, Pudney J, Mayer KH. Targeting Trojan Horse leukocytes for HIV prevention. AIDS. 2010;24:163–87.

39. Anderson DJ, Yunis EJ. "Trojan Horse" leukocytes in AIDS. N Engl J Med. 1983;309:984–5.

40. Kolodkin-Gal D, Hulot SL, Korioth-Schmitz B, Gombos RB, Zheng Y, Owuor J, Lifton MA, Ayeni C, Najarian RM, Yeh WW, et al. Efficiency of cell-free and cell-associated virus in mucosal transmission of human immunodeficiency virus type 1 and simian immunodeficiency virus. J Virol. 2013;87:13589–97.

41. Zhu T, Wang N, Carr A, Nam DS, Moor-Jankowski R, Cooper DA, Ho DD. Genetic characterization of human immunodeficiency virus type 1 in blood and genital secretions: evidence for viral compartmentalization and selection during sexual transmission. J Virol. 1996;70:3098–107.

42. Abela IA, Berlinger L, Schanz M, Reynell L, Gunthard HF, Rusert P, Trkola A. Cell-cell transmission enables HIV-1 to evade inhibition by potent CD4bs directed antibodies. PLoS Pathog. 2012;8:e1002634.

43. Duncan CJ, Williams JP, Schiffner T, Gartner K, Ochsenbauer C, Kappes J, Russell RA, Frater J, Sattentau QJ. High-multiplicity HIV-1 infection and neutralizing antibody evasion mediated by the macrophage-T cell virological synapse. J Virol. 2014;88:2025–34.

44. Gombos RB, Kolodkin-Gal D, Eslamizar L, Owuor JO, Mazzola E, Gonzalez AM, Korioth-Schmitz B, Gelman RS, Montefiori DC, Haynes BF, Schmitz JE. Inhibitory effect of individual or combinations of broadly neutralizing antibodies and antiviral reagents against cell-free and cell-to-cell HIV-1 transmission. J Virol. 2015;89:7813–28.

45. Li H, Zony C, Chen P, Chen BK. Reduced Potency and incomplete neutralization of broadly neutralizing antibodies against cell-to-cell transmission of HIV-1 with transmitted founder Envs. J Virol. 2017;91:e02425–16.

46. Malbec M, Porrot F, Rua R, Horwitz J, Klein F, Halper-Stromberg A, Scheid JF, Eden C, Mouquet H, Nussenzweig MC, Schwartz O. Broadly neutralizing antibodies that inhibit HIV-1 cell to cell transmission. J Exp Med. 2013;210:2813–21.

47. Reh L, Magnus C, Schanz M, Weber J, Uhr T, Rusert P, Trkola A. Capacity of broadly neutralizing antibodies to inhibit HIV-1 cell-cell transmission is strain- and epitope-dependent. PLoS Pathog. 2015;11:e1004966.

48. Schiffner T, Sattentau QJ, Duncan CJ. Cell-to-cell spread of HIV-1 and evasion of neutralizing antibodies. Vaccine. 2013;31:5789–97.

49. Martin N, Welsch S, Jolly C, Briggs JA, Vaux D, Sattentau QJ. Virological synapse-mediated spread of human immunodeficiency virus type 1 between T cells is sensitive to entry inhibition. J Virol. 2010;84:3516–27.

50. Massanella M, Puigdomenech I, Cabrera C, Fernandez-Figueras MT, Aucher A, Gaibelet G, Hudrisier D, Garcia E, Bofill M, Clotet B, Blanco J. Antigp41 antibodies fail to block early events of virological synapses but inhibit HIV spread between T cells. AIDS. 2009;23:183–8.

51. McCoy LE, Groppelli E, Blanchetot C, de Haard H, Verrips T, Rutten L, Weiss RA, Jolly C. Neutralisation of HIV-1 cell-cell spread by human and llama antibodies. Retrovirology. 2014;11:83.

52. Parsons MS, Lloyd SB, Lee WS, Kristensen AB, Amarasena T, Center RJ, Keele BF, Lifson JD, LaBranche CC, Montefiori D, et al. Partial efficacy of a broadly neutralizing antibody against cell-associated SHIV infection. Sci Transl Med. 2017;9:eaaf1483.

53. Salle B, Brochard P, Bourry O, Mannioui A, Andrieu T, Prevot S, Dejucq-Rainsford N, Dereuddre-Bosquet N, Le Grand R. Infection of macaques after vaginal exposure to cell-associated simian immunodeficiency virus. J Infect Dis. 2010;202:337–44.

54. Parsons MS, Cromer D, Davenport MP, Kent SJ. HIV reactivation after partial protection by neutralizing antibodies. Trends Immunol. 2018;39:359–66.

55. Poignard P, Sabbe R, Picchio GR, Wang M, Gulizia RJ, Katinger H, Parren PW, Mosier DE, Burton DR. Neutralizing antibodies have limited effects on the control of established HIV-1 infection in vivo. Immunity. 1999;10:431–8.

56. Trkola A, Kuster H, Rusert P, Joos B, Fischer M, Leemann C, Manrique A, Huber M, Rehr M, Oxenius A, et al. Delay of HIV-1 rebound after cessation of antiretroviral therapy through passive transfer of human neutralizing antibodies. Nat Med. 2005;11:615–22.

57. Mehandru S, Vcelar B, Wrin T, Stiegler G, Joos B, Mohri H, Boden D, Galovich J, Tenner-Racz K, Racz P, et al. Adjunctive passive immunotherapy in human immunodeficiency virus type 1-infected individuals treated with antiviral therapy during acute and early infection. J Virol. 2007;81:11016–31.

58. Klein F, Halper-Stromberg A, Horwitz JA, Gruell H, Scheid JF, Bournazos S, Mouquet H, Spatz LA, Diskin R, Abadir A, et al. HIV therapy by a combination of broadly neutralizing antibodies in humanized mice. Nature. 2012;492:118–22.

59. Horwitz JA, Halper-Stromberg A, Mouquet H, Gitlin AD, Tretiakova A, Eisenreich TR, Malbec M, Gravemann S, Billerbeck E, Dorner M, et al. HIV-1 suppression and durable control by combining single broadly neutralizing antibodies and antiretroviral drugs in humanized mice. Proc Natl Acad Sci U S A. 2013;110:16538–43.

60. Scheid JF, Horwitz JA, Bar-On Y, Kreider EF, Lu CL, Lorenzi JC, Feldmann A, Braunschweig M, Nogueira L, Oliveira T, et al. HIV-1 antibody

3BNC117 suppresses viral rebound in humans during treatment interruption. Nature. 2016;535:556–60.

61. Halper-Stromberg A, Lu CL, Klein F, Horwitz JA, Bournazos S, Nogueira L, Eisenreich TR, Liu C, Gazumyan A, Schaefer U, et al. Broadly neutralizing antibodies and viral inducers decrease rebound from HIV-1 latent reservoirs in humanized mice. Cell. 2014;158:989–99.

62. Lu CL, Murakowski DK, Bournazos S, Schoofs T, Sarkar D, Halper-Stromberg A, Horwitz JA, Nogueira L, Golijanin J, Gazumyan A, et al. Enhanced clearance of HIV-1-infected cells by broadly neutralizing antibodies against HIV-1 in vivo. Science. 2016;352:1001–4.

63. Chung AW, Alter G. Dissecting the antibody constant region protective immune parameters in HIV infection. Future Virol. 2014;9:397–414.

64. Hogarth PM, Pietersz GA. Fc receptor-targeted therapies for the treatment of inflammation, cancer and beyond. Nat Rev Drug Discov. 2012;11:311–31.

65. Moraru M, Black LE, Muntasell A, Portero F, Lopez-Botet M, Reyburn HT, Pandey JP, Vilches C. NK cell and Ig interplay in defense against herpes simplex virus type 1: epistatic interaction of CD16A and IgG1 allotypes of variable affinities modulates antibody-dependent cellular cytotoxicity and susceptibility to clinical reactivation. J Immunol. 2015;195:1676–84.

66. Vidarsson G, Dekkers G, Rispens T. IgG subclasses and allotypes: from structure to effector functions. Front Immunol. 2014;5:520.

67. Shields RL, Lai J, Keck R, O'Connell LY, Hong K, Meng YG, Weikert SH, Presta LG. Lack of fucose on human IgG1 N-linked oligosaccharide improves binding to human Fcgamma RIII and antibody-dependent cellular toxicity. J Biol Chem. 2002;277:26733–40.

68. Chung AW, Crispin M, Pritchard L, Robinson H, Gorny MK, Yu X, Bailey-Kellogg C, Ackerman ME, Scanlan C, Zolla-Pazner S, Alter G. Identification of antibody glycosylation structures that predict monoclonal antibody Fc-effector function. AIDS. 2014;28:2523–30.

69. Ahmad A, Menezes J. Antibody-dependent cellular cytotoxicity in HIV infections. Faseb J. 1996;10:258–66.

70. Kramski M, Schorcht A, Johnston AP, Lichtfuss GF, Jegaskanda S, De Rose R, Stratov I, Kelleher AD, French MA, Center RJ, et al. Role of monocytes in mediating HIV-specific antibody-dependent cellular cytotoxicity. J Immunol Methods. 2012;384:51–61.

71. Worley MJ, Fei K, Lopez-Denman AJ, Kelleher AD, Kent SJ, Chung AW. Neutrophils mediate HIV-specific antibody-dependent phagocytosis and ADCC. J Immunol Methods. 2018;457:41–52.

72. Tjiam MC, Sariputra L, Armitage JD, Taylor JP, Kelleher AD, Tan DB, Lee S, Fernandez S, French MA. Control of early HIV-1 infection associates with plasmacytoid dendritic cell-reactive opsonophagocytic IgG antibodies to HIV-1 p24. AIDS. 2016;30:2757–65.

73. Forthal DN, Landucci G, Bream J, Jacobson LP, Phan TB, Montoya B. FcgammaRIIa genotype predicts progression of HIV infection. J Immunol. 2007;179:7916–23.

74. Sanders LA, Feldman RG, Voorhorst-Ogink MM, de Haas M, Rijkers GT, Capel PJ, Zegers BJ, van de Winkel JG. Human immunoglobulin G (IgG) Fc receptor IIA (CD32) polymorphism and IgG2-mediated bacterial phagocytosis by neutrophils. Infect Immun. 1995;63:73–81.

75. Wang W, Erbe AK, Hank JA, Morris ZS, Sondel PM. NK cell-mediated antibody-dependent cellular cytotoxicity in cancer immunotherapy. Front Immunol. 2015;6:368.

76. Cartron G, Dacheux L, Salles G, Solal-Celigny P, Bardos P, Colombat P, Watier H. Therapeutic activity of humanized anti-CD20 monoclonal antibody and polymorphism in IgG Fc receptor FcgammaRIIIa gene. Blood. 2002;99:754–8.

77. Poonia B, Kijak GH, Pauza CD. High affinity allele for the gene of FCGR3A is risk factor for HIV infection and progression. PLoS ONE. 2010;5:e15562.

78. Forthal DN, Gabriel EE, Wang A, Landucci G, Phan TB. Association of Fcgamma receptor IIIa genotype with the rate of HIV infection after gp120 vaccination. Blood. 2012;120:2836–42.

79. Ackerman ME, Mikhailova A, Brown EP, Dowell KG, Walker BD, Bailey-Kellogg C, Suscovich TJ, Alter G. Polyfunctional HIV-specific antibody responses are associated with spontaneous HIV control. PLoS Pathog. 2016;12:e1005315.

80. Chung AW, Ghebremichael M, Robinson H, Brown E, Choi I, Lane S, Dugast AS, Schoen MK, Rolland M, Suscovich TJ, et al. Polyfunctional

Fc-effector profiles mediated by IgG subclass selection distinguish RV144 and VAX003 vaccines. Sci Transl Med. 2014;6:228ra38.

81. Chung AW, Kumar MP, Arnold KB, Yu WH, Schoen MK, Dunphy LJ, Suscovich TJ, Frahm N, Linde C, Mahan AE, et al. Dissecting polyclonal vaccine-induced humoral immunity against HIV using systems serology. Cell. 2015;163:988–98.

82. Barouch DH, Alter G, Broge T, Linde C, Ackerman ME, Brown EP, Borducchi EN, Smith KM, Nkolola JP, Liu J, et al. Protective efficacy of adenovirus-protein vaccines against SIV challenges in rhesus monkeys. Science. 2015;349:320–4.

83. Richardson SI, Chung AW, Natarajan H, Mabvakure B, Mkhize NN, Garrett N, Abdool Karim S, Moore PL, Ackerman ME, Alter G, Morris L. HIV-specific Fc effector function early in infection predicts the development of broadly neutralizing antibodies. PLoS Pathog. 2018;14:e1006987.

84. Tudor D, Yu H, Maupetit J, Drillet AS, Bouceba T, Schwartz-Cornil I, Lopalco L, Tuffery P, Bomsel M. Isotype modulates epitope specificity, affinity, and antiviral activities of anti-HIV-1 human broadly neutralizing 2F5 antibody. Proc Natl Acad Sci U S A. 2012;109:12680–5.

85. Shen R, Drelichman ER, Bimczok D, Ochsenbauer C, Kappes JC, Cannon JA, Tudor D, Bomsel M, Smythies LE, Smith PD. GP41-specific antibody blocks cell-free HIV type 1 transcytosis through human rectal mucosa and model colonic epithelium. J Immunol. 2010;184:3648–55.

86. Klein K, Veazey RS, Warrier R, Hraber P, Doyle-Meyers LA, Buffa V, Liao HX, Haynes BF, Shaw GM, Shattock RJ. Neutralizing IgG at the portal of infection mediates protection against vaginal simian/human immunodeficiency virus challenge. J Virol. 2013;87:11604–16.

87. Watkins JD, Sholukh AM, Mukhtar MM, Siddappa NB, Lakhashe SK, Kim M, Reinherz EL, Gupta S, Forthal DN, Sattentau QJ, et al. Anti-HIV IgA isotypes: differential virion capture and inhibition of transcytosis are linked to prevention of mucosal R5 SHIV transmission. AIDS. 2013;27:F13–20.

88. Astronomo RD, Santra S, Ballweber-Fleming L, Westerberg KG, Mach L, Hensley-McBain T, Sutherland L, Mildenberg B, Morton G, Yates NL, et al. Neutralization Takes precedence over IgG or IgA Isotype-related functions in mucosal HIV-1 antibody-mediated protection. EBioMedicine. 2016;14:97–111.

89. Lopez E, Shattock R, Kent SJ, Chung AW. The multi-faceted nature of immunoglobulin A and its complex role in HIV. AIDS Res Hum Retroviruses. 2018. https://doi.org/10.1089/AID.2018.0099.

90. Boudreau JE, Hsu KC. Natural killer cell education and the response to infection and cancer therapy: stay tuned. Trends Immunol. 2018;39:222–39.

91. Williams AP, Bateman AR, Khakoo SI. Hanging in the balance. KIR and their role in disease. Mol Interv. 2005;5:226–40.

92. Braud VM, Allan DS, O'Callaghan CA, Soderstrom K, D'Andrea A, Ogg GS, Lazetic S, Young NT, Bell JI, Phillips JH, et al. HLA-E binds to natural killer cell receptors CD94/NKG2A, B and C. Nature. 1998;391:795–9.

93. Anfossi N, Andre P, Guia S, Falk CS, Roetynck S, Stewart CA, Breso V, Frassati C, Reviron D, Middleton D, et al. Human NK cell education by inhibitory receptors for MHC class I. Immunity. 2006;25:331–42.

94. Kim S, Sunwoo JB, Yang L, Choi T, Song YJ, French AR, Vlahiotis A, Piccirillo JF, Cella M, Colonna M, et al. HLA alleles determine differences in human natural killer cell responsiveness and potency. Proc Natl Acad Sci U S A. 2008;105:3053–8.

95. Parsons MS, Zipperlen K, Gallant M, Grant M. Killer cell immunoglobulin-like receptor 3DL1 licenses CD16-mediated effector functions of natural killer cells. J Leukoc Biol. 2010;88:905–12.

96. Fauriat C, Ivarsson MA, Ljunggren HG, Malmberg KJ, Michaelsson J. Education of human natural killer cells by activating killer cell immunoglobulin-like receptors. Blood. 2010;115:1166–74.

97. Gooneratne SL, Center RJ, Kent SJ, Parsons MS. Functional advantage of educated KIR2DL1(+) natural killer cells for anti-HIV-1 antibody-dependent activation. Clin Exp Immunol. 2016;184:101–9.

98. Gooneratne SL, Richard J, Lee WS, Finzi A, Kent SJ, Parsons MS. Slaying the Trojan horse: natural killer cells exhibit robust anti-HIV-1 antibody-dependent activation and cytolysis against allogeneic T cells. J Virol. 2015;89:97–109.

99. Kristensen AB, Kent SJ, Parsons MS. Contribution of NK cell education to both direct and anti-HIV-1 antibody-dependent NK cell functions. J Virol. 2018;92:e02146–17.

100. Parsons MS, Loh L, Gooneratne S, Center RJ, Kent SJ. Role of education and differentiation in determining the potential of natural killer cells to respond to antibody-dependent stimulation. AIDS. 2014;28:2781–6.

101. Isitman G, Lisovsky I, Tremblay-McLean A, Parsons MS, Shoukry NH, Wainberg MA, Bruneau J, Bernard NF. Natural killer cell education does not affect the magnitude of granzyme B delivery to target cells by antibody-dependent cellular cytotoxicity. AIDS. 2015;29:1433–43.

102. Cohen GB, Gandhi RT, Davis DM, Mandelboim O, Chen BK, Strominger JL, Baltimore D. The selective downregulation of class I major histocompatibility complex proteins by HIV-1 protects HIV-infected cells from NK cells. Immunity. 1999;10:661–71.

103. Solana R, Tarazona R, Gayoso I, Lesur O, Dupuis G, Fulop T. Innate immunosenescence: effect of aging on cells and receptors of the innate immune system in humans. Semin Immunol. 2012;24:331–41.

104. Lopez-Verges S, Milush JM, Pandey S, York VA, Arakawa-Hoyt J, Pircher H, Norris PJ, Nixon DF, Lanier LL. CD57 defines a functionally distinct population of mature NK cells in the human CD56dimCD16 + NK-cell subset. Blood. 2010;116:3865–74.

105. Lopez-Verges S, Milush JM, Schwartz BS, Pando MJ, Jarjoura J, York VA, Houchins JP, Miller S, Kang SM, Norris PJ, et al. Expansion of a unique CD57(+)NKG2Chi natural killer cell subset during acute human cytomegalovirus infection. Proc Natl Acad Sci U S A. 2011;108:14725–32.

106. Wu Z, Sinzger C, Frascaroli G, Reichel J, Bayer C, Wang L, Schirmbeck R, Mertens T. Human cytomegalovirus-induced NKG2C(hi) CD57(hi) natural killer cells are effectors dependent on humoral antiviral immunity. J Virol. 2013;87:7717–25.

107. Heath J, Newhook N, Comeau E, Gallant M, Fudge N, Grant M. NKG2C(+)CD57(+) natural killer cell expansion parallels cytomegalovirus-specific CD8(+) T cell evolution towards senescence. J Immunol Res. 2016;2016:7470124.

108. Veillette M, Coutu M, Richard J, Batraville LA, Dagher O, Bernard N, Tremblay C, Kaufmann DE, Roger M, Finzi A. The HIV-1 gp120 CD4-bound conformation is preferentially targeted by antibody-dependent cellular cytotoxicity-mediating antibodies in sera from HIV-1-infected individuals. J Virol. 2015;89:545–51.

109. Veillette M, Richard J, Pazgier M, Lewis GK, Parsons MS, Finzi A. Role of HIV-1 envelope glycoproteins conformation and accessory proteins on ADCC responses. Curr HIV Res. 2016;14:9–23.

110. Alsahafi N, Richard J, Prevost J, Coutu M, Brassard N, Parsons MS, Kaufmann DE, Brockman M, Finzi A. Impaired downregulation of NKG2D ligands by Nef proteins from elite controllers sensitizes HIV-1-infected cells to antibody-dependent cellular cytotoxicity. J Virol. 2017;91:e00109–17.

111. Parsons MS, Richard J, Lee WS, Vanderven H, Grant MD, Finzi A, Kent SJ. NKG2D acts as a co-receptor for natural killer cell-mediated anti-HIV-1 antibody-dependent cellular cytotoxicity. AIDS Res Hum Retroviruses. 2016;32:1089–96.

112. Prevost J, Richard J, Medjahed H, Alexander A, Jones J, Kappes JC, Ochsenbauer C, Finzi A. Incomplete downregulation of CD4 expression affects HIV-1 Env conformation and ADCC responses. J Virol. 2018;92:e00484–18.

113. Arias JF, Heyer LN, von Bredow B, Weisgrau KL, Moldt B, Burton DR, Rakasz EG, Evans DT. Tetherin antagonism by Vpu protects HIV-infected cells from antibody-dependent cell-mediated cytotoxicity. Proc Natl Acad Sci U S A. 2014;111:6425–30.

114. Richard J, Prevost J, Baxter AE, von Bredow B, Ding S, Medjahed H, Delgado GG, Brassard N, Sturzel CM, Kirchhoff F, et al. Uninfected bystander cells impact the measurement of HIV-specific antibody-dependent cellular cytotoxicity responses. MBio. 2018;9:e00358–18.

3

Predominant envelope variable loop 2-specific and gp120-specific antibody-dependent cellular cytotoxicity antibody responses in acutely SIV-infected African green monkeys

Quang N. Nguyen[1†], David R. Martinez[1,2†], Jonathon E. Himes[1], R. Whitney Edwards[1,3], Qifeng Han[1], Amit Kumar[1], Riley Mangan[1], Nathan I. Nicely[1], Guanhua Xie[1], Nathan Vandergrift[1], Xiaoying Shen[1], Justin Pollara[1,3] and Sallie R. Permar[1,2,4,5*]

Abstract

Background: The initial envelope (Env)-specific antibody response in acutely HIV-1-infected individuals and simian immunodeficiency virus (SIV)-infected rhesus monkeys (RMs) is dominated by non-neutralizing antibodies targeting Env gp41. In contrast, natural primate SIV hosts, such as African green monkeys (AGMs), develop a predominant Env gp120-specific antibody response to SIV infection. However, the fine-epitope specificity and function of SIV Env-specific plasma IgG, and their potential role on autologous virus co-evolution in SIV-infected AGMs and RMs remain unclear.

Results: Unlike the dominant linear gp41-specific IgG responses in RMs, SIV-infected AGMs demonstrated a unique linear variable loop 2 (V2)-specific plasma IgG response that arose concurrently with high gp120-directed antibody-dependent cellular cytotoxicity (ADCC) activity, and SIVsab-infected cell binding responses during acute infection. Moreover, SIV variants isolated from SIV-infected AGMs exhibited high amino acid mutation frequencies within the Env V1V2 loop compared to those of RMs. Notably, the linear V2-specific IgG epitope in AGMs overlaps with an analogous region of the HIV V2 loop containing the K169 mutation epitope identified in breakthrough viruses from RV144 vaccinees.

Conclusion: Vaccine-elicited Env V2-specific IgG responses have been proposed as an immune correlate of reduced risk in HIV-1/SIV acquisition in humans and RMs. Yet the pathways to elicit these potentially-protective V2-specific IgG responses remain unclear. In this study, we demonstrate that SIV-infected AGMs, which are the natural hosts of SIV, exhibited high plasma linear V2-specific IgG binding responses that arose concurrently with SIV Env gp120-directed ADCC-mediating, and SIV-infected cell plasma IgG binding responses during acute SIV infection, which were not present in acutely SIV-infected RMs. The linear V2-specific antibody response in AGMs targets an overlapping epitope of the proposed site of vaccine-induced immune pressure defined in the moderately protective RV144 HIV-1 vaccine trial. Identifying host factors that control the early elicitation of Env V2-specific IgG and ADCC antibody responses in

*Correspondence: sallie.permar@duke.edu
†Quang N. Nguyen and David R. Martinez contributed equally to this work
[2] Department of Molecular Genetics and Microbiology, Duke University School of Medicine, Durham, NC, USA
Full list of author information is available at the end of the article

these natural SIV hosts could inform vaccination strategies aimed at rapidly inducing potentially-protective HIV-1 Env-specific responses in humans.

Keywords: SIV, Linear peptide antibody responses, Natural SIV host, African green monkey, Rhesus monkey, Antibody response, ADCC, Envelope, gp120, gp41

Background

The HIV-1 Env glycoprotein contains multiple vulnerable epitopes targeted by potent broad neutralizing antibodies (bNAbs) [1]. However, the elicitation of HIV gp120-specific bNAbs by current Env vaccination strategies is not yet feasible [2, 3]. Thus, HIV vaccine candidates currently in clinical testing focus on the elicitation of antibody specificities and functions identified as potential immune correlates of reduced infection risk in human and non-human primate vaccine efficacy studies. Immune analyses from the HVTN 505 phase IIb vaccine trial, which utilized an HIV Env gp140 protein boost immunogen and failed to show efficacy, demonstrated that the vaccine-elicited humoral responses primarily targeted HIV Env gp41 without identifiable antiviral functions [4]. Similarly, in the setting of HIV-1 infection, the initial antibody response against HIV Env is also dominated by Env gp41-specific IgG responses that are ineffective at controlling viremia [5, 6]. Interestingly, in the moderately-efficacious RV144 HIV-1 Env vaccine efficacy trial, Env-specific IgG responses targeting the variable loop 1 and 2 (V1V2) were found to be associated with reduced HIV acquisition risk [7]. The following sieve analysis of the breakthrough virus variants localized the site of vaccine-induced immune pressure to two amino acid residue positions within V2 loop [8–10]. Moreover, the V2 epitope that was associated with immune escape in RV144 vaccinees spans the region capable of engaging the gut-homing integrin receptor $\alpha4\beta7$, which has been implicated in the trafficking of immune cells to the gut associated lymphoid tissue, and the enhancement of cell-to-cell HIV transmission [11–13]. Furthermore, the HIV Env V2-specific IgG responses in RV144 vaccinees mediated ADCC activity [14, 15]. Notably, V2-specific IgG responses were also associated with a reduced risk of SIVmac251 acquisition in RMs that received a similar vaccine regimen to that in the RV144 HIV-1 trial [16]. While these types of V2-specific IgG responses are a major clinical endpoint of HIV vaccination, our understanding of factors that control the elicitation of V2-specific IgG responses and ADCC function by existing vaccination strategies remains limited [3, 17].

Previous studies have investigated the proportion of SIV Env-specific IgG responses in the setting of infection in natural and non-natural SIV hosts. Antibody responses in acute SIV infection of RMs—a non-natural SIV host species and model of AIDS pathogenesis—predominantly target the SIV Env gp41 region [18–20]. Moreover, in SIV infected RMs, Env-specific IgG autologous virus neutralizing responses do not arise until approximately 1 year post-infection [18]. In contrast, AGMs—which are thought to have co-evolved with SIV for at least 30,000 years—sustain a non-pathogenic SIV infection, and do not exhibit a predominant gp41-specific IgG response over the course of infection [18, 19, 21]. SIV Env-specific IgG responses in chronically SIV-infected AGMs more frequently target gp120 epitopes compared to SIV-infected RMs [20]. While previous studies reported that B cell depletion in SIV-infected AGMs has no appreciable effect in disease progression outcome [22], it has also been shown that SIV-associated B cell dysfunction is associated with pathogenic SIV infection, and not in non-pathogenic SIV infection in natural SIV hosts [19, 23]. Moreover, we previously demonstrated that SIV Env gp120-specific IgG monoclonal antibodies (mAbs) isolated from chronically SIV-infected AGMs mediated robust virus capture activity, and ADCC—an antibody function that has been associated with delayed progression to AIDS in RMs [20, 24]. Moreover, SIV Env gp120-specific mAbs in chronically SIV-infected AGMs exhibited higher binding levels against SIV-infected $CD4^+$ target cells compared to gp41-specific antibodies [20]. In this study, we further explore the kinetics of ADCC and SIV-infected cell binding responses, the fine epitope-specificity of the early Env-specific IgG responses in AGMs and RMs, and their potential role in autologous virus evolution at key vulnerable Env sites. A deeper understanding of the fine-specificity, kinetics, and antiviral function of gp120-specific IgG responses in AGMs may help guide future HIV vaccination strategies aimed at eliciting potentially-protective Env-specific IgG responses in humans.

Results

Kinetics of SIV Env-specific plasma IgG binding response in SIV-infected AGMs and RMs

We previously showed that SIV-infected AGMs have a predominant gp120-specific antibody response compared to SIV-infected RMs [18]. In contrast, SIV-infected RMs have a more focused gp140-specific antibody response compared to SIV-infected AGMs [18]. We set out to further investigate the early acute kinetics of the gp120-specific IgG responses in AGMs and RMs by examining plasma

IgG binding against the autologous SIVsab92018ivTF/SIVmac251 Env gp120 proteins in both species. Prior to SIV infection, AGM and RM plasma IgG exhibited relatively low binding against SIV Env proteins (Fig. 1). By 3 wpi, AGMs had higher magnitude SIV Env-specific IgG binding responses to the autologous SIV gp120 compared to RMs (logED$_{50}$ median in AGMs vs. RMs: 3.0 vs. 2.3, FDR $p = 0.032$) (Fig. 1). By 15 weeks post-infection (wpi) and 1 year post-infection (1 ypi), there was no difference in plasma gp120-specific binding in SIVsab92018ivTF and SIVmac251-infected AGMs and RMs (Fig. 1).

Linear SIV Env peptide-specific plasma IgG binding responses in SIV-infected AGMs and RMs

To map the fine-epitope specificity of SIV Env-specific IgG responses in SIV-infected AGMs and RMs, we measured plasma IgG responses against a linear overlapping peptide library spanning the entire species-specific SIVsab92018WT/SIVmac239 Env gp160 for each species. SIV Env linear peptide-specific plasma IgG binding responses were undetectable prior to infection (Fig. 2a). By 15 wpi, both species demonstrated strong plasma antibody responses against peptides analogous to the HIV gp120-gp41 fusion domain, gp41 immunodominant region, and the N-terminal region of gp41 cytoplasmic tail (Fig. 2a) [5]. Notably, by 15 wpi, RM plasma demonstrated high IgG binding against peptides of the variable loop 1 (V1) and variable loop 3 (V3) regions as well as binding to a large number of peptides within the gp41 subunit, including those of the membrane-proximal external region (MPER), which remained high binding responses at 1 ypi (Fig. 2a). In addition to an appreciable linear V3-specific IgG response by 15 wpi (Fig. 2a), 3 of 6 AGMs (AGMs 90, 93, 94) exhibited strong linear V2-specific IgG response

that was markedly undetectable in all RMs (Fig. 2b). By 1 ypi, all AGMs had a high plasma IgG binding response against the linear V2 epitopes, yet this response remained undetectable in RMs (Fig. 2b). To more closely examine the kinetics of V2-specific IgG response in AGMs, we assessed AGM plasma IgG binding to the overlapping peptide library spanning SIVsab Env gp160 at earlier time-points during acute SIV infection. No appreciable plasma IgG binding to linear V2 peptides was detected at 3 wpi (Fig. 2c). Interestingly, in 3 of 6 SIV-infected AGMs (AGMs 90, 93, 94) plasma IgG binding responses against 3 overlapping linear V2 peptides appeared by 6 wpi (Fig. 2c).

Autologous and heterologous V1V2- and linear V2-specific plasma IgG binding responses in SIV-infected AGMs and RMs

Understanding the development of the predominant V2-specific IgG responses in AGMs is of interest, as it remains unclear how to elicit HIV V1V2-specific IgG responses that correlated with reduced HIV acquisition risk in the moderately protective RV144 vaccine trial [7–10]. To account for the few existing amino acid (AA) differences in the overlapping SIVsab92018WT and SIVmac239 V2 peptide libraries tested (peptides 40–42, and 42–44, respectively) compared to the AGM and RM challenge viruses, we measured AGM and RM plasma IgG binding against linear peptides that cover the same V2 region and directly match the AA sequence of the SIVsab92018ivTF (SFAMAGYRRDVKKNYSTVWYDQE) and SIVmac251 (KFNMTGLKRDKTKEYNETWYSTD) challenge viruses. SIV-infected AGMs exhibited high plasma IgG binding against the linear V2 SIVsab92018ivTF peptide at 15 wpi (median binding OD, 1.35 [range,

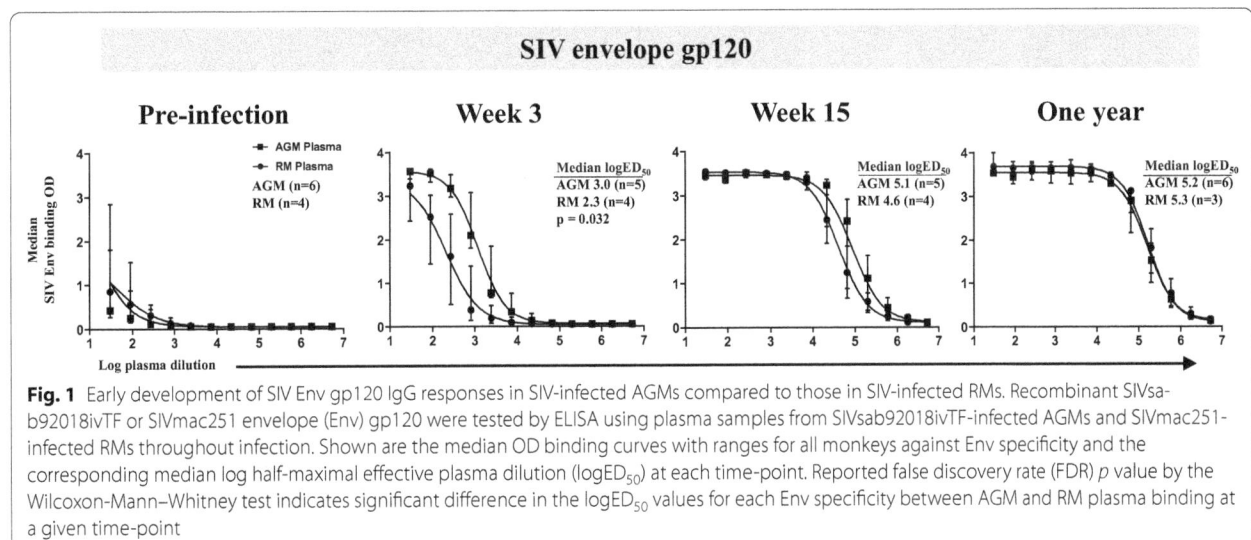

Fig. 1 Early development of SIV Env gp120 IgG responses in SIV-infected AGMs compared to those in SIV-infected RMs. Recombinant SIVsab92018ivTF or SIVmac251 envelope (Env) gp120 were tested by ELISA using plasma samples from SIVsab92018ivTF-infected AGMs and SIVmac251-infected RMs throughout infection. Shown are the median OD binding curves with ranges for all monkeys against Env specificity and the corresponding median log half-maximal effective plasma dilution (logED$_{50}$) at each time-point. Reported false discovery rate (FDR) p value by the Wilcoxon-Mann–Whitney test indicates significant difference in the logED$_{50}$ values for each Env specificity between AGM and RM plasma binding at a given time-point

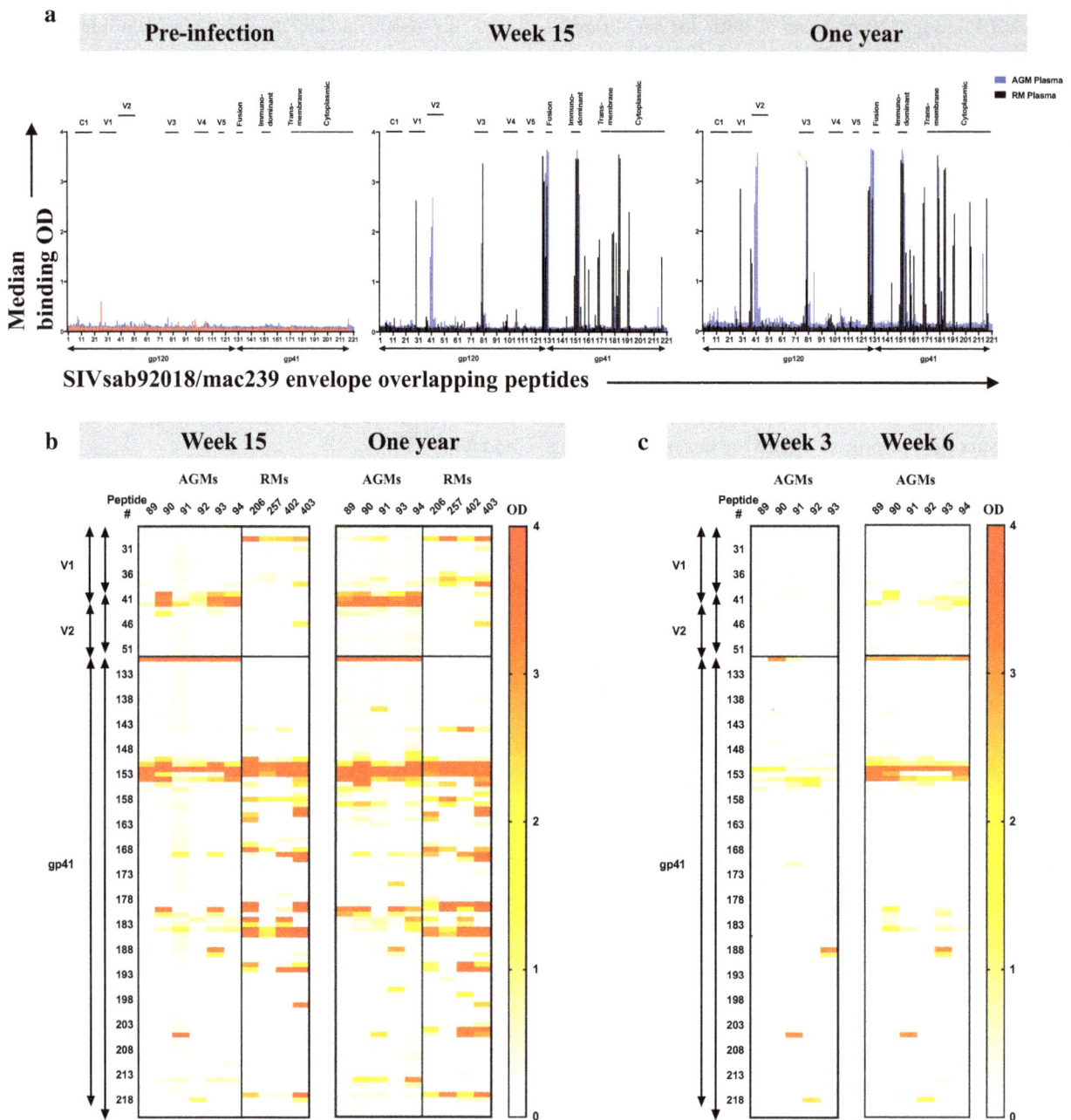

Fig. 2 Distinct pattern of SIV Env linear peptide-specific plasma IgG responses in AGMs and RMs. Plasma samples from SIVsab92018ivTF-infected AGMs and SIVmac251-infected RMs during acute and chronic infection were tested against species-specific overlapping linear peptides spanning SIV envelope (Env) gp160 by ELISA. **a** Each peak represents the median plasma binding levels of all monkeys against each peptide across Env gp160. Each block represents the plasma binding level of **b** AGMs and RMs at week 15 and 1 year against each peptide within the V1, V2, and gp41 regions, or **c** AGMs at week 3 and week 6. Linear V2-specific plasma IgG response emerged at week 6 in AGMs. At week 15, AGM plasma showed a unique binding to a cluster of peptides in the V2 and V3 loops that increased in magnitude through chronic infection in addition to binding clusters nearby the gp120/gp41 fusion domain and immunodominant region of Env gp41

0.34–2.54]) and 1 ypi (median binding OD, 2.76 [range, 2.22–3.11]) (Fig. 3a), whereas RM plasma remained non-reactive against the linear V2 SIVmac251 peptide (median binding OD, 0.04 [range, 0.02–0.11] at 1 ypi) (Fig. 3b).

To examine the cross-reactivity of the predominant V2- and V1V2-specific IgG responses in SIV-infected AGMs, we assessed binding responses to both autologous and heterologous SIVmac and HIV-1 linear V2 peptides and

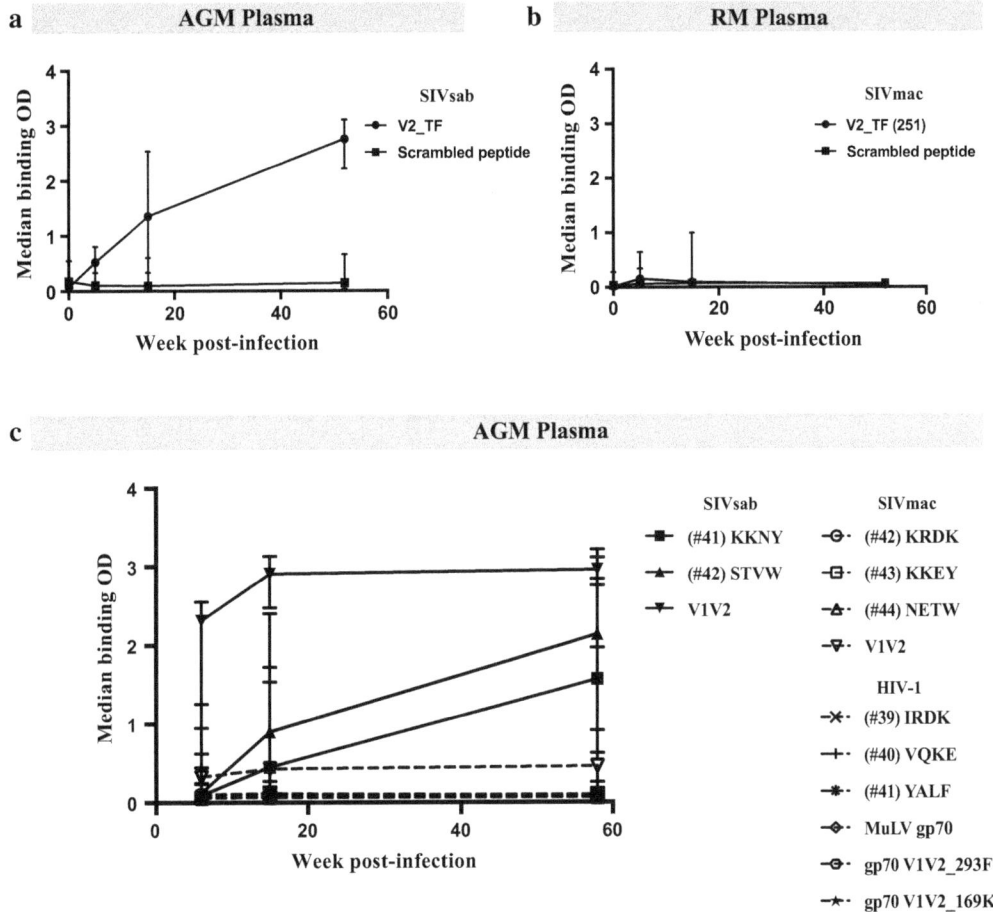

Fig. 3 Autologous and heterologous V1V2- and linear V2-specific plasma IgG binding responses in SIV-infected AGMs. Autologous SIVsab92018ivTF and SIVmac251 linear V2 peptides were tested by ELISA using plasma samples from **a** SIVsab92018ivTF-infected AGMs (n = 5 for 15 wpi, and n = 6 for all other time-points), and **b** SIVmac251-infected RMs (n = 3 for 5 wpi, and n = 4 for all other time-points) throughout infection. **c** Heterologous plasma linear V2-specific IgG binding in 6 SIVsab92018ivTF-infected AGMs was assessed against SIVsab92018WT, and SIVmac239 and HIV-1 Consensus subtype B (ConB) overlapping linear V2 peptides with (#) indicate peptide number, and the last four amino acids from each peptide. Cross-reactivity of AGM V1V2-specific plasma IgG binding was also tested using SIVsab92018ivTF, and SIVmac251 and HIV-1 ConB V1V2 proteins by ELISA. Shown are the median OD binding curves with range for all monkeys against Env specificity at each time-point

V1V2 proteins. The V2-specific IgG response in AGMs was not cross-reactive with heterologous V2 linear SIV and HIV peptides or V1V2 proteins (Fig. 3c). However, SIV-infected AGM plasma demonstrated strong IgG binding to the autologous SIVsab Env V1V2 protein as early as 6 wpi (median binding OD, 2.3 [range, 0.6–2.6]) and this response increased in magnitude (median binding OD, 2.9 [range, 2.5–3.1]) by 15 wpi, and (median binding OD, 3.0 [range, 2.8–3.2]) by 1 ypi.

SIV Env mutation frequency of autologous circulating viruses isolated from plasma of SIV-infected AGMs and RMs

To explore the potential role of the predominant gp120- and V1V2-specific IgG binding responses in AGMs and gp41-specific IgG responses in RMs on autologous viral evolution, we examined the Env gp160 AA sequence variability of single genome Env variants isolated from plasma of SIVsab92018ivTF-infected AGMs at 22 wpi and 1 ypi, and SIVmac251-infected RMs at 18 wpi and 1 ypi. Plasma SIV Env variants from both species demonstrated appreciable mutation frequency in the region of gp120 V4 loop at 1 ypi (Fig. 4a). Yet, the Env variants isolated from SIV-infected RMs exhibited high variability in Env gp41 region, compared to Env variants from SIV-infected AGMs (Fig. 4a). By 1 ypi, Env variants in RMs also showed appreciable sequence variability in a region near the V3 and V5 loops (Fig. 4a). In contrast, plasma Env variants isolated from AGMs showed high sequence variability within C1 region that increased in frequency throughout infection compared to those of SIV-infected RMs (Fig. 4a). Moreover, plasma SIVsab Env variants in AGMs accumulated higher mutation frequencies within

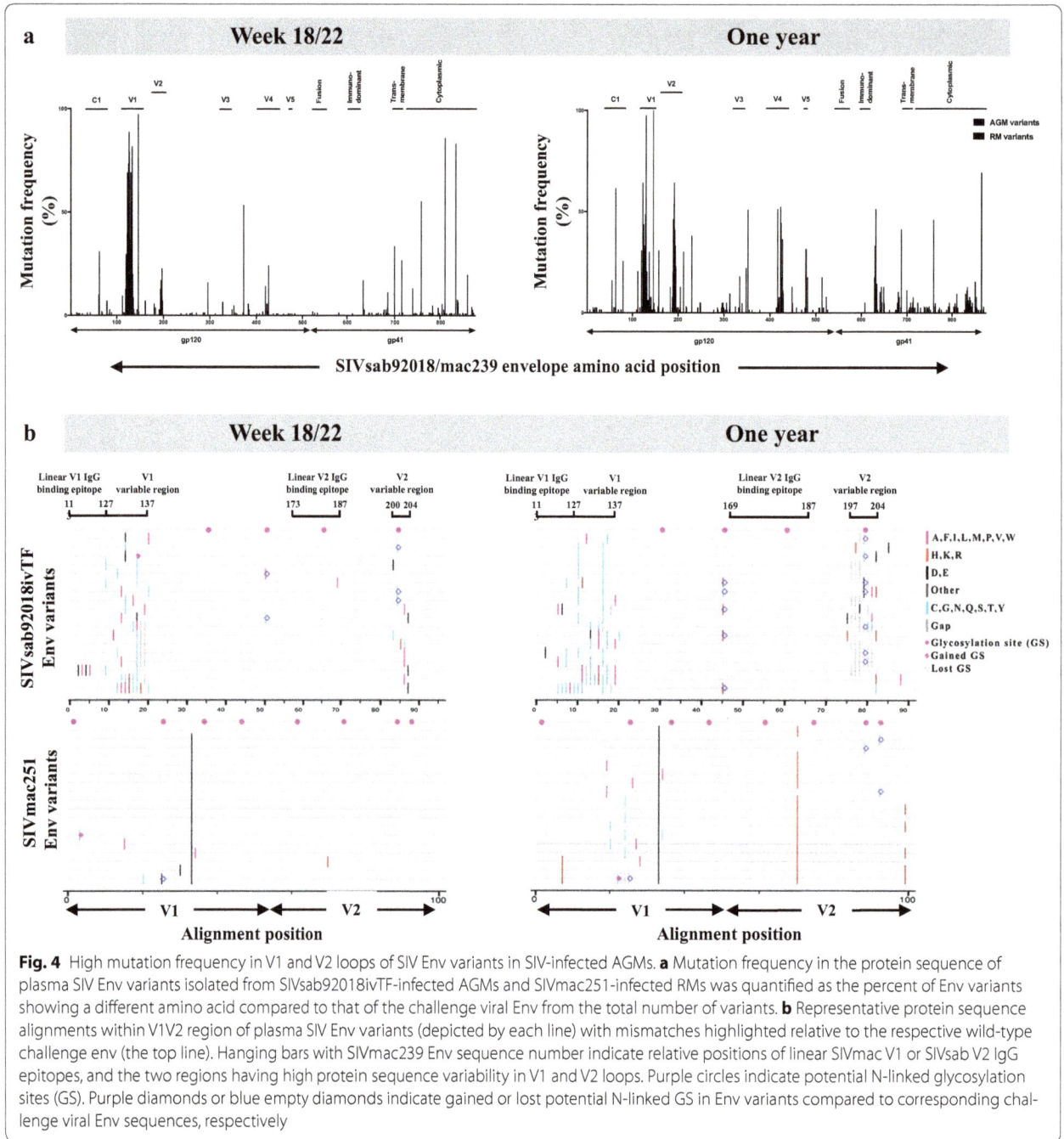

Fig. 4 High mutation frequency in V1 and V2 loops of SIV Env variants in SIV-infected AGMs. **a** Mutation frequency in the protein sequence of plasma SIV Env variants isolated from SIVsab92018ivTF-infected AGMs and SIVmac251-infected RMs was quantified as the percent of Env variants showing a different amino acid compared to that of the challenge viral Env from the total number of variants. **b** Representative protein sequence alignments within V1V2 region of plasma SIV Env variants (depicted by each line) with mismatches highlighted relative to the respective wild-type challenge env (the top line). Hanging bars with SIVmac239 Env sequence number indicate relative positions of linear SIVmac V1 or SIVsab V2 IgG epitopes, and the two regions having high protein sequence variability in V1 and V2 loops. Purple circles indicate potential N-linked glycosylation sites (GS). Purple diamonds or blue empty diamonds indicate gained or lost potential N-linked GS in Env variants compared to corresponding challenge viral Env sequences, respectively

V1 (mutation frequency mean in AGM vs. RM variants, 5.4 vs. 0.22% at 22 or 18 wpi, and 6.7 vs. 3.5% at 1 ypi, respectively), and V2 loops (mutation frequency mean in AGM vs. RM variants, 1.8 vs. 0.086% at 22 or 18 wpi, and 5.9 vs. 3.2% at 1 ypi, respectively) compared to RM Env variants over the course of infection (Fig. 4b). Particularly, AGM plasma SIVsab Env variants exhibited high sequence variability at AA residue positions 127–137 within the V1 loop, and 200–204 within the V2 loop at

22 wpi and at 197–204 within the V2 loop at 1 ypi (SIV-mac239 Env number sequence) (Fig. 4b). The high mutation frequency regions within SIVsab92018ivTF V2 are both near the epitope of the high magnitude linear V2-specific responses and within the vicinity of an analogous region of the HIV V2 loop where the K169 mutation hotspot was identified in breakthrough viruses isolated from HIV RV144 vaccinees (Fig. 4b) [9]. This SIVsab V2 loop site of high sequence variability is also near the

analogous putative gut-homing receptor α4β7-binding motif identified in the HIV-1 Env (Fig. 4b) [11].

As N-linked glycans on Env can evolve in response to the autologous virus-specific IgG responses, we also assessed the N-linked glycosylation pattern in SIV plasma Env variants. AGM SIVsab Env plasma variants exhibited a relatively high loss of predicted N-linked GS motifs within the V2 variable region compared to RM SIVmac Env variants (percent of variants exhibiting a GS loss in AGMs vs. RMs: 35% at 22 wpi and 69% at 1 ypi vs. 0% at 18 wpi and 16% at 1 ypi, respectively) at equivalent AA positions (SIVmac239 Env position 202) (Fig. 4b). SIVsab Env variants also showed a 7 and 31% loss of predicted GS motifs (SIVmac239 Env position 167) at 22 wpi and 1 ypi, respectively, within the V1 loop. A loss in GS motifs within the corresponding V1 region was not observed in SIVmac Env variants (Fig. 4b). However, RM SIVmac Env variants isolated at 1 ypi had 30 and 16% loss of predicted GS motifs within the V5 loop that were not observed in AGM SIVsab Env variants from 1 ypi (SIVmac239 Env positions 476 and 479, respectively).

ADCC kinetics of plasma IgG responses in SIV-infected AGMs and RMs

ADCC-mediating IgG responses and IgG targeting linear V2 epitopes were associated with a decreased risk of HIV-1 infection in the RV144 vaccine trial [25]. To explore the ADCC function of Env gp120-predominant antibody responses and their relationship to the early development of linear V2-specific IgG responses in AGMs, we evaluated the kinetics of plasma Env-specific ADCC responses in AGMs compared to those of RMs. ADCC activity was not detected in AGMs or RMs prior to SIV infection (Fig. 5a, b). As early as 6 wpi in AGMs and 5 wpi in RMs, high ADCC activity was detected against SIV Env gp140-coated cells in both species (ADCC titer as reciprocal plasma dilution median in AGMs vs. RMs: 52,225 [range, 36,931–90,286] vs. 61,826 [range, 54,503–64,725], raw $p = 0.71$, FDR $p = 0.95$) (Fig. 5a). Gp140-specific IgG-mediated ADCC activity increased in both species by 15 wpi in AGMs and 17 wpi in RMs (ADCC titer median in AGMs vs. RMs: 89,851 [range, 64,474–317,680] vs. 409,600 [range, 409,600–409,600], raw $p = 0.024$, FDR $p = 0.063$) (Fig. 5a). Interestingly, SIV-infected AGMs demonstrated high magnitude ADCC activity against SIV Env gp120-coated cells at 6 wpi, and this response was remarkably undetectable in acutely SIV-infected RMs (ADCC titer median in AGMs: 949.3 [range, 319–3746], raw $p = 0.024$, FDR $p = 0.063$) (Fig. 5b). Importantly, the more rapid development of gp120-specific ADCC-mediating response in AGMs arose concurrently with the gp120 and V2 loop-specific antibody responses in AGMs, which are distinct from

that in SIV-infected RMs. Yet, both AGMs and RMs had comparable ADCC-mediating gp120-specific IgG responses by 15 or 17 wpi (ADCC titer median in AGMs vs. RMs: 11,169 [range, 4867–25,125] vs. 13,120 [range, 6036–23,722], raw $p = 0.90$, FDR $p = 1$) (Fig. 5b).

Plasma IgG binding to SIV-infected CD4+ T cells

To examine the infected cell binding activity of the early acute SIV Env-specific IgG response in AGMs and RMs, we measured the binding of Env-specific IgG to CD4+ T cells infected with SIVsab92018ivTF and SIVmac251 infectious molecular clones (IMC). For all experiments, we obtained high levels of infection with > 55% (range, 56–82% p24/p27+) of cells being infected for both viruses. Env-specific IgG plasma responses in AGMs recognized SIV-infected CD4+ target cells more effectively and earlier in acute time points compared to RM plasma (median % FITC positivity in AGMs vs. RMs, 40.8% [range, 29.3–55.6%] vs. 1.0% [range, 0.1–1.1%] at week 6 or 5, raw $p = 0.0095$, FDR $p = 0.057$; 72.5% [range, 58.6–78.3%] vs. 23.2% [range, 17.3–24.6%] at week 15 or 17, raw $p = 0.0095$, FDR $p = 0.057$, respectively) (Fig. 5c).

Limited contribution of linear V2 epitopes to early ADCC and autologous SIV neutralizing responses in SIV-infected AGMs

Given the early development of ADCC and neutralizing activity that arose concurrently with the linear V2-specific plasma IgG binding response in AGMs during acute SIV infection, we sought to define potential contribution of the linear V2-specific IgG response to early gp120-directed functional responses that are unique to AGMs. With a SIVsab linear V2 peptide-coated IgG depletion column of AGM plasma, we achieved an enriched $76 \pm 4.4\%$ (mean and SD) depletion of linear V2-specific antibodies compared to $53 \pm 8.4\%$ (mean and SD) depletion with a scrambled peptide-coated column. We then compared the gp120-specific ADCC and autologous neutralizing function of AGM V2 and scrambled peptide-depleted plasma at 6 and 15 wpi, respectively [18]. Despite a reduction in ADCC activity compared to that of non-depleted plasma (median ADCC titers for non-depleted vs. V2-depleted response, 949.3 [range, 318.8–3746] vs. 314.4 [range, 100–576.3], raw $p = 0.031$, FDR $p = 0.063$; non-depleted vs. scrambled peptide-depleted response, 294.6 [range, 100–679.5], raw $p = 0.031$, FDR $p = 0.063$), we observed similar ADCC antibody titers in linear V2 peptide and scrambled peptide-depleted plasma at 6 wpi (raw $p = 1$, FDR $p = 1$) (Fig. 5d). Similarly, we observed an equivalent decrease in plasma SIVsab neutralizing activity following the linear V2 and scrambled peptide-depletion of AGM plasma at 15 wpi (median ID_{50} for non-depleted vs. V2-depleted activity,

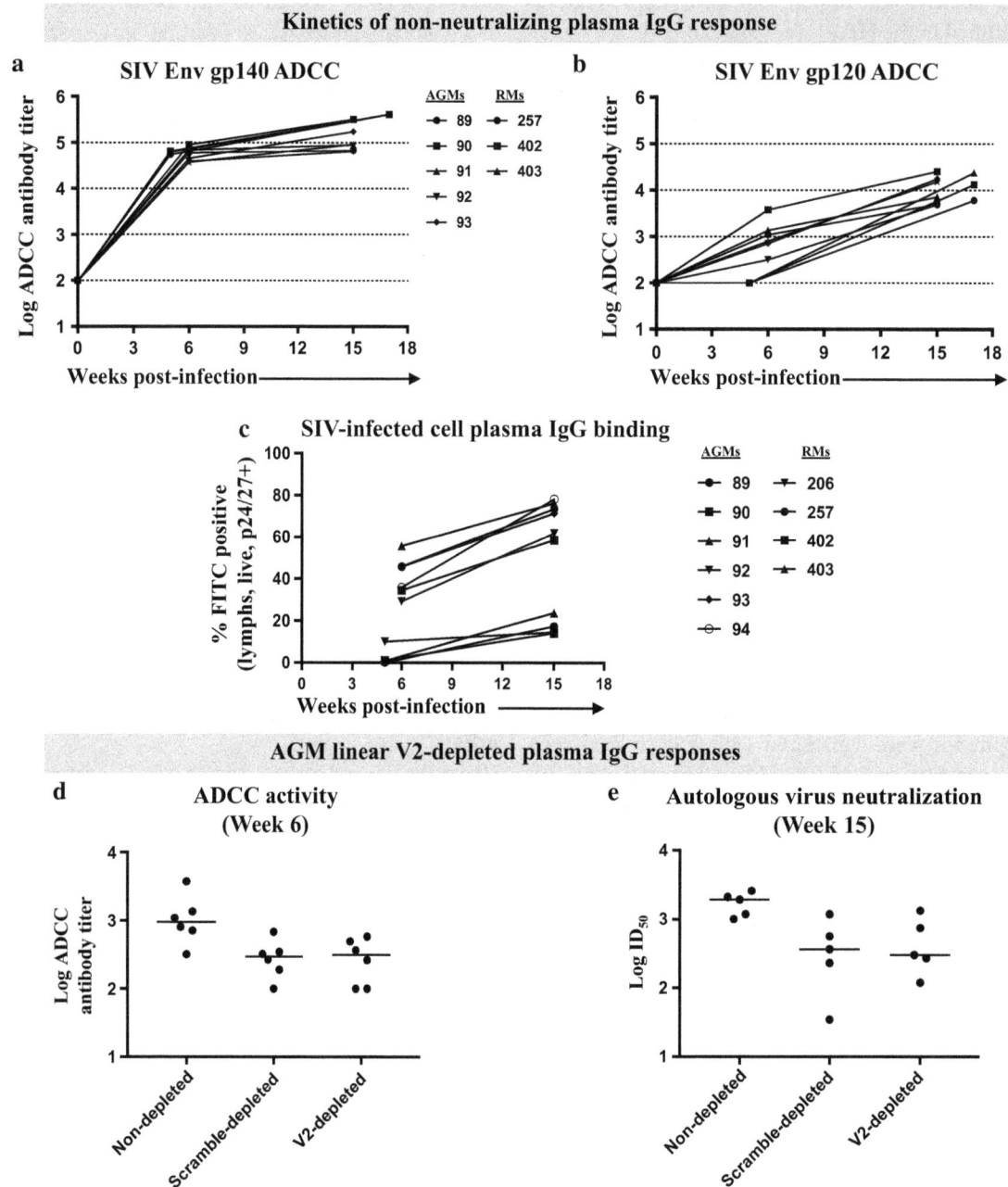

Fig. 5 Early development of SIV Env gp120-directed plasma IgG ADCC and SIV-infected cell binding in AGMs. ADCC activity against the autologous challenge SIV envelope (Env) **a** gp140 and **b** gp120-coated cells of plasma IgG from SIVsab92018ivTF-infected AGMs and SIVmac251-infected RMs prior to infection, at week 6 (AGM) or 5 (RM), and 15 (AGM) or 17 (RM) was quantified as ADCC antibody titers. **c** Binding to SIV-infected cells was measured as % FITC positivity after week 0 background subtraction. **d** Plasma gp120-specific ADCC responses (median shown) after depletion with a linear V2 peptide or scrambled peptide in SIV-infected AGMs at week 6. **e** Neutralizing responses (median shown) in SIVsab92018ivTF-infected AGMs against the autologous challenge virus at week 15 after depletion with a linear V2 peptide and scrambled peptide

1933 [range, 1007–2592] vs. 303 [range, 120–1340], raw $p = 0.13$, FDR $p = 0.19$; non-depleted vs. scrambled peptide-depleted activity, 367 [range, 35–1184], raw $p = 0.063$, FDR $p = 0.11$; scrambled peptide-depleted vs. V2-depleted activity, raw $p = 1$, FDR $p = 1$) (Fig. 5e). AGM and RM plasma IgG binding to scrambled peptide was negligible (median binding OD, 0.21 [range, 0.15–0.25], and 0.08 [range, 0.04–0.12], respectively).

Discussion

Vaccine-elicited V2-specific IgG responses that mediate ADCC activity have been proposed as an immune correlate of reduced HIV-1 infection risk in the moderately protective RV144 vaccine efficacy trial [3, 17, 26]. However, factors controlling the elicitation of V2-specific IgG responses capable of mediating ADCC are not well established. We previously reported that natural SIV hosts, AGMs, have a SIV Env gp120-biased antibody response to SIV infection, and rapidly develop autologous neutralizing antibodies, which are unique from both SIV-infected RMs and HIV-infected human non-natural hosts [18–20]. In this study, we identified that the distinct plasma linear V2-specific IgG responses arose at 6 wpi in 50% of all AGMs, which were markedly undetectable in all RMs. Moreover, acutely SIV-infected AGMs mediated a more rapid development of gp120-directed ADCC activity, and SIV-infected cell binding response compared to SIV-infected RMs. In addition, single genome Env variant analyses demonstrated an increase in AA mutation frequency, and a high loss of predicted N-linked GS within the V1 and V2 loops of SIVsab Env variants over time. Interestingly, the target of linear V2-specific plasma IgG binding responses in AGMs localized to an equivalent HIV V2 loop epitope near residues that were associated with immune escape from the potentially-protective V2-specific IgG responses in RV144 vaccinees [8, 9]. This SIVsab linear V2 epitope is also in close vicinity of the putative binding motif of the gut-homing receptor $\alpha 4\beta 7$ in HIV-1 Env, underlining the potential importance of the V2 loop region for virus infectivity and escape from humoral responses in the natural SIV hosts.

In this study, we found that SIV-infected AGMs exhibited a predominant SIV Env gp120-directed response very early during acute SIV infection compared to the RM counterparts. To further examine the gp120/gp41 antibody differential antibody responses in these species, we measured their SIV Env linear peptide-specific IgG binding responses against overlapping SIVsab92018WT and SIVmac239 peptide libraries spanning Env gp160, respectively. Interestingly, we observed higher binding responses against linear V2 peptides in AGMs but not in RMs. Given that a few AA differences occur in these overlapping peptide libraries compared to the SIVsab92018ivTF and SIVmac251 challenge viruses, we also tested AGM and RM plasma IgG binding against linear V2 peptides matching the challenge viruses. AGMs showed higher magnitude linear V2-specific IgG binding against the linear V2 SIVsab92018ivTF peptide compared to RM plasma binding to linear V2 SIVmac251 peptide, suggesting that the observed binding differences against linear V2 peptides in AGMs and RMs are not due differences in the AA sequences between the SIV

Env overlapping peptide library and the SIV challenge viruses. While the mechanism of the predominant, early plasma linear V2-specific IgG response in AGMs remains unclear, it is possible that AGMs mediate a higher frequency of SIV linear-epitope specific responses given their lower frequency of SIV immune-complex trapping by follicular dendritic cells in germinal centers [27, 28].

We observed that V1 and V2 loops of SIVsab variants had higher mutation frequencies compared to SIVmac variants isolated from RMs. This high Env mutation frequency in the V1V2 region has also been reported in SIVsab isolates from naturally SIV-infected AGMs [29, 30]. Therefore, it is plausible that the early development of predominant gp120-specific and high magnitude V2-specific IgG responses in AGMs may influence the unique Env mutation pattern observed within the V1V2 loop of autologous SIVsab circulating viruses [25, 31, 32]. It is also worth noting that the hypervariable loops of HIV-1 have long been suspected to influence conformational state changes in Env [33]. In addition, mutations within V1 or V2 loop could influence the conformation of nearby epitopes via glycan shielding [31, 32, 34, 35].

Comparisons in SIV and HIV Env-specific antibody responses are admittedly limited by a lack of SIV Env trimer crystal structures [32, 36–38]. The structure of a core SIV gp120 monomer has been determined and differed significantly in the orientation of its inner and outer domains compared to HIV gp120 monomers, suggesting a differing functional SIV Env trimer arrangement ([39]). Nevertheless, SIV V1V2 has been recognized to correspond to HIV-1 V1V2, and the SIV and HIV V2 loops share certain structural motifs, specifically the [ED] [VLI] motif and a lysine-rich motif that appears as K[KV] QK in HIV and KK (alternately, K[KT]K) in SIV [29, 36, 37, 40]. In fact, an RV144 vaccine regimen utilizing SIV gp120 as the immunogen elicited V2 loop-specific IgG responses that were associated with protection against SIVmac251 in RMs [16]. Furthermore, V2-specific antibody responses were inversely correlated with peak and set-point viral loads in SIV-infected RMs [41]. Thus, the V2 loop in HIV and SIV may share immunogenic and functional characteristics that are capable of eliciting potentially-protective IgG responses in non-human primates.

Vaccine-elicited V2-specific IgG responses from the RV144 vaccine efficacy trial may have mediated protection through an ADCC mechanism [7, 9, 15]. In addition to the previously reported early kinetics of autologous virus neutralizing responses in AGMs [18], we observed an early SIV Env gp120-specific ADCC response in AGMs compared to RMs. Moreover, AGM plasma IgG showed higher SIV-infected cell binding activity compared to RM plasma, suggesting that AGM

SIV Env-specific IgG responses may better recognize epitopes exposed on infected cells. Similar functional immune profiles using AGM sera have been observed in previous studies of naturally SIV-infected AGMs [42, 43]. These results suggest that AGM SIV Env-reactive plasma IgG can mediate robust non-neutralizing antiviral functions and increased infected cell binding activity during early acute SIV infection compared to RM plasma antibodies. Intriguingly, we observed similar ADCC activity in V2 and scrambled peptide-depleted AGM plasma, suggesting that other sites within SIVsab gp120 may mediate the early acute ADCC responses. However, it should be noted that there was non-specific IgG depletion in the scrambled peptide depletion experiments [44]. Furthermore, vaccine-elicited antibody responses in the RV144 efficacy trial were mapped to both conformational and linear V2 epitopes, suggesting that V2-specific IgG responses with anti-viral activity may not only target linear V2 epitopes [9, 14]. Interestingly, it has been shown that conformational epitope recognition of SIV Env-specific antibody responses differs greatly between nonpathogenic and pathogenic SIV infections in natural SIV hosts [23]. Thus, ADCC-mediating IgG responses in humans and AGMs may target both linear V2 and conformational gp120 epitopes within HIV and SIV Env.

Conclusion

We have demonstrated that acutely SIV-infected AGMs develop high magnitude plasma linear V2-specific IgG responses that arise concurrently with ADCC-mediating and SIV-infected cellular binding responses targeting gp120 epitopes. Yet, these early plasma linear V2-specific and gp120-specific IgG responses with ADCC activity were undetectable in RMs. Moreover, the antibody responses targeting either the linear V2 or other non-linear gp120 variable loop epitopes that are generated more quickly in AGMs than those in RMs could contribute to the observed faster accumulation of diversity of autologous circulating viruses within the V1V2 loop in SIV-infected AGMs. Our findings support the potential use of AGMs as an alternative non-human primate model for HIV-1 vaccine development, particularly for the evaluation of immunogens that target high magnitude neutralizing and non-neutralizing gp120-specific IgG responses. A greater understanding of host immune factors that lead to the unique functional gp120-specific IgG responses in these natural SIV hosts may provide valuable insights for future HIV vaccine immunogen design.

Methods

Nonhuman primates and sample collection

Six female AGMs (*Chlorocebus sabaeus*) and four female Indian RMs (*Macaca mulatta*) between four and 11 years

of age were intravenously inoculated with, infectious molecular clones of SIVsab92018ivTF, or SIVmac251.30 virus isolate, respectively [19, 20, 45]. All four RMs maintained high-level viremia compared to those of AGMs over the course of infection [18]. Blood was collected in EDTA tubes at 0, 2, 3, 5, 6, 15, 17, and 18 (RMs) or 22 (AGMs) weeks post-infection (wpi), and again at 1 year post-infection (ypi) in both species, and plasma was then isolated. Animals were housed and maintained according to the *Guide for the Care and Use of Laboratory Animals* [46].

HIV/SIV Env protein and peptides

To assess the fine-specificity of SIV Env-specific plasma IgG binding responses in AGMs and RMs, we tested plasma samples for IgG binding to recombinant SIVsab92018ivTF Env gp120, [47] SIVmac251 Env gp120, [47] HIV-1 murine leukemia virus (MuLV) gp70_His6/Mon (293F), gp70 V1V2 CaseA subtype B (293F), gp70 V1V2 CaseA2 subtype B (169 K), and [48] SIVsab92018ivTF or SIVmac251 V1V2 proteins [18]. To examine Env linear peptide IgG binding responses, we used the SIVagm Sabaeus 92018 (Cat #10451), SIVmac239 (Cat #6883, AAA47637.1), and HIV-1 ConB (Cat #9480) Env peptide sets obtained through the NIH NIAID AIDS Reagent Program, Division of AIDS in addition to SIVsab92018ivTF V2 peptide (SFAMAGYRRDVKKNYSTVWYDQE) and SIVmac251 V2 peptide (KFNMTGLKRDKTKEYNETWYSTD) (CPC Scientific, Sunnyvale, CA). SIVmac239 Env peptide regions were annotated based on the HIV-2/SIV protein annotations from HIV Sequence Compendium 2016 [49]. To annotate the regions for SIVsab92018 Env overlapping peptide, its sequence was aligned with SIVmac239 (M33262) using the HIVAlign tool (https://www.hiv.lanl.gov/content/sequence/VIRALIGN/viralign.html). An additional table file details the information of both SIVsab92018 and SIVmac239 Env overlapping peptides for each Env region (see Additional file 1).

HIV/SIV Env-specific IgG binding enzyme-linked immunosorbent assays (ELISAs)

To assess SIV Env-specific plasma IgG binding kinetics, plasma samples from SIVsab92018ivTF-infected AGMs and SIVmac251-infected RMs were tested for IgG binding to recombinant SIVsab92018ivTF or SIVmac251 Env gp120 proteins at the following time-points: 0, 3, 15 wpi, and 1 ypi according to sample availability. To measure linear SIV Env peptide-specific plasma IgG binding responses, plasma samples from SIV-infected AGMs and RMs from 0, 3, 6, 15 wpi, and 1 ypi were tested for IgG binding to SIVsab92018WT and SIVmac239 overlapping linear peptide libraries, respectively. To confirm similar IgG responses to the autologous linear V2 peptides, plasma samples from SIV-infected AGMs and RMs at 5, 15 wpi, and 1 ypi were tested against SIVsab92018ivTF and SIVmac251 linear V2 peptides, respectively. To examine the magnitude and cross-reactivity of the heterologous linear V2 and V1V2 protein-specific plasma IgG binding, plasma samples from SIV-infected AGMs at 6, 15 wpi, and 1 ypi were serially diluted from a 1:100 starting dilution and tested against SIVmac239 and HIV-1 Consensus Subtype B (ConB) overlapping linear V2 peptides, and SIVsab92018ivTF, SIVmac251, and HIV-1 V1V2 proteins. The SIV Env/peptide-specific IgG binding ELISAs were carried out with Env proteins or peptides diluted to 3 μg/mL in 0.1 M sodium bicarbonate, and coated on plates for 1 h. Plasma samples were diluted at 1:100. Plates were washed and blocked with SuperBlock (4% whey protein, 15% goat serum, and 0.5% Tween 20 diluted in 1X phosphate-buffered saline (PBS)) at room temperature for 1 h. Plasma from chronically SIV-infected AGMs and RMs were used as positive controls. Influenza hemagglutinin-specific mAb CH65 [50] and an anti-respiratory syncytial virus antibody, Pavilizumab (Medimmune, Inc, Quakertown, PA), were used as negative controls. Scrambled peptides and species-specific SIV Env gp140 proteins were used as additional negative and positive controls, respectively. Horseradish peroxidase (HRP)-conjugated polyclonal goat anti-monkey IgG (gamma chain) antibody (Rockland Immunochemicals, Gilbertsville, PA) was added and incubated for 1 h at 1:10,000 dilution. Plates were washed and developed with SureBlue reserve TMB substrate for 5 min, and the reaction was stopped by adding an equal volume of TMB stop solution (KPL, Gaithersburg, MD). Optical densities (ODs) were measured at 450 nm using a Spectramax Plus spectrophotometer (Molecular Devices, Sunnyvale, CA). A line of best fit calculated by a 4-parameter logistic curve was used to interpolate the log half-maximal effective plasma dilution (log ED_{50}) using GraphPad Prism 7 (Graph Pad, La Jolla, CA).

Peptide depletion and SIV neutralization assays

To deplete linear V2-specific IgG responses, CNBr-activated Sepharose 4B columns (GE Healthcare, Pittsburgh, PA) were coated with 2 mg of SIVsab92018WT V2 peptide (SFAMAGYRRDVKKNYSTVWDDQE) (CPC Scientific, Sunnyvale, CA), and a scrambled peptide of similar length according to manufacturer's guidelines. AGM plasma samples were run through the columns, and the flow-through was run for a total of 10 times. Depletion efficiency of linear V2 peptide-specific antibodies was quantified as the percent depletion, which equals 1- ((OD of peptide-depleted V2 binding/OD of non-depleted V2 binding) * 100). Non-depleted, linear V2 peptide-depleted, and scrambled peptide-depleted

plasma samples from SIVsab92018ivTF-infected AGMs at 15 wpi were tested against SIVsab92018ivTF infectious molecular clone (IMC) in the TZM-bl cell neutralization assay [18]. In brief, samples were serially diluted in duplicate, and incubated with virus (50,000 relative light unit [RLU] equivalents) for 1 h at 37 °C. Cells were added at a density of 10,000 cells per well, and incubated for 48 h at 37 °C + 5% CO_2. A reduction in luciferase activity was quantified by the Brightglow Luciferase detection system (Promega, Madison, WI). The sample dilution at which a 50% RLU reduction was observed was defined as the inhibitory dilution (ID_{50}).

ADCC assay

We used the GranToxiLux (GTL) ADCC assay to measure the ADCC activity of whole plasma samples, linear V2 peptide-depleted plasma IgG, and/or scrambled peptide-depleted plasma IgG isolated from SIVsab92018ivTF-infected AGMs and SIVmac251-infected RMs at 0, 6 (AGMs) or 5 (RMs), and 15 (AGMs) or 17 (RMs) wpi as described previously [51]. The CEM.NKR$_{CCR5}$ target cells [52] were coated with recombinant SIVsab92018ivTF/SIVmac251 gp120, or avi-tagged gp140 Env representing the same virus isolates. Cryopreserved human peripheral blood mononuclear cells from an HIV-seronegative donor with the 158F/F polymorphic variant of Fcγ receptor 3A served as effector cells [53]. Plasma samples were tested using 4-fold serial dilutions starting at 1:100 dilution. Data were analyzed using FlowJo 9.8.2 (Tree Star Inc., Ashland, OR). The % Granzyme B (GzB) activity was defined as the percentage of cells positive for proteolytically active GzB out of the total viable target cell population. Final results were calculated after subtracting the background % GzB activity observed in wells containing effector and target cells in the absence of plasma or IgG samples. Plasma ADCC antibody titers were determined by interpolating the plasma dilutions that intersect the positive cut-off (8% GzB activity) using Graph Pad Prism 7 (Graph Pad, La Jolla CA).

Plasma IgG binding to Env on the surface of SIV-infected CD4$^+$ cells

Indirect surface staining was used to evaluate the ability of SIV Env-specific plasma IgG from AGMs and RMs to bind the surface of CEM.NKR$_{CCR5}$ CD4$^+$ T cells [54] infected with SIVsab92018ivTF or SIVmac251. Infections with replication competent infectious molecular clone virus (IMC) were performed using DEAE-Dextran as described previously [51, 55]. At 48 h postinfection, the infected CEM.NKR$_{CCR5}$ cells were incubated with a 1:100 dilution of plasma for 2 h at 37 °C and then stained with a vital dye (Live/Dead Fixable Aqua Dead Cell Stain; Invitrogen) to exclude nonviable cells from subsequent analyses. Primary Ab binding was detected by secondary labeling with fluorescein isothiocyanate (FITC)-conjugated goat anti-rhesus IgG (SouthernBiotech Inc., Birmingham, AL), and SIV-infected cells were identified by staining for intracellular expression of p24/27 (KC57-RD1; Beckman Coulter) using standard methods. Binding was quantified as % of live, p24/27 positive, FITC positive cells after subtracting the background binding of week 0 samples. Mock-infected cells were used to establish negative gates.

Single genome amplification (SGA) and sequencing of plasma SIV env variants

SIV env variants from SIVsab92018ivTF-infected AGM plasma samples at 22 and 52 wpi (n = 4, 71 variants, and n = 3, 39 variants, respectively), [56] and SIVmac251-infected RM plasma samples at 18 and 50 wpi (n = 4, 107 variants; and n = 3, 67 variants, respectively) were amplified and sequenced using limiting dilution PCR [56]. For this study, SGAs isolated from AGMs and RMs were aligned against sequences of the corresponding wild-type SIVsab92018 and SIVmac251 using Seaview [57]. For SIVsab92018WT Env sequence (871 amino acid (AA)), the regions include constant region 1 (C1) (54 AA), V1 (42 AA), V2 (45 AA), and gp41 (345 AA). For SIVmac251 Env sequence (876 AA), the regions include C1 (49 AA), V1 (58 AA), V2 (43 AA), and gp41 (348 AA). Mutation frequency of Env variants at each time-point was calculated as the percent of variants with different AA compared to respective SIVsab/mac virus Env sequence at each residue within a defined Env region. Mutations in Env variants were graphically represented in relationship to their respective challenge Env using Highlighter tool (https://www.hiv.lanl.gov/content/sequence/HIGH-LIGHT/highlighter_top.html). Analysis of N-linked glycosylation sites (GS) (Nx[ST] pattern) of plasma Env variants were performed using N-GlycoSite tool (https://www.hiv.lanl.gov/content/sequence/GLYCOSITE/glycosite.html).

Statistical analysis

Wilcoxon-Mann–Whitney was used to compare the Env protein-specific plasma IgG binding $logEC_{50}$ values between AGMs and RMs (Fig. 1). The exact Wilcoxon Rank Sum test was used to compare the gp140 and gp120 ADCC titers in AGMs and RMs (Fig. 5a, b), and the % infected cells in AGMs and RMs (Fig. 5c). The Wilcoxon Signed-Rank test to compare the non-depleted and V2/scrambled peptide depleted ADCC activity (Fig. 5d), and neutralizing activity (Fig. 5e). All analyses were adjusted for multiple comparisons by false discovery rate (FDR) p value correction.

Authors' contributions

QNN, DRM, SRP designed, analyzed, interpreted the data, and wrote the manuscript; JEH and QNN performed and analyzed peptide binding ELISA; DRM, RM and QH performed and analyzed protein binding ELISA; DRM performed and analyzed depletion and neutralization data; RWE and JP performed and analyzed ADCC and virus binding data; QNN and AK analyzed virus envelope variant analysis; NIN and XS contributed important insights for the interpretation and discussion of the results. All authors read and approved the final manuscript.

Author details

[1] Duke Human Vaccine Institute, Duke University School of Medicine, Durham, NC, USA. [2] Department of Molecular Genetics and Microbiology, Duke University School of Medicine, Durham, NC, USA. [3] Department of Surgery, Duke University School of Medicine, Durham, NC, USA. [4] Department of Pediatrics, Duke University School of Medicine, Durham, NC, USA. [5] Department of Immunology, Duke University School of Medicine, Durham, NC, USA.

Acknowledgements

We thank Thomas Jeffries Jr. and Robert Parks for their technical expertise; Kevin Saunders and Melissa Cooper for providing HIV-1 V1V2 proteins; Josh Eudailey for processing stool bacterial lysates; and Meng Chen for statistical advice. The funders had no role in study design, data collection and interpretation, or the decision to submit the work for publication.

Competing interests

The authors declare that they have no competing interests.

Funding

Support for this work was provided by an R01 grant to Sallie R. Permar from the National Institutes of Health (NIH grant 5R01AI106380-04). David R. Martinez is supported by an ASM Robert D. Watkins Graduate Research Fellowship, an NIH NIAID Ruth L. Kirschstein National Research Service Award F31 F31AI127303, and a Burroughs Wellcome Graduate Diversity Enrichment Award.

References

1. Kwong PD, Mascola JR. Human antibodies that neutralize HIV-1: identification, structures, and B cell ontogenies. Immunity. 2012;37:412–25.
2. Haynes BF, Mascola JR. The quest for an antibody-based HIV vaccine. Immunol Rev. 2017;275:5–10.
3. Pollara J, Easterhoff D, Fouda GG. Lessons learned from human HIV vaccine trials. Curr Opin HIV AIDS. 2017;12:216–21.
4. Williams WB, Liao H-X, Moody MA, Kepler TB, Alam SM, Gao F, Wiehe K, Trama AM, Jones K, Zhang R, et al. Diversion of HIV-1 vaccine–induced immunity by gp41-microbiota cross-reactive antibodies. Science. 2015;349:aab1253.
5. Tomaras GD, Yates NL, Liu P, Qin L, Fouda GG, Chavez LL, Decamp AC, Parks RJ, Ashley VC, Lucas JT, et al. Initial B-cell responses to transmitted human immunodeficiency virus type 1: virion-binding immunoglobulin M (IgM) and IgG antibodies followed by plasma anti-gp41 antibodies with ineffective control of initial viremia. J Virol. 2008;82:12449–63.
6. Liao HX, Chen X, Munshaw S, Zhang R, Marshall DJ, Vandergrift N, Whitesides JF, Lu X, Yu JS, Hwang KK, et al. Initial antibodies binding to HIV-1 gp41 in acutely infected subjects are polyreactive and highly mutated. J Exp Med. 2011;208:2237–49.
7. Haynes BF, Gilbert PB, McElrath MJ, Zolla-Pazner S, Tomaras GD, Alam SM, Evans DT, Montefiori DC, Karnasuta C, Sutthent R, et al. Immune-correlates analysis of an HIV-1 vaccine efficacy trial. N Engl J Med. 2012;366:1275–86.
8. Rolland M, Edlefsen PT, Larsen BB, Tovanabutra S, Sanders-Buell E, Hertz T, deCamp AC, Carrico C, Menis S, Magaret CA, et al. Increased HIV-1 vaccine efficacy against viruses with genetic signatures in Env V2. Nature. 2012;490:417–20.
9. Karasavvas N, Billings E, Rao M, Williams C, Zolla-Pazner S, Bailer RT, Koup RA, Madnote S, Arworn D, Shen X, et al. The thai phase III HIV type 1 vaccine trial (RV144) regimen induces antibodies that target conserved regions within the V2 loop of gp120. AIDS Res Hum Retrovir. 2012;28:1444–57.
10. Zolla-Pazner S, deCamp AC, Cardozo T, Karasavvas N, Gottardo R, Williams C, Morris DE, Tomaras G, Rao M, Billings E, et al. Analysis of V2 antibody responses induced in vaccinees in the ALVAC/AIDSVAX HIV-1 vaccine efficacy trial. PLoS ONE. 2013;8:e53629.
11. Tassaneetrithep B, Tivon D, Swetnam J, Karasavvas N, Michael NL, Kim JH, Marovich M, Cardozo T. Cryptic determinant of α4β7 binding in the V2 loop of HIV-1 gp120. PLoS ONE. 2014;9:e108446.
12. Ansari AA, Reimann KA, Mayne AE, Takahashi Y, Stephenson ST, Wang R, Wang X, Li J, Price AA, Little DM, et al. Blocking of α4β7 gut-homing integrin during acute infection leads to decreased plasma and gastrointestinal tissue viral loads in simian immunodeficiency virus-infected rhesus macaques. J Immunol. 2011;186:1044–59.
13. Peachman KK, Karasavvas N, Chenine AL, McLinden R, Rerks-Ngarm S, Jaranit K, Nitayaphan S, Pitisuttithum P, Tovanabutra S, Zolla-Pazner S, et al. Identification of new regions in HIV-1 gp120 variable 2 and 3 loops that bind to α4β7 integrin receptor. PLoS ONE. 2015;10:e0143895.
14. Bonsignori M, Pollara J, Moody MA, Alpert MD, Chen X, Hwang KK, Gilbert PB, Huang Y, Gurley TC, Kozink DM, et al. Antibody-dependent cellular cytotoxicity-mediating antibodies from an HIV-1 vaccine efficacy trial target multiple epitopes and preferentially use the VH1 gene family. J Virol. 2012;86:11521–32.
15. Pollara J, Bonsignori M, Moody MA, Liu P, Alam SM, Hwang KK, Gurley TC, Kozink DM, Armand LC, Marshall DJ, et al. HIV-1 vaccine-induced C1 and V2 Env-specific antibodies synergize for increased antiviral activities. J Virol. 2014;88:7715–26.
16. Vaccari M, Gordon SN, Fourati S, Schifanella L, Liyanage NP, Cameron M, Keele BF, Shen X, Tomaras GD, Billings E, et al. Adjuvant-dependent innate and adaptive immune signatures of risk of SIVmac251 acquisition. Nat Med. 2016;22:762–70.
17. Kim JH, Excler JL, Michael NL. Lessons from the RV144 Thai phase III HIV-1 vaccine trial and the search for correlates of protection. Annu Rev Med. 2015;66:423–37.
18. Amos JD, Himes JE, Armand L, Gurley TC, Martinez DR, Colvin L, Beck K, Overman RG, Liao HX, Moody MA, Permar SR. Rapid development of gp120-focused neutralizing B Cell responses during acute simian immunodeficiency virus infection of African green monkeys. J Virol. 2015;89:9485–98.
19. Amos JD, Wilks AB, Fouda GG, Smith SD, Colvin L, Mahlokozera T, Ho C, Beck K, Overman RG, DeMarco CT, et al. Lack of B cell dysfunction is associated with functional, gp120-dominant antibody responses in breast milk of simian immunodeficiency virus-infected African green monkeys. J Virol. 2013;87:11121–34.
20. Zhang R, Martinez DR, Nguyen QN, Pollara J, Arifin T, Stolarchuk C, Foulger A, Amos JD, Parks R, Himes JE, et al. Envelope-specific B-cell populations in African green monkeys chronically infected with simian immunodeficiency virus. Nat Commun. 2016;7:12131.
21. Chahroudi A, Bosinger SE, Vanderford TH, Paiardini M, Silvestri G. Natural SIV hosts: showing AIDS the door. Science. 2012;335:1188–93.
22. Gaufin T, Pattison M, Gautam R, Stoulig C, Dufour J, MacFarland J, Mandell D, Tatum C, Marx MH, Ribeiro RM, et al. Effect of B-cell depletion on viral replication and clinical outcome of simian immunodeficiency virus infection in a natural host. J Virol. 2009;83:10347–57.
23. Brocca-Cofano E, Kuhrt D, Siewe B, Xu C, Haret-Richter GS, Craigo J, Labranche C, Montefiori DC, Landay A, Apetrei C, Pandrea I. Pathogenic correlates of simian immunodeficiency virus-associated B cell dysfunction. J Virol. 2017;91:e01051-17.
24. Banks ND, Kinsey N, Clements J, Hildreth JE. Sustained antibody-dependent cell-mediated cytotoxicity (ADCC) in SIV-infected macaques correlates with delayed progression to AIDS. AIDS Res Hum Retrovir. 2002;18:1197–205.
25. Liao HX, Bonsignori M, Alam SM, McLellan JS, Tomaras GD, Moody MA, Kozink DM, Hwang KK, Chen X, Tsao CY, et al. Vaccine induction of antibodies against a structurally heterogeneous site of immune pressure within HIV-1 envelope protein variable regions 1 and 2. Immunity. 2013;38:176–86.
26. Hsu DC, O'Connell RJ. Progress in HIV vaccine development. Hum Vaccin Immunother. 2017;13:1018–30.
27. Brenchley JM, Vinton C, Tabb B, Hao XP, Connick E, Paiardini M, Lifson JD, Silvestri G, Estes JD. Differential infection patterns of CD4+ T cells and lymphoid tissue viral burden distinguish progressive and nonprogressive lentiviral infections. Blood. 2012;120:4172–81.
28. Beer B, Scherer J, zur Megede J, Norley S, Baier M, Kurth R. Lack of dichotomy between virus load of peripheral blood and lymph nodes during long-term simian immunodeficiency virus infection of African green monkeys. Virology. 1996;219:367–75.
29. Baier M, Dittmar MT, Cichutek K, Kurth R. Development of vivo of genetic variability of simian immunodeficiency virus. Proc Natl Acad Sci USA. 1991;88:8126–30.
30. Müller MC, Saksena NK, Nerrienet E, Chappey C, Hervé VM, Durand JP, Legal-Campodonico P, Lang MC, Digoutte JP, Georges AJ. Simian immunodeficiency viruses from central and western Africa: evidence for a new species-specific lentivirus in tantalus monkeys. J Virol. 1993;67:1227–35.
31. Shen G, Upadhyay C, Zhang J, Pan R, Zolla-Pazner S, Kong XP, Hioe CE. Rationally targeted mutations at the V1V2 domain of the HIV-1 envelope to augment virus neutralization by anti-V1V2 monoclonal antibodies. PLoS ONE. 2015;10:e0141233.
32. Jiang X, Totrov M, Li W, Sampson JM, Williams C, Lu H, Wu X, Lu S, Wang S, Zolla-Pazner S, Kong XP. Rationally designed immunogens targeting HIV-1 gp120 V1V2 induce distinct conformation-specific antibody responses in rabbits. J Virol. 2016;90:11007–19.
33. Moscoso CG, Xing L, Hui J, Hu J, Kalkhoran MB, Yenigun OM, Sun Y, Paavolainen L, Martin L, Vahlne A, et al. Trimeric HIV Env provides epitope occlusion mediated by hypervariable loops. Sci Rep. 2014;4:7025.
34. Ly A, Stamatatos L. V2 loop glycosylation of the human immunodeficiency virus type 1 SF162 envelope facilitates interaction of this protein with CD4 and CCR5 receptors and protects the virus from neutralization by anti-V3 loop and anti-CD4 binding site antibodies. J Virol. 2000;74:6769–76.
35. Losman B, Bolmstedt A, Schønning K, Björndal A, Westin C, Fenyö EM, Olofsson S. Protection of neutralization epitopes in the V3 loop of oligomeric human immunodeficiency virus type 1 glycoprotein 120 by N-linked oligosaccharides in the V1 region. AIDS Res Hum Retrovir. 2001;17:1067–76.

36. Zanetti G, Briggs JA, Grünewald K, Sattentau QJ, Fuller SD. Cryo-electron tomographic structure of an immunodeficiency virus envelope complex in situ. PLoS Pathog. 2006;2:e83.

37. Hu G, Liu J, Taylor KA, Roux KH. Structural comparison of HIV-1 envelope spikes with and without the V1/V2 loop. J Virol. 2011;85:2741–50.

38. Bohl C, Bowder D, Thompson J, Abrahamyan L, Gonzalez-Ramirez S, Mao Y, Sodroski J, Wood C, Xiang SH. A twin-cysteine motif in the V2 region of gp120 is associated with SIV envelope trimer stabilization. PLoS ONE. 2013;8:e69406.

39. Chen B, Vogan EM, Gong H, Skehel JJ, Wiley DC, Harrison SC. Structure of an unliganded simian immunodeficiency virus gp120 core. Nature. 2005;433:834–41.

40. Cole KS, Alvarez M, Elliott DH, Lam H, Martin E, Chau T, Micken K, Rowles JL, Clements JE, Murphey-Corb M, et al. Characterization of neutralization epitopes of simian immunodeficiency virus (SIV) recognized by rhesus monoclonal antibodies derived from monkeys infected with an attenuated SIV strain. Virology. 2001;290:59–73.

41. Guo J, Zuo T, Cheng L, Wu X, Tang J, Sun C, Feng L, Chen L, Zhang L, Chen Z. Simian immunodeficiency virus infection evades vaccine-elicited antibody responses to V2 region. J Acquir Immune Defic Syndr. 2015;68:502–10.

42. Lozano Reina JM, Favre D, Kasakow Z, Mayau V, Nugeyre MT, Ka T, Faye A, Miller CJ, Scott-Algara D, McCune JM, et al. Gag p27-specific B- and T-cell responses in Simian immunodeficiency virus SIVagm-infected African green monkeys. J Virol. 2009;83:2770–7.

43. Norley SG, Kraus G, Ennen J, Bonilla J, König H, Kurth R. Immunological studies of the basis for the apathogenicity of simian immunodeficiency virus from African green monkeys. Proc Natl Acad Sci USA. 1990;87:9067–71.

44. Martinez DR, Vandergrift N, Douglas AO, McGuire E, Bainbridge J, Nicely NI, Montefiori DC, Tomaras GD, Fouda GG, Permar SR. Maternal binding and neutralizing IgG responses targeting the C terminal region of the V3 loop are predictive of reduced peripartum HIV-1 transmission risk. J Virol. 2017;91:e02422-16.

45. Permar SR, Kang HH, Carville A, Mansfield KG, Gelman RS, Rao SS, Whitney JB, Letvin NL. Potent simian immunodeficiency virus-specific cellular immune responses in the breast milk of simian immunodeficiency virus-infected, lactating rhesus monkeys. J Immunol. 2008;181:3643–50.

46. National Research Council. Guide for the care and use of laboratory animals. Washington, DC: National Academy Press; 1996.

47. Gnanadurai CW, Pandrea I, Parrish NF, Kraus MH, Learn GH, Salazar MG, Sauermann U, Töpfer K, Gautam R, Münch J, et al. Genetic identity and biological phenotype of a transmitted/founder virus representative of nonpathogenic simian immunodeficiency virus infection in African green monkeys. J Virol. 2010;84:12245–54.

48. Yates NL, Liao HX, Fong Y, deCamp A, Vandergrift NA, Williams WT, Alam SM, Ferrari G, Yang ZY, Seaton KE, et al. Vaccine-induced Env V1–V2 IgG3 correlates with lower HIV-1 infection risk and declines soon after vaccination. Sci Transl Med. 2014;6:228ra239.

49. Foley B, Leitner T, Apetrei C, Hahn B, Mizrachi I, Mullins J, Rambaut A, Wolinsky S, Korber B. HIV sequence compendium 2016. LA-UR-16-25625 edition. Los Alamos: Los Alamos National Laboratory, Theoretical Biology and Biophysics; 2016. p. 2016.

50. Whittle JR, Zhang R, Khurana S, King LR, Manischewitz J, Golding H, Dormitzer PR, Haynes BF, Walter EB, Moody MA, et al. Broadly neutralizing human antibody that recognizes the receptor-binding pocket of influenza virus hemagglutinin. Proc Natl Acad Sci USA. 2011;108:14216–21.

51. Pollara J, Hart L, Brewer F, Pickeral J, Packard BZ, Hoxie JA, Komoriya A, Ochsenbauer C, Kappes JC, Roederer M, et al. High-throughput quantitative analysis of HIV-1 and SIV-specific ADCC-mediating antibody responses. Cytometry A. 2011;79:603–12.

52. Trkola A, Matthews J, Gordon C, Ketas T, Moore JP. A cell line-based neutralization assay for primary human immunodeficiency virus type 1 isolates that use either the CCR5 or the CXCR4 coreceptor. J Virol. 1999;73:8966–74.

53. Koene HR, Kleijer M, Algra J, Roos D, von dem Borne AE, de Haas M. Fc gammaRIIIa-158V/F polymorphism influences the binding of IgG by natural killer cell Fc gammaRIIIa, independently of the Fc gammaRIIIa-48L/R/H phenotype. Blood. 1997;90:1109–14.

54. Ferrari G, Pollara J, Kozink D, Harms T, Drinker M, Freel S, Moody MA, Alam SM, Tomaras GD, Ochsenbauer C, et al. An HIV-1 gp120 envelope human monoclonal antibody that recognizes a C1 conformational epitope mediates potent antibody-dependent cellular cytotoxicity (ADCC) activity and defines a common ADCC epitope in human HIV-1 serum. J Virol. 2011;85:7029–36.

55. Edmonds TG, Ding H, Yuan X, Wei Q, Smith KS, Conway JA, Wieczorek L, Brown B, Polonis V, West JT, et al. Replication competent molecular clones of HIV-1 expressing Renilla luciferase facilitate the analysis of antibody inhibition in PBMC. Virology. 2010;408:1–13.

56. Ho C, Wu S, Amos JD, Colvin L, Smith SD, Wilks AB, Demarco CT, Brinkley C, Denny TN, Schmitz JE, et al. Transient compartmentalization of simian immunodeficiency virus variants in the breast milk of african green monkeys. J Virol. 2013;87:11292–9.

57. Gouy M, Guindon S, Gascuel O. SeaView version 4: a multiplatform graphical user interface for sequence alignment and phylogenetic tree building. Mol Biol Evol. 2010;27:221–4.

HIV latency reversing agents act through Tat post translational modifications

Georges Khoury[1], Talia M. Mota[1,2], Shuang Li[3], Carolin Tumpach[2], Michelle Y. Lee[1], Jonathan Jacobson[1], Leigh Harty[1], Jenny L. Anderson[2], Sharon R. Lewin[2,4] and Damian F. J. Purcell[1*]

Abstract

Background: Different classes of latency reversing agents (LRAs) are being evaluated to measure their effects in reactivating HIV replication from latently infected cells. A limited number of studies have demonstrated additive effects of LRAs with the viral protein Tat in initiating transcription, but less is known about how LRAs interact with Tat, particularly through basic residues that may be post-translationally modified to alter the behaviour of Tat for processive transcription and co-transcriptional RNA processing.

Results: Here we show that various lysine and arginine mutations reduce the capacity of Tat to induce both transcription and mRNA splicing. The lysine 28 and lysine 50 residues of Tat, or the acetylation and methylation modifications of these basic amino acids, were essential for Tat transcriptional control, and also for the proviral expression effects elicited by histone deacetylase inhibitors (HDACi) or the bromodomain inhibitor JQ1. We also found that JQ1 was the only LRA tested that could induce HIV mRNA splicing in the absence of Tat, or rescue splicing for Tat lysine mutants in a BRD4-dependent manner.

Conclusions: Our data provide evidence that Tat activities in both co-transcriptional RNA processing together with transcriptional initiation and processivity are crucial during reactivation of latent HIV infection. The HDACi and JQ1 LRAs act with Tat to increase transcription, but JQ1 also enables post-transcriptional mRNA splicing. Tat residues K28 and K50, or their modifications through acetylation or methylation, are critical for LRAs that function in conjunction with Tat.

Keywords: HIV latency, LRA, Tat, Post-translational modification, Splicing

Background

The major barrier to a cure for HIV is long lived latently infected memory CD4+ T-cells that persist on antiretroviral therapy (ART) [1]. One strategy being investigated to eliminate latency is to activate virus production from latency in the presence of ART so that no further rounds of infection occur, and it was speculated that the cell would then die either through immune mediated clearance or virus induced cytolysis [1]. Epigenetic modifiers including histone deacetylase inhibitors (HDACi) have been used to reverse latency in vitro and in vivo [2–7].

Although clinical trials of these agents in HIV-infected individuals on ART demonstrated modest increases in cell-associated unspliced HIV mRNA (US RNA), indicative of the initiation of viral transcription, when used alone, these studies failed to show a reduction in the frequency of latently infected cells as measured by HIV DNA [2–7]. Understanding how different classes of latency reversing agents (LRAs) affect distinct aspects of virus production post integration is needed to define the optimal compounds to efficiently reverse latency.

Tat is a critical viral protein required to transactivate viral transcriptional elongation and splicing [8–13]. In active HIV replication, Tat undergoes various post-translational modifications including acetylation and methylation. Depending on which residue is modified and the type of modification it carries, the behaviour of

*Correspondence: dfjp@unimelb.edu.au
[1] Department of Microbiology and Immunology, The Peter Doherty Institute for Infection and Immunity, University of Melbourne, Melbourne, Australia
Full list of author information is available at the end of the article

Tat changes to regulate its activity [14–27]. These multiple modifications provide an interconnected regulatory network that enables Tat to control viral transcription, elongation, and splicing throughout viral replication [14–27]. These modifications differ depending on the cellular environment, specifically the activation state of the cell [16], and thus should differ during active replication in activated cells versus latent infection in resting cells. Moreover, these modifications may differ under the influence of LRAs as a limited number of studies have demonstrated additive effects of LRAs with the viral protein Tat in initiating transcription [28]. However, less is known about how LRAs interact with Tat, particularly through basic residues that may be post-translationally modified to alter the behaviour of Tat.

In this study, we generated a series of Tat mutants to determine their effects on viral transcription and/or splicing. We investigated the effects of Tat mutants on the activity of a panel of LRAs and found that post translational modifications of different lysine residues of Tat are important for its activity with different LRAs, with differing abilities to actively initiate transcription and/or splicing.

Results

A novel in vitro model using fluorescent reporter proteins to test the impact of interventions on HIV transcription and splicing

A potent LRA is required for efficient reactivation and clearance of latent proviruses. To investigate the ability of LRAs to induce HIV-1 transcription and splicing, we determined the effects of LRAs alone or in combination with full-length wild-type (WT) Tat101 given Tat's important role in splicing and transcription [8].

To this end, we developed an in vitro model that can distinguish between unspliced and spliced viral products by the expression of EGFP and DsRed fluorescent proteins respectively (Fig. 1a). Briefly, a subgenomic reporter construct pLTR.gp140/EGFP.RevΔ38/DsRed, which derives from the authentic env2 mRNA [29], was constructed to allow the detection of LTR-driven 'unspliced' or 'spliced' products by flow cytometry. This construct expresses HIV-1 Env, Rev and small amounts of Vpu proteins [30, 31]. In this system if the mRNA remains unspliced, it would express Env (gp140) fused to EGFP (Fig. 1a). If splicing occurs across splice donor 4 and splice acceptor 7 (D4A7), the spliced mRNA encodes a non-functional Rev protein truncated at amino acid 38 fused to DsRed fluorescent protein (Δ38Rev-DsRed).

To test that this model measures unspliced and spliced viral products, HEK293T cells were co-transfected with the reporter and a plasmid containing rev (pRev) to facilitate the nuclear export of Rev response element

(RRE)-containing unspliced mRNA, in the presence or absence of pTat101. Flow cytometry was used to measure each fluorescent colour using the gating strategy shown for a representative sample (Fig. 1b) out of five independent experiments, each performed in triplicate (Fig. 1c–e). For cells transfected with the reporter and pRev without Tat, a mean of 8.03 and 0.39% of cells expressed EGFP and DsRed respectively, indicating that there was basal transcription from the LTR but only a low efficiency of splicing at D4A7 without Tat (Fig. 1c–e, minus sample). The addition of WT Tat101 (100 ng pTat) enabled a significant increase in transcription (31.7% EGFP+; $p = 0.0076$) (Fig. 1c) and splicing (21.6% DsRed+; n = 5, Paired T test, $p = 0.0015$) (Fig. 1d). To control for Tat-induced increases in transcription and for transfection efficiency, we also measured the percentage of spliced product versus total product (spliced/(spliced + unspliced) × 100). A significant increase in spliced product was observed in the presence of WT Tat compared to cells only and DMSO ($p = 0.0004$; n = 5; Paired T test) (Fig. 1e).

Latency reversing agents change the behaviour of Tat during reactivation from the LTR

Using the same reporter system, we investigated the effects of a panel of LRAs on LTR-driven transcription and splicing in the absence and presence of WT Tat. Transfected cells were treated with the two HDACi vorinostat (VOR) and panobinostat (PAN), the bromodomain inhibitor JQ1, the methyltransferase inhibitor chaetocin (CTN), the anti-alcoholic disulfiram (DIS) and the T cell activation stimuli phorbol myristate acetate/phytohaemagglutinin (PMA/PHA), with concentrations at the maximum tolerated doses to preserve cell viability (Additional file 1: Fig. S1). Cells were then harvested at 48 h post-transfection for flow cytometry analysis.

Without Tat, both PAN and JQ1 were the only LRAs that significantly increased the expression of EGFP (1.68 and 1.69 FC over DMSO respectively; n = 5, 2-way ANOVA across LRAs, $p < 0.05$) indicative of unspliced transcripts (Fig. 2a). However, this increase was modest compared to Tat when added in trans (3.27 FC over DMSO, 2-way ANOVA, $p = 0.0001$) (Fig. 2a). Moreover, in the absence of Tat, JQ1 was the only LRA that increased the proportion of spliced product to a similar level as WT Tat (3.44 and 3.92 FC over DMSO respectively; n = 5, 2-way ANOVA, $p = 0.0001$) (Fig. 2b).

In the presence of Tat101, while JQ1 and both HDACi significantly increased the levels of EGFP (1.2 and 1.3 FC over DMSO respectively, $p < 0.05$) (Fig. 2c), only JQ1 significantly increased the proportion of spliced product when compared to DMSO (Fig. 2d; n = 5, 2-way ANOVA across all LRAs). Similar results were obtained using Tat86 from the HIV NL4-3 strain (data not shown).

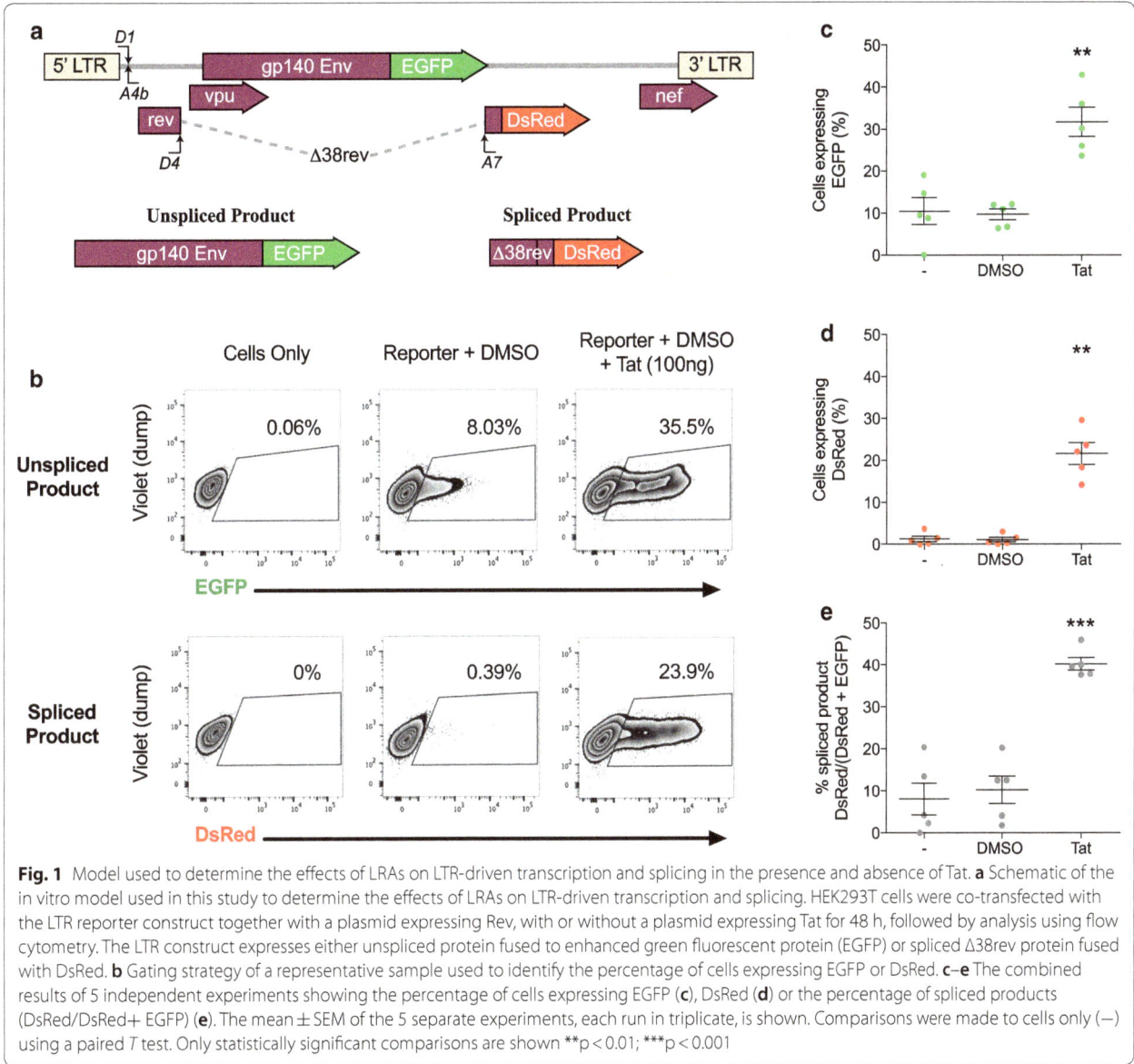

Fig. 1 Model used to determine the effects of LRAs on LTR-driven transcription and splicing in the presence and absence of Tat. **a** Schematic of the in vitro model used in this study to determine the effects of LRAs on LTR-driven transcription and splicing. HEK293T cells were co-transfected with the LTR reporter construct together with a plasmid expressing Rev, with or without a plasmid expressing Tat for 48 h, followed by analysis using flow cytometry. The LTR construct expresses either unspliced protein fused to enhanced green fluorescent protein (EGFP) or spliced Δ38rev protein fused with DsRed. **b** Gating strategy of a representative sample used to identify the percentage of cells expressing EGFP or DsRed. **c–e** The combined results of 5 independent experiments showing the percentage of cells expressing EGFP (**c**), DsRed (**d**) or the percentage of spliced products (DsRed/DsRed+ EGFP) (**e**). The mean ± SEM of the 5 separate experiments, each run in triplicate, is shown. Comparisons were made to cells only (−) using a paired T test. Only statistically significant comparisons are shown **p < 0.01; ***p < 0.001

Taken together, these data demonstrate that different classes of LRAs have differential effects on HIV transcription and splicing. In addition, while Tat alone is the most potent activator of LTR-driven transcription, Tat can also have an additive effect with HDACi and JQ1 on transcription, and with JQ1 alone on splicing.

Accumulation of HIV spliced RNA following JQ1 treatment

To validate the effect of JQ1 on HIV-1 transcription and splicing, we performed similar experiments but also evaluated the changes in viral RNA levels following treatment with JQ1 in the presence or absence of Tat (Fig. 3, Additional file 2: Fig. S2). Transfected cells were harvested at 24 h to capture the peak of RNA expression. Most cells were used for RNA quantification by droplet digital PCR (ddPCR, Fig. 3), while a small portion of cells were also analysed by flow cytometry (Additional file 2: Fig. S2). For ddPCR, a specific probe spanning D4-A7 splice sites was used to quantify the spliced RNAs (Fig. 3a, *rev* primer–probe). Unspliced (US) transcripts were detected by a primer–probe set specific to gp140 Env ORF (Fig. 3a, *env* primer–probe set). Additionally, we quantified all viral RNAs initiated from the HIV long terminal repeat (LTR) by targeting a common region of viral transcripts (Fig. 3a, virus primer–probe).

Both JQ1 alone and Tat alone increased the levels of US (3.16 and 6.65 FC over DMSO) as well as spliced RNA (19.75 and 19.33 FC over DMSO), while no significant

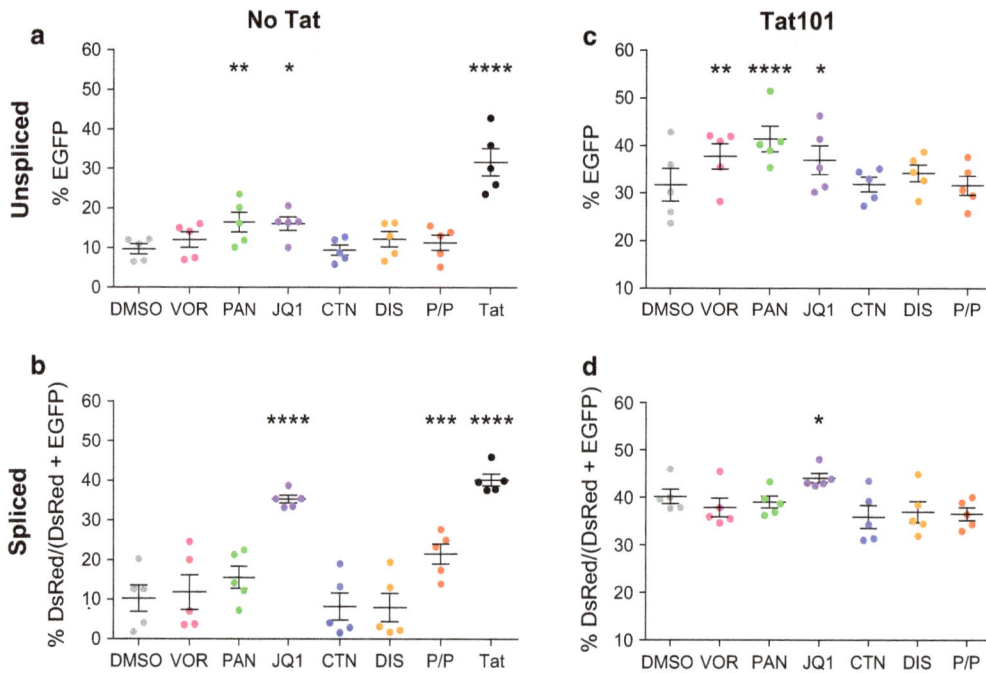

Fig. 2 JQ1 but not HDACi can increase splicing in the absence and presence of Tat. HEK293T cells were co-transfected with the pLTR.gp140/EGFP.RevΔ38/DsRed splicing reporter together with a plasmid expressing Rev, in the absence (**a**, **b**) or presence (**c**, **d**) of 100 ng of pTat101 (AD8)-Flag expression plasmid and then treated with a panel of LRAs or DMSO diluent control (n = 5). EGFP (unspliced) and DsRed (spliced) expression were measured using flow cytometry. Comparisons of each condition to DMSO were made using 2-way ANOVA test. Only statistically significant comparisons are shown *p < 0.05; **p < 0.01; ***p < 0.001; ****p < 0.0001. The black lines represent the mean ± SEM. DMSO (1:5000), VOR = vorinostat (0.5 μM), PAN = panobinostat (30 nM), JQ1 (+) (1 μM), CTN = chaetocin (30 nM), DIS = disulfiram (500 nM), or PMA/PHA = phorbol myristate acetate/phytohaemagglutinin (10 nM PMA, 10 μg/mL PHA)

change was detected in the level of total viral RNA following JQ1 treatment (Fig. 3b). As we observed previously in Fig. 2, the combination of Tat and JQ1 increased the levels of US and spliced RNAs (Fig. 3b) confirming the ability of JQ1 and Tat to turn on HIV transcription and splicing. Moreover, the RNA analysis revealed consistent changes in RNA transcription and splicing that was mirrored by the EGFP and DsRed protein expression in this model following treatment with JQ1: a 2.5-fold increase in both US/all viral RNA and %EGFP+, and 18.5-fold increase in spliced/all viral RNA and %spliced product (compare Fig. 3c, d and Additional file 2: Fig. S2A, S2C). This indicates that EGFP and DsRed expressing cells well reflect the ability of JQ1 to induce HIV transcription and splicing at D4A7. These results also confirm the ability to use the splicing reporter pLTR.gp140/EGFP. RevΔ38/DsRed in high throughput assays where we can accurately measure by flow cytometry the effect of LRAs on HIV transcription and splicing.

To determine whether this was a global effect on cellular RNA transcription, we also looked at changes in *RPP30*, *IPO8* and *TBP* RNA levels following each treatment (Additional file 3: Fig. S3A) and saw no statistically

significant changes in HIV RNA fold changes when normalized to all 3 references genes (Additional file 3: Fig. S3B). We next evaluated whether the effect of JQ1 was a general splicing effect or specific to HIV D4A7 sites by looking at the alternative splicing pattern of multiple human pre-mRNA including *CD46*, *ATF2* and ABI-interactor (*ABI1*) by RT-PCR using specific primers of adjacent exons. A reduction in *CD46* exon 13 (Fig. 4a) and *ATF2* exon 6 (Fig. 4b) inclusions was observed following treatment with JQ1. In addition, *ABI1* exon 8 exclusion and exon 9 inclusion were favoured in the presence of JQ1 (Fig. 4c) suggesting a global effect of JQ1 on alternative splicing. Finally to determine whether the increase in HIV D4-A7 splicing was due to changes in the availability of splicing factors, we also looked at changes in hnRNP protein levels following JQ1 treatment. An increase in PTB coupled with a decrease in hnRNP A1 levels was observed (Fig. 4d).

Overall, these data demonstrate that JQ1 treatment leads to a significant accumulation of HIV spliced RNA. This was consistent with an increase in the ability of JQ1 to drive both HIV-1 transcription but more profoundly splicing, potentially due to a decrease in splicing

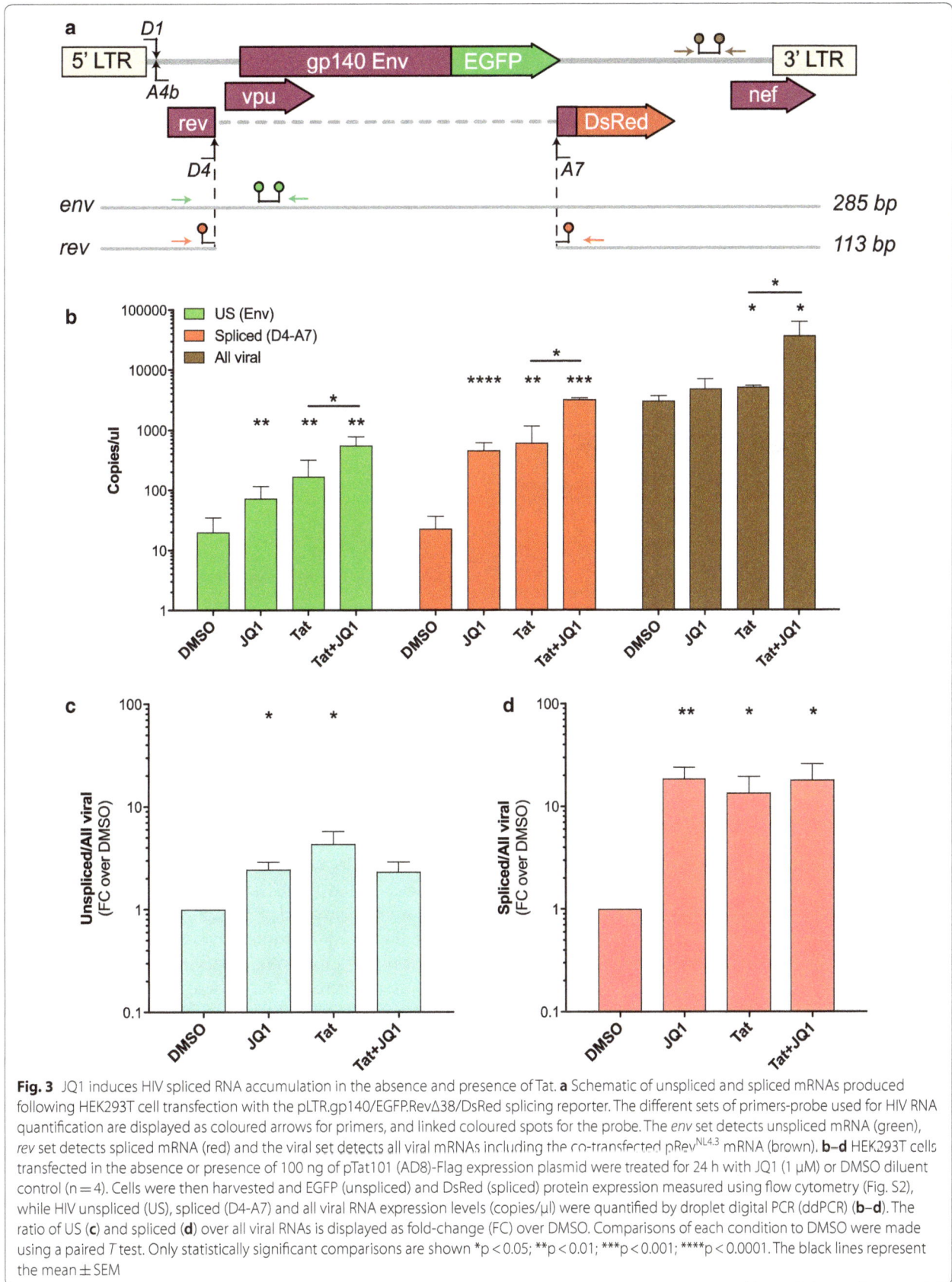

Fig. 3 JQ1 induces HIV spliced RNA accumulation in the absence and presence of Tat. **a** Schematic of unspliced and spliced mRNAs produced following HEK293T cell transfection with the pLTR.gp140/EGFP.RevΔ38/DsRed splicing reporter. The different sets of primers-probe used for HIV RNA quantification are displayed as coloured arrows for primers, and linked coloured spots for the probe. The *env* set detects unspliced mRNA (green), *rev* set detects spliced mRNA (red) and the viral set detects all viral mRNAs including the co-transfected pRev[NL4.3] mRNA (brown). **b–d** HEK293T cells transfected in the absence or presence of 100 ng of pTat101 (AD8)-Flag expression plasmid were treated for 24 h with JQ1 (1 μM) or DMSO diluent control (n = 4). Cells were then harvested and EGFP (unspliced) and DsRed (spliced) protein expression measured using flow cytometry (Fig. S2), while HIV unspliced (US), spliced (D4-A7) and all viral RNA expression levels (copies/μl) were quantified by droplet digital PCR (ddPCR) (**b–d**). The ratio of US (**c**) and spliced (**d**) over all viral RNAs is displayed as fold-change (FC) over DMSO. Comparisons of each condition to DMSO were made using a paired *T* test. Only statistically significant comparisons are shown *p < 0.05; **p < 0.01; ***p < 0.001; ****p < 0.0001. The black lines represent the mean ± SEM

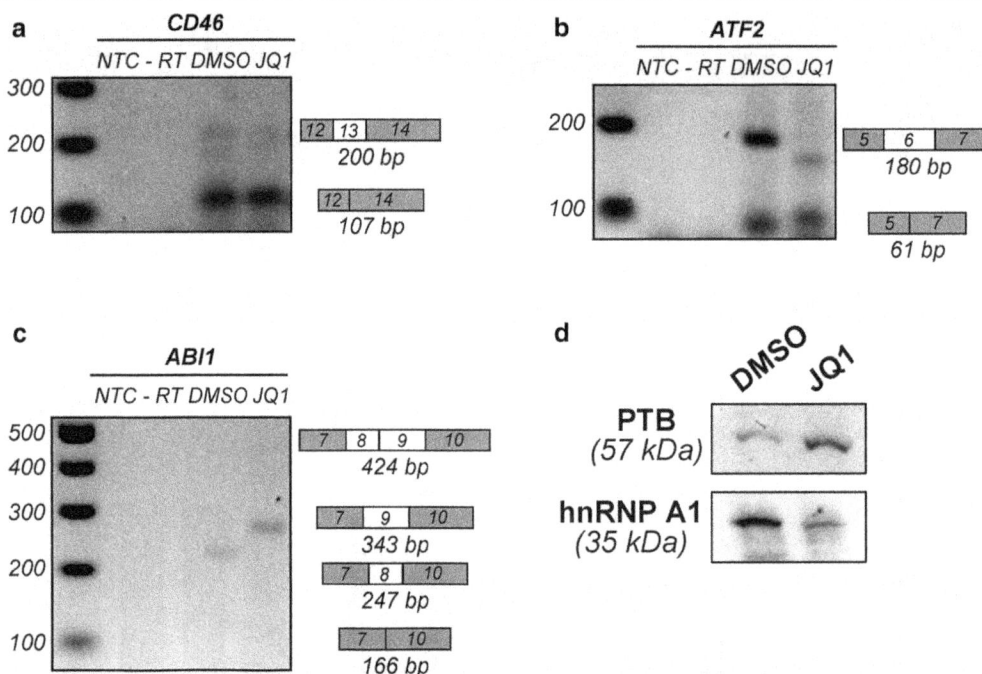

Fig. 4 JQ1 affects alternative splicing by modulating hnRNP protein levels. Alternative splicing pattern of *CD46* (**a**), *ATF2* (**b**) and *ABI1* (**c**) in HEK293T cells following 24 h of JQ1 (1 μM) or DMSO treatment. Inclusion and exclusion of exons are indicated on the right of the gel with white boxes, while grey boxes represent constitutively included exons. NTC = No Template Control, -RT corresponds to minus reverse transcriptase control. **d** Western Blot analysis of splicing factors following treatment with JQ1 or DMSO diluent control

inhibitory factors such as hnRNP A1 and an increase in RNA binding proteins facilitating RNA nuclear export like PTB.

Mutations in lysine and arginine residues in Tat101 reduce HIV transcription and splicing efficiency

Transactivation of the HIV-1 LTR by Tat is a tightly controlled process that is heavily reliant on post-translational modifications (PTMs) of both Tat and P-TEFb [16]. These PTMs serve to fine-tune Tat function allowing its interaction with different cofactors at specific stages of transcription. Several Lysine (K) and Arginine (R) residues in the transactivation and RNA binding domains of Tat are modified (Fig. 5a). To measure the effect of PTMs on HIV transcription and splicing, we introduced a variety of mutations in the basic K or R residues of Tat, using site-directed mutagenesis to change these residues into Alanine (A). The Tat proteins included a C-terminal flag-tag, which allowed their detection by Western blot using an anti-Flag antibody (Fig. 5b). Each mutant or wild-type (WT) Tat was first transfected into HEK293T cells and Western blot confirmed similar expression levels of these mutants as WT Tat (Fig. 5b).

Next, we investigated the effects of these mutations on LTR-driven transcription alone (without splicing) by transfecting each mutant into TZMbl cells that contain a luciferase reporter under the control of HIV LTR. Cells were harvested 48 h later and luciferase expression was measured and represented as a percentage of expression relative to WT Tat (Fig. 5c). Mutations of K28, K50 and K50-51 to alanine significantly reduced the ability of Tat to transactivate transcription from the LTR, while no effect was observed following K71 and R53 mutations (n = 5; Paired T test).

Similar results were obtained when Tat mutants were co-transfected with the splicing reporter construct to assess effects on splicing (Fig. 6). In this set of experiments, these same mutants also exhibited statistically significant reductions in the proportion of spliced product (Fig. 6; n = 5; Paired T test). These data demonstrate that mutations to specific lysine residues within Tat significantly inhibit the efficiency of Tat in driving transcription and splicing at D4A7.

Lysine 28 and 50 mutants reduce LTR-driven transcription in the presence of LRAs

Next, to investigate whether Tat PTMs affect LTR-driven transcription with commonly used LRAs, we co-transfected each mutant into HEK293T with the splicing reporter described above and then treated the cells with the LRA panel or DMSO diluent control.

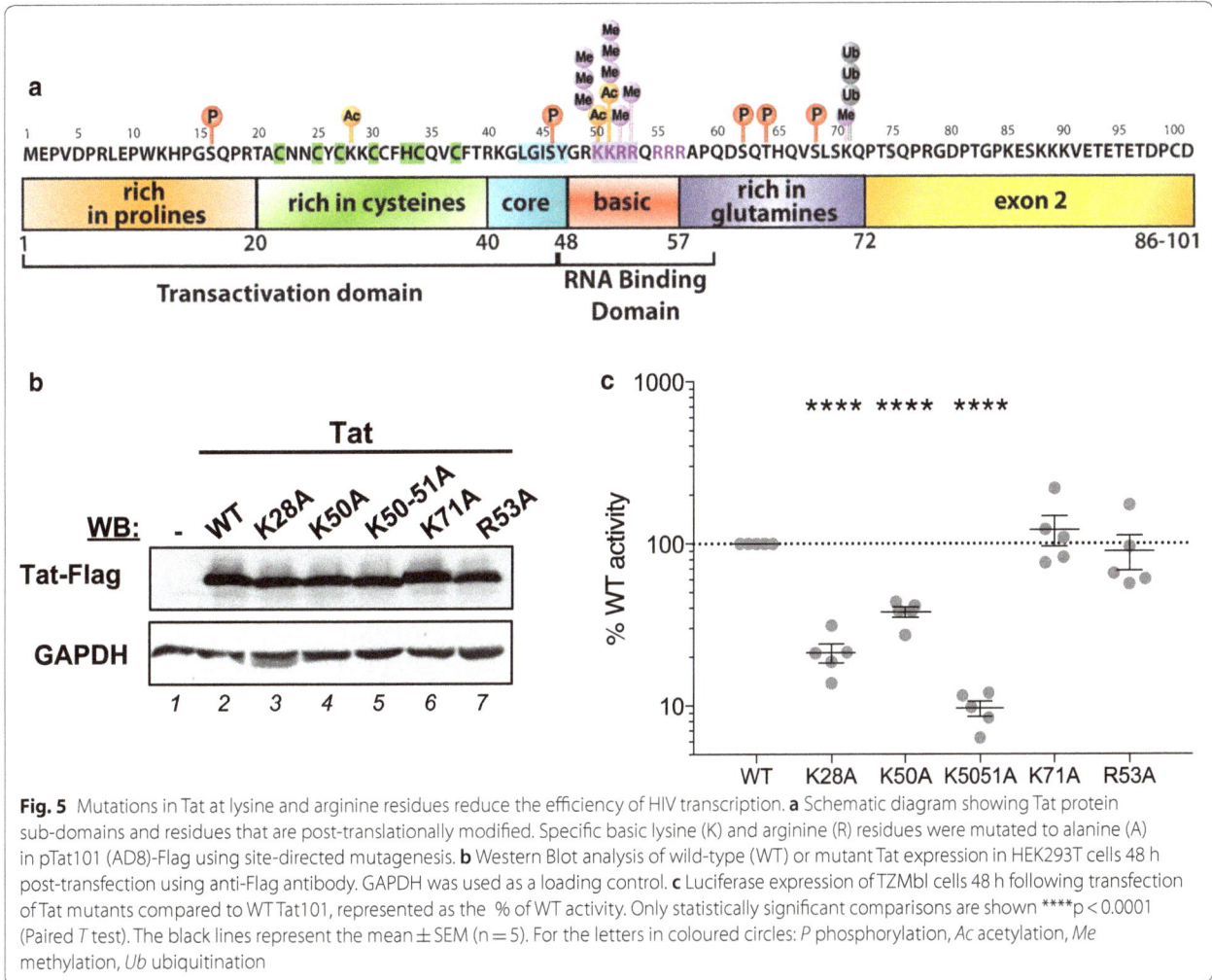

Fig. 5 Mutations in Tat at lysine and arginine residues reduce the efficiency of HIV transcription. **a** Schematic diagram showing Tat protein sub-domains and residues that are post-translationally modified. Specific basic lysine (K) and arginine (R) residues were mutated to alanine (A) in pTat101 (AD8)-Flag using site-directed mutagenesis. **b** Western Blot analysis of wild-type (WT) or mutant Tat expression in HEK293T cells 48 h post-transfection using anti-Flag antibody. GAPDH was used as a loading control. **c** Luciferase expression of TZMbl cells 48 h following transfection of Tat mutants compared to WT Tat101, represented as the % of WT activity. Only statistically significant comparisons are shown ****$p < 0.0001$ (Paired T test). The black lines represent the mean ± SEM (n = 5). For the letters in coloured circles: P phosphorylation, Ac acetylation, Me methylation, Ub ubiquitination

To assess the effects of Tat PTMs on transcription (EGFP+ cells), statistical comparisons of EGFP+ cells were made to DMSO+ Tat101 with or without the designated mutation (Additional file 4: Fig. S4). VOR, PAN and JQ1 had statistically significant activity with WT Tat101 (Additional file 4: Fig. S4A; n = 5; 2-way ANOVA test across all LRAs). However, VOR and JQ1 lost this significant activity with the K28A and K50A mutants compared to their respective DMSO control (Additional file 4: Fig. S4B and S4C). In contrast, Tat K50/51A retained its activity with HDACi and JQ1, and gained a modest but statistically significant enhancement of activity with PMA/PHA (Additional file 4: Fig. S4C). The pattern was different with the K71A and R53A mutants, where PAN and JQ1 retained their ability to induce transcription, but this ability was lost with VOR (Additional file 4: Fig. S4E-F). These data suggest that Tat K28 and K50, or the post translational

modifications that these basic amino acids acquire, are essential for Tat action with VOR and JQ1 in driving transcription.

JQ1 promotes HIV D4-A7 splicing with or without WT Tat101 and its various mutants in a splicing reporter system

To assess the effects of the Tat mutants on HIV splicing (DsRed cells), the HEK293T cells transfected and treated with a panel of LRAs above were analysed by flow cytometry for the percentage of cells expressing DsRed. The fold change in the proportion of spliced product [spliced/(spliced + unspliced)/WT] of Tat mutants relative to WT Tat101+ DMSO is represented in Fig. 7. Although both PAN and JQ1 increased the percentage of cells expressing the unspliced EGFP product without or with WT Tat (Fig. 2), only JQ1 consistently increased the proportion of DsRed spliced product in the absence of Tat (Fig. 7a) and with each Tat mutant (Fig. 7b–f; n = 5; 2-way ANOVA

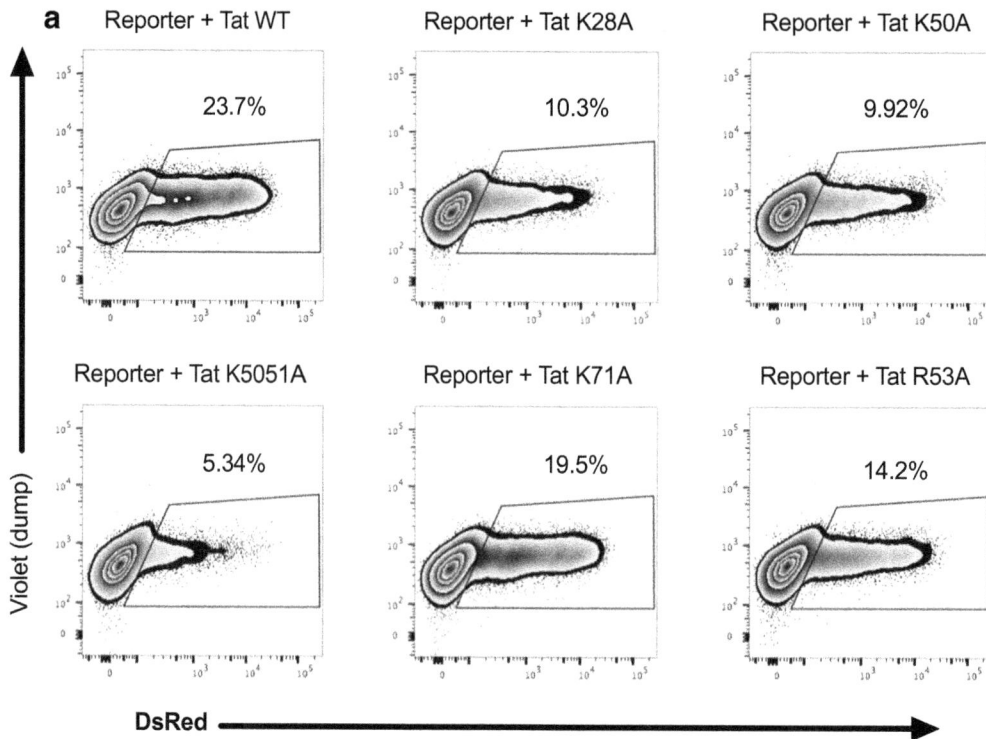

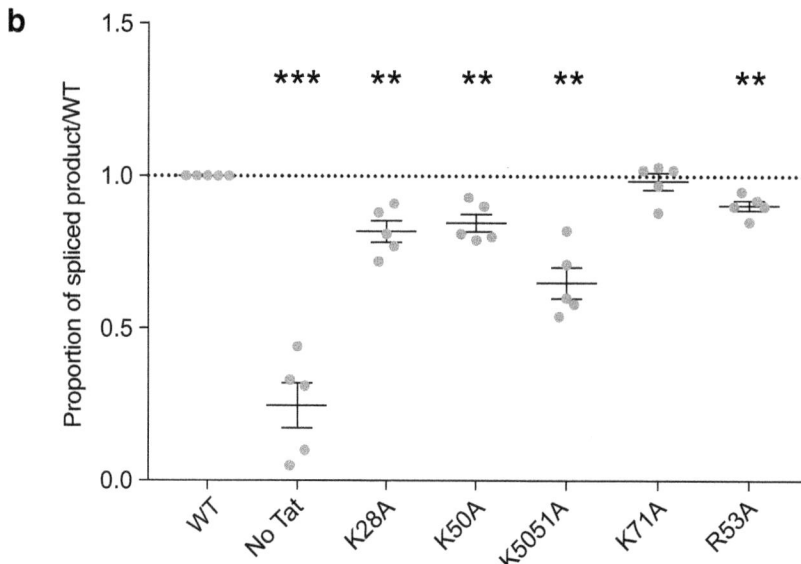

Fig. 6 Specific mutations within Tat reduce HIV D4-A7 splicing. HEK293T cells were co-transfected with the pLTR.gp140/EGFP.RevΔ38/DsRed splicing reporter, 20 ng of pRev and 100 ng of pTat101 without (WT) or with specific mutations (K28A, K50A, K50/51A, K71A and R53A). Cells were harvested at 48 h and DsRed expression was quantified by flow cytometry. **a** A representative example of the gating strategy used to identify % DsRed positive cells that represent spliced product. **b** The proportion of spliced product [DsRed/(DsRed + EGFP) × 100] relative to WT Tat is shown from n = 5 independent experiments, each conducted in triplicate. Comparisons of each condition to DMSO were made using a Paired T test. Only statistically significant comparisons are shown **p < 0.01; ***p < 0.001. The black lines represent the mean ± SEM

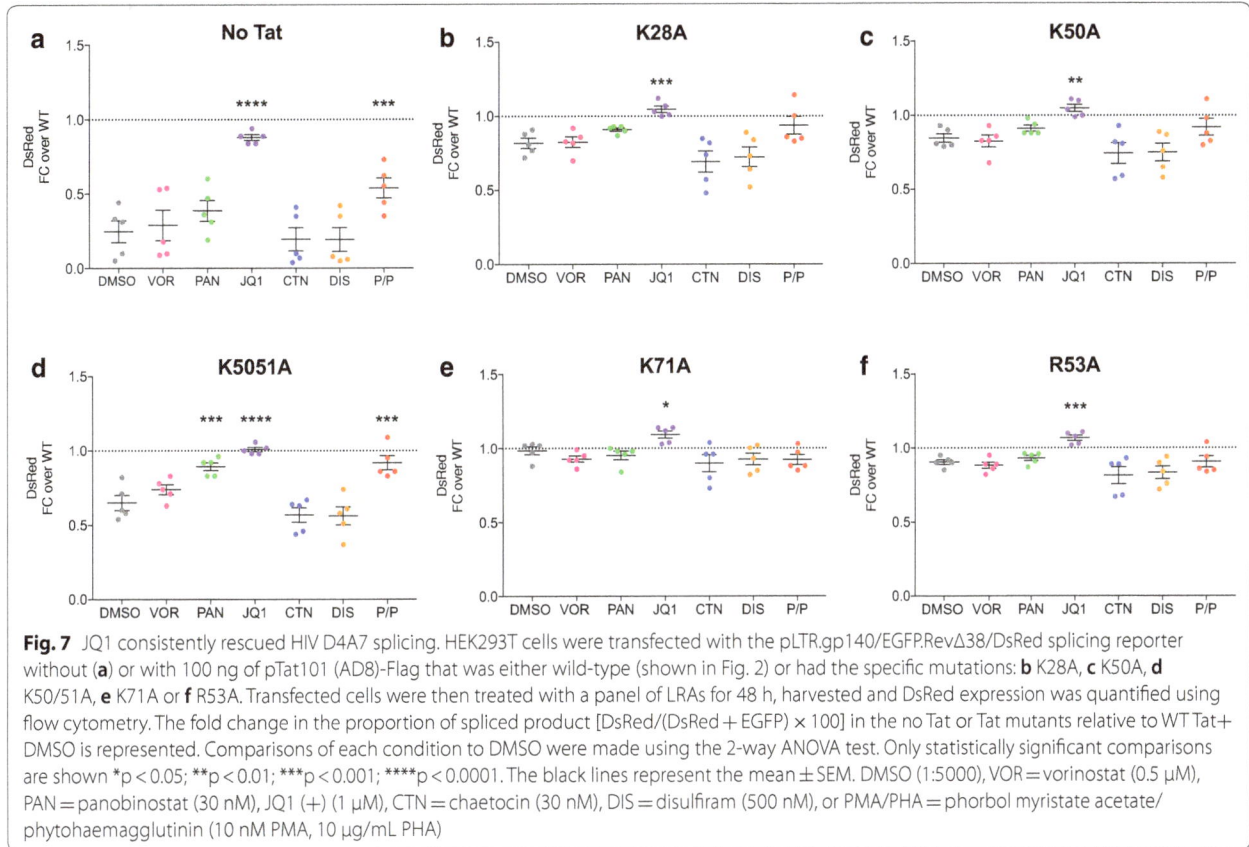

Fig. 7 JQ1 consistently rescued HIV D4A7 splicing. HEK293T cells were transfected with the pLTR.gp140/EGFP.RevΔ38/DsRed splicing reporter without (**a**) or with 100 ng of pTat101 (AD8)-Flag that was either wild-type (shown in Fig. 2) or had the specific mutations: **b** K28A, **c** K50A, **d** K50/51A, **e** K71A or **f** R53A. Transfected cells were then treated with a panel of LRAs for 48 h, harvested and DsRed expression was quantified using flow cytometry. The fold change in the proportion of spliced product [DsRed/(DsRed + EGFP) × 100] in the no Tat or Tat mutants relative to WT Tat+ DMSO is represented. Comparisons of each condition to DMSO were made using the 2-way ANOVA test. Only statistically significant comparisons are shown *p < 0.05; **p < 0.01; ***p < 0.001; ****p < 0.0001. The black lines represent the mean ± SEM. DMSO (1:5000), VOR = vorinostat (0.5 μM), PAN = panobinostat (30 nM), JQ1 (+) (1 μM), CTN = chaetocin (30 nM), DIS = disulfiram (500 nM), or PMA/PHA = phorbol myristate acetate/phytohaemagglutinin (10 nM PMA, 10 μg/mL PHA)

test across all LRAs). We directly compared these changes to DMSO (Fig. 8a), and displayed the difference in activity of JQ1 within each mutant and found statistically significant differences compared to WT Tat101. Although in each mutant, JQ1 enabled a statistically significant increase in the proportion of spliced product compared to DMSO that was always greater than WT activity (Fig. 8a; n = 5; Paired T test), when compared to WT Tat101 this difference was significantly higher for all mutants except K71A (Fig. 8b; n = 5; Paired T test). Taken together, these data show that the presence of WT Tat or JQ1 alone can both enable HIV RNA splicing to a similar degree, and when a specific Tat mutation reduces splicing efficiency (Fig. 6b), only JQ1 could rescue splicing (Figs. 7, 8). Thus, JQ1 may act directly or indirectly with Tat, and independently of the basic K or R residues of Tat, to enable HIV RNA splicing.

BRD4 mediates JQ1 effect on HIV D4-A7 RNA splicing

In the absence of Tat, Bromodomain-containing protein 4 (BRD4), an acetylated histone binding protein with 2 bromodomains (BRD) that recognise acetylated lysine residues, plays an important role during transcriptional elongation by interacting and activating P-TEFb (positive transcription elongation factor b) [32, 33]. On the other

hand, BRD4 can negatively impact HIV transcription via P-TEFb sequestration [34]. As JQ1 inhibits BRD4 activity by binding competitively to acetyl-lysine recognition motifs and releasing P-TEFb, we hypothesised that JQ1 might influence HIV transcription and splicing through BRD4. To further elucidate the interplay of JQ1 and BRD4 in regard to the transcriptional and splicing regulation of HIV RNA, we analysed the expression of HIV using the splicing reporter system after stimulation with 2 enantiomers of JQ1; S (+) and R (−) forms (Fig. 9).

As expected, treatment with JQ1 (−) analogue that does not interact with any bromodomain [35] abolished the JQ1 (+) effect on HIV transcription (Fig. 9a). Interestingly, as shown in Fig. 9b, a specific activation of HIV D4-A7 splicing with JQ1 (+), but not with the stereoisomer control JQ1 (−), was also observed in all cases (p = 0.0151; n = 3; Friedman nonparametric test) suggesting a role of BRD4 in mediating HIV D4-A7 RNA splicing via JQ1 (+).

Discussion

A variety of LRAs are currently being investigated ex vivo and in vivo for their efficacy to induce virus production from latently infected rCD4+ T cells. However, not much is known about how these LRAs affect different aspects essential for the additive effect between LRAs and Tat on transcription. Interestingly, K28 and K50 are highly conserved across HIV-1 and SIV [19]. These same Tat residues, in addition to R53, were also required for efficient RNA splicing. Additionally, in the presence of K28A, K50A, and K50/51A mutations that deny acetylation at these positions, JQ1 alone could rescue this defect in splicing. These data suggest that JQ1 can induce HIV RNA splicing independently of Tat, yet when Tat is present these residues are not essential. It is unclear if this positive activity of JQ1 and Tat extends to other alternatively spliced cellular RNAs.

Suboptimal levels of Tat protein or Tat function facilitate the maintenance of HIV latency where the addition of exogenous or co-transfected Tat can efficiently reactivate virus production from latent HIV [10, 36–40]. It remains unknown if Tat expression and appropriate post-translational modification can be induced by LRAs in rCD4+ T cells, particularly since the long non-coding RNA NRON, which is highly expressed in rCD4+ T cells, can target Tat for degradation [11]. Our results suggest that the Tat residues K28, K50 and K51, or the modifications that these basic amino acids acquire from cellular factors, are essential for Tat mediated HIV transcription and splicing.

When WT Tat is expressed in the context of latent infection, we show that some LRAs more potently induce HIV transcription, than in the absence of Tat. This is due to the multifaceted behaviour of how Tat is controlled, in part, by the cellular environment and the ability of Tat to be post-translationally modified by a variety of cellular factors at different stages of the viral life cycle [14–27]. Although the effects of post-translational modifications on Tat are well characterised, it remains difficult to determine the exact trajectory of Tat in its feedback loop with regard to subcellular location, at what stage in viral replication and by what cellular factor/s that Tat is modified during the viral life cycle. Given these modifications can have positive or negative behaviour-changing effects on Tat function that can be transient or permanent, it makes sense that LRAs, which can act directly or indirectly on lysine or arginine residues, may enable the accumulation of a pool of modified Tat with altered behaviour that may change how Tat interacts and functions during latency reversal [14–27] (see schematic in Fig. 10).

HDACi can modestly activate transcription and their activity is enhanced in the presence of Tat, which could be due to the fact that Tat transactivation through the LTR is intricately controlled by lysine acetylation [14]. In particular, the acetylation of K28 is mediated by host histone acetyltransferases (HATs) p300, which strengthens the binding of Tat to the transactivation response (TAR) RNA element within the LTR to promote

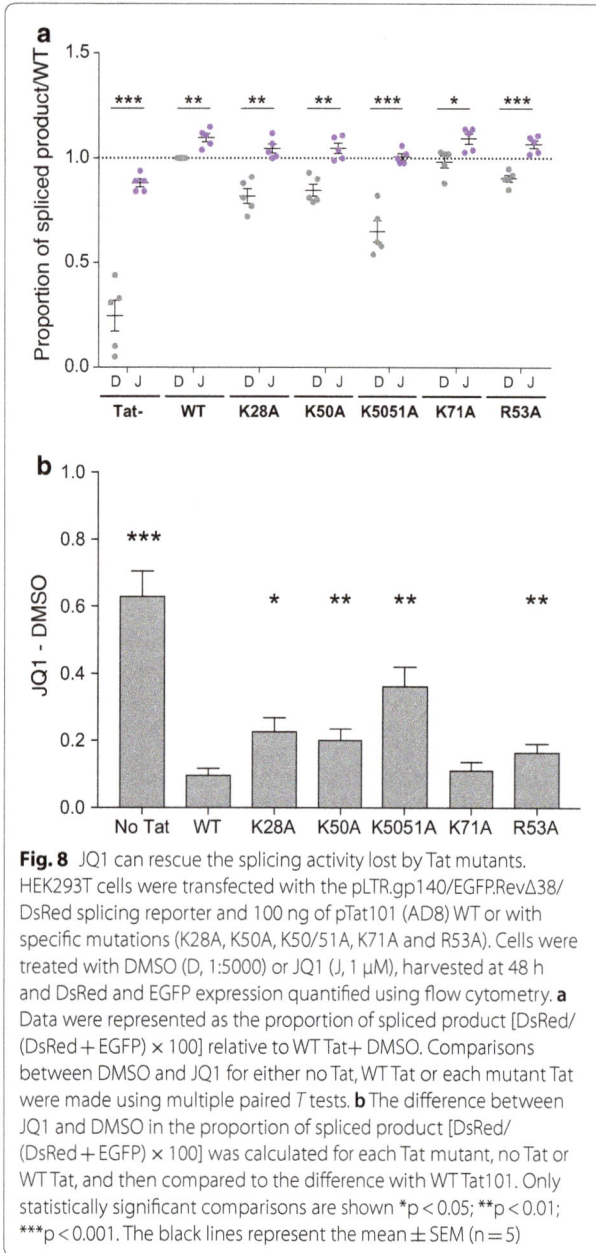

Fig. 8 JQ1 can rescue the splicing activity lost by Tat mutants. HEK293T cells were transfected with the pLTR.gp140/EGFP.RevΔ38/DsRed splicing reporter and 100 ng of pTat101 (AD8) WT or with specific mutations (K28A, K50A, K50/51A, K71A and R53A). Cells were treated with DMSO (D, 1:5000) or JQ1 (J, 1 µM), harvested at 48 h and DsRed and EGFP expression quantified using flow cytometry. **a** Data were represented as the proportion of spliced product [DsRed/(DsRed + EGFP) × 100] relative to WT Tat + DMSO. Comparisons between DMSO and JQ1 for either no Tat, WT Tat or each mutant Tat were made using multiple paired T tests. **b** The difference between JQ1 and DMSO in the proportion of spliced product [DsRed/(DsRed + EGFP) × 100] was calculated for each Tat mutant, no Tat or WT Tat, and then compared to the difference with WT Tat101. Only statistically significant comparisons are shown *p < 0.05; **p < 0.01; ***p < 0.001. The black lines represent the mean ± SEM (n = 5)

of the viral replication cycle, such as the behaviour of Tat protein in transcription and splicing. Given the ability of Tat to be post-translationally modified and the possibility that these modifications may differ under the influence of LRAs, we were interested to investigate how different classes of LRAs acted in combination with Tat.

In agreement with previous studies by Caputi's team [8], our data show that wild-type (WT) Tat101 expression induced a change in HIV-1 splicing pattern, increasing the use of A7 3′ss and thus the expression of *rev* mRNAs. We also showed that the Tat K28 and K50/51 residues are

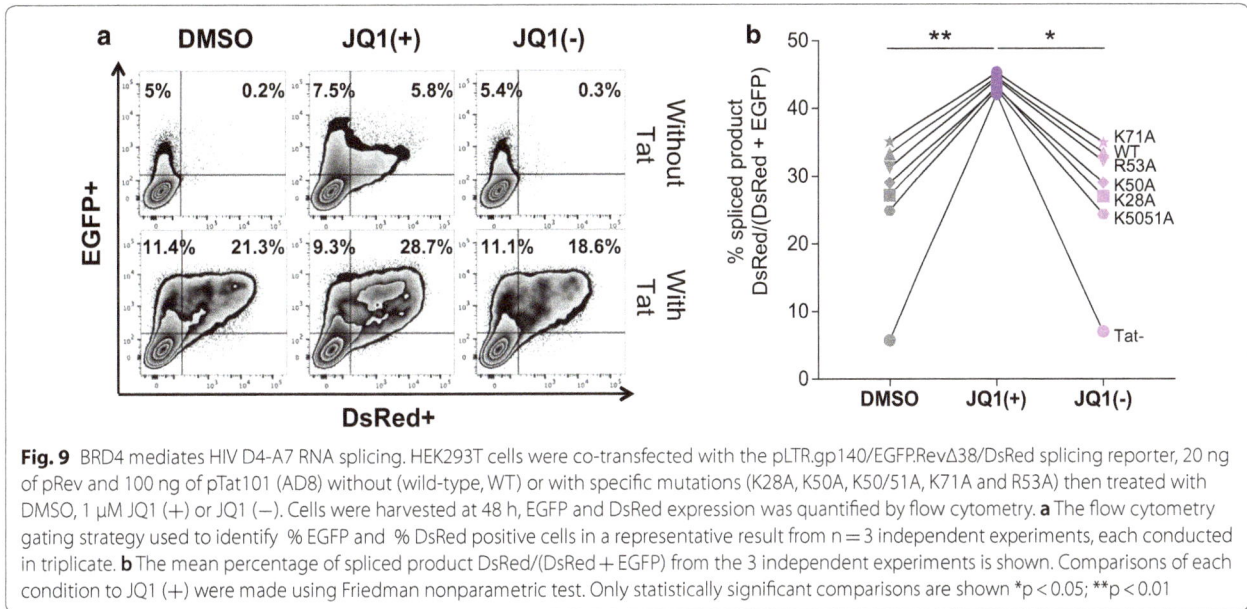

Fig. 9 BRD4 mediates HIV D4-A7 RNA splicing. HEK293T cells were co-transfected with the pLTR.gp140/EGFP.RevΔ38/DsRed splicing reporter, 20 ng of pRev and 100 ng of pTat101 (AD8) without (wild-type, WT) or with specific mutations (K28A, K50A, K50/51A, K71A and R53A) then treated with DMSO, 1 μM JQ1 (+) or JQ1 (−). Cells were harvested at 48 h, EGFP and DsRed expression was quantified by flow cytometry. **a** The flow cytometry gating strategy used to identify % EGFP and % DsRed expressing cells in a representative result from n = 3 independent experiments, each conducted in triplicate. **b** The mean percentage of spliced product DsRed/(DsRed + EGFP) from the 3 independent experiments is shown. Comparisons of each condition to JQ1 (+) were made using Friedman nonparametric test. Only statistically significant comparisons are shown *p < 0.05; **p < 0.01

transcription [19, 21, 22]. Yet when K50 is acetylated by p300, this interaction enables the dissociation of the Tat•P-TEFb•TAR complex to transfer Tat onto the elongating RNA Pol II [19, 21]. Tat is hypothesized to control elongation rates by orchestrating the phosphorylation of the C-terminal domain (CTD) of RNA Pol II to enable the association and dissociation of transcribing RNAs and RNA-associated factors throughout elongation, as well as the control of the processivity and pausing of RNA Pol II to regulate viral splicing [8, 41, 42]. Given that the additive effect on transcription between HDACi and Tat is lost with the K28A and K50A mutants, we propose a model where HDACi act by promoting the acetylation of K28 and K50 to enhance transactivation by Tat-mediated assembly of the transcription complex (Fig. 10). However, acetylation of Tat at K28 may continuously promote the Tat:TAR interaction in a way that precludes splicing.

Using our in vitro model system to assess transcription and splicing, while JQ1 had a similar activity to HDACi in enhancing transcription, JQ1 also had a unique additional action in enabling splicing in the presence and absence of Tat101. JQ1 can act in both a Tat-dependent [43–46] and Tat-independent [47] manner to reverse latency, where the Tat-independent activity of JQ1 is crucial given that Tat protein is scarce in latency [10]. The positive effects of JQ1 on HIV splicing may be explained by its ability either to alter the level of *trans*-acting factors such as hnRNPs (heterogeneous nuclear ribonucleoproteins), which are involved in alternative splicing, mRNA stability, transcriptional and translational regulation [48], or to initiate the upregulation of the CDK9 subunit of P-TEFb [49] and AFF4 [44], as well as host genes

crucial for chromatin reorganization and genes that influence posttranslational modifications of Tat [44]. We demonstrated that the lysine residues at K28, K50, and K50/51 were critical for splicing but JQ1 was able to rescue this defect. Our finding highlights the usefulness of compounds like JQ1 in situations where there are forms of Tat in the latent provirus that have attenuated activity, as defective proviruses rapidly accumulate during acute infection and shape the proviral landscape [50–52]. Therefore, bromodomain inhibitors may be more attractive compounds than HDACi for latency reversal.

JQ1 binds competitively to acetyl-lysine recognition domains as in BRD4 [34]. Besides its role in transcriptional elongation, the bromodomain protein BRD4 is involved in alternative splicing regulation as it interacts with JMJD6 (JmjC domain containing protein 6) that mediates 5′ hydroxylation of U2AF65, a major component of the spliceosomal complex important for 3′ splice site recognition [53, 54]. BRD4 can also regulate splicing following a heat shock response, as an increase in intron retention was observed upon BRD4 depletion [55]. Following JQ1 treatment, the expression of various host proteins is altered, including hnRNP A1 and PTB, which are known regulators of HIV-1 splicing and nuclear export of viral RNAs. HIV splice acceptor sites usage is strongly dependent on SR and hnRNP proteins [56–59]. Through cooperative binding to enhancer (ESE3) and silencer (ESS3a, ISS) elements nearby the viral A7 splice site, hnRNP A1, a known regulator of HIV-1 splicing, modulates *tat* and *rev* mRNA production [60]. Additionally, a lack of PTB (polypyrimidine tract-binding protein), also known as hnRNP I in resting CD4+ T cells has been

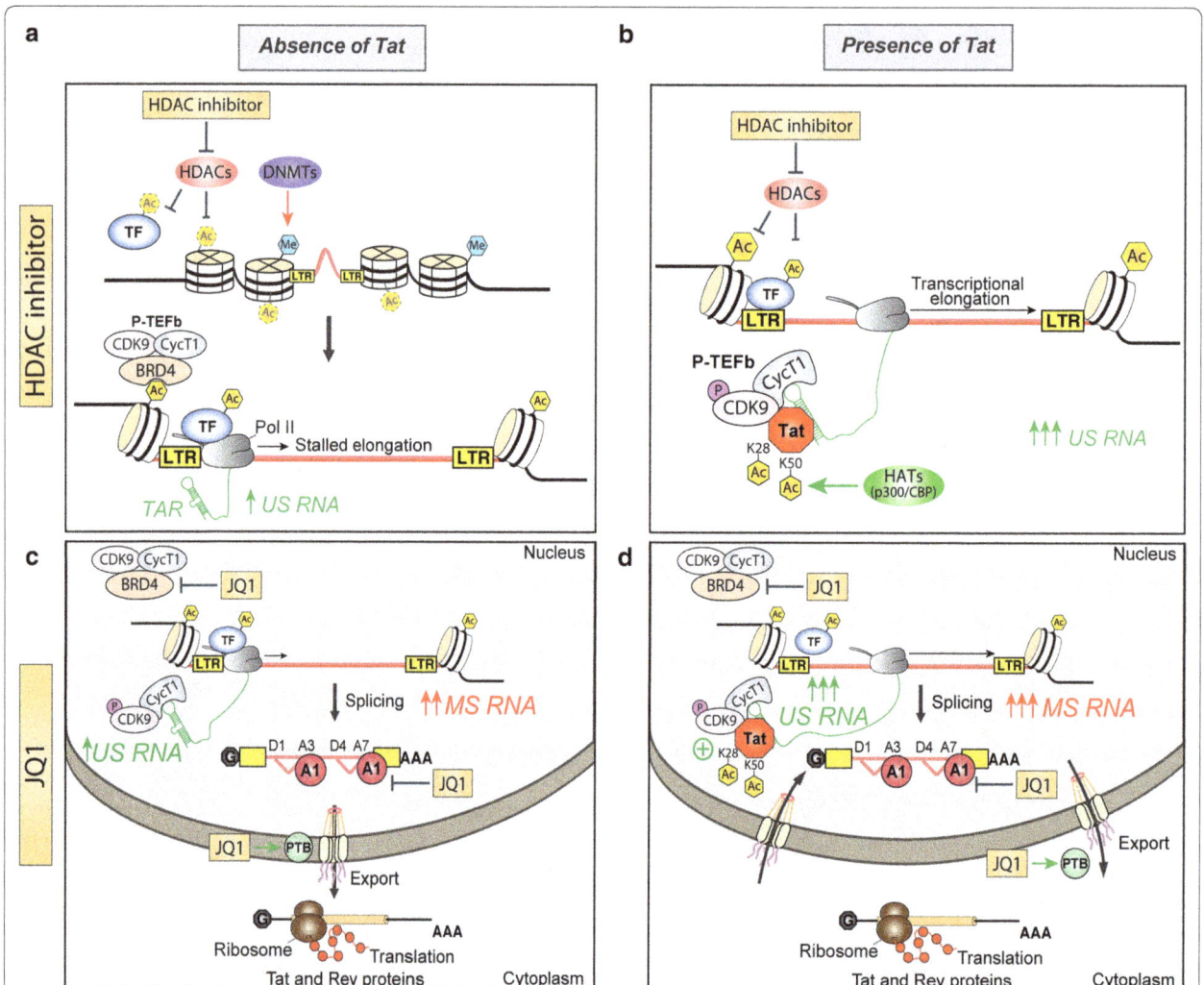

Fig. 10 Proposed model of the effects of LRAs in combination with Tat on inducing HIV-1 transcription and splicing. **a** During latency, the nucleosomes surrounding the proviral 5′LTR are subject to repressive epigenetic modifications such as histone methylation and deacetylation induced by DNA methyltransferases (DNMT) and histone deacetylases (HDAC), respectively. Upon treatment with HDACi, histone acetylation by histone acetyltransferase (HAT) would induce chromatin decondensation and transcription factor (TF) mobilisation to the RNA polymerase II (Pol II). This subsequently relieves the transcriptional repression at the 5′LTR resulting in expression of low levels of HIV US RNA. **b** Tat expression can induce transcription elongation from quiescent LTR promoters by recruiting the positive transcription elongation factor b (P-TEFb), which comprises CDK9 and Cyclin T1 (CycT1), to the stalled RNA Pol II at the viral promoter. Acetylation of Tat lysine 28 (K28) by PCAF is required for high affinity binding of Tat to the TAR/SEC (Super elongation complex). In combination with Tat, HDACi such as vorinostat and panobinostat can reactivate latent proviruses by increasing the pool of active P-TEFb through CDK9 T-loop phosphorylation. **c** HIV expression may be further restricted by inefficient splicing and defects in nuclear export of multiply spliced HIV RNAs (MS RNA). Moreover, Bromodomain containing proteins such as BRD4 can compete with Tat for binding to P-TEFb. BRD inhibitor treatment (JQ1) may block the activity of BRD4, leading to release of P-TEFb and activation of HIV expression. Given our results, we suggest that JQ1 would further antagonise latency by enhancing HIV splicing through downregulation of hnRNP A1 levels, as well as promoting the export of MS RNAs to the cytoplasm by upregulating PTB expression. **d** Upon the initial rounds of Tat and Rev production following JQ1 treatment and P-TEFb release, Tat would enable transcriptional elongation through a strong positive feedback loop creating a pool of US HIV RNA that would be exported efficiently through Rev binding to the Rev-Responsive Element (RRE)

implicated in nuclear retention of multiply spliced RNAs during latency [61]. An increase in the levels of PTB following JQ1 treatment would allow efficient export and expression of multiply spliced RNAs encoding for Tat and Rev. Given that changes in the balance of splicing can perturb viral replicative fitness and infectivity [29,

62], these alterations in splicing factors may have a major impact on the efficiency of virus production from latency. Whether through splicing and/or export, the ability of PTB to revert nuclear retention of multiply spliced RNAs in rCD4+ from patients on cART [61] indicates an mRNA processing restriction mechanism that is in place in rCD4+ T cells affecting Tat and Rev expression during latency. In fact, a new study revealed a series of blocks to HIV proximal elongation, distal transcription/polyadenylation (completion) and splicing (D4-A7) in CD4+ T cells from HIV infected patients on ART [63]. As viral Tat and Rev proteins play crucial roles in transcription initiation-elongation and nuclear export, multiply spliced transcripts (*tat* and *rev* mRNAs) may be of increased utility as a marker for viral rebound in patients after cART interruption [64] than unspliced RNA, which have been mainly used in clinical trials.

Recent study from Ott's group has revealed that a short isoform of BRD4 promotes latency by engaging repressive SWI/SNF chromatin-remodelling complexes, which could be reversed by JQ1 treatment [65]. In synergy with protein kinase C (PKC) agonists such as Bryostatin-1, bromodomain and extra-terminal domain inhibitors (BETis) like JQ1, UMB-136 and OTX015 constitute highly effective LRA combinations capable of inducing robust increase in HIV mRNA expression, comparable to CD3/CD28 antibodies stimulation, in rCD4 T cells from infected individuals on ART without inducing global T cell activation. This reactivation occurs through binding of BETis with the long isoform of BRD4 and release of P-TEFb [46, 66–69]. In agreement with these previous reports, our data revealed JQ1 ability to induce BRD4 dependent HIV-1 transcription and D4-A7 RNA splicing.

Given the difficulty in measuring Tat protein and Tat activity ex vivo, there are several limitations in this study. We chose HEK293T cells to use the splicing reporter system given the feasibility of transfecting these cells with the multiple plasmids required to clearly visualize EGFP and DsRed expression, which proved more difficult in a T-cell line such as Jurkats. It would be interesting to test these Tat mutants and LRAs in the context of full-length virus in a primary cell model of latency or ex vivo given the different landscape of cellular factors in rCD4+ T cells compared to a cancer cell line that affect the capacity of a cell to reactivate a latent provirus. Differences in the availability of host transcription, elongation and splicing factors in a rCD4+ T cell may augment the results observed in this study. Primary resting cells lack sufficient levels of transcription and elongation factors that mainly remain in inhibitory complexes in the cytoplasm [70–72]. We predict our results may be more pronounced ex vivo given P-TEFb, which exists in very low levels in rCD4+ T cells [45, 73] can be released from its inhibitory complex with 7SK snRNP and HEXIM1 with the addition of an HDACi, JQ1 or Tat protein [45, 49, 72, 74, 75]. Finally, we did not specifically address whether these same effects on transcription and splicing are relevant in other cellular reservoirs such as long lived

infected macrophages, or whether they can induce replication competent virus by measuring HIV RNA production in culture supernatant.

Conclusions

A lack of Tat is important in maintaining latency in resting CD4+ T-cells and therefore Tat is not readily available during the initial reactivation of provirus. This will limit the potency of some LRAs, such as HDACi, which fail to induce splicing in the absence of Tat. In contrast, JQ1 which also acts in combination with Tat to activate transcription, can enable splicing even in the absence of Tat. In conclusion, the potency of an LRA to induce virus production is enhanced if Tat is present, as certain agents may work directly or indirectly through posttranslational modifications of Tat. Strategies to increase Tat expression during latency reversal should be explored to fully activate the viral replication cycle and further enhance the potency of LRAs.

Methods
Tat101 mutants
Tat101^{AD8}—Flag was inserted into pcDNA3.1 (−) vector (Invitrogen) cleaved by *Xba*I and *EcoR*I. Site-directed mutagenesis was used to insert alanine substitutions or conservative mutations at particular locations to remove Lysine or Arginine function within Tat (see Additional file 5: Table S1 for oligonucleotide sequences for each mutant). Mutagenesis PCR was performed using High-Fidelity PCR DNA Polymerase (Promega) according to the manufacturer's instructions. The PCR reaction was performed as following: 98 °C 5 min, 30 cycles of 98 °C 30 s, 50 °C 30 s, 72 °C 7 min, and a final 72 °C 10 min. After treatment with *Dpn*I (NEB), amplified PCR product was purified with DNA gel extraction (Macherey–nagel nucleospin gel) and transformed into TOP10 competent *E. Coli* bacteria. Sequencing analysis confirmed the accuracy of cloning.

Immunoblotting
HEK293T cells transfected with WT and mutants Tat plasmids, and then treated with JQ1 (1 µM) or DMSO diluent control, were lysed with RIPA buffer (50 mM Tris–HCl pH8, 150 mM NaCl, 1% IgePal, 1 mM EDTA) supplemented with protease inhibitor cocktail (Roche), followed by sonication and centrifugation at 12,000xg for 15 min at 4 °C. The amount of proteins in the cell lysate was determined by Bradford assay (BioRad). Equal amounts of each sample were loaded on 12.5% SDS-PAGE, transferred to a nitrocellulose membrane (0.45 µm BioRad) then blocked in 5% milk-PBS-T (0.1% Tween-20) for 1 h at room temperature. Blots were

probed with anti-Flag (ab1162, abcam, 1/2500°), anti-GAPDH (#14C10, cell signalling, 1/1000°), anti-PTBP1 (clone 7, ThermoFischer Scientific, #325000, 1/500°) and anti-hnRNP A1 (clone 9H10, Santa Cruz, sc-56700, 1/25°). After several washes, the membrane was incubated with either 1/5000° goat anti-rabbit IgG (H+L) HRP (Invitrogen, Cat. No. 656120) or goat anti-mouse IgG (H+L) HRP (Invitrogen, Cat. No. 626520) for 1 h at RT. Blots were developed using Supersignal west pico chemiluminescent substrate (ThermoFisher Scientific) and visualized using the MF-ChemiBis 3.2 imaging system (DNR).

Splicing reporter experiments

Splicing reporter experiments with pLTR.gp140/EGFP.RevΔ38/DsRed were performed as previously described [30, 31]. Briefly, 2×10^4 HEK293T cells (human embryonic kidney cells that stably express the SV40 large T antigen; American Tissue Culture Collection) were seeded per well into 96-well plates with DMEM (Gibco)+10% FBS with Penicillin (100U/ml)/Streptomycin (100 µg/ml) and cultured overnight. Cells were then transfected in the absence of antibiotics using Lipofectamine 2000 (ThermoFisher) with 400 ng of an LTR-driven splicing reporter pLTR.gp140/EGFP.RevΔ38/DsRed, 20 ng of pRev$^{NL4.3}$, with or without wild type or mutant pTat101^{AD8} in triplicate wells per experiment on 5 separate occasions for n=5. A matched empty tat vector pcDNA3.1 (−) was used for experiments without Tat. Cells were incubated for 5 h prior to treatment with DMSO (1:5000, #67-68-S Merck), vorinostat (0.5 µM, #10009929 Cayman Chemical or #S1047 Selleck Chemicals), panobinostat (30 nM, #P180500 TRC or #S1030 Selleck Chemicals), JQ1 (+) (1 µM, #11187 Cayman Chemical or #S7110 Selleck Chemicals), JQ1 (−) (1 µM, #11232 Cayman Chemical), chaetocin (30 nM, #C9492 Sigma), disulfiram (500 nM, #D3374 LKT or #S1680 Selleck Chemicals), or PMA/PHA (10 nM PMA, #16561-29-8 Sigma-Aldrich/10 µg/mL PHA, #HA15/R30852701 Remel). Cells were harvested at 48 h, stained with LIVE/DEAD Fixable Dead Cell Stain (Near-IR, Thermo Fisher Scientific) and then assessed for EGFP and DsRed expression by flow cytometry (LSRII, BD Biosciences). Optimal compensation was achieved using HEK293T cells expressing the individual fluorescent protein. A minimum of 10.000 viable cell events per sample was acquired. Data was analysed using *FlowJo version 10.0.8*. The gating strategy includes exclusion of debris and selection of single cells based on forward and side scatter. Size selected cells were subgated using the live/dead marker, followed by the identification of unspliced and spliced products as positive for EGFP and DsRed, respectively. For that, live cells were gated on EGFP and DsRed versus "dump channel" (violet). The CellTiter 96 Aqueous One Solution Cell Proliferation Assay (Promega) was also used following manufacturer's instructions to determine the toxicity of the LRAs.

Quantitative PCR of viral and human RNA species

Total RNA was extracted from cells using TRIzol (Invitrogen) following manufacturer instructions followed by RQ1 RNase-Free DNase (Promega, 2 U/µg) treatment for 30 min at 37 °C. One µg of DNase treated RNA was reverse-transcribed using Omniscript-reverse transcriptase (Qiagen), d(T)15 and random hexamer primers following the manufacturers specifications. HIV US, spliced and all viral RNA (copies/µl) were quantified by ddPCR. Briefly, the ddPCR reaction consisted of 12 µl $2 \times$ ddPCR super mix for probes (no dUTP, Bio-Rad); 900 nM of each primer; 250 nM probe (FAM-MGBNFQ, Applied Biosystems, Additional file 5: Table S1) and 0.8-80 ng cDNA into a 24 µl final volume. Ribonuclease P/MRP 30 kDa (RPP30, dHsaCPE5038241), importin8 (IPO8, dHsaCPE5044719) and TATA-binding protein (TBP, dHsaCPE5058363) were used as reference genes (HEX, Bio-Rad) in multiplexed reactions with the HIV quantification. Following droplets generation (15,000-18,000 on average), thermal cycling was conducted as follows: 95 °C for 10 min, 40 cycles of 94 °C for 30 s and 60 °C for 60 s, followed by 98 °C for 10 min (ramp rate 2 °C/s for each step) on a C1000 Touch Thermal cycler (Bio-Rad). The droplets were subsequently read by a QX200 droplet-reader (Bio-Rad) and the data were analysed with *QuantaSoft 1.7.4 software*. A minus reverse transcriptase control (−RT) was included for each sample. The positive droplets were designated based on the −RT and the no template controls (NTC). Data of the triplicate wells per experiment were merged and the mean of the 4 independent assays was determined. The synthesized cDNA (10 ng) was also used as a template for semi-quantitative RT-PCR reactions to access exon inclusion and exclusion isoforms of *CD45-exon13*, *ATF2-exon6* and *ABI1-exon8,9* using primers listed in Additional file 5: Table S1. PCR products were resolved on a 2% agarose gel (TBE 1×) and visualized on a Syngene GBox imaging system.

TZMbl experiments

TZMbl cells (NIH AIDS Reagent Program) were seeded into 96-well plates in DMEM (Gibco)+10% FBS with Penicillin (100U/ml)/Streptomycin (100 µg/ml) and cultured overnight. Cells were then transfected in the absence of antibiotics using Lipofectamine 2000 (ThermoFisher) with or without WT or mutant pTat101^{AD8} (100 ng) in triplicates wells on 5 separate occasions for n = 5. Cells were harvested at 48 h and lysed with 35 μl of 1 × Passive Lysis Buffer (PLB, Promega), incubated for 5 min at RT before 5ul of each well was transferred to a CoStar 96-well white plate. The luciferase assay was performed as per the manufacturer's protocol (Promega) by addition of 25 μl of LARII and quantified on a FLUOStar Omega microplate reader (BMG Labtech, Ortenburg, Germany).

Statistical analyses

GraphPad PRISM version 7 software was used for statistical analyses. Paired *T* tests and 2-way ANOVA were used to compare values to DMSO and across all LRAs, as indicated.

Additional files

Additional file 1: Figure S1. Cellular toxicity of LRAs. The CellTiter 96 Aqueous One Solution Cell Proliferation MTS assay was used to measure the toxicity of a panel of LRAs on HEK293T cells over a range of concentrations (31.25 to 1000 nM) for 48 h. VOR = vorinostat; PAN = panobinostat; CTN = chaetocin; DIS = disulfiram. The lines represent the mean + SD (n = 2)

Additional file 2: Figure S2. JQ1 increases EGFP and DsRed expression from an LTR-driven splicing reporter in the absence and presence of Tat. HEK293T cells were transfected with the pLTR.gp140/EGFP.RevΔ38/DsRed splicing reporter in the absence or presence of 100 ng of pTat101 (AD8)-Flag expression plasmid and then treated for 24 h with JQ1 (1 μM) or DMSO diluent control. Cells were harvested and portion analysed for either the percentage of cells expressing EGFP (unspliced, **A.**) or DsRed (spliced, **B.**) using flow cytometry, or HIV unspliced (US), spliced (D4-A7) and all viral RNA expression levels (copies/ul) by droplet digital PCR (ddPCR) (Fig. 3). The fold-change (FC) over DMSO of Live+ EGFP+ (**A.**), Live + DsRed + (**B.**) and percentage of spliced product DsRed/ (DsRed + EGFP) (**C.**) were determined. Comparisons of each condition to DMSO were made using a paired *T* test. Only statistically significant comparisons are shown **p < 0.01; ***p < 0.001; ****p < 0.0001. The black lines represent the mean ± SEM (n = 4)

Additional file 3: Figure S3. Cellular and HIV RNA levels following JQ1 treatment. **A.** Absolute quantification of *RPP30*, *IPO8* and *TBP* cellular mRNAs (copies/μl) were performed using total RNAs derived from transfected HEK293T cells with the pLTR.gp140/EGFP.RevΔ38/DsRed splicing reporter in the absence and presence of 100 ng of pTat101 (AD8)-Flag expression plasmid and treated with JQ1 (1 μM) or DMSO diluent control. **B.** HIV unspliced (US), spliced (D4-A7) and all viral RNA expression levels (copies/ul) were quantified by droplet digital PCR (ddPCR) and normalized over the 3 reference genes. Comparisons of each condition to DMSO were made using a paired *T* test. Only statistically significant comparisons are shown *p < 0.05; **p < 0.01; ***p < 0.001; ****p < 0.0001. The black lines represent the mean ± SEM (n = 4)

Additional file 4: Figure S4. Some Tat mutants reduce the additive effect with LRAs on transcription. HEK293T cells were transfected with the pLTR.gp140/EGFP.RevΔ38/DsRed splicing reporter and 100 ng of pTat101 (AD8)-Flag with specific mutations; K28A (**A.**), K50A (**B.**), K50/51A (**C.**), K71A (**D.**), R53A (**E.**) and were treated with a panel of LRAs. Cells were harvested at 48 h and EGFP expression from the US mRNA was quantified using flow cytometry and represented as % EGFP positive cells. Comparisons of each condition to DMSO were made using 2-way ANOVA test. Only statistically significant comparisons are shown * p < 0.05; ** p < 0.01; *** p < 0.001; **** p < 0.0001. The black lines represent the mean ± SEM (n = 5). DMSO (1:5000), VOR = vorinostat (0.5 μM), PAN = panobinostat (30 nM), JQ1 (+) (1 μM), CTN = chaetocin (30 nM), DIS = disulfiram (500 nM), or PMA/PHA = phorbol myristate acetate/phytohaemagglutinin (10 nM PMA, 10 μg/mL PHA)

Authors' contributions

GK TMM DFJP conceived and designed the study. GK TMM SL CT MYL JJ LH performed the experiments. GK TMM analysed the data. GK and TMM interpreted the data. GK TMM JLA SRL DFJP contributed important intellectual discussion. GK TMM SRL DFJP wrote the manuscript. All authors read and approved the final manuscript.

Author details

[1] Department of Microbiology and Immunology, The Peter Doherty Institute for Infection and Immunity, University of Melbourne, Melbourne, Australia. [2] The Peter Doherty Institute for Infection and Immunity, Royal Melbourne Hospital, University of Melbourne, Melbourne, Australia. [3] School of Life Sciences, Peking University, Beijing, China. [4] Department of Infectious Diseases, Alfred Health and Monash University, Melbourne, Australia.

Acknowledgements

We thank the DMI Flow Facility staff for their advice and generous assistance in maintaining the flow cytometer used in this study.

Competing interests

The authors declare that they have no competing interests.

Funding

This work was supported by project grant APP1129320, and program grant APP1052979 from the NHMRC of Australia. SRL is an NHMRC practitioner fellow and is supported by the National Institutes for Health Delaney AIDS Research Enterprise (DARE U19 AI096109), and the American Foundation for AIDS Research.

References

1. Deeks SG, Lewin SR, Ross AL, Ananworanich J, Benkirane M, Cannon P, Chomont N, Douek D, Lifson JD, Lo YR, et al. International AIDS Society global scientific strategy: towards an HIV cure 2016. Nat Med. 2016;22:839–50.
2. Archin NM, Liberty AL, Kashuba AD, Choudhary SK, Kuruc JD, Crooks AM, Parker DC, Anderson EM, Kearney MF, Strain MC, et al. Administration of vorinostat disrupts HIV-1 latency in patients on antiretroviral therapy. Nature. 2012;487:482–5.
3. Archin NM, Bateson R, Tripathy MK, Crooks AM, Yang K-H, Dahl NP, Kearney MF, Anderson EM, Coffin JM, Strain MC, et al. HIV-1 expression within resting CD4+ T cells after multiple doses of vorinostat. J Infect Dis. 2014;210:728–35.
4. Elliott JH, Wightman F, Solomon A, Ghneim K, Ahlers J, Cameron MJ, Smith MZ, Spelman T, McMahon J, Velayudham P, et al. Activation of HIV transcription with short-course vorinostat in HIV-infected patients on suppressive antiretroviral therapy. PLoS Pathog. 2014;10:E1004473.
5. Rasmussen TA, Tolstrup M, Brinkmann CR, Olesen R, Erikstrup C, Solomon A, Winckelmann A, Palmer S, Dinarello C, Buzon M, et al. Panobinostat, a histone deacetylase inhibitor, for latent-virus reactivation in HIV-infected patients on suppressive antiretroviral therapy: a phase 1/2, single group, clinical trial. Lancet HIV. 2014;1:e13–21.

6. Søgaard OS, Graversen ME, Leth S, Olesen R, Brinkmann CR, Nissen SK, Kjaer AS, Schleimann MH, Denton PW, Hey-Cunningham WJ, et al. The depsipeptide romidepsin reverses HIV-1 latency in vivo. PLoS Pathog. 2015;11:E1005142.

7. Leth S, Schleimann MH, Nissen SK, Højen JF, Olesen R, Graversen ME, Jørgensen S, Kjær AS, Denton PW, Mørk A, et al. Combined effect of Vacc-4x, recombinant human granulocyte macrophage colony-stimulating factor vaccination, and romidepsin on the HIV-1 reservoir (REDUC): a single-arm, phase 1B/2A trial. Lancet HIV. 2016;3:e463–72.

8. Jablonski JA, Amelio AL, Giacca M, Caputi M. The transcriptional transactivator Tat selectively regulates viral splicing. Nucleic Acids Res. 2009;38:1249–60.

9. Karn J, Stoltzfus CM. Transcriptional and posttranscriptional regulation of HIV-1 gene expression. Cold Spring Harb Perspect Med. 2012;2:a006916.

10. Razooky BS, Pai A, Aull K, Rouzine IM, Weinberger LS. A hardwired HIV latency program. Cell. 2015;160:990–1001.

11. Li J, Chen C, Ma X, Geng G, Liu B, Zhang Y, Zhang S, Zhong F, Liu C, Yin Y, et al. Long noncoding RNA NRON contributes to HIV-1 latency by specifically inducing Tat protein degradation. Nat Commun. 2016;7:11730.

12. Pace MJ, Graf EH, Agosto LM, Mexas AM, Male F, Brady T, Bushman FD, O'Doherty U. Directly infected resting CD4+ T cells can produce HIV Gag without spreading infection in a model of HIV latency. PLoS Pathog. 2012;8:15.

13. Graf EH, Pace MJ, Peterson BA, Lynch LJ, Chukwulebe SB, Mexas AM, Shaheen F, Martin JN, Deeks SG, Connors M, et al. Gag-positive reservoir cells are susceptible to HIV-specific cytotoxic T lymphocyte mediated clearance. PLoS ONE. 2013;8:e71879.

14. He M, Zhang L, Wang X, Huo L, Sun L, Feng C, Jing X, Du D, Liang H, Liu M, et al. Systematic analysis of the functions of lysine acetylation in the regulation of Tat activity. PLoS ONE. 2013;8:e67186.

15. Ott M, Schnölzer M, Garnica J, Fischle W, Emiliani S, Rackwitz HR, Verdin E. Acetylation of the HIV-1 Tat protein by p300 is important for its transcriptional activity. Curr Biol. 1999;9:1489–92.

16. Ott M, Geyer M, Zhou Q. The control of HIV transcription: keeping RNA polymerase II on track. Cell Host Microbe. 2011;10:426–35.

17. Pagans S, Kauder SE, Kaehlcke K, Sakane N, Schroeder S, Dormeyer W, Trievel RC, Verdin E, Schnolzer M, Ott M. The cellular lysine methyltransferase Set7/9-KMT7 binds HIV-1 TAR RNA, monomethylates the viral transactivator Tat, and enhances HIV transcription. Cell Host Microbe. 2010;7:234–44.

18. Sakane N, Kwon HS, Pagans S, Kaehlcke K, Mizusawa Y, Kamada M, Lassen KG, Chan J, Greene WC, Schnoelzer M, Ott M. Activation of hiv transcription by the viral Tat protein requires a demethylation step mediated by lysine-specific demethylase 1 (LSD1/KDM1). PLoS Pathog. 2011;7:e1002184.

19. Kiernan RE, Vanhulle C, Schiltz L, Adam E, Xiao H, Maudoux F, Calomme C, Burny A, Nakatani Y, Jeang KT, et al. HIV-1 Tat transcriptional activity is regulated by acetylation. EMBO J. 1999;18:6106–18.

20. Col E, Caron C, Seigneurin-Berny D, Gracia J, Favier A, Khochbin S. The histone acetyltransferase, hGCN5, interacts with and acetylates the HIV transactivator. Tat J Biol Chem. 2001;276:28179–84.

21. Kaehlcke K, Dorr A, Hetzer-Egger C, Kiermer V, Henklein P, Schnoelzer M, Loret E, Cole PA, Verdin E, Ott M. Acetylation of Tat defines a CyclinT1-independent step in HIV transactivation. Mol Cell. 2003;12:167–76.

22. Dorr A, Kiermer V, Pedal A, Rackwitz HR, Henklein P, Schubert U, Zhou MM, Verdin E, Ott M. Transcriptional synergy between Tat and PCAF is dependent on the binding of acetylated Tat to the PCAF bromodomain. EMBO J. 2002;21:2715–23.

23. Huo L, Li D, Sun X, Shi X, Karna P, Yang W, Liu M, Qiao W, Aneja R, Zhou J. Regulation of Tat acetylation and transactivation activity by the microtubule-associated deacetylase HDAC6. J Biol Chem. 2011;286:9280–6.

24. Van Duyne R, Easley R, Wu W, Berro R, Pedati C, Klase Z, Kehn-Hall K, Flynn EK, Symer DE, Kashanchi F. Lysine methylation of HIV-1 Tat regulates transcriptional activity of the viral LTR. Retrovirology. 2008;5:40.

25. Xie B, Invernizzi CF, Richard S, Wainberg MA. Arginine methylation of the human immunodeficiency virus type 1 Tat protein by PRMT6 negatively affects Tat interactions with both cyclin T1 and the Tat transactivation region. J Virol. 2007;81:4226–34.

26. Sivakumaran H, van der Horst A, Fulcher AJ, Apolloni A, Lin M-H, Jans DA, Harrich D. Arginine methylation increases the stability of human immunodeficiency virus type 1 Tat. J Virol. 2009;83:11694–703.

27. Ali I, Ramage H, Boehm D, Dirk LMA, Sakane N, Hanada K, Pagans S, Kaehlcke K, Aull K, Weinberger L, et al. The HIV-1 Tat protein is monomethylated at lysine-71 by the lysine methyltransferase KMT7. J Biol Chem. 2016;291:16240.

28. Tang X, Lu H, Dooner M, Chapman S, Quesenberry PJ, Ramratnam B. Exosomal Tat protein activates latent HIV-1 in primary, resting CD4+ T lymphocytes. JCI Insight. 2018;3:e95676.

29. Purcell DF, Martin MA. Alternative splicing of human immunodeficiency virus type 1 mRNA modulates viral protein expression, replication, and infectivity. J Virol. 1993;67:6365–78.

30. Anderson JL, Johnson AT, Howard JL, Purcell DFJ. Both linear and discontinuous ribosome scanning are used for translation initiation from bicistronic human immunodeficiency virus type 1 env mRNAs. J Virol. 2007;81:4664–76.

31. Alexander MR, Wheatley AK, Center RJ, Purcell DFJ. Efficient transcription through an intron requires the binding of an Sm-type U1 snRNP with intact stem loop II to the splice donor. Nucleic Acids Res. 2010;38:3041–53.

32. Yang Z, Yik JHN, Chen R, He N, Moon KJ, Ozato K, Zhou Q. Recruitment of P-TEFb for stimulation of transcriptional elongation by the bromodomain protein Brd4. Mol Cell. 2005;19:535–45.

33. Moon KJ, Mochizuki K, Zhou M, Jeong HS, Brady JN, Ozato K. The bromodomain protein Brd4 is a positive regulatory component of P-TEFb and stimulates RNA polymerase II-dependent transcription. Mol Cell. 2005;19:523–34.

34. Bisgrove DA, Mahmoudi T, Henklein P, Verdin E. Conserved P-TEFb-interacting domain of BRD4 inhibits HIV transcription. Proc Natl Acad Sci. 2007;104:13690–5.

35. Filippakopoulos P, Qi J, Picaud S, Shen Y, Smith WB, Fedorov O, Morse EM, Keates T, Hickman TT, Felletar I, et al. Selective inhibition of BET bromodomains. Nature. 2010;468:1067–73.

36. Sonza S, Mutimer HP, O'Brien K, Ellery P, Howard JL, Axelrod JH, Deacon NJ, Crowe SM, Purcell DFJ. Selectively reduced Tat mRNA heralds the decline in productive human immunodeficiency virus type 1 infection in monocyte-derived macrophages. J Virol. 2002;76:12611–21.

37. Kuhn AN, van Santen MA, Schwienhorst A, Urlaub H, Lührmann R. Stalling of spliceosome assembly at distinct stages by small-molecule inhibitors of protein acetylation and deacetylation. RNA (New York, NY). 2009;15:153–75.

38. Cannon P, Kim SH, Ulich C, Kim S. Analysis of Tat function in human immunodeficiency virus type 1-infected low-level-expression cell lines U1 and ACH-2. J Virol. 1994;68:1993–7.

39. Emiliani S, Van Lint C, Fischle W, Paras P, Ott M, Brady J, Verdin E. A point mutation in the HIV-1 Tat responsive element is associated with postintegration latency. Proc Natl Acad Sci USA. 1996;93:6377–81.

40. Lu HK, Gray LR, Wightman F, Ellenberg P, Khoury G, Cheng WJ, Mota TM, Wesselingh S, Gorry PR, Cameron PU, et al. Ex vivo response to histone deacetylase (HDAC) inhibitors of the HIV long terminal repeat (LTR) derived from HIV-infected patients on antiretroviral therapy. PLoS ONE. 2014;9:e113341.

41. Bentley DL. Rules of engagement: co-transcriptional recruitment of pre-mRNA processing factors. Curr Opin Cell Biol. 2005;17:251–6.

42. Kornblihtt AR. Promoter usage and alternative splicing. Curr Opin Cell Biol. 2005;17:262–8.

43. Li Z, Guo J, Wu Y, Zhou Q. The BET bromodomain inhibitor JQ1 activates HIV latency through antagonizing Brd4 inhibition of Tat-transactivation. Nucleic Acids Res. 2013;41:277–87.

44. Banerjee C, Archin N, Michaels D, Belkina AC, Denis GV, Bradner J, Sebastiani P, Margolis DM, Montano M. BET bromodomain inhibition as a novel strategy for reactivation of HIV-1. J Leukoc Biol. 2012;92:1147–54.

45. Bartholomeeusen K, Xiang Y, Fujinaga K, Peterlin BM. Bromodomain and extra-terminal (BET) bromodomain inhibition activate transcription via transient release of Positive Transcription Elongation Factor b (P-TEFb) from 7SK small nuclear ribonucleoprotein. J Biol Chem. 2012;287:36609–16.

46. Darcis G, Kula A, Bouchat S, Fujinaga K, Corazza F, Ait-Ammar A, Delacourt N, Melard A, Kabeya K, Vanhulle C, et al. An in-depth comparison of latency-reversing agent combinations in various in vitro and ex vivo HIV-1 latency models identified bryostatin-1+JQ1 and ingenol-B+JQ1 to potently reactivate viral gene expression. PLoS Pathog. 2015;11:e1005063.

47. Boehm D, Calvanese V, Dar RD, Xing S, Schroeder S, Martins L, Aull K, Li PC, Planelles V, Bradner JE, et al. BET bromodomain-targeting compounds reactivate HIV from latency via a Tat-independent mechanism. Cell Cycle. 2013;12:452–62.

48. Geuens T, Bouhy D, Timmerman V. The hnRNP family: insights into their role in health and disease. Hum Genet. 2016;135:851–67.

49. Jamaluddin M, Hu P, Jan Y, Siwak E, Rice A. Short communication: the broad-spectrum histone deacetylase inhibitors vorinostat and panobinostat activate latent HIV in CD4 (+) T cells in part through phosphorylation of the T-loop of the CDK9 subunit of P-TEFb. AIDS Res Hum Retrovir. 2016;32:169–73.

50. Bruner KM, Murray AJ, Pollack RA, Soliman MG, Laskey SB, Capoferri AA, Lai J, Strain MC, Lada SM, Hoh R, et al. Defective proviruses rapidly accumulate during acute HIV-1 infection. Nat Med. 2016;22:1043–9.

51. Imamichi H, Dewar RL, Adelsberger JW, Rehm CA, O'Doherty U, Paxinos EE, Fauci AS, Lane HC. Defective HIV-1 proviruses produce novel protein-coding RNA species in HIV-infected patients on combination antiretroviral therapy. Proc Natl Acad Sci. 2016;113:8783–8.

52. Pollack RA, Jones RB, Pertea M, Bruner KM, Martin AR, Thomas AS, Capoferri AA, Beg SA, Huang SH, Karandish S, et al. Defective HIV-1 proviruses are expressed and can be recognized by cytotoxic T lymphocytes, which shape the proviral landscape. Cell Host Microbe. 2017;21(494–506):e4.

53. Rahman S, Sowa ME, Ottinger M, Smith JA, Shi Y, Harper JW, Howley PM. The Brd4 extraterminal domain confers transcription activation independent of pTEFb by recruiting multiple proteins, including NSD3. Mol Cell Biol. 2011;31:2641–52.

54. Webby CJ, Wolf A, Gromak N, Dreger M, Kramer H, Kessler B, Nielsen ML, Schmitz C, Butler DS, Yates JR, et al. Jmjd6 catalyses lysyl-hydroxylation of U2AF65, a protein associated with RNA splicing. Science. 2009;325:90–3.

55. Hussong M, Kaehler C, Kerick M, Grimm C, Franz A, Timmermann B, Welzel F, Isensee J, Hucho T, Krobitsch S, Schweiger MR. The bromodomain protein BRD4 regulates splicing during heat shock. Nucleic Acids Res. 2017;45:382–94.

56. Zahler AM, Damgaard CK, Kjems J, Caputi M. SC35 and heterogeneous nuclear ribonucleoprotein A/B proteins bind to a juxtaposed exonic splicing enhancer/exonic splicing silencer element to regulate HIV-1 Tat exon 2 splicing. J Biol Chem. 2004;279:10077–84.

57. Ropers D, Ayadi L, Gattoni R, Jacquenet S, Damier L, Branlant C, Stévenin J. Differential effects of the SR proteins 9G8, SC35, ASF/SF2, and SRp40 on the utilization of the A1 to A5 splicing sites of HIV-1 RNA. J Biol Chem. 2004;279:29963–73.

58. Amendt BA, Si ZH, Stoltzfus CM. Presence of exon splicing silencers within human immunodeficiency virus type 1 Tat exon 2 and Tat-rev exon 3: evidence for inhibition mediated by cellular factors. Mol Cell Biol. 1995;15:4606–15.

59. Si ZH, Amendt BA, Stoltzfus CM. Splicing efficiency of human immunodeficiency virus type 1 Tat RNA is determined by both a suboptimal 3' splice site and a 10 nucleotide exon splicing silencer element located within Tat exon 2. Nucleic Acids Res. 1997;25:861–7.

60. Marchand V, Mereau A, Jacquenet S, Thomas D, Mougin A, Gattoni R, Stevenin J, Branlant C. A Janus splicing regulatory element modulates HIV-1 Tat and rev mRNA production by coordination of hnRNP A1 cooperative binding. J Mol Biol. 2002;323:629–52.

61. Lassen KG, Ramyar KX, Bailey JR, Zhou Y, Siliciano RF. Nuclear retention of multiply spliced HIV-1 RNA in resting CD4+ T cells. PLoS Pathog. 2006;2:0650–61.

62. Ja J. Caputi M. Role of cellular RNA processing factors in human immunodeficiency virus type 1 mRNA metabolism, replication, and infectivity. J Virol. 2009;83:981–92.

63. Yukl SA, Kaiser P, Kim P, Telwatte S, Joshi SK, Vu M, Lampiris H, Wong JK. HIV latency in isolated patient CD4+ T cells may be due to blocks in HIV transcriptional elongation, completion, and splicing. Sci Transl Med. 2018;10:eaa9927.

64. Fischer M, Joos B, Hirschel B, Bleiber G, Weber R, Günthard HF. Cellular viral rebound after cessation of potent antiretroviral therapy predicted by levels of multiply spliced HIV-1 RNA encoding nef. J Infect Dis. 2004;190:1979–88.

65. Conrad RJ, Fozouni P, Thomas S, Sy H, Zhang Q, Zhou MM, Ott M. The short isoform of BRD4 promotes HIV-1 latency by engaging repressive SWI/SNF chromatin-remodeling complexes. Mol Cell. 2017;67(1001–1012):e6.

66. Zhu J, Gaiha GD, John SP, Pertel T, Chin CR, Gao G, Qu H, Walker BD, Elledge SJ, Brass AL. Reactivation of Latent HIV-1 by Inhibition of BRD4. Cell Rep. 2012;2:807–16.

67. Laird GM, Bullen CK, Rosenbloom DIS, Martin AR, Hill AL, Durand CM, Siliciano JD, Siliciano RF. Ex vivo analysis identifies effective HIV-1 latency: reversing drug combinations. J Clin Invest. 2015;125:1901–12.

68. Huang H, Liu S, Jean M, Simpson S, Huang H, Merkley M, Hayashi T, Kong W, Rodríguez-Sánchez I, Zhang X, et al. A novel bromodomain inhibitor reverses HIV-1 latency through specific binding with BRD4 to promote Tat and P-TEFb association. Front Microbiol. 2017;8:1035.

69. Lu P, Qu X, Shen Y, Jiang Z, Wang P, Zeng H, Ji H, Deng J, Yang X, Li X, et al. The BET inhibitor OTX015 reactivates latent HIV-1 through P-TEFb. Sci Rep. 2016;6:24100.

70. Williams SA, Chen LF, Kwon H, Ruiz-Jarabo CM, Verdin E, Greene WC. NF-κB p50 promotes HIV latency through HDAC recruitment and repression of transcriptional initiation. EMBO J. 2006;25:139–49.

71. Zhong H, May MJ, Jimi E, Ghosh S. The phosphorylation status of nuclear NF-κB determines its association with CBP/p300 or HDAC-1. Mol Cell. 2002;9:625–36.

72. Cho S, Schroeder S, Kaehlcke K, Kwon HS, Pedal A, Herker E, Schnoelzer M, Ott M. Acetylation of cyclin T1 regulates the equilibrium between active and inactive P-TEFb in cells. EMBO J. 2009;28:1407–17.

73. Chiang K, Sung T-L, Rice AP. Regulation of cyclin T1 and HIV-1 replication by MicroRNAs in resting CD4+ T lymphocytes. J Virol. 2012;86:3244–52.

74. Contreras X, Schweneker M, Chen C-S, McCune JM, Deeks SG, Martin J, Peterlin BM. Suberoylanilide hydroxamic acid reactivates HIV from latently infected cells. J Biol Chem. 2009;284:6782–9.

75. Barboric M, Yik JHN, Czudnochowski N, Yang Z, Chen R, Contreras X, Geyer M, Peterlin BM, Zhou Q. Tat competes with HEXIM1 to increase the active pool of P-TEFb for HIV-1 transcription. Nucleic Acids Res. 2007;35:2003–12.

CD8$^+$ T cells specific for conserved, cross-reactive Gag epitopes with strong ability to suppress HIV-1 replication

Hayato Murakoshi[1†], Chengcheng Zou[1†], Nozomi Kuse[1], Tomohiro Akahoshi[1], Takayuki Chikata[1], Hiroyuki Gatanaga[1,3], Shinichi Oka[1,3], Tomáš Hanke[2,4] and Masafumi Takiguchi[1*]

Abstract

Background: Development of AIDS vaccines for effective prevention of circulating HIV-1 is required, but no trial has demonstrated definitive effects on the prevention. Several recent T-cell vaccine trials showed no protection against HIV-1 acquisition although the vaccines induced HIV-1-specific T-cell responses, suggesting that the vaccine-induced T cells have insufficient capacities to suppress HIV-1 replication and/or cross-recognize circulating HIV-1. Therefore, it is necessary to develop T-cell vaccines that elicit T cells recognizing shared protective epitopes with strong ability to suppress HIV-1. We recently designed T-cell mosaic vaccine immunogens tHIVconsvX composed of 6 conserved Gag and Pol regions and demonstrated that the T-cell responses to peptides derived from the vaccine immunogens were significantly associated with lower plasma viral load (pVL) and higher CD4$^+$ T-cell count (CD4 count) in HIV-1-infected, treatment-naive Japanese individuals. However, it remains unknown T cells of which specificities have the ability to suppress HIV-1 replication. In the present study, we sought to identify more T cells specific for protective Gag epitopes in the vaccine immunogens, and analyze their abilities to suppress HIV-1 replication and recognize epitope variants in circulating HIV-1.

Results: We determined 17 optimal Gag epitopes and their HLA restriction, and found that T-cell responses to 9 were associated significantly with lower pVL and/or higher CD4 count. T-cells recognizing 5 of these Gag peptides remained associated with good clinical outcome in 221 HIV-1-infected individuals even when comparing responders and non-responders with the same restricting HLA alleles. Although it was known previously that T cells specific for 3 of these protective epitopes had strong abilities to suppress HIV-1 replication in vivo, here we demonstrated equivalent abilities for the 2 novel epitopes. Furthermore, T cells against all 5 Gag epitopes cross-recognized variants in majority of circulating HIV-1.

Conclusions: We demonstrated that T cells specific for 5 Gag conserved epitopes in the tHIVconsvX have ability to suppress replication of circulating HIV-1 in HIV-1-infected individuals. Therefore, the tHIVconsvX vaccines have the right specificity to contribute to prevention of HIV-1 infection and eradication of latently infected cells following HIV-1 reactivation.

Keywords: HIV-1, Gag, CTL, Vaccine, Conserved epitope

---

*Correspondence: masafumi@kumamoto-u.ac.jp

†Hayato Murakoshi and Chengcheng Zou contributed equally to this work

[1] Center for AIDS Research, Kumamoto University, 2-2-1 Honjo, Chuo-ku, Kumamoto 860-0811, Japan

Full list of author information is available at the end of the article

Background

Development of effective vaccines against HIV-1 is the best hope for controlling the AIDS epidemic, but no trials has yet showed definitive effect on prevention of HIV-1 infection. Although the RV144 trial in Thailand showed weak protection against HIV-1 most likely through generation of non-neutralizing antibodies [1–7], the outcome of this vaccine trial remains to be reproduced [8, 9]. The STEP study of a candidate T-cell vaccine induced low frequency responses in 77% of vaccine recipients and showed no protection against HIV-1 acquisition [10, 11]. Although a sieve effect of break-through viruses was described, overall, the vaccine-elicited CD8$^+$ T cells had insufficient capacity to suppress HIV-1 replication. There is no simple functional or phenotypic T-cell marker consistently associated with HIV-1 control. The protective capacity of CD8$^+$ T cells likely comes from multiple attributes including specificity, breadth, quality, quantity and being at the right time at the right place. Targeting protective epitopes is one of the key traits.

Our strategy for induction of effective responses is to focus the CD8$^+$ T cells on the highly functionally conserved regions of the HIV-1 proteome [12, 13]. To further improve their efficacy, vaccine immunogens tHIVconsvX consist of 6 protein regions from Gag and Pol with high coverage of known protective epitopes and employ a bivalent mosaic (two versions of each region, which differ in approximately 1/10 amino acids) to maximize the match of the vaccine to the global circulating viruses. Indeed, using overlapping 15-mer peptides derived from the tHIVconsvX immunogens, we demonstrated the correlation of both the total magnitude and breadth of the tHIVconsvX-specific T-cell responses to lower plasma viral load (pVL) and higher CD4$^+$ T-cell count (CD4 count) in a cohort of 120 treatment-naïve, HIV-1-positive patients in Japan [14].

Numerous studies have showed that CD8$^+$ T cell targeting of HIV-1 Gag linked to viral load or disease outcome in HIV-1 infection [15–17]. The mechanism of this effect may involve that the viral genome is delivered into the cell in a ribonucleoprotein complex composed largely of Gag after infection, so that Gag epitopes can be processed, presented on the cell surface and finally recognized by Gag-specific CD8$^+$ T cells within a few hours of infection before Nef-mediated down-regulation takes place [18–20].

We previously showed association of CD8$^+$ T cells specific for several Gag and Pol epitopes with significantly lower pVL and higher CD4 count in chronically HIV-1-infected Japanese patients [21]. The majority of these CD8$^+$ T cells recognized conserved or cross-recognized mutated epitopes mostly on the Gag protein. Half of these T cells were restricted by 2 protective alleles,

HLA-B*52:01 or HLA-B*67:01, while the remaining recognized peptides presented by HLA-A*02:06, HLA-B*40:02, or HLA-B*40:06.

In the present study, we determined fine specificities and HLA-restriction of CD8$^+$ T-cell responses specific for the two Gag conserved regions of the candidate tHIVconsvX vaccine and extended the protective correlations to clinical outcome in 221 treatment-naïve HIV-1-positive patients. The study identified additional CD8$^+$ T cells specific for Gag conserved epitopes with strong ability to suppress HIV-1 replication. Thus, Gag-specific CD8$^+$ T cells induced by the tHIVconsvX vaccine have the potential to significantly contribute to prevention of HIV-1 infection and eradication of latently infected cells.

Results

T-cell responses to the conserved regions of Gag were protective

We previously showed in 120 treatment-naive HIV-1$^+$ Japanese patients that CD8$^+$ T-cell responses specific for the conserved regions of the tHIVconsvX immunogen were protective [14]. Here, we focused on the two vaccine conserved regions of Gag, since the responses to Gag had the strongest effect on the suppression of HIV-1 replication in most previous studies [15–17]. We analyzed additional 80 treatment-naive HIV-1-positive patients and reanalyzed the data together from 200 individuals for the magnitude and breadth of CD8$^+$ T-cell responses to 3 pools of the Gag 15-mer peptides (Pools 1, 2, and 3). The magnitude and breadth of the T-cell responses to Pools 2 and 3, and particularly responses to Pool 3, were significantly correlated with high CD4 count and low pVL, whereas those to Pool 1 were not (Fig. 1 and Additional file 1: Fig. S1). These results suggest that T cells specific for peptides within Pools 2 and 3 contribute to the suppression of HIV-1 replication.

Mapping the CD8$^+$ T-cell Gag-specificity to optimal epitopes

We found that 89 and 59 individuals recognized 15-mer peptides in Pools 2 and 3, respectively. Of these, we selected 50 and 53 based on sufficient PBMC sample availability for the fine definition of optimal epitopes. Pools 2 and 3 included peptide pairs derived from the bivalent mosaic and one single peptide common between the two mosaics. By using an IFN-γ ELISPOT assay, we found T-cell responses to 12 peptide pairs in Pool 2 (Fig. 2a) and 10 peptide pairs and one common peptide in Pool 3 (Fig. 3a) in at least one individual. These 15-mer peptides contained sequences of previously reported epitopes; 13 epitopes in Pool 2 and 10 in Pool 3 (Figs. 2b and 3b). Upon inspection of the subjects' HLA, most of the responders had the reported restricting

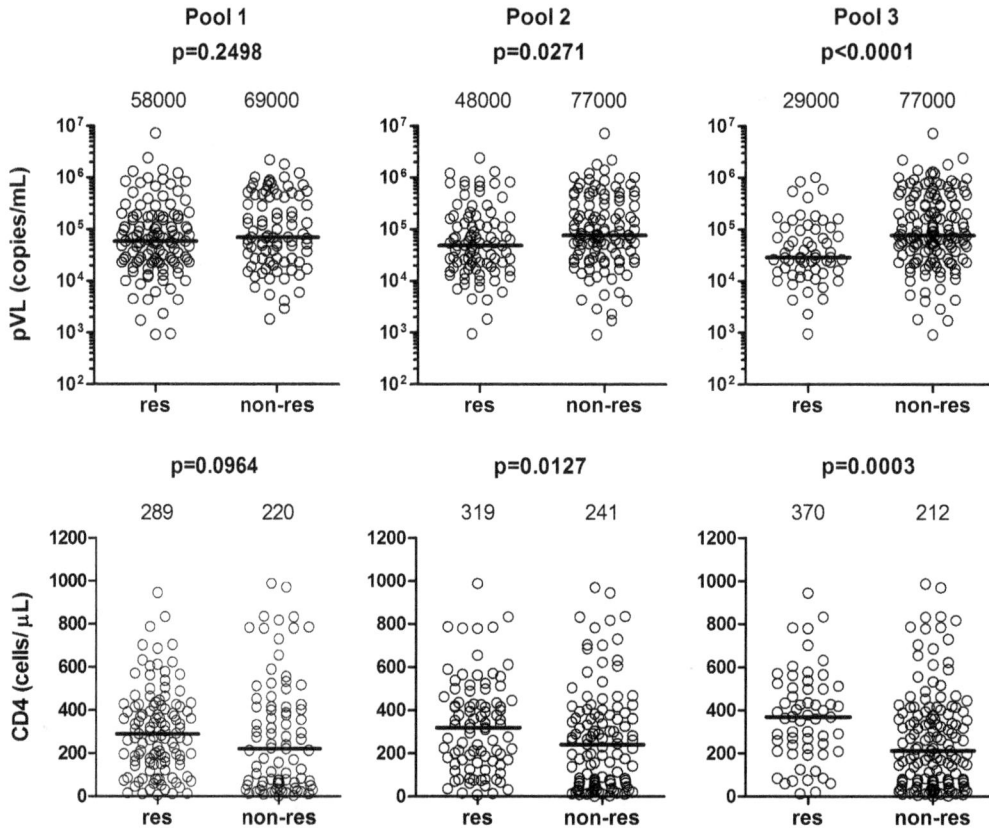

Fig. 1 Correlation of T-cell responses to Gag conserved peptides of tHIVconsvX. Correlation of T-cell responses to Gag conserved peptides of tHIVconsvX with pVL and CD4 count. T-cell responses to Gag peptide Pools 1, 2 and 3 derived from vaccine immunogen tHIVconsvX were enumerated using an IFN-γ ELISPOT assay in 200 HIV-1-infected Japanese individuals. Comparison of pVL and CD4 count between responders and non-responders to the Gag peptides was statistically analyzed using the Mann-Whitney test. The value in each figure represents the median of pVL and CD4 count

alleles (Figs. 2b and 3b). However, responders to 15-mer peptides C48/49, C052/053, C054/055, C113/114, or C125/126 did not have the matching restricting HLA alleles, indicating that their CD8$^+$ T cells may recognize novel, previously unreported epitopes.

Next, we sought to define these novel epitopes and their HLA restriction. We did not pursue the epitope in C48/49 since only one responder to this peptide pair was detected in the 50 tested individuals. The responder KI-1020 had T cells specific for the C052/053 and C054/055 peptide pairs, while KI-1102 and KI-1114 had responses to C125/126 and C113/114 peptides, respectively (Fig. 4a). To define the HLA restriction, subjects' PBMCs were first expanded with each peptide pair for 12–14 days and these STCL were tested in ICS assay using either C1R or 721.221 cells stably transfected with all subject's HLA class I molecules and pulsed with the peptides. The results showed that both T-cell responses to the C052/053 and C054/055 15-mer peptide pairs were restricted by HLA-A*26:02 and responses to the

C113/114 and C125/126 peptides were restricted by HLA-A*33:03 and HLA-A*02:06, respectively (Fig. 4b).

We next narrowed the optimal epitopes by using overlapping 11-mer and further truncated peptides. Both the C052/053 STCL and C054/055 STCL recognized both Gag 11-121 and Gag 11-122 peptides (Fig. 4c), suggesting that all the STCL were specific for the same epitope. Analysis using truncated peptides showed that the optimal peptide was TLQEQIGWM (TM9) (Fig. 4d) restricted by HLA-A*26:02. This epitope has not been previously reported. The C113/114 STCL and C125/126 STCL recognized Gag 11-200 and Gag 11-214/215, respectively (Fig. 4c). Again using truncated peptides, we identified previously unreported epitopes HIAKN-CRAPR (HR10) and RQANFLGKI (RI9) as the optimal peptides presented by HLA-A*33:03 and HLA-A*02:06, respectively (Fig. 4d). Thus, we identified three novel candidate peptides for the Los Alamos National Laboratory HIV Sequence Database (LANL-HSD; www.hiv.lanl.gov) 'A' list of well-defined epitopes.

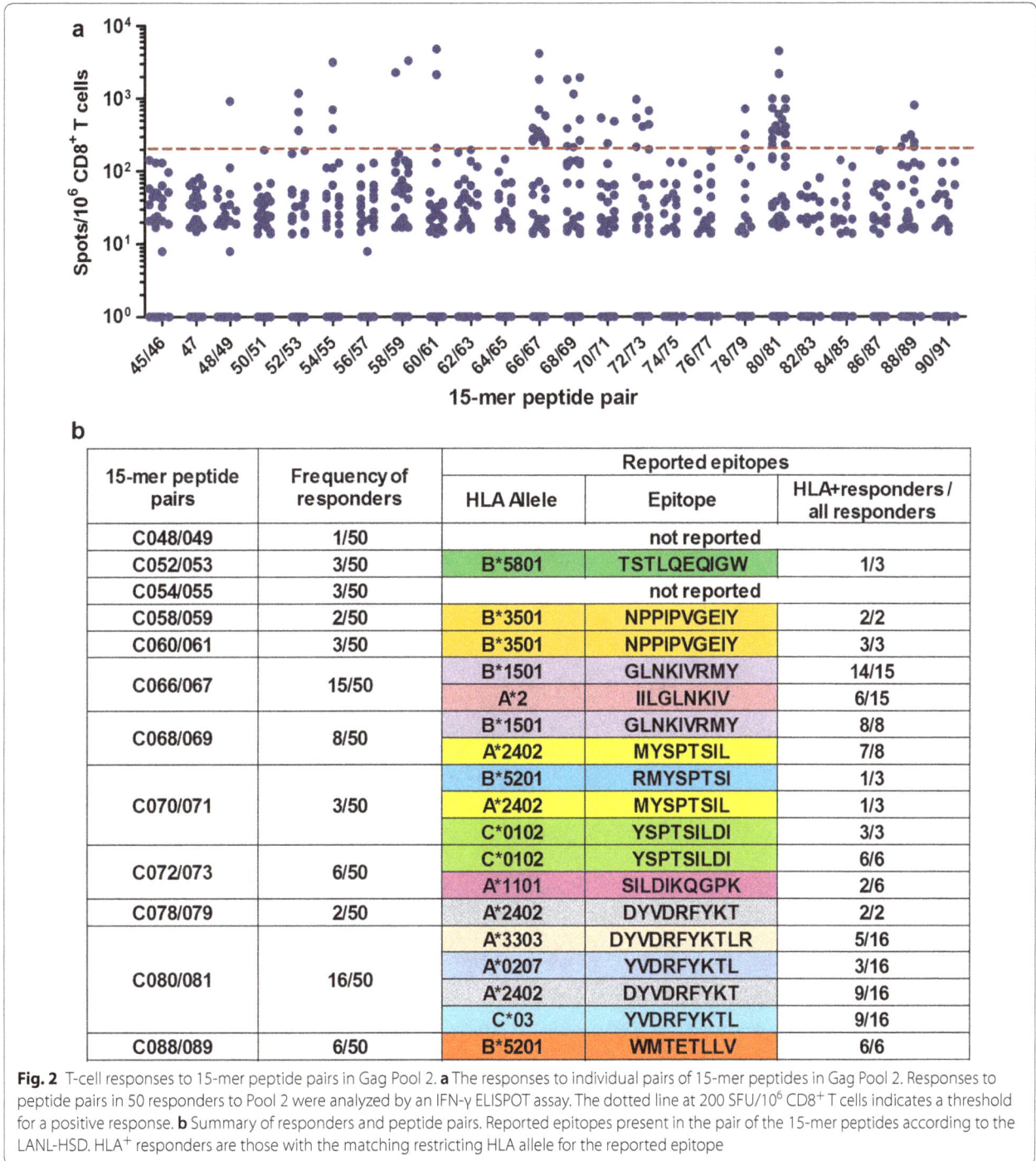

Fig. 2 T-cell responses to 15-mer peptide pairs in Gag Pool 2. **a** The responses to individual pairs of 15-mer peptides in Gag Pool 2. Responses to peptide pairs in 50 responders to Pool 2 were analyzed by an IFN-γ ELISPOT assay. The dotted line at 200 SFU/10^6 CD8$^+$ T cells indicates a threshold for a positive response. **b** Summary of responders and peptide pairs. Reported epitopes present in the pair of the 15-mer peptides according to the LANL-HSD. HLA$^+$ responders are those with the matching restricting HLA allele for the reported epitope

CD8$^+$ T cells recognizing Gag conserved epitopes are protective in vivo

As described in above (Figs. 2b and 3b), T cells specific for 23 reported and 3 novel HIV-1 epitopes recognize tHIVconsvX-derived Gag peptides in HIV-1-infected patients in Japan. To investigate further these T-cell responses, we selected 221 individuals whose PBMCs were available for this analysis. Thus, T cells specific for epitopes SK10/HLA-A*11:01 and KR9/HLA-A*31:01 were not detected in any patients. CD8$^+$ T-cells responses recognizing epitopes DT9/HLA-A*24:02, ML8/HLA-A*24:02, NY10/HLA-B*35:01, NL11/HLA-B*67:01, IV9/HLA-A*02, YL9/HLA-A*02:07 and TW10/HLA-B*58:01 were only detected in 1 or 2 patients

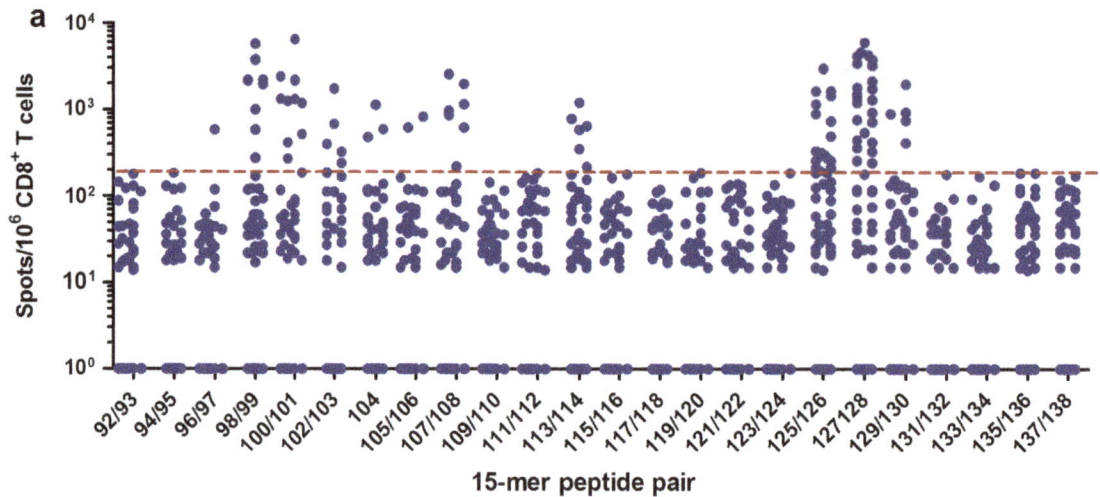

Fig. 3 T-cell responses to 15-mer peptide pairs in Gag Pool 3. **a** The responses to individual pairs of 15-mer peptides in Gag Pool 3. Responses to peptide pairs in 53 responders to Pool 3 were analyzed by an IFN-γ ELISPOT assay. The dotted line at 200 SFU/10⁶ CD8⁺ T cells indicates a threshold for a positive response. **b** Summary of responders and peptide pairs. Reported epitopes included in the pair of the 15-mer peptides are shown according to the LANL-HSD. HLA⁺ responders are those with the matching restricting HLA allele for the reported epitope

(Table 1) and were excluded from further statistical analysis because of the small number of responders. The analysis of CD8⁺ T-cell responses to 9 epitopes with sufficient number of responders showed a significant association with lower pVL and/or higher CD4 count relative to non-responders to these epitopes. T cells specific for the WV8/HLA-B*52:01, RI8/HLA-B*52:01 and AA9/HLA-A*02:06 epitopes were previously shown to inhibit HIV-1 in vivo [21, 22]. Therefore, the present study in treatment-naïve, HIV-1-positive patients newly identified

T cells specific for 6 epitopes FS8/HLA-A*02:01, TL8/HLA-B*40:02, KL9/HLA-C*08, RI9/HLA-A*02:06, TM9/HLA-A*26:02 and HR10/HLA-A*33:03, that could effectively suppress HIV-1 replication (Table 1).

We further analyzed the association of responses to these 9 epitopes with lower pVL and/or higher CD4 count in individuals having the epitopes' restricting HLA molecules. We again confirmed that responders to the WV8/HLA-B*52:01, RI8/HLA-B*52:01 or AA9/HLA-A*02:06 epitopes had significantly lower

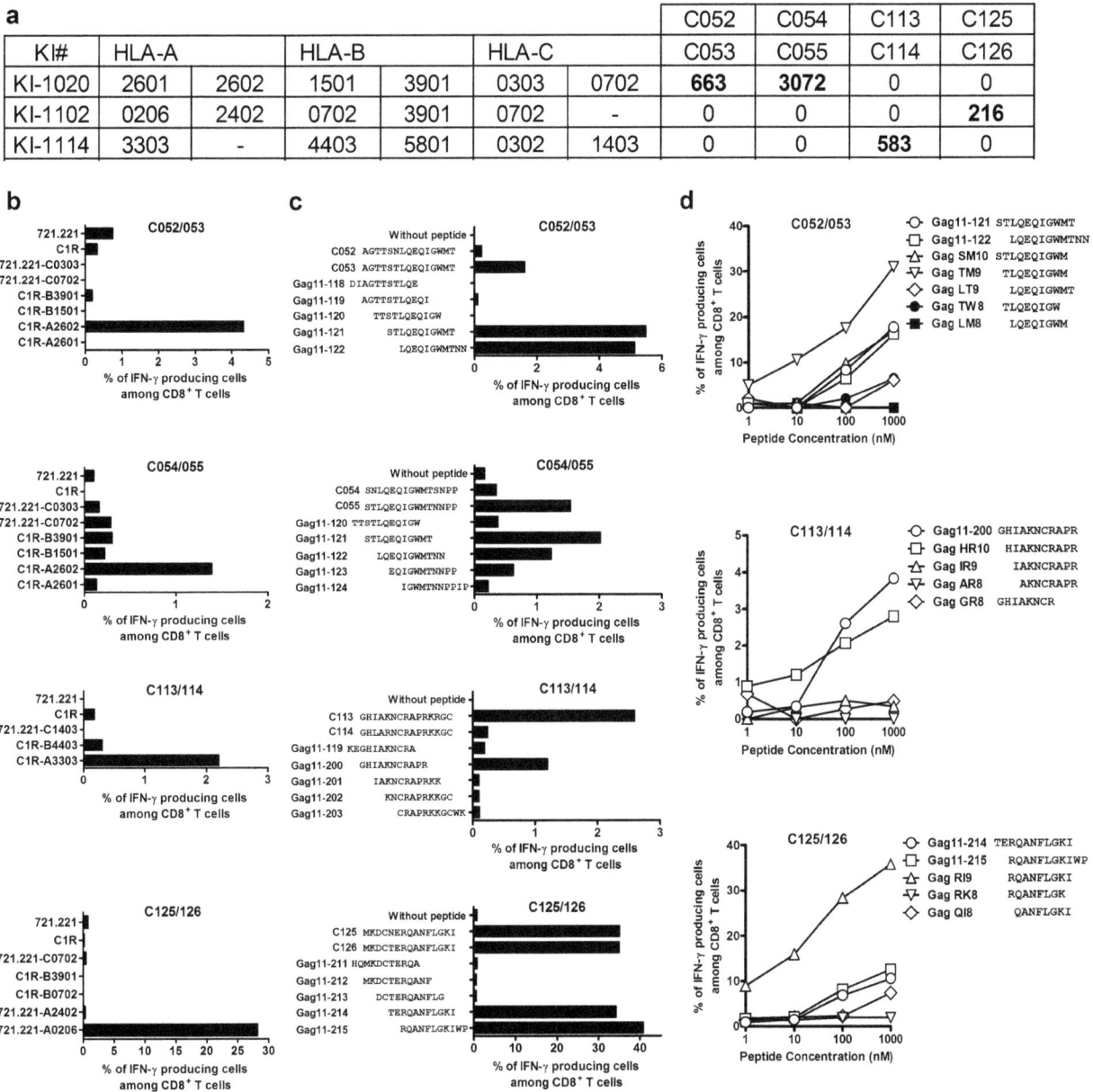

Fig. 4 Identification of novel T-cell Gag epitopes. **a** T-cell responses to peptide pairs in individuals KI-1020, KI-1102, and KI-1114, who did not have matching HLA alleles for previously reported epitopes. **b** HLA restriction. Responses by STCL stimulated with C1R or 721.221 cells expressing individual HLA molecule shared by the responders and pulsed with the peptide pair were analyzed by ICS assay. C052/053 and C054/055 peptides were analyzed by using the T cells derived from KI-1020, while C113/114 and C125/126 by using the T cells from KI-1114 and KI-1102, respectively. **c** Identification of 11-mer HIV-1 clade B overlapping peptides recognized by the HLA-A*26:02-, HLA-A*33:03-, or HLA-A*02:06-restricted T cells. The responses by STCL expanded with C052/053, C054/055, C113/114, or C125/126 peptide pairs to the corresponding stimulator cells pre-pulsed with 11-mer HIV-1 clade B-derived overlapping peptides across the parental 15-mer were analyzed in ICS assay. **d** Identification of optimal peptides. The STCL responses stimulated with peptide pairs C052/053, C113/114, or C125/126 to the corresponding stimulator cells C1R-A2602, C1R-A3303, or 721.221-A0206 pre-pulsed with individual truncated peptides were analyzed by ICS assay

pVL than non-responders with the same HLA alleles, while responders to WV8 and RI8 also had significantly higher CD4 count than the non-responders (Additional file 2: Fig. S2). Responders to HR10/HLA-A*33:03 and TL8/HLA-B*40:02 had significantly both lower pVL and higher CD4 count than the non-responders (Fig. 5a). Thus overall, responses to epitopes WV8, RI8, AA9, HR10, and TL8 exhibited signs of better clinical outcome.

Table 1 Association of CTL responses to Gag epitopes with pVL and CD4 count

Epitope	Sequence	HLA	Frequency		Median of pVL		Median of CD4		P value[b]	
			Res	Non-res	Res	Non-res	Res	Non-res	pVL	CD4
IV9	IILGLNKIV	A*02	2	219	–	–	–	–	–	–
FS8	FLGKIWPS	A*02:01	3	218	910,000	55,500	629	274	0.9882	*0.012*
AA9	ATLEEMMTA	A*02:06	16	205	22,500	58,000	388	269	*0.0057*	0.1788
YL9	YVDRFYKTL	A*02:07	2	219	–	–	–	–	–	–
SK10	SILDIKQGPK	A*11:01	0	221	–	–	–	–	–	–
AK11	ACQGVGGPGHK	A*11:01	4	217	36,500	56,000	450	274	0.3586	0.1277
DT9	DYVDRFYKT	A*24:02	1	220	–	–	–	–	–	–
ML8	MYSPTSIL	A*24:02	1	220	–	–	–	–	–	–
KR9	KIWPSHKGR	A*31:01	0	221	–	–	–	–	–	–
IK10	IAKNCRAPRK	A*31:01	9	212	67,000	55,500	325	275	0.4332	0.7564
DR11	DYVDRFYKTLR	A*33:03	5	216	55,000	56,000	185	279	0.5951	0.3866
GL9	GPGHKARVL	B*07:02	3	218	38,000	56,500	646	274	0.402	0.0741
GY9	GLNKIVRMY	B*15:01	13	208	100,000	55,000	269	285	0.6736	0.8588
NY10	NPPIPVGEIY	B*35:01	1	220	–	–	–	–	–	–
TL8	TERQANFL	B*40:02	23	198	45,000	59,500	416	275	0.1029	*0.0392*
WV8	WMTETLLV	B*52:01	22	199	39,500	58,000	405	269	*0.0481*	*0.0006*
RI8	RMYSPTSI	B*52:01	31	190	43,000	59,500	389	264	*0.0414*	*0.0005*
TW10	TSTLQEQIGW	B*58:01	2	219	–	–	–	–	–	–
NL11	NPDCKTILRAL	B*67:01	1	220	–	–	–	–	–	–
YI9	YSPTSILDI	C*01:02	10	211	123,000	55,000	214	281	0.0919	0.159
KL9	KALGPAATL	C*03	9	212	24,000	56,000	307	275	0.368	0.7865
YL9	YVDRFYKTL	C*03	5	216	76,000	55,500	224	285	0.7639	0.6464
KL9	KALGPAATL	C*08	13	208	24,000	58,000	320	274	*0.0228*	0.64
RI9[a]	RQANFLGKI	A*02:06	4	217	15,000	57,000	319	274	*0.009*	0.9741
TM9[a]	TLQEQIGWM	A*26:02	7	214	39,000	57,500	410	274	*0.032*	0.0921
HR10[a]	HIAKNCRAPR	A*33:03	9	212	4900	58,000	416	273	*0.0002*	*0.0196*

[a] New epitope

[b] Statistically analyzed differences in pVL or CD4 count between responders and non-responders by Mann–Whitney test. Italics indicates that differences were statistically significant

We also analyzed the impact of the total breadth (number of recognized epitopes) and magnitude of the T-cell responses to 5 protective epitopes AA9, TL8, WV8, RI8, and HR10 on clinical outcome and found their very strong negative and positive association with respective pVL (breadth: $p < 1 \times 10^{-4}$, r $= -0.37$; magnitude: $p < 1 \times 10^{-4}$, r $= -0.40$) and CD4 count (breadth: $p < 1 \times 10^{-4}$, r$=0.44$; magnitude: $p < 1 \times 10^{-4}$, r$=0.44$), respectively (Fig. 5b and Additional file 3: Fig. S3).

TL8- and HR10-specific T cells suppress HIV-1 replication in vitro

We next investigated the ability of T cells specific for the reported TL8/HLA-B*40:02 [23, 24] and novel HR10/A*33:03 epitopes to suppress HIV-1 replication *in vitro*. We established T-cell lines specific for TL8 and HR10 from PBMCs of individuals KI-1391 (HLA-B*40:02[+]) and KI-1320 (HLA-A*33:03[+]), respectively, by

FACS sorting using the HLA/peptide tetrameric complexes (Fig. 6a). TL8- and HR10-specific T-cell lines were effectively stimulated by peptide-pulsed and HIV-1-infected target cells 721.221/HLA-B*40:02 and 721.221/HLA-A*33:03, respectively, but not uninfected or HLA-untransfected 721.221 cells (Fig. 6b). These T-cell lines efficiently suppressed HIV-1 replication in vitro (Fig. 6c). This HIV-1-inhibitory activity concurs with their improved clinical outcome.

Gag-specific CD8[+] T cells cross-recognize epitope variants

Our previous study showed that CD8[+] T cells specific for conserved epitopes WV8/HLA-B*52:01 and AA9/HLA-A*02:06 recognized 97 and 90%, respectively, of the circulating viruses in Japan. In contrast, RI8/HLA-B*52:01-specific T cells selected escape mutations, which were present in approximately 27% of the circulating HIV-1 variants [21]. Consensus sequences of HR10/

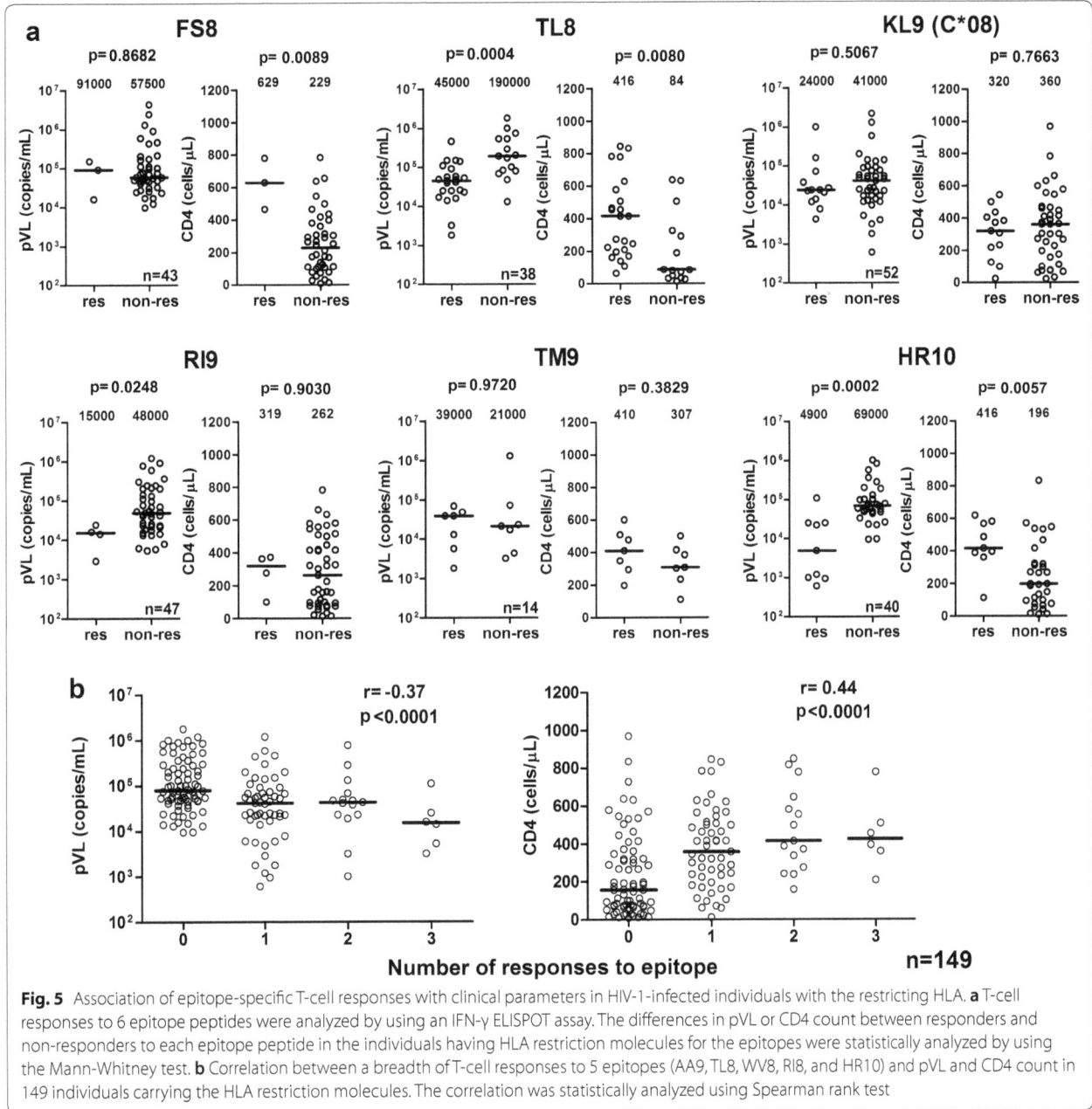

Fig. 5 Association of epitope-specific T-cell responses with clinical parameters in HIV-1-infected individuals with the restricting HLA. **a** T-cell responses to 6 epitope peptides were analyzed by using an IFN-γ ELISPOT assay. The differences in pVL or CD4 count between responders and non-responders to each epitope peptide in the individuals having HLA restriction molecules for the epitopes were statistically analyzed by using the Mann-Whitney test. **b** Correlation between a breadth of T-cell responses to 5 epitopes (AA9, TL8, WV8, RI8, and HR10) and pVL and CD4 count in 149 individuals carrying the HLA restriction molecules. The correlation was statistically analyzed using Spearman rank test

HLA-A*33:03 and TL8/HLA-B*40:02 were found in approximately 60% of circulating viruses in the present Japanese cohort. We therefore analyzed cross-recognition of mutant epitopes by CD8$^+$ T cells recognizing the two conserved Gag epitopes, HR10 and TL8. Three mutants for each of these epitopes were detected in >5% of circulating viruses (Fig. 7a). We therefore assessed the recognition of these mutant epitope peptides by using the IFN-γ ELISPOT assay. Three TL8 mutant peptides were cross-recognized by T cells in 5 HIV-1-infected HLA-B*40:02$^+$ patients with the TL8-specific

responses, although the recognition of the 1D mutation was reduced (Fig. 7b). Indeed in a dose response analysis, the stimulation of the TL8-specific T-cell line by the 1D mutant peptide was severely reduced (Fig. 7c). The HLA-B*40:02-associated mutation in Gag T427N ($p − 1.0 \times 10^{-9}$, $q − 3.2 \times 10^{-6}$) was found within the TL8/HLA-B*40:02 epitope [25], suggesting that this mutation represented an escape from CD8$^+$ T-cell recognition. Nevertheless, the TL8-1N mutated peptide was cross-recognized in all of the 5 tested individuals including 2 having the TL8-1N mutant viruses (Additional file 4:

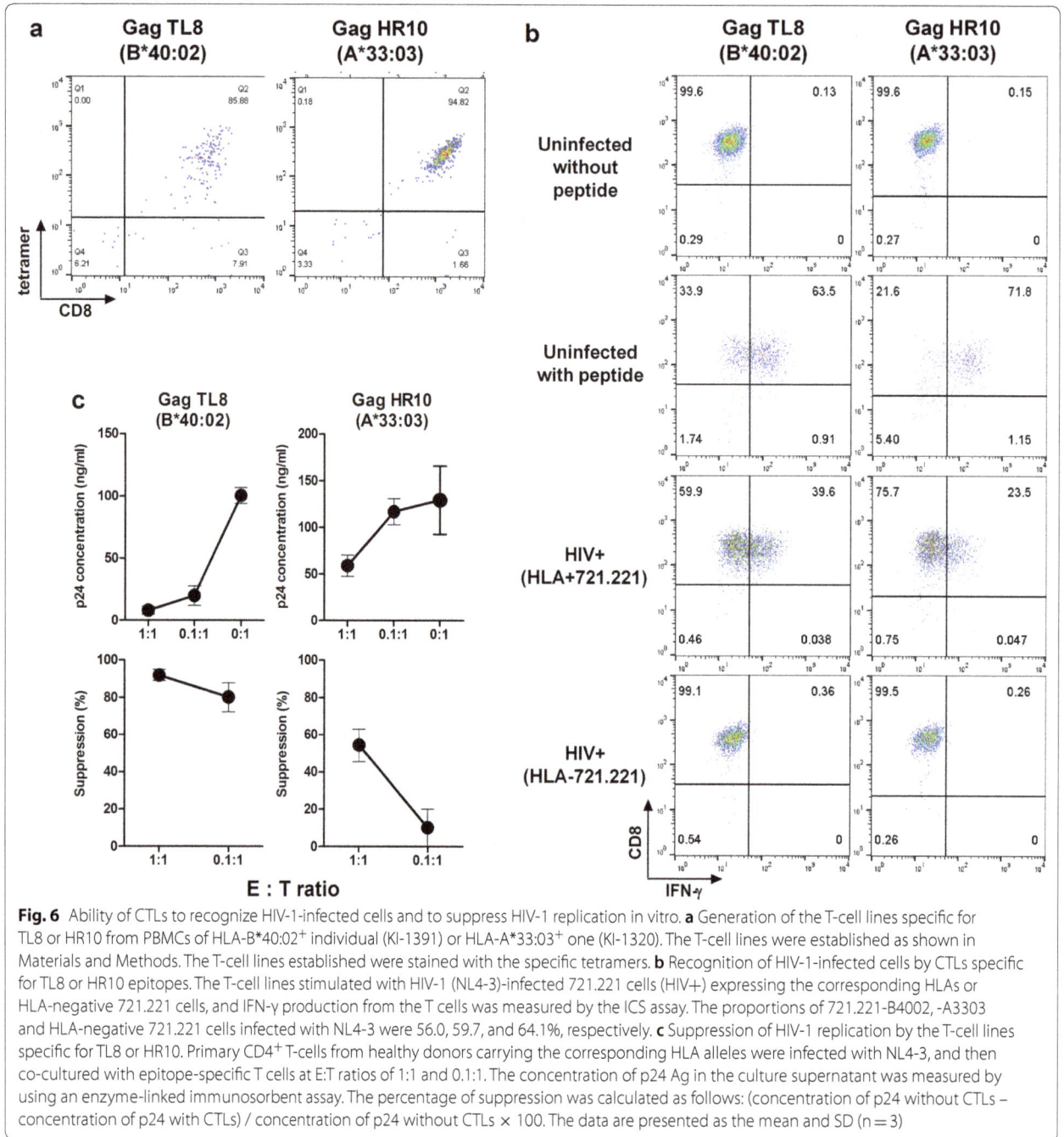

Fig. 6 Ability of CTLs to recognize HIV-1-infected cells and to suppress HIV-1 replication in vitro. **a** Generation of the T-cell lines specific for TL8 or HR10 from PBMCs of HLA-B*40:02[+] individual (KI-1391) or HLA-A*33:03[+] one (KI-1320). The T-cell lines were established as shown in Materials and Methods. The T-cell lines established were stained with the specific tetramers. **b** Recognition of HIV-1-infected cells by CTLs specific for TL8 or HR10 epitopes. The T-cell lines stimulated with HIV-1 (NL4-3)-infected 721.221 cells (HIV+) expressing the corresponding HLAs or HLA-negative 721.221 cells, and IFN-γ production from the T cells was measured by the ICS assay. The proportions of 721.221-B4002, -A3303 and HLA-negative 721.221 cells infected with NL4-3 were 56.0, 59.7, and 64.1%, respectively. **c** Suppression of HIV-1 replication by the T-cell lines specific for TL8 or HR10. Primary CD4[+] T-cells from healthy donors carrying the corresponding HLA alleles were infected with NL4-3, and then co-cultured with epitope-specific T cells at E:T ratios of 1:1 and 0.1:1. The concentration of p24 Ag in the culture supernatant was measured by using an enzyme-linked immunosorbent assay. The percentage of suppression was calculated as follows: (concentration of p24 without CTLs – concentration of p24 with CTLs) / concentration of p24 without CTLs × 100. The data are presented as the mean and SD (n = 3)

Fig. S4). Similarly, the HR10-2L mutant peptide was cross-recognized by T cells in all 5 HIV-1-infected HLA-A*33:03[+] individuals who were not infected with HR10-2L or HR10-4R mutant viruses (Additional file 4: Fig. S4), whereas HR10-2L4R and/or HR10-4R mutant peptides were cross-recognized by T cells in patients KI-1002 and KI-1320. HR10-specific T cells from KI-1320 confirmed cross-recognition of these mutant peptides (Fig. 7c). Thus, CD8[+] T-cells responses specific for TL8 and HR10

epitopes can recognize 70–75% of the circulating HIV-1 isolates in Japan.

Discussion

Unique vaccine immunogens tHIVconsvX were assembled, which use 2 Gag and 4 Pol conserved regions to focus T-cell responses on the most vulnerable regions (not full-size proteins and not epitopes) of HIV-1 with the bi-valent mosaic design providing the vaccine with a

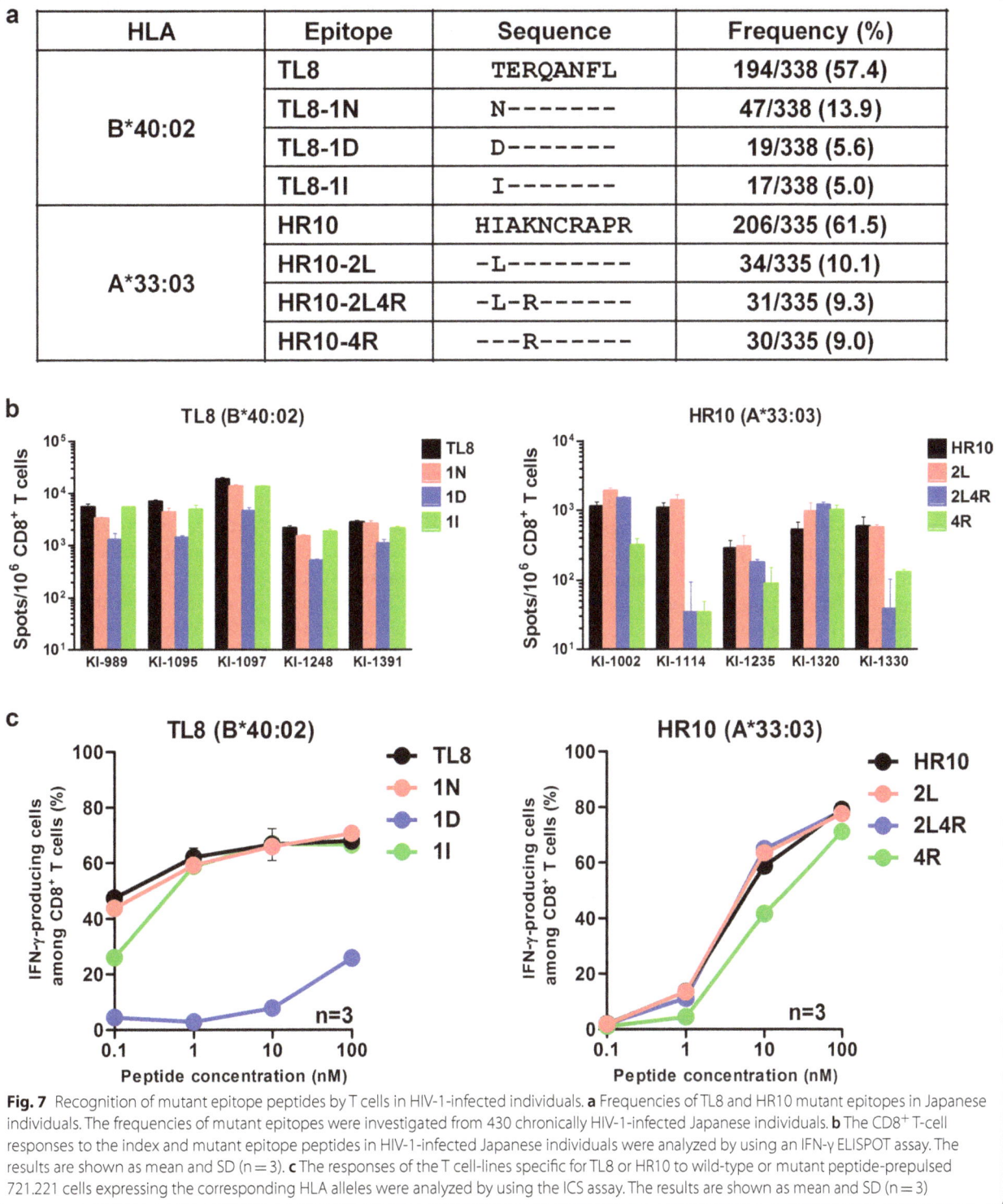

a

HLA	Epitope	Sequence	Frequency (%)
B*40:02	TL8	TERQANFL	194/338 (57.4)
	TL8-1N	N-------	47/338 (13.9)
	TL8-1D	D-------	19/338 (5.6)
	TL8-1I	I-------	17/338 (5.0)
A*33:03	HR10	HIAKNCRAPR	206/335 (61.5)
	HR10-2L	-L--------	34/335 (10.1)
	HR10-2L4R	-L-R------	31/335 (9.3)
	HR10-4R	---R------	30/335 (9.0)

Fig. 7 Recognition of mutant epitope peptides by T cells in HIV-1-infected individuals. **a** Frequencies of TL8 and HR10 mutant epitopes in Japanese individuals. The frequencies of mutant epitopes were investigated from 430 chronically HIV-1-infected Japanese individuals. **b** The CD8+ T-cell responses to the index and mutant epitope peptides in HIV-1-infected Japanese individuals were analyzed by using an IFN-γ ELISPOT assay. The results are shown as mean and SD (n = 3). **c** The responses of the T cell-lines specific for TL8 or HR10 to wild-type or mutant peptide-prepulsed 721.221 cells expressing the corresponding HLA alleles were analyzed by using the ICS assay. The results are shown as mean and SD (n = 3)

high match to global HIV-1 variants. To date, the immunogenicity of these regions was demonstrated in preclinical studies [14, 26]. Importantly, we were previously able to show that CD8+ T-cell responses to 10 peptide pools derived from the two tHIVconsvX mosaic immunogens correlated significantly with low pVL and high CD4 count in 120 treatment-naïve, HIV-1-infected Japanese patients [14]. In the present study, we focused on

Gag-specific CD8$^+$ T-cells because of their strong contribution to favorable clinical outcome. We defined a number of optimal epitopes and their HLA restriction, which were recognized by CD8$^+$ T cells specific for the Gag conserved regions of tHIVconsvX. Furthermore, we demonstrated that 9 Gag-specific CD8$^+$ T-cell responses were significantly associated with low pVL and/or high CD4 count in an extended 221-patient cohort of treatment-naïve patients, implying that T cells specific for these 9 epitopes may contribute to suppression of HIV-1 replication in these individuals. To increase the analysis sensitivity and further endorse the ability of these CD8$^+$ T-cell responses to suppress HIV-1 replication, we confirmed the association of these T-cells with good clinical parameters among the individuals carrying the appropriate HLA restriction molecules. Finally, we identified 5 Gag epitope-specific protective CD8$^+$ T-cell responses and showed a strong association of the magnitude and the breadth of the responses to the 5 epitopes with favorable pVL or CD4 count, indicating again that the responses to 5 Gag epitopes are beneficial. Although escape mutants were selected by the RI8-specific T cells and these HIV-1 mutants accumulated in the Japanese population [21], 70% of circulating HIV-1 still contain variants of the RI8 epitope recognized by RI8-elicited T cells.

It has now been well documented that not all CD8$^+$ T-cell responses contribute to the suppression of HIV-1 replication equally [14, 15, 21, 27]. Mothe et al. showed that the T-cell responses to forty-eight 18-mer overlapping peptides associated with low viral load in South Africa, Peru, and Spain cohorts [27]. These 18-mer overlapping peptides covering Gag, Pol, Nef, and Vif regions include 59 optimal defined epitopes in the LANL-HSD. The tHIVconsvX immunogen contains most of these; 19 in Gag and 14 in Pol. In the present study, we identified CD8$^+$ T cells specific for 5 Gag conserved epitopes with the ability to suppress HIV-1 replication in Japanese individuals. These CD8$^+$ T cells are restricted by HLA-B*52:01, HLA-A*02:06, HLA-A*33:03, and HLA-B*40:02, and at least one of these four alleles are shared in approximately 70% of Japanese population [28]. Since at least one of these alleles is also found in 45% of Chinese [29], 35% of Vietnamese [30], 40% of Thai [31], 50% of Indian [32], and 65% of Korean [33], we hypothesize that if indeed effective, the tHIVconsvX vaccine could be deployed in all these countries; the vaccine would be universal.

To confirm whether the 5 Gag epitopes were recognized by specific T cells as conserved epitopes, we analyzed cross-recognitions of mutant epitopes among the subtype B using the IFN-γ ELISPOT assay. Notably, the circulating viruses carry epitopes with a perfect 9/9 amino acid match or cross-recognized variations in 70–97% isolates from the Japanese population and

46–97% of subtype B viruses (LANL-HSD) and were recognized by T cells specific for 4 epitopes WV8, AA9, TL8, and HR10, though escape mutants selected by the RI8-specific T cells were detected in 27% of the circulating virus in the Japanese cohort [21]. These results suggest that the 4 epitopes are functionally conserved at least among the subtype B viruses. We further analyzed HLA-associated mutations within these six epitopes and found HLA-B*40:02-associated Gag mutation T427N within the HLA-B*40:02/TL8 epitope [25], suggesting that this mutant is accumulated in the HLA-B*40:02$^+$ Japanese individuals. However, since mutant Gag epitope TL8-1N was cross-recognized by CD8$^+$ T cells in 5 individuals with HLA-B*40:02 (Fig. 7b), TL8-1N may elicit a new T-cell repertoire specific for the 1N mutant or cross-recognizing this mutant. CD8$^+$ T-cells responses specific for TL8 and HR10 epitopes can recognize 70–75% of the circulating HIV-1 isolates in Japan while those specific for WV8, AA9, and RI8 did recognized > 70% of them.

We previously demonstrated that three HLA-B*52:01-, two HLA-B*67:01-, and one HLA-B*02:06-restricted CD8$^+$ T cells specific for Gag epitopes had a strong ability to suppress HIV-1 replication in the Japanese population [21]. The present study demonstrated that CD8$^+$ T cells specific for additional 2 Gag epitopes also contribute to the suppression of HIV-1. Although contained in the tHIVconsvX vaccines, T cells specific for MI8 restricted by HLA-B*52:01 [21], and TL9 and NL11 restricted by HLA-B*67:01 [21] were not identified in this study. This may be explained by the fact that MI8 and TL9 are included in Pool 1 and that the HLA-B*67:01 is a rare allele found in only 4 out of 221 patients involved in the present study. These findings suggest that Japanese individuals vaccinated with the tHIVconsvX vaccines may respond to 8 Gag epitopes and suppress better HIV-1 replication by killer T cells (Additional file 5: Fig. S5).

The present work supports the hypothesis that the CD8$^+$ T-cell responses, which the tHIVconsvX vaccines aim to elicit, have a real chance to contribute to the suppression of HIV-1 replication *in vivo* in Japan and other Asian populations both in the context of prevention of HIV-1 infection complementing neutralizing antibodies and in HIV cure by eradicating latently infected cells after HIV-1 reactivation. These results warrantee timely testing of this target immunogen strategy in the clinic.

Methods

Subjects

All treatment-naïve Japanese individuals chronically infected with HIV-1 subtype B were recruited from the National Center for Global Health and Medicine. This study was approved by the ethics committees of Kumamoto University and the National Center for Global

Health and Medicine. Informed consent was obtained from all individuals according to the Declaration of Helsinki. Plasma and PBMCs were separated from whole blood. HLA types of the individuals were determined by standard sequence-based genotyping.

Peptides

The mosaic proteins maximize the coverage of potential T-cell epitopes for the global circulating viruses. We generated three pools containing pairs of 15-mer Gag peptides overlapped by 11 amino acids covering two mosaic regions in the tHIVconsvX. Each pool contains 17 to 23 pairs of the 15-mer peptides. Pool 1, 2, and 3 cover Gag 133-231, Gag 221-327, and Gag 317-363/391-459, respectively [14]. The sequences of the 15-mer peptides in each Pool are shown in Additional file 6: Fig. S6. The 15-mer peptides derived from the tHIVconsvX mosaics were generously provided by the International AIDS Vaccine Initiative. Shorter mapping peptides were synthesized by utilizing an automated multiple peptide synthesizer and purified by high-performance liquid chromatography (HPLC). Purity of all peptides (>90%) was examined by HPLC and mass spectrometry.

Cell lines

C1R cells expressing HLA-A*26:01 (C1R-A2601), HLA-A*26:02 (C1R-A2602), HLA-A*33:03 (C1R-A3303), HLA-B*07:02 (C1R-B0702), HLA-B*15:01 (C1R-B1501), HLA-B*39:01 (C1R-B3901), or HLA-B*44:03 (C1R-B4403) were previously generated by transfecting these genes into C1R cell lines [21, 34–39]. 721.221 cells expressing CD4 molecules and HLA-C*03:03 (721.221-C0303) were generated by transfecting the genes into the 721.221 cell line. 721.221 cells expressing CD4 molecules and HLA-A*02:06 (721.221-A0206), HLA-A*24:02 (721.221-A2402), HLA-A*33:03 (721.221-A3303), HLA-B*40:02 (721.221-B4002), HLA-C*14:03 (721.221-C1403), or HLA-C*07:02 (721.221-C0702) were previously generated [21, 40–43]. All cell lines were cultured in RPMI 1640 medium containing 10% FCS medium (R10) with 0.15 mg/ml hygromycin B.

Expansion of HIV-1-specific T cells from HIV-1-infected individuals

PBMCs from KI-1020, KI-1102, and KI-1114 were incubated with 1 µM 15-mer peptide pairs (C052/053 or C054/055, C113/114, and C125/126, respectively) and cultured for 12-14 days to induce peptide-specific short-term cell lines (STCL).

Intracellular cytokine staining (ICS) assay

C1R and 721.221 cells prepulsed with each peptide or 721.221 cells infected with the HIV-1, strain NL4-3, were added to the effector STCLs in a 96-well plate and incubated for 2 h at 37 °C. Brefeldin A (10 µg/ml) was then added and the cells were incubated further for 4 h, fixed with 4% paraformaldehyde and incubated in permeabilization buffer [0.1% saponin–10% FBS–phosphate-buffered saline (PBS)] after staining with allophycocyanin (APC)-labeled anti-CD8 monoclonal antibody (mAb) (Dako, Glostrup, Denmark). Thereafter, the cells were stained with fluorescein isothiocyanate (FITC)-labeled anti-interferon γ (IFN-γ) mAb (BD Bioscience, CA). The percentage of IFN-γ-producing cells among the CD8+ T-cell population was determined by flow cytometry.

IFN-γ enzyme-linked immunospot (ELISPOT) assay

1×10^5 PBMCs from HIV-1-positive individuals and peptides were added to 96-well polyvinylidene plates (Millipore, Bedford, MA) that had been precoated with 5 µg/ml anti-IFN-γ mAb; 1-D1K (Mabtech, Stockholm, Sweden). Peptide pools or 15-mer peptide pairs were used at a concentration of 1 µM whereas optimal epitope peptides at a concentration of 100 nM in this assay. The plates were then incubated for 16 h at 37 °C before the addition of biotinylated anti-IFN-γ mAb (Mabtech) at 1 µg/ml at room temperature for 90 min, streptavidin-conjugated alkaline phosphatase (Mabtech) for at room temperature 60 min. Individual cytokine-producing cells were visualized as dark spots after a 20-min reaction with 5-bromo-4-chloro-3-indolyl phosphate and nitro blue tetrazolium in the presence of an alkaline phosphatase-conjugated substrate (Bio-Rad, Richmond, CA, USA). The spots were counted with an Eliphoto-Counter (Minerva Teck, Tokyo, Japan). The frequencies of the responding cells were represented as spot-forming units (SFU)/10^6 CD8+ T cells by measuring frequency of CD8+ T cells using a flow cytometry. A mean+5 SD of the SFUs of samples (N=3) from 12 HIV-1-naïve individuals for the peptide pool was 115 SFU/10^6 CD8+ T cells. Therefore, we defined a positive ELISPOT response as larger than 200 SFU/10^6 CD8+ T cells to exclude false positive.

Establishment of T-cell lines specific for TL8 and HR10 peptides using HLA/peptide tetramer complexes

To establish T-cell lines specific for TL8 and HR10 peptides, HLA-B*40:02/TL8 or HLA-A*33:03/HR10 tetrameric complexes (tetramers) were synthesized as previously described [44]. Briefly, PBMCs of HLA-B*40:02+ individual (KI-1391) and HLA-A*33:03+ one (KI-1320) were stained with PE-conjugated specific tetramers at a concentration of 100 nM at 37 °C for 30 min. The cells were then washed twice with R10, followed by staining with FITC-conjugated anti-CD8 mAb and 7-AAD at 4 °C for 30 min. The CD8+ T cells specific for the TL8 and HR10 peptides were then sorted by the

FACSAria. The sorted cells were stimulated with 100 nM of the corresponding epitope peptides and then cultured for 12–14 days to induce T cell lines specific for TL8 and HR10. To confirm purities of the specific T cells, the cell lines were analyzed by using the specific tetramers.

In vitro virus inhibition assay

The ability of HIV-1-specific CTLs to suppress HIV-1 replication was examined as previously described [45, 46]. CD4$^+$ T cells isolated from PBMCs of healthy donors carrying HLA-B*40:02 or -A*33:03 were infected with NL4-3 and then the infected cells were co-cultured with epitope-specific T-cell lines at E:T ratios of 1:1 and 0.1:1. On day 3–4 post infection, the concentration of p24 Ag in the culture supernatant was measured by using an enzyme-linked immunosorbent assay.

Statistical analyses

Two-tailed Mann–Whitney's test was performed for comparison of two groups. Correlations between magnitudes and breadths of T cell responses and pVL or CD4 count were statistically analyzed using Spearman rank test. P values < 0.05 were considered to be statistically significant.

Additional files

Additional file 1: Fig. S1. Correlation of the magnitudes of the Gag responses with pVL and CD4 count. T-cell responses to Gag peptide Pools 1, 2 and 3 derived from vaccine immunogen tHIVconsvX were enumerated using an IFN-γ ELISPOT assay in 200 HIV-1-infected Japanese individuals. Correlation coefficients (r) and p-values were determined by using the Spearman rank correlation test.

Additional file 2: Fig. S2. Association of the T-cell responses to AA9, WV8, or RI8 with pVL or CD4 count. T-cell responses to the 3 epitope peptides were analyzed by using the IFN-γ ELISPOT assay. The differences in pVL or CD4 count between responders and non-responders to each epitope peptide in the individuals having HLA restriction molecules for the epitopes were statistically analyzed by using the Mann-Whitney test.

Additional file 3: Fig. S3. Correlation between a total magnitude of T-cell responses to 5 epitopes and pVL and CD4 count. T-cell responses to 5 epitope peptides (AA9, TL8, WV8, RI8, and HR10) were analyzed in 149 individuals carrying the HLA restriction molecules by using the IFN-γ ELISPOT assay. Correlation coefficients (r) and p-values were determined by using the Spearman rank correlation test.

Additional file 4: Fig. S4. HIV-1 sequences within Gag TL8 and Gag HR10 epitopes in HIV-1-infected individuals. HIV-1 sequences within Gag TL8 and Gag HR10 were analyzed in HIV-1-infected individuals tested in Figure 7b. Mutant positions are highlighted in red.

Additional file 5: Fig. S5. Location of the 8 Gag CTL epitopes in the tHIVconsvX. The tHIVconsvX vaccine is composed of 2 Gag and 4 Pol conserved fragments. The two complementing mosaic immunogens corresponding to the 6 conserved regions are used in this vaccine. HLA-B*67:01-restricted TL9-specific, HLA-B*52:01-restricted MI8-specific, and HLA-B*67:01-restricted NL11-specific CTLs also have strong abilities to suppress HIV-1 replication in vivo (highlighted in green, Murakoshi et al., 2015).

Additional file 6: Fig. S6. List of 15-mer overlapping peptide pairs in Pools 1-3. Pool 1, 2, and 3 cover Gag133-231, Gag221-327, and Gag317-363 / 391-459, respectively.

Authors' contributions

HM wrote the manuscript, performed assays, and analyzed assay results. CZ performed assays and analyzed assay results. NK, TA and TC performed assays. HG and SO collected samples and clinical data from patients. TH provided the overlapping 15-mer peptides derived from the tHIVconsvX immunogens and contributed to writing the manuscript. MT designed the study, oversaw the experiments, analyzed all of the data, and wrote and edited the manuscript. All authors read and approved the final manuscript.

Author details

[1] Center for AIDS Research, Kumamoto University, 2-2-1 Honjo, Chuo-ku, Kumamoto 860-0811, Japan. [2] International Research Center of Medical Sciences, Kumamoto University, Kumamoto, Japan. [3] AIDS Clinical Center, National Center for Global Health and Medicine, Tokyo, Japan. [4] The Jenner Institute, University of Oxford, Old Road Campus Research Building, Roosevelt Drive, Oxford, UK.

Acknowledgements

Not applicable.

Competing interests

The authors declare that they have no competing interests.

Funding

This research was supported by grants-in-aid (15fk0410019h0001, 16fk0410202h0002, and17fk0410302h0003) for AIDS Research from AMED and by grants-in-aid (26293240, 17K10021) for scientific research from the Ministry of Education, Science, Sports, and Culture, Japan. C.Z. was supported by the China Scholarship Council (CSC) scholarship. The funders had no role in study design, data collection and interpretation, or the decision to submit the work for publication.

References

1. Rerks-Ngarm S, Pitisuttithum P, Nitayaphan S, Kaewkungwal J, Chiu J, Paris R, et al. Vaccination with ALVAC and AIDSVAX to prevent HIV-1 infection in Thailand. N Engl J Med. 2009;361:2209–20.
2. Haynes BF, Gilbert PB, McElrath MJ, Zolla-Pazner S, Tomaras GD, Alam SM, et al. Immune-correlates analysis of an HIV-1 vaccine efficacy trial. N Engl J Med. 2012;366:1275–86.
3. Rolland M, Edlefsen PT, Larsen BB, Tovanabutra S, Sanders-Buell E, Hertz T, et al. Increased HIV-1 vaccine efficacy against viruses with genetic signatures in Env V2. Nature. 2012;490:417–20.
4. Liao HX, Bonsignori M, Alam SM, McLellan JS, Tomaras GD, Moody MA, et al. Vaccine induction of antibodies against a structurally heterogeneous site of immune pressure within HIV-1 envelope protein variable regions 1 and 2. Immunity. 2013;38:176–86.
5. Chung AW, Kumar MP, Arnold KB, Yu WH, Schoen MK, Dunphy LJ, et al. Dissecting polyclonal vaccine-induced humoral immunity against HIV using systems serology. Cell. 2015;163:988–98.
6. Yates NL, Liao HX, Fong Y, deCamp A, Vandergrift NA, Williams WT, et al. Vaccine-induced Env V1-V2 IgG3 correlates with lower HIV-1 infection risk and declines soon after vaccination. Sci Transl Med. 2014;6:228ra239.
7. McMichael AJ, Haynes BF. Lessons learned from HIV-1 vaccine trials: new priorities and directions. Nat Immunol. 2012;13:423–7.
8. Gray GE, Allen M, Moodie Z, Churchyard G, Bekker LG, Nchabeleng M, et al. Safety and efficacy of the HVTN 503/Phambili study of a clade-B-based HIV-1 vaccine in South Africa: a double-blind, randomised, placebo-controlled test-of-concept phase 2b study. Lancet Infect Dis. 2011;11:507–15.

9. Hammer SM, Sobieszczyk ME, Janes H, Karuna ST, Mulligan MJ, Grove D, et al. Efficacy trial of a DNA/rAd5 HIV-1 preventive vaccine. N Engl J Med. 2013;369:2083–92.

10. Buchbinder SP, Mehrotra DV, Duerr A, Fitzgerald DW, Mogg R, Li D, et al. Efficacy assessment of a cell-mediated immunity HIV-1 vaccine (the Step Study): a double-blind, randomised, placebo-controlled, test-of-concept trial. Lancet. 2008;372:1881–93.

11. McElrath MJ, De Rosa SC, Moodie Z, Dubey S, Kierstead L, Janes H, et al. HIV-1 vaccine-induced immunity in the test-of-concept Step Study: a case-cohort analysis. Lancet. 2008;372:1894–905.

12. Hanke T. Conserved immunogens in prime-boost strategies for the next-generation HIV-1 vaccines. Expert Opin Biol Ther. 2014;14:601–16.

13. Letourneau S, Im EJ, Mashishi T, Brereton C, Bridgeman A, Yang H, et al. Design and pre-clinical evaluation of a universal HIV-1 vaccine. PLoS ONE. 2007;2:e984.

14. Ondondo B, Murakoshi H, Clutton G, Abdul-Jawad S, Wee EG, Gatanaga H, et al. Novel conserved-region T-cell mosaic vaccine with high global HIV-1 coverage is recognized by protective responses in untreated infection. Mol Ther. 2016;24:83242.

15. Kiepiela P, Ngumbela K, Thobakgale C, Ramduth D, Honeyborne I, Moodley E, et al. CD8+ T-cell responses to different HIV proteins have discordant associations with viral load. Nat Med. 2007;13:46–53.

16. Klein MR, van Baalen CA, Holwerda AM, Kerkhof Garde SR, Bende RJ, Keet IP, et al. Kinetics of Gag-specific cytotoxic T lymphocyte responses during the clinical course of HIV-1 infection: a longitudinal analysis of rapid progressors and long-term asymptomatics. J Exp Med. 1995;181:1365–72.

17. Ogg GS, Jin X, Bonhoeffer S, Dunbar PR, Nowak MA, Monard S, et al. Quantitation of HIV-1-specific cytotoxic T lymphocytes and plasma load of viral RNA. Science. 1998;279:2103–6.

18. Chen DY, Balamurugan A, Ng HL, Cumberland WG, Yang OO. Epitope targeting and viral inoculum are determinants of Nef-mediated immune evasion of HIV-1 from cytotoxic T lymphocytes. Blood. 2012;120:100–11.

19. Kloverpris HN, Payne RP, Sacha JB, Rasaiyaah JT, Chen F, Takiguchi M, et al. Early antigen presentation of protective HIV-1 KF11Gag and KK10Gag epitopes from incoming viral particles facilitates rapid recognition of infected cells by specific CD8+ T cells. J Virol. 2013;87:2628–38.

20. Sacha JB, Chung C, Rakasz EG, Spencer SP, Jonas AK, Bean AT, et al. Gag-specific CD8+ T lymphocytes recognize infected cells before AIDS-virus integration and viral protein expression. J Immunol. 2007;178:2746–54.

21. Murakoshi H, Akahoshi T, Koyanagi M, Chikata T, Naruto T, Maruyama R, et al. Clinical control of HIV-1 by cytotoxic T cells specific for multiple conserved epitopes. J Virol. 2015;89:5330–9.

22. Chikata T, Murakoshi H, Koyanagi M, Honda K, Gatanaga H, Oka S, et al. Control of HIV-1 by an HLA-B*52:01-C*12:02 Protective Haplotype. J Infect Dis. 2017;216:1415–24.

23. Sabbaj S, Bansal A, Ritter GD, Perkins C, Edwards BH, Gough E, et al. Cross-reactive CD8+ T cell epitopes identified in US adolescent minorities. J Acquir Immune Defic Syndr. 2003;33:426–38.

24. Borthwick N, Lin Z, Akahoshi T, Llano A, Silva-Arrieta S, Ahmed T, et al. Novel, in-natural-infection subdominant HIV-1 CD8+ T-cell epitopes revealed in human recipients of conserved-region T-cell vaccines. PLoS ONE. 2017;12:e0176418.

25. Chikata T, Carlson JM, Tamura Y, Borghan MA, Naruto T, Hashimoto M, et al. Host-specific adaptation of HIV-1 subtype B in the Japanese population. J Virol. 2014;88:4764–75.

26. Wee EG, Ondondo B, Berglund P, Archer J, McMichael AJ, Baltimore D, et al. HIV-1 conserved mosaics delivered by regimens with integration-deficient DC-Targeting lentiviral vector induce robust T cells. Mol Ther. 2017;25:494–503.

27. Mothe B, Llano A, Ibarrondo J, Daniels M, Miranda C, Zamarreno J, et al. Definition of the viral targets of protective HIV-1-specific T cell responses. J Transl Med. 2011;9:208.

28. Ikeda N, Kojima H, Nishikawa M, Hayashi K, Futagami T, Tsujino T, et al. Determination of HLA-A, -C, -B, -DRB1 allele and haplotype frequency in Japanese population based on family study. Tissue Antigens. 2015;85:252–9.

29. Qin Qin P, Su F, Xiao Yan W, Xing Z, Meng P, Chengya W, et al. Distribution of human leucocyte antigen-A, -B and -DR alleles and haplotypes at high resolution in the population from Jiangsu province of China. Int J Immunogenet. 2011;38:475–81.

30. Hoa BK, Hang NT, Kashiwase K, Ohashi J, Lien LT, Horie T, et al. HLA-A, -B, -C, -DRB1 and -DQB1 alleles and haplotypes in the Kinh population in Vietnam. Tissue Antigens. 2008;71:127–34.

31. Kupatawintu P, Pheancharoen S, Srisuddee A, Tanaka H, Tadokoro K, Nathalang O. HLA-A, -B, -DR haplotype frequencies in the Thai Stem Cell Donor Registry. Tissue Antigens. 2010;75:730–6.

32. Rani R, Marcos C, Lazaro AM, Zhang Y, Stastny P. Molecular diversity of HLA-A, -B and -C alleles in a North Indian population as determined by PCR-SSOP. Int J Immunogenet. 2007;34:201–8.

33. Huh JY, Yi DY, Eo SH, Cho H, Park MH, Kang MS. HLA-A, -B and -DRB1 polymorphism in Koreans defined by sequence-based typing of 4128 cord blood units. Int J Immunogenet. 2013;40:515–23.

34. Satoh M, Takamiya Y, Oka S, Tokunaga K, Takiguchi M. Identification and characterization of HIV-1-specific CD8+ T cell epitopes presented by HLA-A*2601. Vaccine. 2005;23:3783–90.

35. Kawashima Y, Satoh M, Oka S, Shirasaka T, Takiguchi M. Different immunodominance of HIV-1-specific CTL epitopes among three subtypes of HLA-A*26 associated with slow progression to AIDS. Biochem Biophys Res Commun. 2008;366:612–6.

36. Hossain MS, Tomiyama H, Inagawa T, Ida S, Oka S, Takiguchi M. Identification and characterization of HLA-A*3303-restricted, HIV type 1 Pol- and Gag-derived cytotoxic T cell epitopes. AIDS Res Hum Retroviruses. 2003;19:503–10.

37. Falk K, Rotzschke O, Takiguchi M, Gnau V, Stevanovic S, Jung G, et al. Peptide motifs of HLA-B58, B60, B61, and B62 molecules. Immunogenetics. 1995;41:165–8.

38. Ogawa A, Tokunaga K, Nakajima F, Kikuchi A, Karaki S, Kashiwase K, et al. Identification of the gene encoding a novel HLA-B39 subtype. Two amino acid substitutions on the beta-sheet out of the peptide-binding floor form a novel serological epitope. Hum Immunol. 1994;41:241–7.

39. Kato N, Kikuchi A, Kano K, Egawa K, Takiguchi M. Molecular analysis of a novel HLA-A33 subtype associated with HLA-B44. Tissue Antigens. 1993;41:211–3.

40. Watanabe K, Murakoshi H, Tamura Y, Koyanagi M, Chikata T, Gatanaga H, et al. Identification of cross-clade CTL epitopes in HIV-1 clade A/E-infected individuals by using the clade B overlapping peptides. Microbes Infect. 2013;15:874–86.

41. Koizumi H, Iwatani T, Tanuma J, Fujiwara M, Izumi T, Oka S, et al. Escape mutation selected by Gag28-36-specific cytotoxic T cells in HLA-A*2402-positive HIV-1-infected donors. Microbes Infect. 2009;11:198–204.

42. Lin Z, Kuroki M, Kuse N, Sun X, Akahoshi T, Qi Y, et al. HIV-1 Control by NK Cells via Reduced Interaction between KIR2DL2 and HLA-C *12:02/C *14:03. Cell Rep. 2016;17:2210–20.

43. Watanabe T, Murakoshi H, Gatanaga H, Koyanagi M, Oka S, Takiguchi M. Effective recognition of HIV-1-infected cells by HIV-1 integrase-specific HLA-B *4002-restricted T cells. Microbes Infect. 2011;13:160–6.

44. Akahoshi T, Chikata T, Tamura Y, Gatanaga H, Oka S, Takiguchi M. Selection and accumulation of an HIV-1 escape mutant by three types of HIV-1-specific cytotoxic T lymphocytes recognizing wild-type and/or escape mutant epitopes. J Virol. 2012;86:1971–81.

45. Tomiyama H, Akari H, Adachi A, Takiguchi M. Different effects of Nef-mediated HLA class I down-regulation on human immunodeficiency virus type 1-specific CD8(+) T-cell cytolytic activity and cytokine production. J Virol. 2002;76:7535–43.

46. Tomiyama H, Fujiwara M, Oka S, Takiguchi M. Cutting Edge: Epitope-dependent effect of Nef-mediated HLA class I down-regulation on ability of HIV-1-specific CTLs to suppress HIV-1 replication. J Immunol. 2005;174:36–40.

Rapid HIV disease progression following superinfection in an HLA-B*27:05/B*57:01-positive transmission recipient

Jacqui Brener[1]*●, Astrid Gall[2], Jacob Hurst[4], Rebecca Batorsky[5], Nora Lavandier[1], Fabian Chen[6], Anne Edwards[7], Chrissy Bolton[1], Reena Dsouza[1], Todd Allen[5], Oliver G. Pybus[8], Paul Kellam[3,9], Philippa C. Matthews[4] and Philip J. R. Goulder[1]

Abstract

Background: The factors determining differential HIV disease outcome among individuals expressing protective HLA alleles such as HLA-B*27:05 and HLA-B*57:01 remain unknown. We here analyse two HIV-infected subjects expressing both HLA-B*27:05 and HLA-B*57:01. One subject maintained low-to-undetectable viral loads for more than a decade of follow up. The other progressed to AIDS in < 3 years.

Results: The rapid progressor was the recipient within a known transmission pair, enabling virus sequences to be tracked from transmission. Progression was associated with a 12% Gag sequence change and 26% Nef sequence change at the amino acid level within 2 years. Although next generation sequencing from early timepoints indicated that multiple CD8+ cytotoxic T lymphocyte (CTL) escape mutants were being selected prior to superinfection, < 4% of the amino acid changes arising from superinfection could be ascribed to CTL escape. Analysis of an HLA-B*27:05/B*57:01 non-progressor, in contrast, demonstrated minimal virus sequence diversification (1.1% Gag amino acid sequence change over 10 years), and dominant HIV-specific CTL responses previously shown to be effective in control of viraemia were maintained. Clonal sequencing demonstrated that escape variants were generated within the non-progressor, but in many cases were not selected. In the rapid progressor, progression occurred despite substantial reductions in viral replicative capacity (VRC), and non-progression in the elite controller despite relatively high VRC.

Conclusions: These data are consistent with previous studies demonstrating rapid progression in association with superinfection and that rapid disease progression can occur despite the relatively the low VRC that is typically observed in the setting of multiple CTL escape mutants.

Keywords: HIV-1, HLA, CTL response, Transmission pair, Superinfection, Ultra-deep sequencing

Background

Outcome in HIV infection is strongly influenced by the particular HLA alleles that are expressed, the most protective of which are HLA-B*27:05 and HLA-B*57:01 [1, 2]. The mechanism by which these HLA alleles confer protection is related to the presentation of a broad array of epitopes that enable CD8+ cytotoxic T lymphocytes (CTL) to recognise and kill HIV-infected target cells [2, 3]. As HIV-specific CTL are likely to play a critical role in strategies designed to eradicate viral reservoirs [4], it remains important to define what features affect the ability of CTL to be effective in killing virus-infected cells. We here contrast HIV disease outcomes in two HIV-infected subjects expressing both HLA-B*27:05 and HLA-B*57:01. One subject is a typical HIV non-progressor, maintaining viral loads below the level of detection for more than a decade of follow up. The other subject

*Correspondence: jacquibrener@gmail.com
[1] Department of Paediatrics, University of Oxford, Oxford, UK
Full list of author information is available at the end of the article

initially presented the characteristic phenotype of an HLA-B*27:05/57:01-positive HIV-infected subject, with a low viral load (65 copies/ml) and high absolute CD4+ T cell count (950 cells/mm^3), but within 2.7 years had progressed rapidly to AIDS (CD4+ T cell count < 200 cells/mm^3).

Methods

Study subjects

The adult Caucasian transmission pair R096 (HLA-A*02:01/A*11:01 B*13:02/B*51:01 C*03:03 C*06:02) and R097 (HLA-A*11:01/A*24:01 B*27:05/B*57:01 C*02:02 C*06:02) and non-progressor RI088 (HLA-A*01:01/A*03:01 B*27:05/B*57:01 C*02:02 C*06:02) were recruited from the Thames Valley Cohort, UK, previously described [5].

DNA and RNA extraction

Proviral and genomic DNA were extracted for proviral sequencing and HLA-typing respectively, using Pure-Gene reagents according to the manufacturers instructions. Viral plasma RNA was extracted using the Qiamp Viral RNA Mini Kit (Qiagen, UK) according to the manufacturers instructions. For RNA extraction for ultra-deep sequencing, minor modifications to the manufacturers protocol were made, as previously described [6].

HLA-typing

Four digit HLA Class I typing was performed at the CLIA/ASHI accredited laboratory of William Hildebrand, PhD, D (ABHI), University of Oklahoma Health Sciences Center. Locus specific PCR amplification of exons 2 and 3 and heterozygous sequencing were performed from genomic DNA. Ambiguities were resolved by homozygous sequencing [7].

IFN-γ ELISpot assays

Peripheral blood mononuclear cells were tested for responses to 410 18mer overlapping peptides spanning the B clade HIV proteome as previously described [8] using pools of 11–12 peptides followed by confirmatory assays using individual 18mer peptides.

Sanger sequencing of proviral DNA

The *gag* gene was amplified from proviral DNA using a nested touchdown PCR with BioTaq DNA polymerase (Bioline, UK) using the following primers: 5′-CTCTAGCAGTGGCGCCCGAA-3′ and 5′-TCCTTTCCACATTTCCAACAGCC-3′ for the first round PCR and 5′-ACTCGGCTTGCTGAAGTGC-3′ and 5′ CAATTTCTGGCTATGTGCCC-3′ for the second round PCR. Twenty cycles of denaturation at 94 °C for 15 s, annealing at 60 °C for 30 s and elongation at

72 °C for 1 min were performed followed by another 20 cycles with an annealing temperature of 57 °C. Purified PCR product was used to prepare sequencing templates using BigDye Terminator v3.1 reaction mix (Applied Biosystems, UK) and sequenced on an ABI 3730xl DNA Analyzer (Applied Biosystems, UK) by the Department of Zoology Sequencing Facility, University of Oxford. For clonal sequencing, purified PCR product was cloned into TOPO vectors using Zero Blunt TOPO PCR Cloning Kit (Invitrogen, UK) and used to transform chemically competent One Shot TOP10 *E. coli* cells (Invitrogen, UK) according to the manufacturers instructions. Where possible, clones were selected from two independent PCRs to avoid PCR amplification bias. Selected colonies were cultured overnight in LB broth before proceeding with mini-prep plasmid DNA extraction using Montage 96-well plasmid preparation kits (Millipore, US) according to the manufacturers instructions. Plasmid DNA was used for sequencing template preparation as described above.

Ultra-deep sequencing de novo assembly of consensus sequences and minor variant haplotype analysis

The full-length HIV genome was amplified in four fragments from plasma RNA using Superscript III One-Step RT PCR Kit with Platinum Taq High Fidelity enzyme (Invitrogen, UK) as previously described [9]. Sequencing of pooled amplicons was performed using Illumina MiSeq 250 bp paired-end technology. Quality control of reads was performed using QUASR (http://sourceforge.net/projects/quasr/) as previously described [6, 10, 11]. A de novo assembly was constructed using SPAdes version 2.4.0 [12] and a consensus sequence was generated using Abacas version 1.3.1 and MUMmer version 3.2 [13]. Haplotypes in the epitope regions were determined using *Vprofiler* [12] by selecting reads that span the epitope region and which contain only accepted variants.

Phylogenetic analysis and recombination detection

Maximum likelihood phylogenetic trees were constructed using Mega 6.06 software under the General Time Reversible model of nucleotide substitution as determined by jModelTest version 0.1.1 [14] with 1000 bootstrap replicates and viewed using FigTree v1.4.0 software. Recombination analysis was performed using RDP 4.46 (Recombination Detection Programme) [15] and SimPlot 3.5.1 [16].

Generation of recombinant *gag-protease* HIV virions and viral replicative capacity assays (VRC)

Recombinant viral vectors expressing autologous-*gag-protease* sequences from HLA-B*27:05/HLA-B*57:01+ individuals were constructed by transfecting *gag-protease* amplicons into the *Gag-Pro* deleted HIV backbone ΔGag-Pro NL4-3 as previously described [17, 18]. *Gag-protease* was amplified by nested PCR from plasma RNA using previously published primers [18]. The first round amplification was performed using Superscript III One-Step RT PCR Kit with Platinum Taq High Fidelity enzyme (Invitrogen, UK) followed by second round PCR using High Fidelity Platinum (Invitrogen, UK) according to the manufacturers' instructions. PCR product was purified using QIAquick PCR Purification Kit (Qiagen, UK) and sequenced by Sanger sequencing to confirm accurate amplification of the patient-derived *gag-protease* sequence.

The ΔGag-Pro NL4-3 was produced by introducing BstEII restriction enzyme sites on either side of the *gag-protease*-gene in NL4-3, followed by BstEII digest to delete *gag-protease* and allow self ligation of the plasmid [18]. For transfection, the plasmid was linearised by BstEII digest at 60 °C for 2 h. For each transfection, 2.5 μg of purified *gag-protease* amplicon and 10 μg of linearised ΔGag-Pro NL4-3 were co-transfected into 2 million CEM-GXR reporter cells [17, 19] by electroporation (300 V, 500 μF capacitance and infinite resistance). Recombinant viral cultures were expanded over 1 month and viral spread measure by GFP expression detected by flow cytometry. Viral supernatant was collected when > 30% of live cells were infected. Viral RNA extraction and *gag-protease* sequencing confirmed the correct sequence amplification of viral stocks. Viral titres were determined by infection of 1 million CEM-GXR cells with a standardized volume of viral supernatant and examining GFP expression after 48 h.

Viral replicative capacity assays (VRC): CEM-GXR cells were infected in triplicate at a low multiplicity of infection (0.025% GFP+ cells at day 2). GFP expression was monitored daily by flow cytometry over 12 days.

Logistic curve modelling of viral replicative capacity data
Viral growth curves were modeled on the logistic curve function:

$$y = m(x, \theta) + \varepsilon$$
$$= \theta_1 / 1 + \exp\left(-\theta_2 + \theta_3 x\right)$$

where θ_1 represents the asymptotic y point, θ_2 the midpoint, and θ_3 the scaling factor (rate of change) of the curve. Curves were fitted using the nonlinear regression nls function in R version 3.2.1, plotting the best fit logistic growth curve. To assess whether each parameter was statistically different when comparing curves, models were built where one of the parameters was fixed while the others were allowed to vary. A model where all parameters were allowed to vary was then fitted and a statistical

comparisons of parameters was made using ANOVA. The parameters used for the curves in Fig. 4 are shown in Additional file 1: Table 1, together with the statistics for the overall fit and for the separate parameters.

Sequence accession numbers
Sequence data has been deposited in Genbank under the accession numbers MF039091-MF039203.

Results
Rapid progression to AIDS in a transmission recipient expressing HLA-B*27:05/B*57:01
The starting point for this study was the MSM transmission pair R096/R097 (Fig. 1a, b). The transmission recipient, R097, expressed both HLA-B*27:05 and HLA-B*57:01, both of which are strongly associated with slow progression to AIDS. The viral load in R097 at diagnosis (time 0) was 65 HIV RNA copies/ml plasma and the absolute CD4+ T cell count was 950 cells/mm³, reflecting successful immune control of HIV. Over the next 2–3 years, however, despite the co-expression of HLA-B*27:05 and HLA-B*57:01, progression to AIDS (absolute CD4+ T cell < 200 cells/mm³) occurred rapidly, in association with viral loads increasing to > 10⁵ copies/ml. The donor R096 at time 0 had a viral load of 221,839 copies/ml and an absolute CD4+ T cell count of 260 cells/mm³ and initiated antiretroviral therapy (ART) at this time.

To investigate why disease had progressed so rapidly in R097, and to seek evidence to support the clinical history suggesting transmission from R096 to R097, we ultra-deep sequenced the virus in both individuals (Fig. 1c). Tight phylogenetic clustering of the viral sequences at 'time 0' in R096 and R097 strongly supported the notion that R096/R097 were a transmission pair. Viral sequences from R097 post-progression (2.0–3.4 years after 'time 0') clustered separately from the time 0 sequences. Gag sequences in R097 differed by 12% at the amino acid level in the 2 years from 'time 0' and Nef sequences by 26% at the amino acid level over this short time. These changes occurred in the context of a 12.5% nucleotide change across the full-length genome.

The direction of transmission from R096 to R097 was supported by the presence of virus encoding escape mutants in five HLA-B*51:01-restricted CTL epitopes in both subjects (Table 1). Since HLA-B*51:01 is expressed by R096 and not R097, this is consistent with the variant being selected initially in R096 and being transmitted to R097. In four of the HLA-B*51:01-restricted epitopes, the variant we observed was the one most commonly seen in association with HLA-B*51:01, a so-called HLA footprint [for example, I135T within the epitope TAFTIPSI (RT 128-135)] [20–22]. In contrast,

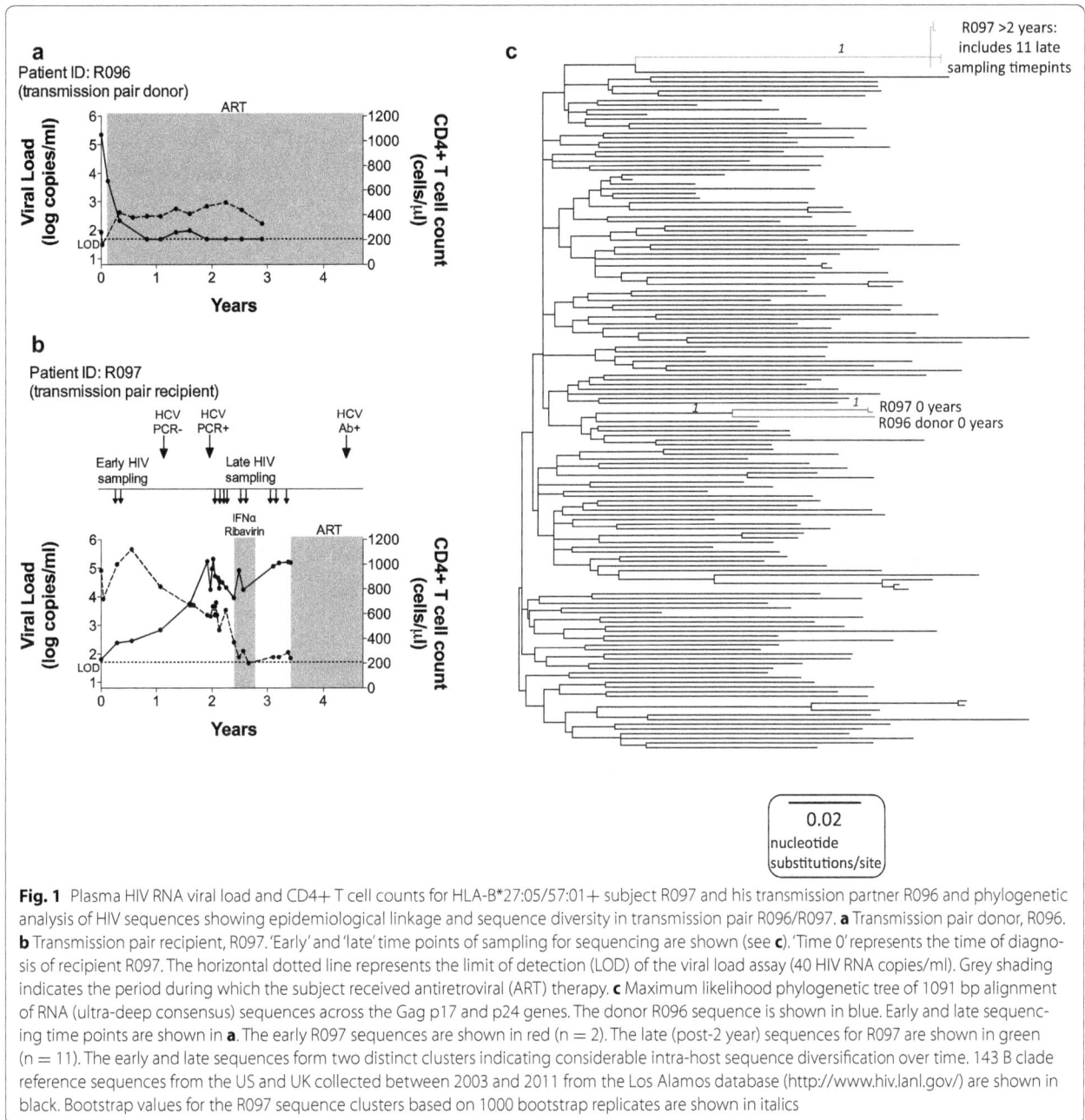

Fig. 1 Plasma HIV RNA viral load and CD4+ T cell counts for HLA-B*27:05/57:01+ subject R097 and his transmission partner R096 and phylogenetic analysis of HIV sequences showing epidemiological linkage and sequence diversity in transmission pair R096/R097. **a** Transmission pair donor, R096. **b** Transmission pair recipient, R097. 'Early' and 'late' time points of sampling for sequencing are shown (see **c**). 'Time 0' represents the time of diagnosis of recipient R097. The horizontal dotted line represents the limit of detection (LOD) of the viral load assay (40 HIV RNA copies/ml). Grey shading indicates the period during which the subject received antiretroviral (ART) therapy. **c** Maximum likelihood phylogenetic tree of 1091 bp alignment of RNA (ultra-deep consensus) sequences across the Gag p17 and p24 genes. The donor R096 sequence is shown in blue. Early and late sequencing time points are shown in **a**. The early R097 sequences are shown in red (n = 2). The late (post-2 year) sequences for R097 are shown in green (n = 11). The early and late sequences form two distinct clusters indicating considerable intra-host sequence diversification over time. 143 B clade reference sequences from the US and UK collected between 2003 and 2011 from the Los Alamos database (http://www.hiv.lanl.gov/) are shown in black. Bootstrap values for the R097 sequence clusters based on 1000 bootstrap replicates are shown in italics

no HLA-B*57:01 or HLA-B*27:05-associated mutants were observed in the 'time 0' sequences in R096 and R097 (Table 2). One variant L268I was shared by R096 and R097 at 'time 0', which lies within the HLA-B*27:05-restricted epitope KRWIILGLNK (Gag 263-272). However, this mutant is an HLA-B*08:01-associated variant flanking the overlapping HLA-B*08:01 epitope EIYKR-WII (Gag 260-267) [22] and thus is likely to have been originally selected in an HLA-B*08:01-positive subject prior to transmission to R096.

Mechanism of distinct phylogenetic clustering of R097 sequences following progression

Comparison of the viral sequences in R097 at 'time 0' and the cluster following progression 2.0–3.4 years later showed dramatic differences, prompting the hypothesis that R097 might have progressed as a consequence of HIV superinfection. To determine whether the dramatic sequence changes observed were likely to be the result of superinfection, or of multiple escape mutations being selected over a short period of time to give the

Table 1 HLA-B*51:01 and HLA-B*13:02 footprints in the recipient R097 sequence

HLA-B*51:01-associated footprints		HLA-B*13:02-associated footprints	
Gag	325NANPDCKTIL334	**Gag**	135VQNLQGQMV143 144HQAI148
R096 0 years	-S--------	R096 0 years	--------- ----
R097 0 years	-S--------	R097 0 years	--------- ----
Pol	63QRPLVTIKI71	**Gag**	429RQANFLGKI437
R096 0 years	-----S--V	R096 0 years	---------
R097 0 years	-----S--V	R097 0 years	---------
Pol	283TAFTIPSI290	**Pol**	113RQYDQILIEI122
R096 0 years	-------T	R096 0 years	------P---
R097 0 years	-------T	R097 0 years	-----VP---
Pol	743LPPVVAKEI751	**Pol**	519DVKQLTEAVQK529
R096 0 years	--S------	R096 0 years	-----------
R097 0 years	--S------	R097 0 years	---Q-------
Pol	768DKCQLKGEAM777	**Vpr**	61IRILQQLLF69
R096 0 years	----------	R096 0 years	---------
R097 0 years	----------	R097 0 years	---------
Vpr	29EAVRHFPRI37	**Nef**	21RRAEPAAD28
R096 0 years	--------P	R096 0 years	--T---EG
R097 0 years	--------P	R097 0 years	--T---EG
		Nef	106RQDILDLWV114
		R096 0 years	---------
		R097 0 years	---------

For each epitope the B clade consensus sequence is represented as the top line. The R096 (donor) sequence is represented on the middle line, and the R097 (recipient) sequence at time 0 on the bottom line. Polymorphisms that represent previously described HLA-associated footprints [22] underlined. Sequences where an HLA-associated footprint does not fall within a described epitope are shaded in grey

appearance of superinfection, we first sought evidence of escape within HLA-B*27:05 and HLA-B*57:01-restricted epitopes selected between 'time 0' and 2.0 years later (Table 2). In patient R097 between 'time 0' and 2.0 years later, we examined 17 HLA-B*27:05/57:01 epitopes previously shown to contain well-characterised footprints [22], and found escape mutants in 12 of these (one mutation being contained in two overlapping HLA-B*27:05 and HLA-B*57:01 epitopes in Vpr). Additional mutants were observed that were selected between 'time 0' and 2.0 years later in HLA-B*27:05/57:01 restricted epitopes, but where HLA footprints have not been described (for example in the HLA-B*27:05 epitope GRRGWEALKY). Thus a proportion of the amino acid differences between the 'time 0' sequence and the viral sequences post progression can be explained by the selection of escape mutants in R097. However this did not distinguish rapid selection of escape mutants from the possibility of superinfection with an HIV variant carrying multiple HLA-B*27:05 and HLA-B*57:01-associated escape variants.

To examine this further, we analysed the timing of selection of escape mutants in R097 using ultra-deep sequencing (Table 3). At 'time 0' in R097, many of the escape variants that had reached fixation 2.0 years later were already present at low frequencies. For example, Gag-A146P was present at 19%, Gag-T242N at 4%,

Gag-R264K at 3%, and Pol-T839N at 50% in R097 at 'time 0', and all were present at 99 or 100% 2.0 years later. Each of these variants were present in 0% of viruses in R096 at 'time 0'. These data are consistent with the rapid increase in frequency of escape mutations in multiple epitopes restricted by HLA-B*27:05 and HLA-B*57:01 in the 2 years after 'time 0', but clearly selection of escape mutants had already been initiated by 'time 0'.

However, two features of the sequence data argue strongly in favour of superinfection having occurred in R097. First, some of the escape mutants selected at 'time 0' and not shared at the 'time 2.0' timepoint, and vice versa, are relatively rare. Examples here are A248E (87% at 'time 0' and 0% at 'time 2.0'), which is a highly effective escape mutant [18], and S148T (0% at 'time 0' and 100% at 'time 2.0'). Both of these mutants are within HLA-B*57:01-restricted CTL epitopes, but they are not selected sufficiently often to be included as HLA-B*57:01-associated 'footprints' [22]. In contrast, many of the HLA-B*27:05/B*57:01-associated escape mutants present both at 'time 0' and 0% at 'time 2.0', such as T242N and R264K, are commonly observed footprints for these HLA alleles [22], and could easily have arisen independently in the two viruses in different subjects expressing HLA-B*27:05/57:01. Second, the number of amino acid differences between the viruses at 'time 0' and

Table 2   Donor R096 and recipient R097 viral sequences encoding HLA-B*27:05/B*57:01-restricted epitopes

HLA-B*57-restricted epitope	
Gag-ISW9	[146]A ISPRTLNAW[155]
R096 0 years	- ---------
R097 0 years	- ---------
R097 2 years	P LT-------
Gag-KF11	[162]KAFSPEVIPMF[172]
R096 0 years	----------
R097 0 years	----------
R097 2 years	----------
Gag-TW10	[240]TSTLQEQIGW[249]
R096 0 years	----------
R097 0 years	--------E-
R097 2 years	--N-------
Pol-ISW9	[399]IVLPEKDSW[407]
R096 0 years	---------
R097 0 years	-Q--D----
R097 2 years	-E-------
Pol-IW9	[530]IATESIVIW[538]
R096 0 years	---------
R097 0 years	---------
R097 2 years	--L------
Pol-SW10	[838]STTVKAACWW[847]
R096 0 years	----------
R097 0 years	-NA-------
R097 2 years	-N--------
Vif-IF9	[31]ISKKAKGWF[39]
R096 0 years	------R-V
R097 0 years	------D--
R097 2 years	T-R---D-R
Vif-HL9	[73]HTGERDWHL[81]
R096 0 years	-----E---
R097 0 years	Q--------
R097 2 years	Q--------
Vpr-AW9/AL10	[30]AVRHFPRIW[38] L[39]
R096 0 years	-------P- -
R097 0 years	-------P- -
R097 2 years	--------- -

HLA-B*57...	
Rev-KY10	[14]KTVRLIKFLY[23]
R096 0 years	---------H
R097 0 years	-----V-R--
R097 2 years	-----V-R--
Nef-KF9	[82]KAAVDLSHF[90]
R096 0 years	-G-L-----
R097 0 years	-G-F---F-
R097 2 years	-G-L-----
Nef-HW9	[116]HTQGYFPDW[124]
R096 0 years	---------
R097 0 years	not resolved
R097 2 years	N--------

HLA-B*27-restricted epitope	
Gag-KK10	[263]KRWIILGLNK[272]
R096 0 years	------I----
R097 0 years	------I----
R097 2 years	-K--------
Gag-QK10	[379]QRGNFRNQRK[388]
R096 0 years	-K--------
R097 0 years	-K--------
R097 2 years	-K--------
Pol-KY9	[901]KRKGGIGGY[909]
R096 0 years	---------
R097 0 years	---------
R097 2 years	---------
Vpr-VL9	[31]VRHFPRIWL[39]
R096 0 years	------P--
R097 0 years	------P--
R097 2 years	---------
Nef-RV10	[105]RRQDILDLWV[114]
R096 0 years	Q---------
R097 0 years	K--E------
R097 2 years	----------

Epitopes showing evidence of CTL driven evolution in R097 are highlighted in grey

at 'time 2.0' across the full-length proteomes numbered 810. Less than 3% of these amino acid changes (19/810) can be ascribed to escape arising within epitopes that are restricted by the HLA alleles expressed by R097. Thus the dramatic sequence changes observed in R097 between 'time 0' and 0% at 'time 2.0' cannot have been driven by CTL escape alone, but are consistent with HIV superinfection.

HCV co-infection as an additional explanation for rapid immunological escape

Having established that HIV superinfection was likely to account for the rapid evolutionary changes in HIV sequences and disease progression in subject R097, we

considered alternative explanations for the uncharacteristic speed of progression in an HLA B*27/B*57-positive individual. At the time of peak HIV viraemia (time 2.0 years) the recipient was diagnosed with hepatitis C virus (HCV) genotype 1a co-infection by PCR (viral load 4.03 log copies/ml), although his HCV antibody test remained negative for a further 2.5 years before he finally seroconverted. An HCV RNA test 10 months earlier (that is, 14 months after 'time 0') had been negative. He went on to receive treatment with IFNα/Ribavirin for 24 weeks, starting 5 months after the HCV diagnosis was made, although this did not result in clearance. Although HCV coinfection typically accelerates disease progression in HIV infection [23], in subject R097, as

Table 3 Ultra-deep RNA sequencing of HLA-B*57:01 and HLA-B*27:05-restricted epitopes and associated compensatory positions from R097 and his transmission partner R096

HLA Class I Restriction and Epitope	B Clade Consensus and Autologous Variants	Donor R096 (HLA-B*13:02/B*51:01)	Recipient R097 (HLA-B*27:05/57:01)											
		0 Years	0 Years	2 Years	2.1 Years	2.2 Years	2.25 Years	2.3 Years	2.4 Years	2.6 Years	2.7 Years	3.1 Years	3.2 Years	3.4 Years
HLA-B*57 Gag-IW9	147ISPRTLNAW155	98	86	0	0	0	0	0	0	0	0	0	2	
	L--------	2	*14*	0	0	0	1	0	0	7	13	9	14	
	LT-------	0	0	99	99	100	50	3	0	7	8	35	44	
	-T-------	0	0	0	0	0	48	96	99	86	78	55	41	
	146A	99	80	0	0	0	0	0	0	0	0	0	0	0
	P	0	*19*	99	99	100	99	99	99	99	99	100	99	76
	S	0	0	0	0	0	0	0	0	0	0	0	0	24
HLA-B*57 Gag-KF11	162KAFSPEVIPMF172	100	100	99	98	100	100	100	100	100	99	100	100	100
HLA-B*57 Gag-TW10	240TSTLQEQIGW249	96	6	0	0	0	0	0	0	0	0	0	0	0
	--------A-	3	0	0	0	0	0	0	0	0	0	0	0	0
	--------E-	0	87	0	0	0	0	0	0	0	0	0	0	0
	--N------	0	*4*	100	100	98	99	98	100	99	99	99	100	100
	--N-----N-	0	*3*	0	0	0	0	0	0	0	0	0	0	0
	219H 223I 226M	100	90	0	0	0	0	0	0	0	0	0	0	0
	H V M	0	*10*	93	94	95	97	97	98	99	99	99	99	99
	H A M	0	0	6	6	4	3	2	2	0	0	0	0	0
HLA-B*27 Gag-KK10	263KRWIILGLNK272	17	5	0	0	1	0	0	0	0	0	0	0	0
	-----I----	83	92	0	0	0	0	0	0	0	0	0	0	0
	-K--------	0	*3*	100	100	99	100	100	100	100	100	100	100	100
	173S	0	0	0	0	0	0	0	0	0	0	0	0	0
	T	98	87	0	0	0	0	0	0	0	0	0	0	0
	A	0	*10*	99	99	99	99	99	99	99	99	99	100	99
HLA-B*57 Pol-SW10	838STTVKAACWW847	98	0	0	0	0	0	3		0	0	0	0	0
	-N--------	0	*50*	74	86	57	69	63		53	60	76	81	100
	--A-------	0	50	0	0	4	0	2		0	0	0	0	0
	-A--------	0	0	24	13	38	30	32		45	39	23	18	0
	-AM-------	0	0	0	0	0	0	0		1	0	0	0	0

Depth of coverage ranges from 46 to 85,000 reads. Epitopes at which predictable footprints [22] are selected in the donor are shown. The early selection of escape and compensatory mutations in the minor variant populations are shown in bold italics

described above, escape mutants in multiple HIV-specific HLA-B*27:05- and HLA-B*57:01-restricted epitopes had already been selected, and the viral load was on an upward trajectory, more than a year prior to the HCV infection. Nonetheless, it is evident that HIV superinfection occurred either simultaneous with, or weeks-to-months before, HCV co-infection. In either case, HCV co-infected is likely to have accelerated the speed of progression to AIDS in this subject.

Lack of sequence diversification in an HLA-B*27:05/57:01-positive non-progressor

To contrast the speed and extent of viral escape in the HLA-B*27:05/57:01-positive rapid progressor, R097, even before superinfection had occurred, with the sequence changes that might be expected in a non-progressor, we analysed *gag* viral sequences over a 10-year period in an ART-naive HLA-B*27:05/57:01-positive individual RI088, whose viral loads remained at < 1000 copies/ml, and at < 40 copies/ml for much of this period (Fig. 2). In this instance, viral sequence diversification was negligible with 1.1% difference in Gag at the amino acid level over 10 years. In contrast, we saw a 12% difference at the amino acid level in Gag over 2 years in the rapid progressor R097. Analysis of viral sequence at the clonal level in RI088 (Table 4, Additional file 2: Figure 1) shows

that escape mutants were generated periodically but not always selected. For example, the most commonly selected variant, T242N, within the HLA-B*57:01 epitope TSTLQEQIGW (Gag 240–249), reached a frequency of 55% 1.4 years after diagnosis, but subsequently declined to 0% (at 3.4 years) before being selected later. Variants within KF11 and KK10 were observed transiently and at low frequencies. The relative lack of sequence change in the virus in RI088 is also reflected in persistence of CTL responses, such as to the HLA-B*27:05-restricted Gag epitope KK10 and the HLA-B*57:01-restricted Nef epitope HW9 (Fig. 3). In contrast, although these same responses are present at 'time 0' in R097, they declined in association with the selection of escape (Fig. 3).

Progression to AIDS in subject R097 associated with increasing viral replicative capacity

One of the mechanisms that has been proposed for HLA-B*27:05 and HLA-B*57:01-mediated protection against progression to HIV disease is the observation that the Gag escape mutations associated with these HLA molecules significantly reduce viral replicative capacity [5, 24–27]. Thus, even if the virus succeeds in evading the effective Gag-specific CTL responses restricted by HLA-B*27:05/57:01, the cost of reduced VRC facilitates maintained control of HIV through other immune responses

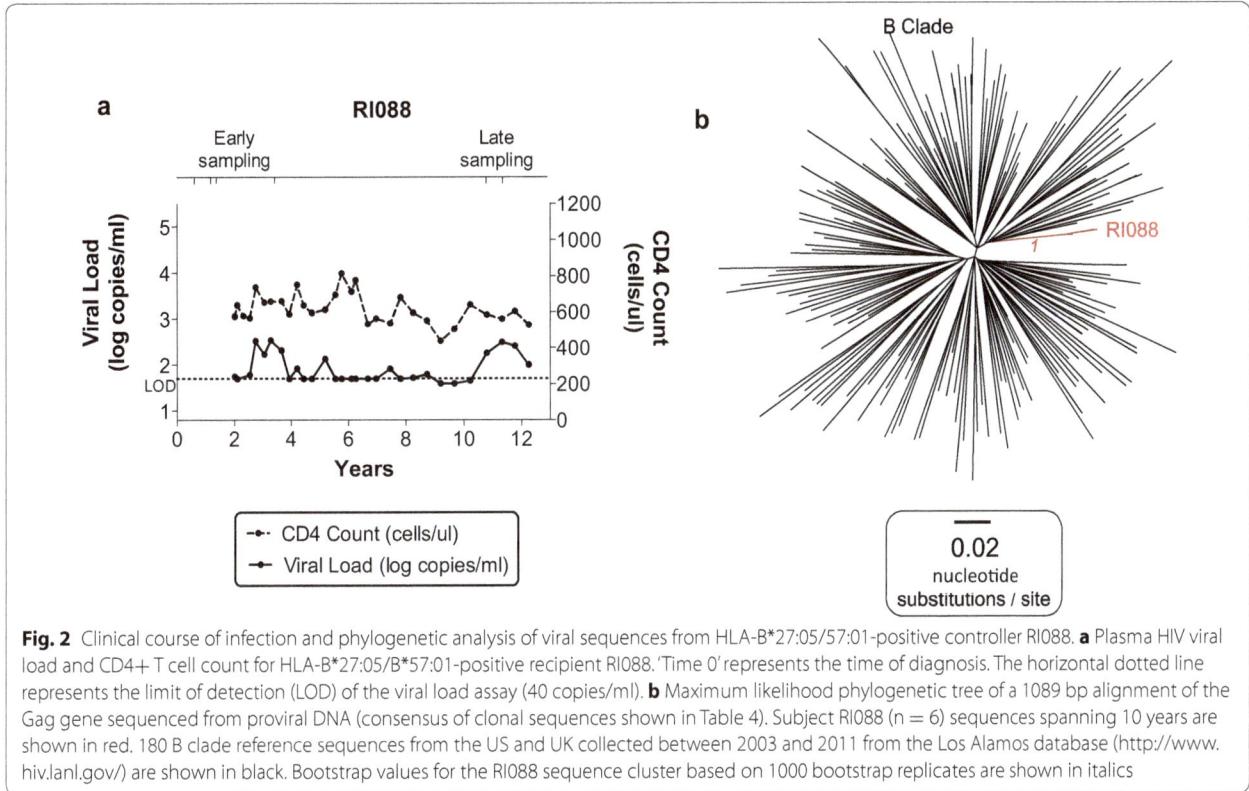

Fig. 2 Clinical course of infection and phylogenetic analysis of viral sequences from HLA-B*27:05/57:01-positive controller RI088. **a** Plasma HIV viral load and CD4+ T cell count for HLA-B*27:05/B*57:01-positive recipient RI088. 'Time 0' represents the time of diagnosis. The horizontal dotted line represents the limit of detection (LOD) of the viral load assay (40 copies/ml). **b** Maximum likelihood phylogenetic tree of a 1089 bp alignment of the Gag gene sequenced from proviral DNA (consensus of clonal sequences shown in Table 4). Subject RI088 (n = 6) sequences spanning 10 years are shown in red. 180 B clade reference sequences from the US and UK collected between 2003 and 2011 from the Los Alamos database (http://www.hiv.lanl.gov/) are shown in black. Bootstrap values for the RI088 sequence cluster based on 1000 bootstrap replicates are shown in italics

Table 4 Clonal Sequencing of HIV proviral DNA at HLA-B*57:01 and HLA-B*27:05-restricted Gag epitopes from controller RI088

Years Since Diagnosis	Number of clones sequenced	Number of Independent PCRs	146A ISPRTLNAW155	%	162KAFSPEVIPMF172	%	240TSTLQEQIGW249	%	263KRWIILGLNK272	%
					HLA-B*57:01-Restricted Epitopes				HLA-B*27:05-Restricted Epitopes	
0.6	17	1	- ----------	100	----------	100	---------- I---------	94 6	----------	100
1.2	17	2	- ---------- P L--------	88 12	---------- ------T--- -------L-- ------M---	82 6 6 6	---------- --N------- ----R-----	82 12 6	----------	100
1.4	20	2	P L-------- - ---------- - T---A---- - -------S--	55 35 5 5	---------- --------T-	95 5	--N------- ----------	55 45	---------- ---V------ ----V-----	90 5 5
3.4	6	1	- ---------- - --T------	83 17	---------- ------M---	83 17	----------	100	----------	100
10.8	26	2	P --A------ P --A---S--	92 8	---------- ----------I	96 4%	--N-------	100	----------	100
11.3	17	2	P --A------	100	---------- --------T- --------V-	88 6% 6%	--N------- --NP------	94 6	----------	100

The number of clones sequenced at each timepoint and number of independent PCR reactions from which PCR product was cloned are given. The percentage of clones with each sequence haplotype is shown. The most prevalent (consensus) epitope sequence is shown in black. Lower frequency variant sequences are shown in grey.

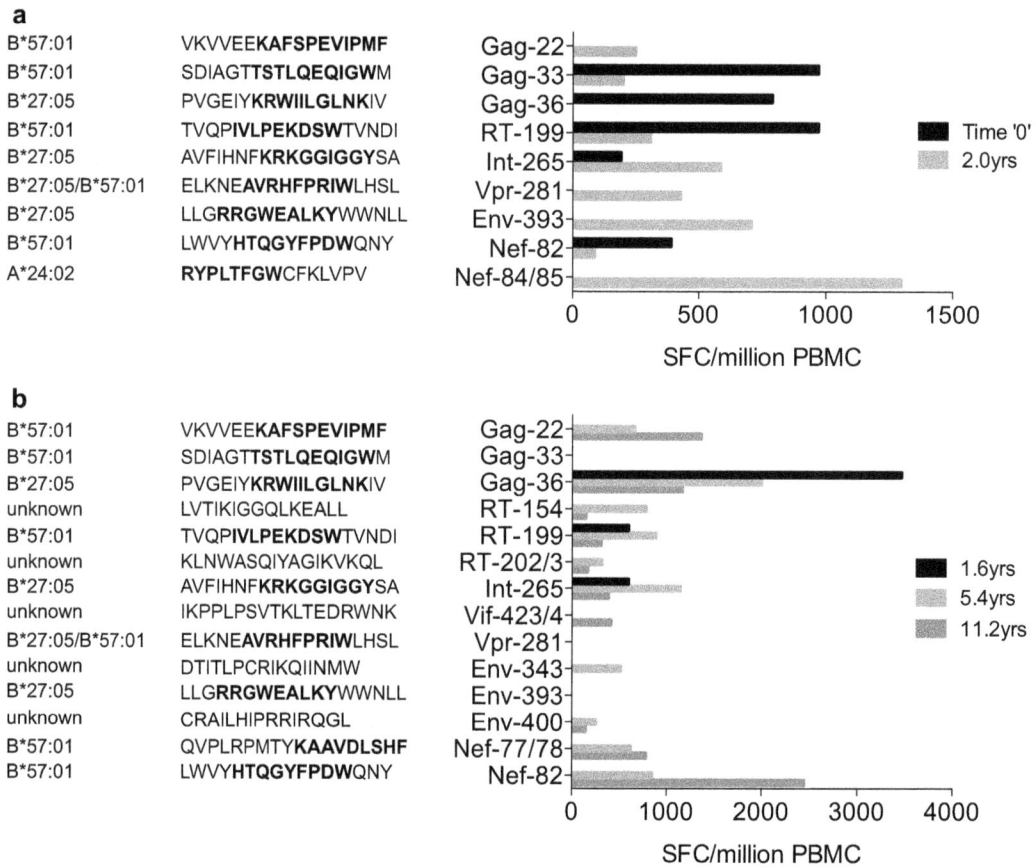

Fig. 3 HIV-specific CTL responses in progressor R097 and in non-progressor RI088. EliSpot assays tested recognition of overlapping 18mer peptides, which together spanned the B clade proteome. The figure includes the full sequence of each 18mer peptide recognised and the HLA restriction where known, with known optimal epitopes shown in bold. **a** EliSpot responses detected in progressor R097 at time 0 (diagnosis) and 2.0 years later. Data shown at 2.0 years are the median of 3 assays undertaken at 1.96, 1.98 and 2.15 years after time 0. No responses were detected to the 18mer peptides containing the epitopes ISPRTLNAW or STTVKAACWW at either timepoint. **b** Responses detected in non-progressor RI088 at the times shown post diagnosis. Selected peptides that were strongly recognized in R097 but not in RI088 are included in panel B

from which the virus has not escaped. However, it is also well-described that reductions in viral replicative capacity resulting from selection of certain escape mutants are typically mitigated, to a varying degree, by selection of alternative escape mutants [28] and the co-selection of compensatory mutants [27, 29–31]. To investigate whether VRC was substantially reduced in the face of the selection of, or superinfection by a virus carrying, multiple Gag escape mutants in R097, we generated chimeric viruses comprising NL4-3 and the autologous *gag-pro* sequence from R097 (Fig. 4a). At 'time 0', when the viral load was low and the CD4+ T cell count was high, the VRC in R097 was substantially lower than both NL4-3 wildtype and 'time 0' R096 virus. However, during the course of progression, the VRC ultimately had increased to an intermediate level (at 3.4 years after 'time 0'), reflecting some successful correction of fitness costs of

escape variants by compensatory mutants or by the selection of alternative, higher fitness escape mutants. In contrast, although in the case of RI088 the transmitted virus was not known, the lack of multiple Gag escape mutants in RI088 appeared to have little impact on VRC compared to wildtype NL4-3 (Fig. 4b). These data are consistent with previous findings that the HLA-B*27:05- and HLA-B*57:01-associated escape mutants in Gag reduce viral replicative capacity, but even a relatively disabled virus can drive rapid progression to AIDS in the absence of effective HIV-specific CD8+ T cell activity.

Discussion

We here describe two HIV-infected adults who express both HLA-B*27:05 and HLA-B*57:01, the most protective HLA class molecules against HIV disease progression, one of whom is a typical long-term non-progressor,

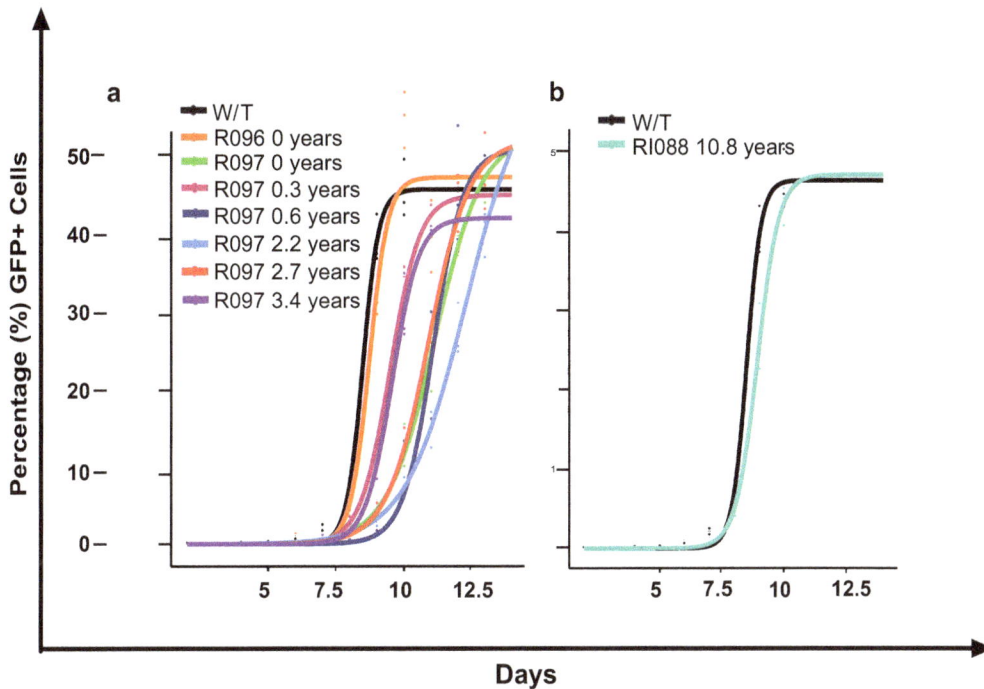

Fig. 4 Viral replicative capacity (VRC) of recombinant viruses produced from autologous *gag-pro* from HLA-B*27:05/B*57:01-positive subjects. VRC of *gag-pro* chimeric virus derived from **a** longitudinal sampling of progressor R097 and his transmission partner R096; and **b** controller RI088. VRC is given by the percentage of infected (GFP-expressing) target cells

maintaining low-to-undetectable viral loads over more than a decade of follow up, whilst the other is a rapid progressor, whose CD4+ T cell decline from immune control of HIV to AIDS occurs within a period of 3 years. In the rapid progressor studied here, we have shown using ultra-deep sequencing that escape mutations were selected in early infection across several of the known HLA-B*27:05 and HLA-B*57:01 epitopes, from the earliest timepoint when the CD4+ T cell count was 950 cells/mm^3 and viral load was 65 copies/ml, preceding loss of immune control. However, the most dramatic viral sequence changes observed in this subject, coincident with rapid progression to AIDS, were associated with superinfection with a virus whose ancestry is substantially different from the original transmitted strain of HIV. Although many of the classical HLA-B*27:05 and HLA-B*57:01 'footprints' [22] were present both pre- and post-superinfection, these commonly arise predictably and independently in individuals expressing these HLA molecules, and > 96% of amino acid changes were unrelated to CTL-driven escape.

In contrast, very little viral sequence change occurred over more than a decade in the non-progressor. Clonal sequencing reveals that escape mutants were generated all of this time, but in the majority of instances these were not selected. Finally, analysis of the viral replicative capacity (VRC) of the viruses in the two subjects revealed that differential rates of progression were not explained by lower VRC in the non-progressor. On the contrary, rapid progression occurred despite reductions in VRC in the subject with progressive disease.

Approximately 16% of Caucasians express HLA-B*27:05 and/or HLA-B*57:01 and ~ 60% of Caucasian elite controllers—approximately 0.3% of infected individuals overall [18]—express one or the other of these alleles [18]. Therefore, only a minority of individuals expressing HLA-B*27:05 and/or HLA-B*57:01—approximately 2%—become elite controllers, for reasons which remain unclear. Factors proposed to explain differential outcome in subjects with matched HLA-B allele expression may be categorised as immunological, genetic and virological. Immunological factors include breadth of the Gag-specific CTL response [3], avidity of the T cell receptor for the peptide-MHC complex [32], and ability of the TCR repertoire to recognise potential escape variants [33]. Genetic factors include the HLA-A and HLA-C [34, 35] and KIR alleles expressed [36], and the presence of CCR5 variants such as the delta-32 mutant [37]. Virological factors include replicative capacity of the transmitted virus and pre-adaptation of the transmitted virus to the HLA class I molecules expressed in the transmission recipient [38–41].

A further influence on HIV disease outcome is the introduction of co-infection with another blood-borne virus. HCV may skew the immunological response to HIV, for example by increasing immune activation [42]. The immunological influence of HCV therapy on HIV is complex, as exemplified by the APRICOT study in which HCV/HIV co-infected patients receiving IFNα had a 1.0 log reduction in HIV viral load, but also a reduction in absolute CD4+ T cell counts [43]. In the patient we describe here, it is likely that intercurrent acute HCV infection (and/or IFN-based therapy) may have contributed to HIV progression. However, this co-infection cannot explain the whole picture as changes in CD4+ T cell count and HIV viral load that herald progression to AIDS were already evident before the HCV infection occurred, and also the extent of the sequence changes observed can only be explained by HIV superinfection.

In the case of the rapid progressor, the observation that several escape mutations were selected very early in the course of infection (prior to 'time 0') illustrates that the presence of a broad HIV-specific immune response does not provide complete protection against escape. Indeed, at the initial timepoint, when the CD4+ T cell count was 950 cells/mm^3 and the HIV viral load was 65 copies/ml, five CTL responses were detectable (Fig. 3). Perhaps more significant is the observation of variants being generated in viral sequences derived from the non-progressor RI088 that did not get selected. Taken together with the data showing the relatively high viral replicative capacity of virus derived from RI088 compared to the R097 viruses, these findings are consistent with the quality of individual key HIV-specific responses being critical to outcome. These two case reports cannot provide definitive information on which specificities are most important to immune control, but are consistent with numerous previous studies indicating that the HLA-B*27:05-KK10 response plays a vital role in immune control of HIV in subjects expressing HLA-B*27:05.

The influence of genetic factors other than the HLA-B type has not been evaluated in these two study subjects. Although HLA-A and HLA-C alleles can influence immune control of HIV, HLA-B alleles have a greater impact than HLA-A or HLA-C [1, 35, 44]. The HLA-A alleles expressed by the progressor (A*11:01/24:02) and non-progressor (A*01:01/03:01) have not been associated with differential disease outcome and the HLA-C alleles expressed (C*02:02/06:02) were the same in both subjects.

The changes in viral replicative capacity over time in R097 are of interest, showing an initial significant decrease in VRC as the B27/57 escape mutants are selected, and then a partial recovery towards the VRC of the original infecting strain from R096. These findings are consistent

with many studies that have shown the ability of the virus to limit the cost of escape mutants either via the selection of alternative escape mutants [28] and/or the co-selection of compensatory mutants [27, 30, 31, 45–50]. However, although the VRC returns towards normal, it remains well below that of the original transmitted virus. In contrast, the VRC of the virus in the elite controller remains very close to the reference NL4-3 despite more than a decade of strong selection pressure on the virus.

Conclusions

The description here of two HIV-infected subjects expressing both HLA-B*27:05 and HLA-B*57:01 with differential disease outcomes demonstrates the rapidity with which progression can occur, even when HIV-specific CTL responses restricted by these protective alleles are present. In this report rapid progression occurred following HIV superinfection. However, only a small minority of subjects expressing protective HLA alleles remain non-progressors. Consistent with previous studies, qualitative aspects of the HIV-specific CTL response are likely to play a critical part in maintaining long-term immune control of HIV infection.

Additional files

Additional file 1: Table 1. The parameters used for the curves shown in Figure 4, together with the statistics for the overall fit and for the separate parameters.

Additional file 2: Fig. 1. Phylogenetic analysis of clonal HIV sequences from RI088. Maximum likelihood phylogenetic tree of 1091bp alignment of clonal DNA sequences across the Gag p17 and p24 genes. RI088 sequences are shown in colour (0.6 years in purple, 1.2 years in pink, 1.4 years in green, 3.4 years in orange, 10.8 years in blue, 11.3 years in red). 143 B B clade reference sequences from the US and UK collected between 2003 and 2011 from the Los Alamos database (https://www.hiv.lanl.gov/) are shown in black. Bootstrap values based on 1000 bootstrap replicates are shown in italics.

Abbreviations

AIDS: acquired immunodeficiency syndrome; ART: antiretroviral therapy; CTL: cytotoxic T lymphocyte; DNA: deoxyribonucleic acid; ELISpot: enzyme-linked immunosorbent spot assay; Gag: group-specific antigen (capsid protein); HCV: hepatitis C virus; HIV: human immunodeficiency virus; HLA: human leukocyte antigen; IFN: interferon; LOD: limit of detection; MHC: major histocompatibility complex; MSM: men who have sex with men; Nef: negative regulatory factor protein; PCR: polymerase chain reaction; RNA: ribonucleic acid; RT: reverse transcription; VRC: viral replicative capacity.

Rapid HIV disease progression following superinfection in an HLA-B*27:05/B*57:01-positive transmission...

85

Authors' contributions

JB carried out experimental work, data analysis and contributed to manuscript preparation. Ultra-deep sequencing was performed in collaboration with AG and PK. AG performed the de novo assembly of consensus sequences. RB performed minor variant sequence haplotype analysis. JH designed the logistic curve models for analysing VRC data. NL contributed to clonal sequencing. FC and AE recruited the study participants. CB and RD contributed to sequence data analysis. OP interpreted phylogenetic data. PM supervised the study and contributed to manuscript preparation. PG conceived and supervised the study and prepared manuscript text. All authors read and approved the final manuscript.

Author details

[1] Department of Paediatrics, University of Oxford, Oxford, UK. [2] Department of Veterinary Medicine, University of Cambridge, Cambridge, UK. [3] Wellcome Trust Sanger Institute, Wellcome Trust Genome Campus, Hinxton, Cambridge, UK. [4] Nuffield Department of Medicine, University of Oxford, Oxford, UK. [5] Ragon Institute of MGH, MIT and Harvard, Boston, MA, USA. [6] Department of Sexual Health, Royal Berkshire Hospital, Reading, UK. [7] Department of GU Medicine, The Churchill Hospital, Oxford University NHS Foundation Trust, Oxford, UK. [8] Department of Zoology, University of Oxford, Oxford, UK. [9] Division of Infection and Immunity, University College London, Gower Street, London, UK.

Acknowledgements

Not applicable.

Competing interests

The authors declare that they have no competing interests.

Funding

This work was funded by grants from the National Institutes of Health (RO1AI46995 to PJRG), the Wellcome Trust (WT104748MA to PJRG), PCM received salary support from NIHR and the Wellcome Trust (Grant Number 110110/Z/15/Z), JB received support from the Commonwealth Scholarship Commission and Oppenheimer Memorial Trust. OP was funded by the ERC under European Research Council Grant Agreement Number 614725-PATHPHYLODYN.

References

1. Pereyra F, Jia X, McLaren PJ, Telenti A, de Bakker PIW, Walker BD, et al. The major genetic determinants of HIV-1 control affect HLA class I peptide presentation. Science (80-). 2010;330:1551–7.
2. Goulder PJR, Walker BD. HIV and HLA class I: an evolving relationship. Immunity. 2012;37:426–40.
3. Kiepiela P, Ngumbela K, Thobakgale C, Ramduth D, Honeyborne I, Moodley E, et al. CD8+ T-cell responses to different HIV proteins have discordant associations with viral load. Nat Med. 2007;13:46–53.
4. Deng K, Pertea M, Rongvaux A, Wang L, Durand CM, Ghiaur G, et al. Broad CTL response is required to clear latent HIV-1 due to dominance of escape mutations. Nature. 2015;517:381–5.
5. Payne RP, Kløverpris H, Sacha JB, Brumme Z, Brumme C, Buus S, et al. Efficacious early antiviral activity of HIV Gag- and Pol-specific HLA-B 2705-restricted CD8+ T cells. J Virol. 2010;84:10543–57.
6. Brener J, Gall A, Batorsky R, Riddell L, Buus S, Leitman E, et al. Disease progression despite protective HLA expression in an HIV-infected transmission pair. Retrovirology. 2015;12:55.
7. Cano P, Klitz W, Mack SJ, Maiers M, Marsh SGE, Noreen H, et al. Common and well-documented HLA alleles: report of the ad-hoc committee of the American Society for Histocompatiblity and Immunogenetics. Hum Immunol. 2007;68:392–417.
8. Addo MM, Yu XG, Rathod A, Cohen D, Eldridge RL, Strick D, et al. Comprehensive epitope analysis of human immunodeficiency virus type 1 (HIV-1)-specific T-cell responses directed against the entire expressed HIV-1 genome demonstrate broadly directed responses, but no correlation to viral load. J Virol. 2003;77:2081–92.
9. Gall A, Ferns B, Morris C, Watson S, Cotten M, Robinson M, et al. Universal amplification, next-generation sequencing and assembly of HIV-1 genomes. J Clin Microbiol. 2012;50:3838–44.
10. Bentley DR, Balasubramanian S, Swerdlow HP, Smith GP, Milton J, Brown CG, et al. Accurate whole human genome sequencing using reversible terminator chemistry. Nature. 2008;456:53–9.
11. Gall A, Morris C, Kellam P. Complete genome sequence of the WHO international standard for HIV-1 RNA determined by deep sequencing. Genome Announc. 2014;2:10–1.
12. Henn MR, Boutwell CL, Charlebois P, Lennon NJ, Power K, Macalalad AR, et al. Whole genome deep sequencing of HIV-1 reveals the impact of early minor variants upon immune recognition during acute infection. PLoS Pathog. 2012;8:e1002529.
13. Kurtz S, Phillippy A, Delcher AL, Smoot M, Shumway M, Antonescu C, et al. Versatile and open software for comparing large genomes. Genome Biol. 2004;5:R12.
14. Posada D. jModelTest: phylogenetic model averaging. Mol Biol Evol. 2008;25:1253–6.
15. Martin DP, Murrell B, Golden M, Khoosal A, Muhire B. RDP4: detection and analysis of recombination patterns in virus genomes. Virus Evol. 2015;1:1.
16. Lole KS, Bollinger RC, Paranjape RS, Gadkari D, Kulkarni SS, Novak NG, et al. Full-length human immunodeficiency virus type 1 genomes from subtype C-infected seroconverters in India, with evidence of intersubtype recombination. J Virol. 1999;73:152–60.
17. Brockman M, Tanzi GO, Walker BD, Allen TM. Use of a novel GFP reporter cell line to examine replication capacity of CXCR4- and CCR5-tropic HIV-1 by flow cytometry. J Virol Methods. 2006;131:134–42.
18. Miura T, Brockman MA, Brumme ZL, Brumme CJ, Pereyra F, Trocha A, et al. HLA-associated alterations in replication capacity of chimeric NL4-3 viruses carrying gag-protease from elite controllers of human immunodeficiency virus type 1. J Virol. 2009;83:140–9.
19. Gervaix A, West D, Leoni LM, Richman DD, Wong-Staal F, Corbeil J. A new reporter cell line to monitor HIV infection and drug susceptibility in vitro. Proc Natl Acad Sci. 1997;94:4653–8.
20. Tomiyama H, Sakaguchi T, Miwa K, Oka S, Iwamoto A, Kaneko Y, et al. Identification of multiple HIV-1 CTL epitopes presented by HLA-B*5101 molecules. Hum Immunol. 1999;60:177–86.
21. Kawashima Y, Pfafferott K, Frater J, Matthews P, Payne R, Addo M, et al. Adaptation of HIV-1 to human leukocyte antigen class I. Nature. 2009;458:641–5.
22. Carlson JM, Brumme CJ, Martin E, Listgarten J, Brockman M, Le AQ, et al. Correlates of protective cellular immunity revealed by analysis of population-level immune escape pathways in HIV-1. J Virol. 2012;86:13202–16.
23. Matthews PC, Geretti AM, Goulder PJR, Klenerman P. Epidemiology and impact of HIV coinfection with hepatitis B and hepatitis C viruses in Sub-Saharan Africa. J Clin Virol. 2014;61:1–14.
24. Martinez-picado J, Prado JG, Fry EE, Pfafferott K, Leslie A, Chetty S, et al. Fitness cost of escape mutations in p24 gag in association with control of human immunodeficiency virus type 1. J Virol. 2006;80:3617–23.
25. Leslie AJ, Pfafferott KJ, Chetty P, Draenert R, Addo MM, Feeney M, et al. HIV evolution: CTL escape mutation and reversion after transmission. Nat Med. 2004;10:282–9.
26. Crawford H, Lumm W, Leslie A, Schaefer M, Boeras D, Prado JG, et al. Evolution of HLA-B*5703 HIV-1 escape mutations in HLA-B*5703-positive individuals and their transmission recipients. J Exp Med. 2009;206:909–21.
27. Schneidewind A, Brockman MA, Yang R, Adam RI, Li B, Le Gall S, et al. Escape from the dominant HLA-B27-restricted cytotoxic T-lymphocyte response in Gag is associated with a dramatic reduction in human immunodeficiency virus type 1 replication. J Virol. 2007;81:12382–93.
28. Goonetilleke N, Liu MKP, Salazar-Gonzalez JF, Ferrari G, Giorgi E, Ganusov VV, et al. The first T cell response to transmitted/founder virus

contributes to the control of acute viremia in HIV-1 infection. J Exp Med. 2009;206:1253–72.

29. Schneidewind A, Brumme ZL, Brumme CJ, Power KA, Reyor LL, O'Sullivan K, et al. Transmission and long-term stability of compensated CD8 escape mutations. J Virol. 2009;83:3993–7.

30. Crawford H, Prado JG, Leslie A, Hué S, Honeyborne I, Reddy S, et al. Compensatory mutation partially restores fitness and delays reversion of escape mutation within the immunodominant HLA-B*5703-restricted Gag epitope in chronic human immunodeficiency virus type 1 infection. J Virol. 2007;81:8346–51.

31. Wright JK, Naidoo VL, Brumme ZL, Prince JL, Claiborne DT, Goulder PJR, et al. Impact of HLA-B*81-associated mutations in HIV-1 gag on viral replication capacity. J Virol. 2012;86:3193–9.

32. Almeida JR, Price D, Papagno L, Arkoub ZA, Sauce D, Bornstein E, et al. Superior control of HIV-1 replication by CD8+ T cells is reflected by their avidity, polyfunctionality, and clonal turnover. J Exp Med. 2007;204:2473–85.

33. Chen H, Ndhlovu ZM, Liu D, Porter LC, Fang JW, Darko S, et al. TCR clono-types modulate the protective effect of HLA class I molecules in HIV-1 infection. Nat Immunol. 2012;13:691–700.

34. Pereyra F, Addo MM, Kaufmann DE, Liu Y, Miura T, Rathod A, et al. Genetic and immunologic heterogeneity among persons who control HIV infec-tion in the absence of therapy. J Infect Dis. 2008;197:563–71.

35. Apps R, Qi Y, Carlson JM, Chen H, Gao X, Thomas R, et al. Influence of HLA-C expression level on HIV control. Science. 2013;340:87–91.

36. Martin MP, Qi Y, Gao X, Yamada E, Martin JN, Pereyra F, et al. Innate partnership of HLA-B and KIR3DL1 subtypes against HIV-1. Nat Genet. 2007;39:733–40.

37. Dean M, Carrington M, Winkler C, Huttley GA, Smith MW, Allikmets R, et al. Genetic restriction of HIV-1 infection and progression to AIDS by a dele-tion allele of the CKR5 structural gene. Science (80-). 1996;273:1856–62.

38. Carlson JM, Du VY, Pfeifer N, Bansal A, Tan VYF, Power K, et al. Impact of pre-adapted HIV transmission. Nat Med. 2016;22:606–13.

39. Claiborne DT, Prince JL, Scully E, Macharia G, Micci L, Lawson B, et al. Replicative fitness of transmitted HIV-1 drives acute immune activation, proviral load in memory CD4+ T cells, and disease progression. Proc Natl Acad Sci. 2015;112:E1480–9.

40. Goepfert PA, Lumm W, Farmer P, Matthews P, Prendergast A, Carlson JM, et al. Transmission of HIV-1 Gag immune escape mutations is associated with reduced viral load in linked recipients. J Exp Med. 2008;205:1009–17.

41. Prince JL, Claiborne DT, Carlson JM, Schaefer M, Yu T, Lahki S, et al. Role of transmitted Gag CTL polymorphisms in defining replicative capacity and early HIV-1 pathogenesis. PLoS Pathog. 2012;8:e1003041.

42. Gonzalez VD, Falconer K, Blom KG, Reichard O, Morn B, Laursen AL, et al. High levels of chronic immune activation in the T-cell compartments of patients coinfected with hepatitis C virus and human immunodeficiency virus type 1 and on highly active antiretroviral therapy are reverted by alpha interferon and ribavirin treatment. J Virol. 2009;83:11407–11.

43. Torriani FJ, Rodriguez-Torres M, Rockstroh JK, Lissen E, Gonzalez-Garcia J, Lazzarin A, et al. Peginterferon Alfa-2a plus ribavirin for chronic hepatitis C virus infection in HIV-infected patients. N Engl J Med. 2004;351:438–50.

44. Kiepiela P, Leslie AJ, Honeyborne I, Ramduth D, Thobakgale C, Chetty S, et al. Dominant influence of HLA-B in mediating the potential co-evolution of HIV and HLA. Nature. 2004;432:769–75.

45. Schneidewind A, Brockman MA, Sidney J, Wang YE, Chen H, Suscovich TJ, et al. Structural and functional constraints limit options for cytotoxic T-lymphocyte escape in the immunodominant HLA-B27-restricted epitope in human immunodeficiency virus type 1 capsid. J Virol. 2008;82:5594–605.

46. Rolland M, Carlson JM, Manocheewa S, Swain JV, Lanxon-Cookson E, Deng W, et al. Amino-acid co-variation in HIV-1 Gag subtype C: HLA-mediated selection pressure and compensatory dynamics. PLoS ONE. 2010;5:e12463.

47. Brockman MA, Brumme ZL, Brumme CJ, Miura T, Sela J, Rosato PC, et al. Early selection in Gag by protective HLA alleles contributes to reduced HIV-1 replication capacity that may be largely compensated for in chronic infection. J Virol. 2010;84:11937–49.

48. Crawford H, Matthews PC, Schaefer M, Carlson JM, Leslie A, Kilembe W, et al. The hypervariable HIV-1 capsid protein residues comprise HLA-driven CD8+ T-cell escape mutations and covarying HLA-independent polymorphisms. J Virol. 2011;85:1384–90.

49. Huang KHG, Goedhals D, Carlson JM, Brockman MA, Mishra S, Brumme ZL, et al. Progression to AIDS in South Africa is associated with both reverting and compensatory viral mutations. PLoS ONE. 2011;6:e19018.

50. Tsai M-H, Muenchhoff M, Adland E, Carlqvist A, Roider J, Cole DK, et al. Paediatric non-progression following grandmother-to-child HIV transmis-sion. Retrovirology. 2016;13:65.

7

Engineering multi-specific antibodies against HIV-1

Neal N. Padte, Jian Yu, Yaoxing Huang and David D. Ho*

Abstract

As increasing numbers of broadly neutralizing monoclonal antibodies (mAbs) against HIV-1 enter clinical trials, it is becoming evident that combinations of mAbs are necessary to block infection by the diverse array of globally circulating HIV-1 strains and to limit the emergence of resistant viruses. Multi-specific antibodies, in which two or more HIV-1 entry-targeting moieties are engineered into a single molecule, have expanded rapidly in recent years and offer an attractive solution that can improve neutralization breadth and erect a higher barrier against viral resistance. In some unique cases, multi-specific HIV-1 antibodies have demonstrated vastly improved antiviral potency due to increased avidity or enhanced spatiotemporal functional activity. This review will describe the recent advancements in the HIV-1 field in engineering monoclonal, bispecific and trispecific antibodies with enhanced breadth and potency against HIV-1. A case study will also be presented as an example of the developmental challenges these multi-specific antibodies may face on their path to the clinic. The tremendous potential of multi-specific antibodies against the HIV-1 epidemic is readily evident. Creativity in their discovery and engineering, and acumen during their development, will be the true determinant of their success in reducing HIV-1 infection and disease.

Keywords: HIV-1, Bispecific antibody, Trispecific antibody, Multi-specific antibody, Neutralizing antibody, Passive immunization

Background

The past decade has introduced a new generation of potent and broad neutralizing monoclonal antibodies (mAbs) against HIV-1 [1–10], several of which have entered the clinic recently [11–17]. This resurgence of promising HIV-1 mAbs has energized the field of passive immunization and propelled the testing of existing mAbs as treatment, particularly because of their long half-lives as compared to existing oral antiretroviral options. The high degree of HIV-1 envelope (Env) diversity, however, requires further improvements to these mAbs to better ensure their clinical utility. For example, viral resistance can rapidly evade antiviral pressure from a single mAb treatment [11, 12, 14, 18, 19], and a large fraction of circulating HIV-1 already exhibit pre-existing resistance to many of the antibodies currently in development [20–22].

HIV-1 mAbs directed to more conserved components of the viral entry process, such as ibalizumab, which binds to the CD4 receptor on T-cells [23], and PRO140, which binds to the CCR5 co-receptor [24], broadly neutralize a greater fraction of circulating HIV-1 than Env-targeting mAbs [20, 25]. Indeed, ibalizumab (Trogarzo®) has recently become the first mAb against HIV-1 to receive FDA approval and is currently indicated for use as salvage therapy in patients whose viruses are resistant to multiple existing antiretroviral drugs [26, 27]. PRO140 is currently in a Phase 2b/3 pivotal trial in heavily treatment-experienced HIV-1 patients [28]. However, these promising antibodies must be used in combination with other antiretroviral agents to limit emerging viral resistance. While the newer generation of Env-targeting mAbs that have recently entered Phase 1 trials are more potent and broad than earlier generations of HIV-1 Env-targeting mAbs, they still face these same issues of viral resistance unless they can be administered in combinations, and this costly undertaking could limit their practical feasibility, particularly in the setting of HIV-1 prevention in

*Correspondence: dho@adarc.org
Aaron Diamond AIDS Research Center, The Rockefeller University, 455
First Avenue, New York, NY 10016, USA

under-resourced nations [29]. Engineering antibodies for greater HIV-1 neutralization and breadth, particular by the creation of bispecific and trispecific antibodies, and for improved in vitro stability and in vivo pharmacokinetics, has the potential to drastically reduce the amount of antibody required for efficacy in humans, and may put the goal of an efficacious HIV-1 prevention and therapeutic antibody strategy within reach.

Engineering mAbs to improve potency and breadth against HIV-1

One strategy to improve HIV-1 mAbs is to use structure-guided design to develop rationally engineered antibody variants with improved antiviral properties. Many of the engineering principles applied to these HIV-1 mAbs were also incorporated into the investigational studies to engineer multi-specific antibodies reviewed in this article, and therefore a short summary of these structure-guided engineering approaches for HIV-1 mAbs will be reviewed first.

Engineering CD4 binding site mAbs

The HIV-1 CD4 binding site antibody NIH45–46 was identified as a more potent clonal variant of VRC01 [6, 10]. Structural studies determined that NIH45–46 lacked a critical interaction to a hydrophobic pocket between the gp120 bridging sheet and outer domain that is typically occupied by a phenylalanine on CD4, and it was reasoned that a hydrophobic residue at position 54 on NIH45–46 could improve its interaction with gp120. After engineering one of a series of hydrophobic residues at this position 54, the variant NIH45–46^{G54W} was found to increase contact with the gp120 bridging sheet and improved its neutralization potency by tenfold [30].

VRC07, another somatic variant of VRC01, was engineered with improved binding to the HIV-1 CD4 binding site by incorporating a histidine mutation at the G54 position of this antibody (the same position as that mutated in NIH45–46^{G54W}). VRC07 was also engineered with several mutations in its light chain to increase solubility and to remove a potential N-linked glycosylation site, which together resulted in a 7.9-fold enhancement in potency as compared to VRC01 and with reduced autoreactivity as compared to NIH45–46^{G54W} [5]. A variant of VRC07-523 engineered to have a longer half-life in vivo (VRC07-523-LS) demonstrated protective efficacy at one-fifth of the dose of VRC01-LS in a non-human primate model, and is currently in Phase 1 clinical evaluation [16].

Engineering MPER binding site mAbs

A similar approach to improve antibody solubility and potency was taken for the gp41 membrane proximal external region (MPER) binding antibody, 10E8 [3]. 10E8 was identified from an HIV-1 infected individual and is one of the broadest antibodies reported to date, neutralizing >95% of circulating HIV-1 strains. However, 10E8 is naturally prone to aggregation, which limited its clinical manufacturability potential. By identifying somatic variants of 10E8 with inherently better solubility, and then using structural data to mutate a hydrophobic patch distal from the binding site of this antibody, a significantly more soluble variant of 10E8 was obtained [31]. Because germline variants often exhibit reduced potency compared to their affinity matured antibody counterparts, residues from 10E8 critical for binding to MPER were then grafted onto this more soluble antibody. The new 10E8 variants retained the improved solubility but now also exhibited potency similar to the originally identified 10E8. The top variants, 10E8v4 and 10E8v5, exhibited improved pharmacokinetic profiles in mice and rhesus macaques as compared to 10E8, and 10E8v5 has been advanced for clinical evaluation [32]. An additional 10E8v4 variant, known as 10E8v4-5R + 100cF, was recently reported to improve the potency of 10E8v4 by an additional ~10-fold using a surface-matrix screening approach [33].

Engineering a CD4-targeting mAb

In addition to engineering antibodies for improved solubility and potency against HIV-1, improved breadth of neutralization against circulating HIV-1 strains has also been demonstrated, which has the potential to erect a higher genetic barrier to viral resistance. The aforementioned CD4-targeting antibody, ibalizumab, already demonstrated favorable potency and breadth against circulating HIV-1 strains [20]. It neutralized 92% of viruses tested in vitro as assessed by $\geq 50\%$ neutralization, but only neutralized 66% of viruses when assessed as $\geq 80\%$ inhibition. This indicated that a significant fraction of circulating viruses may be able to escape complete neutralization. These studies revealed a strong correlation between HIV-1 resistance to ibalizumab and a loss of a V5 glycan on the viral envelope. In a separate study in HIV-1 infected patients in which ibalizumab monotherapy was added to failing drug regimens, a transient decrease in viral load was followed by evolution of resistant HIV-1 variants with a similar loss of a V5 glycosylation site [19]. Taken together with epitope mapping and X-ray crystallography structural studies used to define the ibalizumab-CD4 binding interface [34, 35], it was hypothesized that the loss of the HIV-1 V5 glycan provided the viral envelope more flexibility to circumvent the steric hindrance induced by ibalizumab. To address this deficiency in ibalizumab, a panel of variants was engineered with glycans added to the ibalizumab light chain at positions predicted to sterically fill the empty space created by the loss of V5 glycan in the resistant viruses [36]. These modified glycan variants were able to neutralize HIV-1 strains previously resistant to ibalizumab, and the top variant, known as LM52, neutralized 100% of circulating HIV-1 strains tested as assessed by $\geq 80\%$ neutralization, and at a potency ~ 5- to 10-fold better than wild-type ibalizumab. LM52 is currently in preclinical development in preparation for clinical evaluation [37].

The examples presented above demonstrate how structure-guided approaches and rational design, in combination with germline antibody identification, can improve the potency, breadth and solubility of multiple antibodies against HIV-1, and several of these are currently in preclinical or clinical development. However, even with these improvements, the dynamics of HIV-1 viral replication and the rapid mutation rate of HIV-1 require these antibodies be used in combinations in order to limit the emergence of resistant viruses in a treatment setting and in order to block infection by a diverse range of circulating subtypes in a prevention setting. While such combinations of antibodies are currently being explored [22], the high cost of development and delivery of these biologic combinations has the potential to limit their widespread use, necessitating alternative solutions.

Engineering multi-specific antibodies to improve breadth against HIV-1

The idea that multi-specific antibodies could improve upon the functional activities of single mAbs or combinations of mAbs originated in the cancer therapy field in the mid-1980s, primarily as a way to direct effector cells toward tumor cells [38–40]. As a result, the majority of bispecific antibodies currently under clinical evaluation today are for the treatment of various cancers [41]. The need for multi-specific antibodies for HIV-1 prevention and treatment, however, is readily evident. Multiple HIV-1 targeting epitopes can be incorporated into one antibody-like molecule, allowing for increased neutralization breadth against diverse HIV-1 strains and thereby also erecting a higher genetic barrier for viral resistance. Additionally, the large array of multi-specific antibody formats currently available [42] allow the tailoring of any particular combination of HIV-1 targeting antibody moieties by a number of structural properties such as size, distance, and valency in order to meet the requirements of viral inhibition.

Engineering bispecific antibodies with improved breadth
One example of a bispecific antibody that can enhance neutralization breadth is iMabm36 [43], which inhibits HIV-1 entry by targeting CD4, via ibalizumab (iMab), and the gp120 co-receptor binding site, via the antibody

domain m36. This bispecific antibody is generated by genetically linking m36 to the C-terminus of the ibalizumab heavy chain (Fig. 1a). As stated earlier, ibalizumab neutralizes 66% of viruses when assessed as $\geq 80\%$ inhibition, indicating a significant fraction of circulating viruses may escape complete neutralization by ibalizumab. In contrast, the bispecific antibody iMabm36 neutralized 87% of viruses as defined by $\geq 80\%$ inhibition, indicating a substantial improvement in neutralization breadth. This is attributed to the presence of two distinct HIV-1 entry inhibiting antibody domains within the same molecule. Improved antiviral activity was dependent on both the CD4-binding activity of the iMab component as well as the gp120 coreceptor-binding activity of the m36 component, as knocking out the activity of either of these components within the iMab36 molecule greatly reduced its antiviral activity. The linker length between the m36 antibody domain and the C-terminus of the iMab heavy chain also affected the antiviral activity of the bispecific antibody, suggesting that the flexibility and position of the fused domains relative to one another are also important for the functional activity of iMabm36.

In a separate line of study, a panel of bispecific antibodies was engineered in which one of several gp120-targeting single-chain variable fragments (scFv) was fused to the N-terminus or C-terminus of the ibalizumab heavy chain (Fig. 1b, c) [44]. A number of variations of this format were also engineered, including those which inverted the orientation of variable domains within the scFv (for example, V_H followed by V_L, or V_L followed by V_H), and those which varied the linker lengths between the V_H and V_L domains within each scFv or between the scFv domains and the ibalizumab heavy chain. Interestingly, the binding and neutralization activity of each of these bispecific antibody variants varied widely, and the most optimal format in terms of V_H and V_L orientation and linker lengths differed depending on which HIV-1 Env-targeting scFv was fused to ibalizumab. Therefore, identifying an optimal bispecific antibody format and design, even within the context of structure-guided rational design of HIV-1 antibody-epitope pairings, is still an empirical process.

Ibalizumab fused to gp120 CD4 binding site antibodies, such as VRC01, NIH45–46^{G54W}, or 3BNC60, neutralized > 99% of circulating HIV-1 strains tested, as assessed by $\geq 50\%$ neutralization, and with a geometric mean IC$_{50}$ ranging from 0.025 to 0.031 µg/mL. These bispecific antibodies also neutralized > 97% of strains tested, as assessed by $\geq 80\%$ inhibition, with a geometric mean IC$_{80}$ ranging from 0.076 to 0.092 µg/mL. This significant enhancement in neutralization breadth when ibalizumab was fused to each of these gp120 CD4 binding site antibodies indicates that these sets of parental antibody pairings could prove

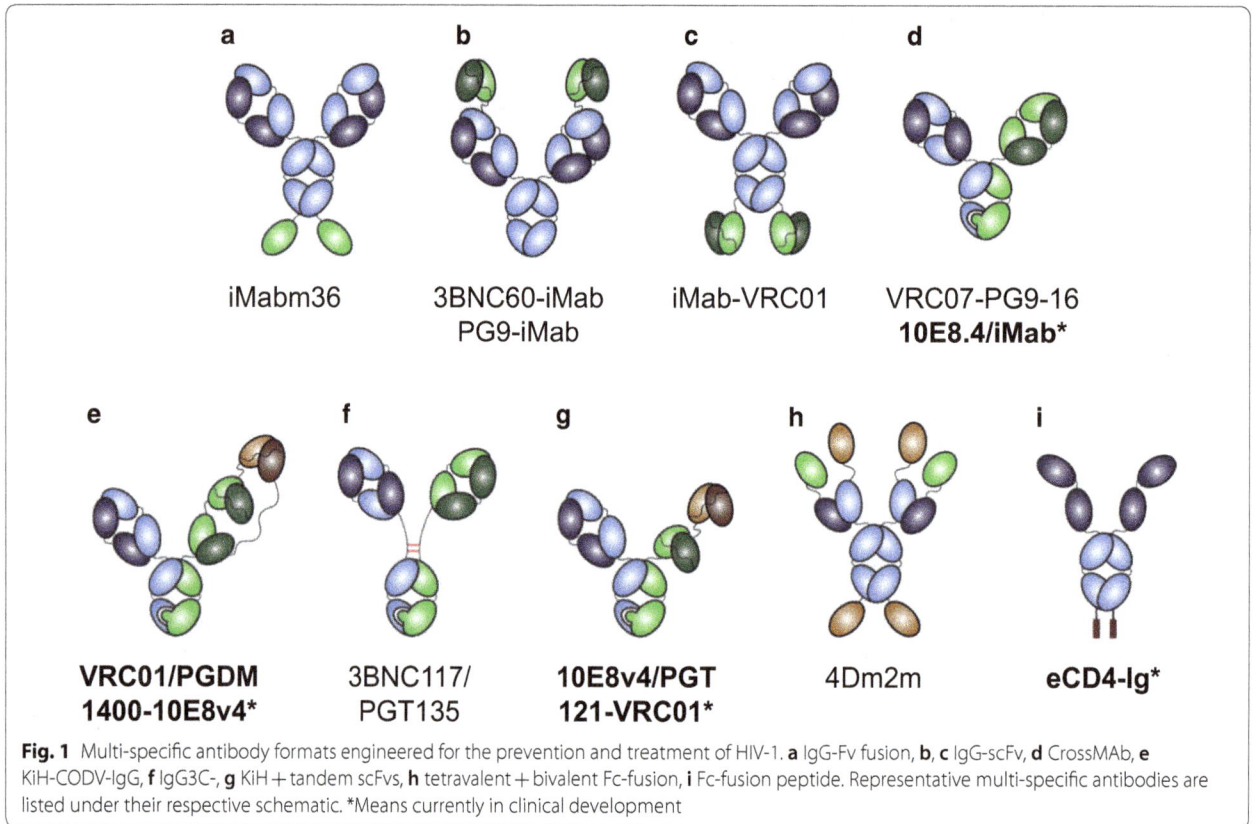

Fig. 1 Multi-specific antibody formats engineered for the prevention and treatment of HIV-1. **a** IgG-Fv fusion, **b, c** IgG-scFv, **d** CrossMAb, **e** KiH-CODV-IgG, **f** IgG3C-, **g** KiH + tandem scFvs, **h** tetravalent + bivalent Fc-fusion, **i** Fc-fusion peptide. Representative multi-specific antibodies are listed under their respective schematic. *Means currently in clinical development

optimal in neutralizing a diverse sequence of circulating HIV-1 strains. Indeed, as mentioned earlier, a strong correlation was observed between HIV-1 resistance to ibalizumab and a loss of a V5 glycan on the viral envelope [20] and, in contrast, resistance to VRC01 involves the presence of bulky V5 residues [45]. Therefore, by combining two antibodies with complimentary resistance profiles into a single bispecific antibody, tremendous enhancements in neutralization breadth at or close to 100% can be achieved.

The CrossMAb format for engineering bispecific antibodies, originally developed by Roche, has also been utilized for HIV-1 antibody development in recent years. The CrossMAb format allows for correct assembly of two heavy chains and two light chains from different antibodies into one bispecific antibody molecule that resembles a typical monoclonal antibody in terms of mass and architecture, and with no artificial linkers required (Fig. 1d) [46]. This is achieved by combining the knob-into-hole technology, which enables heterodimerization of two different heavy chains, and the light chain crossover technology, which ensures correct association of each of the light chains with their cognate heavy chains.

In one study, CrossMAb antibodies targeting four major HIV-1 Env epitopes known to be important for

HIV-1 neutralization, the CD4 binding site, V3 glycan, V1V2, and MPER regions, were engineered [47]. These HIV-1 CrossMAb bispecific antibodies neutralized 95–97% of circulating HIV-1 strains tested, and the most promising candidate from this study, VRC07-PG9-16, neutralized the panel of viruses with a median IC_{50} of 0.055 µg/mL. This represented an improvement in neutralization breadth and coverage over the single parental mAbs from which VRC07-PG9-16 was derived, and was similar in breadth and potency to the co-administration of the two parental mAbs, which was not the case for all of the bispecific antibodies engineered and evaluated.

Engineering trispecific antibodies with improved breadth

It is now well known that the highly dynamic nature of HIV-1 replication in vivo demands treating HIV-1 with three antiretroviral agents simultaneously since viral escape against any single agent is an inevitable consequence of the large number of HIV-1 mutants generated per day within an infected person [48–50]. With this in mind, the continuous evolution of HIV-1 Env during the course of infection also attests to the exceptional selective pressure exerted by naturally elicited virus-specific antibodies [51]. Therefore, trispecific antibodies with the potential to inhibit viral entry with three distinct HIV-1

Env-targeting antibody moieties was of interest. In one study, the trispecific antibodies VRC01/PGDM1400-10E8v4 and N6/PGDM1400-10E8v4 were engineered using a knob-in hole (KiH) heterodimerization technology [52] and a cross-over dual variable immunoglobulin G (CODV-Ig) technology to ensure affinity of each variable region was maintained [53] in order to target the HIV-1 envelope CD4 binding site, MPER and V2 glycan site (Fig. 1e) [54]. Multiple combinations of broadly neutralizing parental antibodies and formats were tested before downselecting VRC01/PGDM1400-10E8v4 and N6/PGDM1400-10E8v4, which demonstrated 98% and > 99% breadth, respectively, as defined by ≥ 50% neutralization. Surface plasmon resonance confirmed that each of the three antibody-targeting domains within VRC01/PGDM1400-10E8v4 had comparable affinities for its HIV-1 Env antigens relative to its parental Fab counterparts. VRC01/PGDM1400-10E8v4 also provided 100% protection to nonhuman primates challenged mucosally with a mixture of two SHIVs, SHIV 325C and SHIV BaLP4, which each had varying sensitivities to two of the parental mAb counterparts of VRC01/PGDM1400-10E8v4, while only 62% and 75% of nonhuman primates administered VRC01 or PGDM1400, respectively, were protected in this model. Therefore, the improvement in neutralization breadth observed by VRC01/PGDM1400-10E8v4 in vitro translated to an improved breadth of protection against SHIV in vivo.

While the bispecific and trispecific antibodies discussed above enhanced HIV-1 neutralization breadth relative to their parental mAb counterparts, they were limited in their ability to enhance potency relative to the parental mAbs provided individually or in combination. This is thought to be due, in part, to the low spike density of gp160 trimers on the surface of HIV-1 [55–57], which may limit the ability of these bispecific and trispecific antibodies to bind to the HIV-1 envelope bivalently (or trivalently in the case of a trispecific antibody) through inter-spike crosslinking. The gp160 trimer spike structure itself may also limit the ability of these multi-specific antibodies to achieve intra-spike crosslinking [55, 56]. While antibodies elicited naturally during HIV-1 infection also typically interact monovalently with the HIV-1 gp160 trimer spike, polyreactive antibodies have been proposed to be positively selected and retained during affinity maturation and can increase their overall apparent affinity for HIV-1 Env through heteroligation [58]. The VRC07-PG9-16 CrossMAb discussed earlier can achieve a potency similar to, but not better than, the most potent of its parental mAbs against any particular virus, and this is thought to be due to an inability of VRC07-PG9-16 to simultaneously bind both of its epitopes on the HIV-1 Env trimer [47]. If multivalent binding of these bispecific

or trispecific antibodies was possible, one could imagine that a significant enhancement in antiviral potency could be gained in addition to enhanced breadth.

Engineering multi-specific antibodies to improve breadth and potency against HIV-1

One study has investigated the importance of this potential for enhanced HIV-1 neutralization by inter- and intra-spike binding by using DNA as a "molecular ruler" that has a HIV-1 Env binding antibody domain conjugated to each end [59]. By increasing or decreasing the number of basepairs (bp) between two Fabs of either 3BNC60 [6] or VRC01 [10], homo-dimer Fabs with different lengths of "reach" were used to probe the distance needed to achieve avidity as opposed to single arm Fab binding. These studies revealed that a length of ~ 60 bp resulted in ~ 100-fold increased potency for either 3BNC60 or VRC01 homo-diFabs against the specific HIV-1 strain tested, likely due to bivalent binding to two CD4 binding sites within a single gp120 trimer. Hetero-diFabs also exhibited enhanced potency as compared to combinations of their monoclonal antibody counterparts. For example, a PG16-3BNC60 diFab, targeting both V1V2 and the CD4 binding site in a single gp120 trimer, enhanced neutralization potency by ~ 100-fold when a 50 bp double-stranded (ds) DNA bridge was used to separate these two Fabs. The 50–60 bp ds DNA bridges in these molecules represent a reach distance of ~ 17–21 nm between the two Fabs in a single molecule, which is longer than the ~ 12–15 nm reach of two Fab arms in a typical IgG molecule [55]. While the molecular flexibility and dynamics that may be associated with an antibody binding to either the open or closed HIV-1 Envelope trimer may somewhat alter these distances in a case-dependent manner, it is generally thought that the reach between the two Fab arms in a HIV-1 multi-specific antibody would need to be larger than that within a typical IgG in order to capture the benefits of avidity and multivalent binding. These DNA diFab constructs provide an elegant method to investigate the science underlying antibody avidity to HIV-1 Env, but are not readily translatable to product development and clinical use.

All of the bispecific antibodies discussed until now have utilized an IgG1 or IgG4 subtype, based on their intended mechanism of action. Another subclass, IgG3, possesses a relatively longer and more flexible hinge domain region [60, 61], which may allow for the greater "reach" needed to achieve bivalent binding of a bispecific antibody against HIV-1 Env. To test this, a small panel of CrossMAb format HIV-1 bispecific antibodies were generated in which the typical IgG1 hinge domain was replaced with a longer and more flexible IgG3 hinge-like region called IgG3C- (Fig. 1f) [62]. One of these

IgG3C- hinge variants that targeted the CD4 binding site and V3 region of the HIV-1 envelope, 3BNC117/PGT135, exhibited both superior breadth (93% as defined by 50% inhibition and 89.1% as defined by 80% inhibition) and superior potency (IC_{50} geometric mean of 0.036 μg/mL and IC_{80} geometric mean of 0.159 μg/mL) relative to its single parental mAbs or the predicted combination of both parental mAbs. Variants in which the IgG3C- hinge length of 3BNC117/PGT135 were decreased resulted in decreased neutralization activity. Combined with structural data modeling 3BNC117 and PGT135 Fabs complexed with the Env trimer, this suggests that the IgG3C- hinge variant of 3BNC117/PGT135 may allow for bivalent binding, enhanced avidity, and ultimately greater potency relative to its parental mAb counterparts. No differences in the pharmacokinetic profile of this bispecific antibody were observed in mice in comparison to typical mAbs, and a 1.5 $\log_{10}$ decrease in viral load was observed in a humanized mouse model for HIV-1 treatment. In comparison, treatment with a mixture of the 3BNC117 and PGT135 parental mAbs yielded very little change in viral loads.

Another study reported the engineering of trispecific antibodies in order to increase "reach" and improve HIV-1 neutralization breadth and potency. Using scFv domains connected in tandem with flexible linkers, different formats of scFv domains targeting the HIV-1 CD4 binding site, V3, and MPER regions were engineered and characterized for their ability to improve antiviral activity and HIV-1 Env binding avidity (Fig. 1g). From these studies, 10E8v4/PGT121-VRC01 emerged as the most promising trispecific antibody candidate, exhibiting 99.5% breadth, as defined by 50% inhibition, an IC_{50} geometric mean of 0.069, and an IC_{80} geometric mean of 0.298 μg/mL [63]. Biolayer interferometry was used to confirm that all three scFv domains in this trispecific antibody could bind to their cognate HIV-1 Env epitopes, and it is suggested that the four-fold enhancement in potency of 10E8v4/PGT121-VRC01 relative to its parental mAbs is due to the cooperative effect of binding to at least two epitopes simultaneously on the HIV-1 Env trimer.

In addition to bispecific and trispecific antibody formats, smaller Fc fusion proteins have also been engineered with the goal of improving potency by enabling bispecific avidity. 4Dm2m is comprised of a single domain of soluble CD4, known as mD1.22, fused to the N- and C-termini of a human IgG1 heavy chain constant region, and an antibody domain targeting the coreceptor binding site on gp120, known as m36.4, fused to the N-terminus of the human antibody light chain constant region via a glycine-serine linker (Fig. 1h) [64, 65]. This bispecific multivalent fusion protein neutralized all HIV-1 isolates tested with a potency about 10-fold higher than the CD4 binding site antibody, VRC01. The authors reasoned that the improvement in potency between 4Dm2m and a variant with m36.4 only at the N-termini, known as 2Dm2m, was due to bivalent binding of both the head and tail m36.4 antibody domains in 4Dm2m and the relative close proximity of the CD4 binding site and coreceptor binding site on gp120.

eCD4-Ig is a fusion of CD4-Ig, which itself is comprised of CD4 domains 1 and 2 fused to Fc, and a small CCR5-mimetic sulfopeptide (Fig. 1i) [66]. eCD4-Ig neutralized 100% of a diverse panel of circulating HIV-1 strains, and could also neutralize HIV-2 strains, and this outstanding antiviral breadth is thought to be due to the relatively well conserved nature of the CD4 binding site and CCR5 coreceptor binding site epitopes on HIV-1 Env. A structural model of eCD4-Ig bound to the HIV-1 Env trimer predicts that both the CD4-Ig and CCR5-mimetic sulfopeptide bind avidly and cooperatively to HIV-1. This would support the high potency of eCD4-Ig, neutralizing a panel of HIV-1 with a geometric mean of < 0.05 μg/mL, as defined by 50% inhibition. eCD4-Ig variants neutralized each particular HIV-1 strain tested with a potency 10- to >200-fold better than CD4-Ig alone. A rhesus version of one of the bispecific fusion variants, known as rh-eCD4-IgG2^{I39N,mim2}, was cloned into an adeno-associated virus serotype 2 (AAV2) vector and, when co-administered with a separate single-stranded AAV vector expressing rhesus tyrosine-protein sulfotransferase to promote rh-eCD4-Ig sulfation, provided 100% protection against repeated SHIV-AD8 challenges. Recently, an improved variant of eCD4-Ig that utilized mD1.22, the stabilized form of CD4 domain 1 discussed earlier, was shown to improve the potency of this bispecific fusion peptide by another 9-fold while maintaining satisfactory production efficiency [67].

The antibodies discussed above demonstrate the principle that engineering multi-specific antibodies against HIV-1 for increased avidity can increase their antiviral potency and breadth. However, the large divergence in HIV-1 Envs and their relative dynamic nature pose a challenge to identifying multi-specific molecules with sufficient reach to consistently interact with target epitopes across diverse HIV-1 strains. Another approach to increase avidity and potency is to exploit the dynamic nature of HIV-1 Env to identify at least two antiviral targets in the overall viral entry process. By investigating the spatiotemporal process of HIV-1 entry, it was plausible that new combinations of bispecific antibody targets could be discovered that were not exclusive to targeting HIV-1 Env.

PG9-iMab and PG16-iMab, comprised of the scFv of the V1V2-targeting PG9 or PG16 mAbs fused to the CD4-targeting mAb ibalizumab, are two such examples

(Fig. 1b) [68]. PG9-iMab and PG16-iMab both exhibited impressive breadth and potency, neutralizing 100% of viruses tested, as defined by 50% inhibition. When defined as 80% inhibition, PG9-iMab still neutralized 100% of viruses while PG16-iMab neutralized 98% of viruses. The enhancement in potency was also remarkable, with PG9-iMab exhibiting an IC_{50} geometric mean of 0.004 μg/mL and an IC_{80} geometric mean of 0.017 μg/mL, and PG16-iMab exhibiting an IC_{50} geometric mean of 0.003 μg/mL and an IC_{80} geometric mean of 0.015 μg/mL. The enhancement in potency was >20-fold compared to the parental mAb ibalizumab and >100-fold compared to the parental mAb PG9 or PG16, and far better than a co-mixture of the two parental mAbs together. Importantly, the ability of PG9-iMab to bind both CD4 on the T cell and V1V2 on HIV-1 Env did not result in any obviously detrimental form of crosslinking that could enhance viral activity in the TZM-bl and PBMC neutralization assays evaluated, but rather only potently and broadly inhibited viral activity. In some cases, the potencies of these bispecific antibodies were improved up to four-logs compared to their parental mAb counterparts. Mechanistic studies determined that the enhanced potency of PG9-iMab required anchoring of this bispecific antibody to CD4 via its ibalizumab component. Additional modeling studies suggest that this anchoring to CD4 positions the PG9 scFv component of PG9-iMab so that it can more easily interact with the V1V2 epitope on the Env of the incoming viral particle. In effect, this increases the local concentration of PG9 scFv precisely at the site where it can exert its antiviral activity.

Interestingly, the enhancement in potency observed with PG9-iMab in this scFv bispecific format was not replicated with other scFv bispecific combinations such as VRC01-iMab, 3BNC60-iMab or 45-46-iMab, which target CD4 via ibalizumab and the HIV-1 Env CD4 binding site via VRC01, 3BNC60, or NIH45−46 scFv domains [44]. However, an enhancement in potency was observed with the CD4- and HIV-1 Env V3-targeting PGT123-iMab, PGT128-iMab and 10-1074-iMab, approaching the level of potency observed with PG9-iMab or PG16-iMab. This suggests that, similar to a preferred accessibility to the HIV-1 Env V1V2 epitope when PG9-iMab and PG16-iMab are anchored to CD4, the HIV-1 Env V3 epitope may be similarly accessible when PGT123-iMab, PGT128-iMab or 10-1074-iMab are bound to CD4 [44].

While several scFv-format bispecific antibodies are currently in development, several properties inherent to this bispecific antibody format must be addressed before they can be advanced into the clinic. For example, the linker fusing the V_H and V_L domains of the scFv moiety, and the linker fusing the scFv moiety to either an IgG-like molecule or another scFv moiety, must be sufficiently flexible so as not to impair the normal folding and function of the binding domains within the bispecific antibody, must be sufficiently stable so as to avoid cleavage and subsequent separation of the antibody binding domains during manufacture or in vivo, and must be sufficiently soluble so as to avoid potential aggregation. The ideal linker length and orientation of the V_H and V_L domains within the scFv moiety may also vary depending on the biophysical properties and mechanism of action of the particular bispecific antibody. All of these properties vary from molecule to molecule, and must be empirically investigated and optimized during the development process. Finally, the unnatural architecture of many scFv-format bispecific antibodies, which may deviate significantly from typical IgG antibodies, or their associated linkers, may create neoantigens or expose cryptic epitopes that may lead to immunogenicity in vivo [69]. While several in silico or in vitro methods may be able to identify potential hotspots of antibody immunogenicity, host immune responses cannot be predicted solely by these methods [70], and the ultimate test of antibody immunogenicity is by clinical study [71].

As discussed earlier, the CrossMAb bispecific antibody format retains more of a native IgG-like structure and avoids the need for foreign linker sequences [46], which may obviate some of the development challenges associated with scFv bispecific antibodies. However, the native-like structure of CrossMAbs may also restrict the "reach," and consequently the avidity, of two HIV-1 Env epitope binding variable domains when incorporated into this format [47]. Directing bispecific antibodies to host cell receptors with one of the CrossMAb arms, however, while targeting the other CrossMAb arm to the HIV-1 envelope, could take advantage of the dynamic nature of the HIV-1 entry process and allow for avidity by binding two HIV-1 entry targets simultaneously, similar to what was achieved with the PG9-iMab scFv format bispecific antibody. One study constructed and characterized a panel of 20 CrossMAb bispecific antibodies in which one arm inhibited HIV-1 by targeting the CD4 receptor or the CCR5 coreceptor via ibalizumab (iMab) or PRO140 (P140) [23, 24], and the other arm targeted the HIV-1 envelope MPER, CD4 binding site, V3 region, V1V2 region, or gp41−gp120 interface via 10E8, 3BNC117, PGT128, PGT145 or PGT151 [1, 3, 6, 8], and an optimal combination was identified which yielded exquisite antiviral potency and breadth [25]. The HIV-1 CrossMAbs 10E8/iMab and 10E8/P140 exhibited IC_{50} geometric means of 0.002 μg/mL and 0.001 μg/mL, respectively, and neutralization breadth (as assessed by ≥50% neutralization) of 100% and 99%, respectively. This represented a synergistic enhancement in potency hundreds of fold greater than those of its parental mAbs, and represented some of the most potent bispecific antibodies against HIV-1 identified to date. Interestingly, a CrossMAb comprised of a CD4-targeting ibalizumab arm and a V1V2-targeting PGT145 arm did not enhance antiviral potency, even though the CD4/V1V2-targeting PG9-iMab yielded a synergistic enhancement in potency in a scFv bispecific format [68]. Based on structural modeling data of the PG9-iMab scFv bispecific antibody discussed earlier, it is possible that the PG9 moiety may not be positioned at the right angle or length to neutralize HIV-1 Env when it is bound to CD4 or CCR5 in a CrossMAb format. Both 10E8/iMab and 10E8/P140 CrossMAbs, similar to the PG9-iMab scFv bispecific antibody, exerted their impressive antiviral activity by anchoring 10E8 near the two receptors HIV-1 utilizes, CD4 and CCR5, essentially placing 10E8 at precisely the right place and right time to bind HIV-1 Env MPER and potently neutralize an incoming viral particle. Indeed, if either the 10E8 or ibalizumab arm in 10E8/iMab (or the 10E8 or PRO140 arm in 10E8/P140) was engineered for reduced binding, the antiviral activity of the mutant bispecific was only as good as the mAb represented by the remaining intact arm within each of the bispecific CrossMAbs. After several rounds of antibody engineering to identify variants of these HIV-1 CrossMAbs with improved physicochemical homogeneity, an optimized variant known as $10E8_{V2.0}$/iMab (renamed 10E8.2/iMab) emerged with improved physicochemical properties, two-fold enhancement in bioavailability, and further improvement in antiviral potency compared to its predecessor (IC_{50} geometric mean of 0.002 μg/mL and IC_{80} geometric mean of 0.006 μg/mL). 10E8.2/iMab also demonstrated impressive antiviral activity in vivo, reducing viral load in HIV-1-infected humanized mice by 1.7 $\log_{10}$ and providing 100% protection against multiple systemic challenges with the tier-2 R5 virus, JR-CSF. Utilizing in vitro neutralization data for 10E8.2/iMab and other HIV-1 mAbs against subtype A, C, and D pseudoviruses, a model of neutralization potency and breadth for single and two mAb combinations predicted that this single bispecific molecule, 10E8.2/iMab, could provide broader and more potent protection across subtypes as compared to all two mAb combinations evaluated [22].

Bispecific antibody development challenges

The impressive potency, breadth and higher barrier against emerging resistant viruses that can be achieved with HIV-1 bispecific or trispecific antibodies warrants their further investigation. In addition, the ability to capture this impressive antiviral activity in a single multi-specific molecule, as opposed to combinations of multiple mAbs, makes the development of HIV-1 bispecific and trispecific antibodies an attractive path

commercially. One HIV-1 multi-specific molecule could achieve the same or better antiviral activity as combinations of multiple mAbs, but the manufacturing, storage, transport and administration costs remain similar to that of a single agent.

However, while the manufacturing process for typical mAbs is relatively mature and established, unexpected manufacturing challenges unique to each bispecific or trispecific antibody format must be overcome in order to make development of these multi-specific molecules a feasible strategy for HIV-1 treatment or prevention. Some of the challenges of scFv format bispecific antibodies were discussed earlier, such as the potential for linker instability, aggregation propensity and potential immunogenicity in vivo due to the difference in architecture between these bispecific molecules and typical IgG antibodies. Additionally, the non-native structure of this bispecific antibody format could result in a poor pharmacokinetic profile in vivo. Other bispecific formats, such as the CrossMAb format, avoid the use of linkers and maintain a more natural IgG antibody architecture while still achieving bispecificity as asymmetric IgG heterodimers. However, because two distinct heavy chains and two distinct light chains are required to produce the desired product, homodimer byproducts or light chain mispairings may arise and must be overcome.

Downstream processes may also possess unique challenges. While typical mAbs are purified using a Protein A resin that binds to the Fc region of the mAb, and then additional purification polishing steps are performed as necessary, bispecific antibodies that utilize asymmetry, such as the CrossMAb format, cannot be distinguished from homodimer impurities since the Fc regions of both the target heterodimer product and the impurity consisting of homodimers would interact equally well with Protein A. These bispecific formats must exploit asymmetry to their advantage in their purification processes as well, for example, by using a kappa light chain with one arm of the intact molecule and a lambda light chain with the other arm of the intact molecule so that successive rounds of purification that capture each of the light chain arms sequentially would allow for purification of the intact molecule [42]. Other purification tools that can take advantage of asymmetry could also be employed, such as engineering each bispecific antibody arm with sufficient differences in isoelectric points so that sequential purification by anion exchange and cation exchange chromatographies would result in purified heterodimers. Additionally, the combination of difficult upstream production procedures for certain complex bispecific antibody formats and multiple downstream purification steps may result in lower final product yields for bispecific antibodies as compared to typical mAbs.

Nonetheless, the tremendous therapeutic potential of HIV-1 bispecific and trispecific antibodies, with evidence of synergistically enhancing antiviral activity by several logs and the potential for drastically lower production costs by containing the therapeutic to a singular molecular entity, necessitate strategies be developed to overcome these challenges. By embarking on a scientifically rigorous approach towards developability and manufacturability that combines elements of quality by design with a deep mechanistic understanding of the specific therapeutic, promising bispecific or trispecific antibodies can overcome these developmental hurdles in order to advance into human testing as novel and potentially powerful therapeutic or prophylactic agents against HIV-1. Indeed, several of these novel candidates are already in clinical development (Figs. 1 and 5). Below, we present a case study of one such bispecific antibody against HIV-1.

Case study: quality by design approach to engineer a HIV-1 bispecific antibody with improved developability properties

As discussed earlier, 10E8.2/iMab [25] is a CrossMAb format bispecific antibody in which one antigen binding arm (iMab) targets the human CD4 receptor via the Fab of the humanized mAb ibalizumab [23], and a second antigen binding arm (10E8.2) targets the HIV-1 Env MPER via a variant of the human mAb 10E8 (Fig. 1d) [3]. The positioning of CD4- and MPER-targeting arms in this CrossMAb format produces a bispecific antibody with exquisitely potent and broad HIV-1 antiviral activity, neutralizing 100% of circulating HIV-1 strains in a 118 multi-clade panel with an IC_{50} geometric mean of 0.002 µg/mL, >97% of this panel with an IC_{80} geometric mean of 0.006 µg/mL, and >98% of a second 200 virus Clade C panel with similar antiviral potencies [25]. 10E8.2/iMab also potently inhibited HIV-1 in vivo, reducing viral load in HIV-1-infected humanized mice by 1.7 log_{10} and providing 100% protection against systemic challenge with a tier-2 R5 virus [25].

Despite this impressive antiviral activity in vitro and in vivo, a short-term "stress test" of 10E8.2/iMab revealed that this bispecific antibody starts to precipitate soon after incubation at 50 °C, suggesting a potential thermoinstability and aggregation propensity of this molecule under certain conditions. Five different CrossMAb format bispecific antibodies are currently in the clinic [72–76], indicating that the CrossMAb technology itself is not the cause of this thermoinstability and aggregation propensity. Additionally, other iMab-based CrossMAbs and the ibalizumab mAb did not exhibit such a high level of thermoinstability, indicating that this arm of 10E8.2/

iMab was likely not causing this issue. However, the parental mAb 10E8 was previously reported to have poor solubility and a tendency to precipitate [77], suggesting that the MPER-binding arm in 10E8.2/iMab was most likely responsible for the insolubility observed at high temperatures. This inherent biophysical property had the potential to limit the further development of this potent bispecific antibody.

Hydrophobic residues constantly or dynamically exposed on the surface of proteins often result in aggregation as protein concentration increases [31, 78]. Therefore, a quality by design (QbD) approach was taken to identify and systematically mutate externally-facing hydrophobic residues on the 10E8.2 arm of 10E8.2/iMab and to replace them with hydrophilic residues in an effort to find a functional variant with improved solubility. Out of 17 antibody variants engineered, hydrophobic to hydrophilic mutations at 6 residues in 10E8.2/iMab retained satisfactory functional activity, and combinations of these 6 mutations were subjected to biophysical characterizations to determine if there was any improvement in solubility.

The apparent solubility of 10E8.4/iMab was determined in comparison to 10E8.2/iMab by formulating both antibodies at identical starting concentrations and subjecting them to ultracentrifugation. At concentrations above 50 mg/mL, 10E8.4/iMab showed consistently higher protein concentrations and solubility over time as compared to 10E8.2/iMab, and the apparent solubility, or maximum concentration achieved, of 10E8.4/iMab was calculated to be >230 mg/mL (Fig. 2a). This improvement in solubility, combined with long-term stability data, strongly suggests that 10E8.4/iMab could be formulated not just for intravenous administration to humans, but also at the higher concentrations required for subcutaneous administration since volume constraints are often a concern for delivery by this latter route. Consequently, 10E8.4/iMab delivery by both of these routes of administration will be evaluated clinically.

The turbidity of 10E8.2/iMab and 10E8.4/iMab at various protein concentrations was also evaluated in order to draw a correlation between these two parameters. While the turbidity of both 10E8.2/iMab and 10E8.4/iMab expectedly increased with protein concentration over time, 10E8.2/iMab showed consistently higher turbidity than 10E8.4/iMab at the same protein concentrations over 100 mg/mL, indicating improved solubility of 10E8.4/iMab (Fig. 2b). 10E8.2/iMab and 10E8.4/iMab were also subjected to a forced degradation analysis to determine their relative protein stabilities under thermal stress-inducing conditions. In addition to an improvement in appearance and decrease in turbidity, 10E8.4/iMab also exhibited better intact molecule purity over

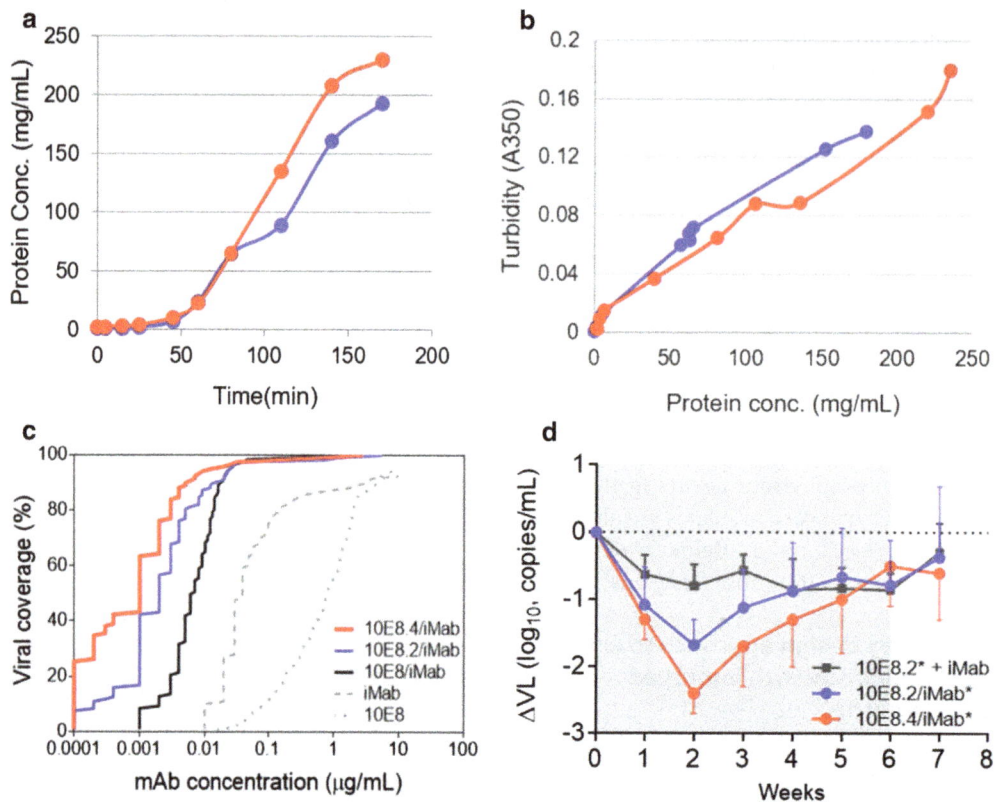

Fig. 2 Improved solubility and antiviral activity of 10E8.4/iMab. **a** Apparent solubility and **b** turbidity of 10E8.4/iMab and its predecessor variant 10E8.2/iMab. **c** Percent of a 118 Tier-2 HIV-1 Env pseudovirus panel neutralized (based on IC_{50} values) by 10E8.4/iMab and its predecessor variants 10E8/iMab and 10E8.2/iMab. Parental mAbs iMab and 10E8 are included for reference. **d** Decrease in viral load by 10E8.4/iMab and its predecessor variant, 10E8.2/iMab, in HIV-1-infected humanized mice. Shaded area indicates the period of weekly antibody administration. Error bars = SD. * = N297A mutant variant of each bispecific antibody. As reported previously [84], this mutation in the Fc region of each bispecific antibody is required for evaluation of non-FcR binding human antibodies in the murine model

time by capillary electrophoresis (CE) SDS-PAGE and fewer aggregation-associated high molecular weight species over time by size exclusion chromatography, indicating its relatively better stability under thermal stress-inducing conditions as compared to 10E8.2/iMab.

In addition to its improved solubility and thermostability, 10E8.4/iMab also exhibited a 2.5-fold enhancement in antiviral potency when tested against the same panel of 118 Tier-2 HIV-1 pseudotyped viruses representing diverse clades and geographic origins described earlier (Fig. 2c). In a humanized mouse model of HIV-1 infection, weekly administrations of 10E8.4/iMab reduced the viral load of HIV-1-infected mice by 2.4 $\log_{10}$ while a maximum mean viral load reduction of ~1.7 $\log_{10}$ was observed in mice treated with 10E8.2/iMab (Fig. 2d).

In summary, in silico analysis of the 10E8.2/iMab sequence and structure for potential aggregation-inducing hotspots revealed a number of residues that could be detrimental for the developability of this potent bispecific antibody for the clinic. A potential setback as a result of these

inherent molecular properties may often not be realized until significant funds and time are exerted for the advancement of a particular therapeutic into the clinic. However, utilizing a QbD approach to systematically mutate each of these hotspot residues individually, and iteratively testing combinations of these engineered variants for improved product quality attributes, led to the identification of a new improved variant, 10E8.4/iMab. While there is always the theoretical risk that engineering new residues into an antibody may result in unanticipated immunogenicity, the likelihood of this is uncertain and cannot be definitively assessed until clinical investigation [71]. Therefore, based on its superior solubility and stability and its further improved potent in vitro and in vivo antiviral activity, 10E8.4/iMab was selected as a clinical lead candidate for further development.

Case study: cell line development of a CrossMAb format HIV-1 bispecific antibody

Cell line development in preparation for reproducible production of a given mAb therapeutic for human use is now an established process, as evidenced by the >85 mAbs approved for commercial use by the US FDA for the treatment of a number of different human diseases [79], and this does not include the many more mAbs that are currently in preclinical and clinical development. The heavy chain and light chain of a given mAb are encoded together on one plasmid that contains an antibiotic resistance selection marker or separately on two plasmids, each with its own unique antibiotic resistance selection marker. These plasmids are then stably transfected into a cell line. After transfection, single clones that produce high titers of the mAb, as determined by Protein A binding to the Fc region of antibody secreted into the supernatant, are selected and further characterized in order to downselect a lead clone for GMP master cell bank production. For the cell line development of 10E8.4/iMab, a modified approach was necessary due to a total of four separate open reading frames (encoding 10E8.4 heavy chain, 10E8.4 light chain, iMab heavy chain, and iMab light chain) that need to be stably transfected. By transient transfection, encoding four different open reading frames in four separate plasmids reproducibly produces CrossMAb bispecific antibodies with >80% intact molecule purity [46]. For stable transfection, however, encoding these four different open reading frames in four separate plasmids was not feasible because the high level of antibiotic selection pressure against four distinct markers would drastically reduce the number of surviving clones that could be screened for high titer-producing antibody levels.

After attempting stable transfection of 10E8.4/iMab encoded in two or three plasmid configurations, and screening for high titer clones by Protein A binding to the Fc region of the secreted antibody, the highest level of intact molecule purity produced from a stable pool of clones was 68.5%, which is too low to support a viable upstream production and downstream purification strategy for clinical development. Analysis by non-reduced CE SDS-PAGE of the impurities present in the supernatant of the top stable pools revealed a significant fraction of heavy chain–heavy chain (HH) and heavy chain–heavy chain–light chain (HHL) impurities present in the clonal supernatant. Theoretically, the knob-in-hole and light chain crossover technologies incorporated into the CrossMAb format should prevent these impurities from being secreted. However, our investigational analyses revealed that, if all four ORFs are not present in the transfection mix, impure byproducts can be readily secreted. For example, transfection of 10E8.4 HC and iMab HC, without their cognate light chains, can be secreted (Fig. 3a), as can 10E8.4 HC, iMab HC and iMab LC impurities (Fig. 3b). Fundamental biological studies of monoclonal antibody secretion indicate that antibody HCs are not typically secreted from cells without their cognate LCs associated, and a closer investigation revealed that the signal for this antibody secretion is associated with close proximity of the CH1 domain of a nascently formed antibody HC with the CL domain of a nascently formed antibody LC in the endoplasmic reticulum [80]. Due to the unique configuration of the light chain crossover technology in CrossMAb antibodies, however, the CL

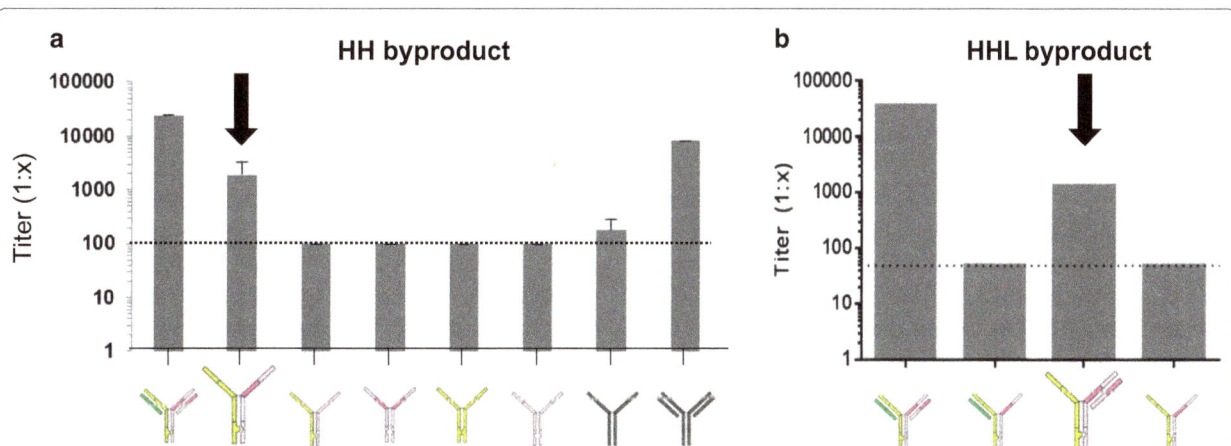

Fig. 3 Secretion of CrossMAb byproducts that could hinder cell line development and clone selection. Detection of the indicated antibody or antibody byproduct in supernatant after transient transfection of ORFs encoding for the antibody chains indicated in the schematics. Protein detection in supernatant was determined by Protein A binding ELISA. Dashed lines indicate the assay limit of detection. Error bars = SD. **a** HH dimer byproducts and **b** HHL impurity byproducts were readily detected in supernatants

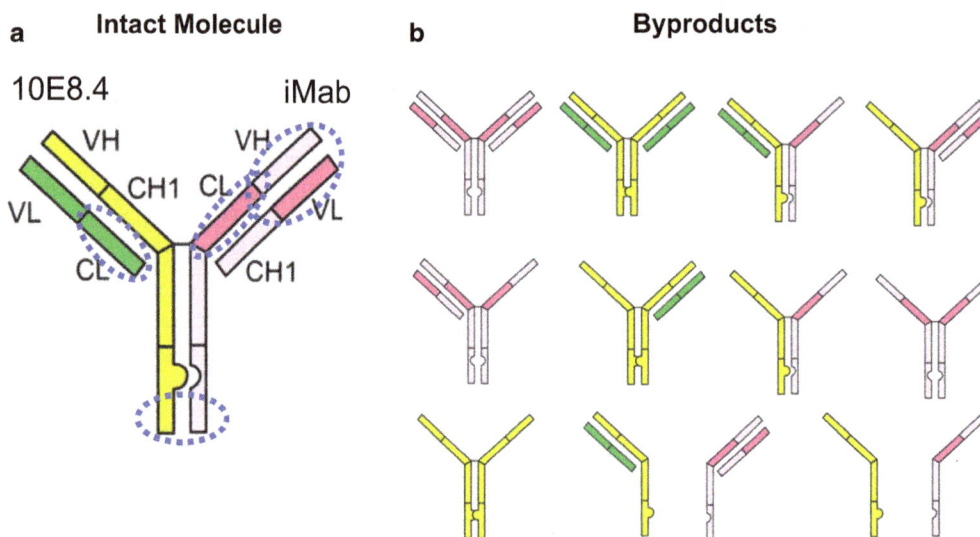

Fig. 4 CrossMab format for bispecific antibody production. Knob-in hole mutations in the CH3 domains favor heterodimer heavy chain formation. CH1-CL crossover in one arm of the CrossMAb favors proper light chain association with its cognate heavy chain. In combination, **a** intact molecule production and secretion is favored and **b** byproduct production and secretion is disfavored. Dashed blue circles indicate target domains that, when detected simultaneously, ensure a greater percentage of intact molecule

of ibalizumab is located on the "heavy chain" (Fig. 4a), and we speculate that the close proximity of this CL in the ibalizumab "heavy chain" and the CH1 domain in the 10E8.4 HC can trigger antibody secretion without their cognate LCs. With consideration to our stable cell line transfection efforts, one can easily envision how overexpression or underexpression of one or more of the four bispecific antibody chains in a stable cell line could allow for permissive secretion of HH or HHL impurities if the missing chain(s) is produced at relatively low levels. Also, since our initial screening strategy, which is commonly used for mAb cell line selection, indiscriminately selected for high-producer clones by Fc-binding to Protein A, it was impossible to differentiate clones producing the intact HHLL molecule from those that produced HHLL along with a mixture of HH and HHL impurities since all of these products would have nearly identical binding properties to Protein A.

To overcome these challenges, we undertook a multi-pronged approach that specifically addressed the unique differences in cell line development between a typical mAb and the 10E8.4/iMab bispecific CrossMAb. We generated new two and three plasmid vector combinations encoding the 10E8.4 HC, 10E8.4 LC, iMab HC and iMab LC in several different permutations, and transiently transfected them at numerous ratios to identify the plasmid combinations and ratios that could give the best percentage of intact molecule purity by transient transfection in order to downselect the most promising set of plasmids and conditions to advance

into stable transfection studies. In all, more than 20 different plasmid configurations and conditions were evaluated. Next, by designing a new screening strategy that recognized four distinct domains of 10E8.4/iMab simultaneously rather than only its singular Fc region, we could select for high titer producing clones with better assurance that they were producing fully intact HHLL molecules rather than byproduct impurities (Fig. 4a). In effect, if we equate identifying a high titer producing clone within a large pool of stably transfected clones to identifying a needle in a haystack, our redesigned screening strategy was a powerfully tuned magnet that could sift through the "hay" of clones to find our high titer producing "needle." To do this, we developed new FRET-based methods to simultaneously detect multiple distinct arms within the 10E8.4/iMab intact molecule, and utilized CE SDS-PAGE as our analytical screening tool to confirm intact molecule purity levels relative to byproduct impurities. If a suitable bispecific ELISA-based method was available that could simultaneously detect both functional antibody arms, this could also be employed. Finally, we plated and screened over five times as many clones as was done for a typical mAb cell line development program in order to ensure that we could identify a suitable lead clone. In effect, now equipped with our powerful screening strategy and magnet, we could increase the size of the haystack in order to ensure that one or more of our needles was contained within it. These laborious efforts proved fruitful, and a final lead cell line clone was identified that produced 10E8.4/iMab at >90% intact molecule purity after a simple 1-step purification and at a titer of >3 g/L. This titer is on par with excellent mAb-producing clones and much better than what is expected for a typical bispecific antibody. Additional polishing steps purified 10E8.4/iMab to >97%, which is well within the range of purity acceptable to advance this novel and potent HIV-1 bispecific antibody into clinical evaluation.

Conclusions

The new generation of broadly neutralizing mAbs against HIV-1 has given the field a new avenue of hope for prophylactic and therapeutic possibilities to reduce the existing HIV-1 burden. In addition to the recent FDA approval of ibalizumab (Trogarzo®) for use as salvage therapy in patients whose viruses are resistant to multiple existing antiretroviral drugs, VRC01 is currently in two Phase 2b efficacy trials for HIV-1 prevention in HIV-1 uninfected men and transgender persons who have sex with men in the United States, Peru, Brazil, and Switzerland (HVTN 704/HPTN 085) and in HIV-1 uninfected sexually active women in seven countries in sub-Saharan Africa (HVTN 703/HPTN 081) [26, 81]. Known as the Antibody Mediated Prevention

(AMP) Studies, the lessons learned from these VRC01 Phase 2b efficacy trials will be of tremendous benefit the field of antibody-mediated HIV-1 prevention. It is clear, however, that drastic improvements to antibody potency and breadth will be required in order to produce a feasible antibody regimen which could be used widespread and which could limit the emergence of viral resistance well known to those in the HIV-1 treatment field. Bispecific and trispecific antibodies offer a new beacon of hope to combat viral resistance by improving neutralization breadth and, in some cases, by drastically improving antiviral potency by orders of magnitude over the best HIV-1 mAbs currently in existence (Fig. 5). However, the development of these HIV-1 multi-specific antibodies is not without its own challenges. The potential for aggregation, immunogenicity and low GMP cell line titers is an issue for any antibody, and these are amplified in cases of multi-specific antibodies due to their unique formats and engineered properties required to create their multi-specificity. In addition to the challenges discussed in this review, other downstream chemistry, manufacturing and controls obstacles such as antibody purification and stability of engineered multi-specific molecules may exist. Further in development, nonclinical challenges, such

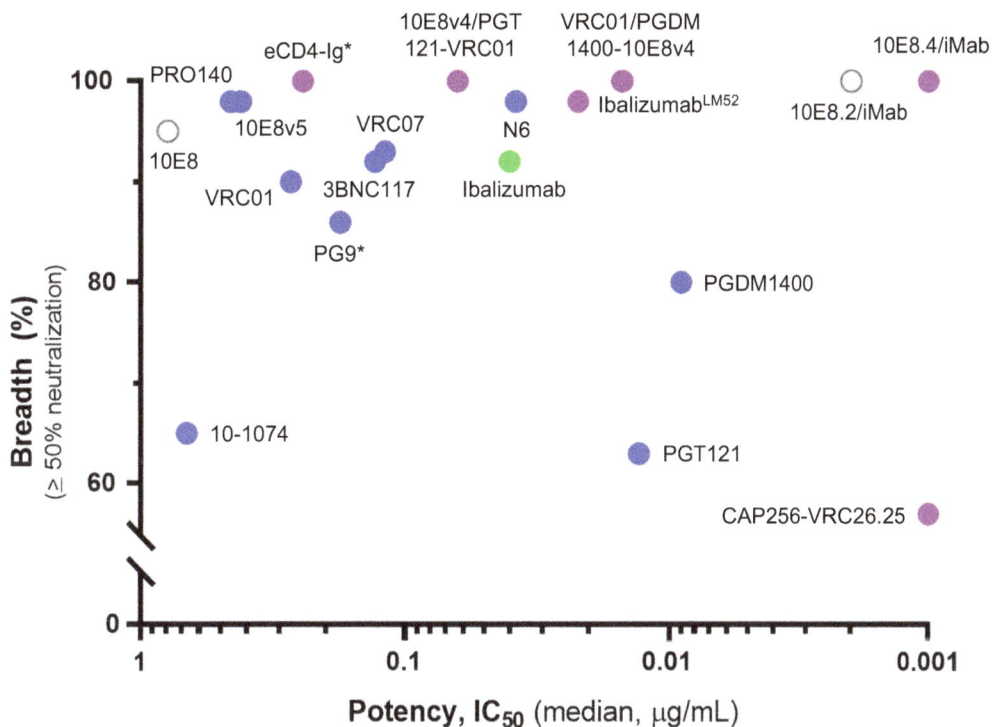

Fig. 5 Antiviral potency and breadth of HIV-1 mAbs and multi-specific Abs. HIV-1 mAbs and multi-specific antibodies that are licensed (green), in clinical trials (blue), or in clinical development (purple). Open circles represent earlier variants of antibodies in development that are presented. *Means antibodies were delivered by AAV. Figure adapted from Xu et al., 2017 and additional published reports [54, 85, 86]

as manufacturing and incorporating parental mAb control groups into GLP toxicology programs in the event that safety signals for a given multi-specific antibody requires further investigation, may also arise [82]. During clinical investigation, pharmacokinetic and anti-drug antibody assays must be able to detect each specificity within a given multi-specific antibody, and therefore reagents or assays that can detect each unique epitope within a given HIV-1 multi-specific antibody are preferred [83].

Despite these challenges, the tremendous opportunities for bispecific and trispecific antibodies against HIV-1 are readily evident. Applying the same creativity and rigor to the development and manufacture of HIV-1 multi-specific antibodies as that which was used for their creation and initial characterization promises to offer to the field a new generation of potent and broad multi-specific antibodies that could be ready to enter the clinic within the same timeframe as a typical mAb. In parallel, the ongoing discovery of ever more potent and broadly neutralizing HIV-1 mAbs continues to provide new and improved foundational starting blocks for incorporation into multi-specific antibodies. How we create and advance these powerful multi-specific antibodies for the prevention and treatment of HIV-1 will only be limited by our imagination, rigor and diligence.

Abbreviations
AAV: adeno-associated virus; bp: basepairs; CE: capillary electrophoresis; CODV-Ig: cross-over dual variable immunoglobulin G; DNA: deoxyribonucleic acid; ds: double-stranded; Env: envelope; HH: heavy chain–heavy chain; HHL: heavy chain–heavy chain–light chain; IC: inhibitory concentration; HIV-1: human immunodeficiency virus 1; KiH: knob-in hole; iMab: ibalizumab; mAb: monoclonal antibody; MPER: membrane proximal external region; P140: PRO140; QbD: quality by design; SHIV: simian human immunodeficiency virus; scFv: single-chain variable fragment.

Authors' contributions
NNP, JY, YH and DDH jointly wrote this review article and conducted or supervised all unpublished studies presented. All authors read and approved the final manuscript.

Acknowledgements
The authors wish to thank Wuxi Biologics for their support in 10E8.2/iMab and 10E8.4/iMab solubility and thermostability studies and 10E8.4/iMab cell line development studies, Christian Klein at Roche Innovation Center Zurich for helpful discussions regarding 10E8.4/iMab cell line development and for information regarding clinical experience with CrossMAbs, Michael Seaman at Beth Israel Deaconess Medical Center, Harvard Medical School for conducting in vitro neutralization studies of 10E8.4/iMab against the multi-clade HIV envelope pseudotyped virus panel, Mili Gajjar for technical assistance with 10E8.4/iMab in vivo studies, Yang Luo for project coordination, Wendy Chen for help with figure preparation, and members of the Ho laboratory for helpful discussions.

Competing interests
JY, YH and DDH are inventors on a patent describing HIV CrossMAbs, including 10E8/iMab and 10E8/P140 and their variants, for HIV-1 prevention and therapy. The rights of this technology for use in HIV-1 therapy have been licensed to TaiMed Biologics, Inc., which also owns the commercial rights to ibalizumab. DDH is the scientific founder of TaiMed Biologics, Inc. and, in this capacity, has equity in the company. DDH is also an inventor on a patent describing LM52, which has been licensed to TaiMed Biologics, Inc.

Consent to participate
Not applicable.

Consent for publication
Not applicable.

Funding
DDH is supported by the Bill and Melinda Gates Foundation's Collaboration for AIDS Vaccine Discovery for the development of bispecific antibodies for HIV-1 prevention under Grants OPP1040731 and OPP1169162.

References
1. Blattner C, Lee JH, Sliepen K, Derking R, Falkowska E, de la Pena AT, Cupo A, Julien JP, van Gils M, Lee PS, et al. Structural delineation of a quaternary, cleavage-dependent epitope at the gp41–gp120 interface on intact HIV-1 Env trimers. Immunity. 2014;40:669–80.
2. Doria-Rose NA, Schramm CA, Gorman J, Moore PL, Bhiman JN, DeKosky BJ, Ernandes MJ, Georgiev IS, Kim HJ, Pancera M, et al. Developmental pathway for potent V1V2-directed HIV-neutralizing antibodies. Nature. 2014;509:55–62.
3. Huang J, Ofek G, Laub L, Louder MK, Doria-Rose NA, Longo NS, Imamichi H, Bailer RT, Chakrabarti B, Sharma SK, et al. Broad and potent neutralization of HIV-1 by a gp41-specific human antibody. Nature. 2012;491:406–12.
4. Mouquet H, Scharf L, Euler Z, Liu Y, Eden C, Scheid JF, Halper-Stromberg A, Gnanapragasam PN, Spencer DI, Seaman MS, et al. Complex-type N-glycan recognition by potent broadly neutralizing HIV antibodies. Proc Natl Acad Sci USA. 2012;109:E3268–77.
5. Rudicell RS, Kwon YD, Ko SY, Pegu A, Louder MK, Georgiev IS, Wu X, Zhu J, Boyington JC, Chen X, et al. Enhanced potency of a broadly neutralizing HIV-1 antibody in vitro improves protection against lentiviral infection in vivo. J Virol. 2014;88:12669–82.
6. Scheid JF, Mouquet H, Ueberheide B, Diskin R, Klein F, Oliveira TY, Pietzsch J, Fenyo D, Abadir A, Velinzon K, et al. Sequence and structural convergence of broad and potent HIV antibodies that mimic CD4 binding. Science. 2011;333:1633–7.
7. Sok D, van Gils MJ, Pauthner M, Julien JP, Saye-Francisco KL, Hsueh J, Briney B, Lee JH, Le KM, Lee PS, et al. Recombinant HIV envelope trimer selects for quaternary-dependent antibodies targeting the trimer apex. Proc Natl Acad Sci USA. 2014;111:17624–9.

8. Walker LM, Huber M, Doores KJ, Falkowska E, Pejchal R, Julien JP, Wang SK, Ramos A, Chan-Hui PY, Moyle M, et al. Broad neutralization coverage of HIV by multiple highly potent antibodies. Nature. 2011;477:466–70.

9. Walker LM, Phogat SK, Chan-Hui PY, Wagner D, Phung P, Goss JL, Wrin T, Simek MD, Fling S, Mitcham JL, et al. Broad and potent neutralizing antibodies from an African donor reveal a new HIV-1 vaccine target. Science. 2009;326:285–9.

10. Wu X, Yang ZY, Li Y, Hogerkorp CM, Schief WR, Seaman MS, Zhou T, Schmidt SD, Wu L, Xu L, et al. Rational design of envelope identifies broadly neutralizing human monoclonal antibodies to HIV-1. Science. 2010;329:856–61.

11. Caskey M, Klein F, Lorenzi JC, Seaman MS, West AP Jr, Buckley N, Kremer G, Nogueira L, Braunschweig M, Scheid JF, et al. Viraemia suppressed in HIV-1-infected humans by broadly neutralizing antibody 3BNC117. Nature. 2015;522:487–91.

12. Caskey M, Schoofs T, Gruell H, Settler A, Karagounis T, Kreider EF, Murrell B, Pfeifer N, Nogueira L, Oliveira TY, et al. Antibody 10-1074 suppresses viremia in HIV-1-infected individuals. Nat Med. 2017;23:185–91.

13. Ledgerwood JE, Coates EE, Yamshchikov G, Saunders JG, Holman L, Enama ME, DeZure A, Lynch RM, Gordon I, Plummer S, et al. Safety, pharmacokinetics and neutralization of the broadly neutralizing HIV-1 human monoclonal antibody VRC01 in healthy adults. Clin Exp Immunol. 2015;182:289–301.

14. Lynch RM, Boritz E, Coates EE, DeZure A, Madden P, Costner P, Enama ME, Plummer S, Holman L, Hendel CS, et al. Virologic effects of broadly neutralizing antibody VRC01 administration during chronic HIV-1 infection. Sci Transl Med. 2015;7:319ra206.

15. A Clinical Trial of PGDM1400 and PGT121 Monoclonal Antibodies in HIV-infected and HIV-uninfected Adults. ClinicalTrials.gov. U.S. National Library of Medicine. https://clinicaltrials.gov/ct2/show/NCT03205917. Accessed 13 May 2018.

16. VRC 605: Safety and Pharmacokinetics of a Human Monoclonal Antibody, VRC-HIVMAB075-00-AB (VRC07-523IS), Administered Intravenously or Subcutaneously to Healthy Adults. ClinicalTrials.gov. U.S. National Library of Medicine. https://clinicaltrials.gov/ct2/show/NCT03015181. Accessed 13 May 2018.

17. A Clinical Trial of the Safety, Pharmacokinetics and Antiviral Activity of PGT121 Monoclonal Antibody (mAb) in HIV-uninfected and HIV-infected Adults. ClinicalTrials.gov. U.S. National Library of Medicine. https://clinicaltrials.gov/ct2/show/NCT02960581. Accessed 13 May 2018.

18. Jacobson JM, Saag MS, Thompson MA, Fischl MA, Liporace R, Reichman RC, Redfield RR, Fichtenbaum CJ, Zingman BS, Patel MC, et al. Antiviral activity of single-dose PRO 140, a CCR5 monoclonal antibody, in HIV-infected adults. J Infect Dis. 2008;198:1345–52.

19. Toma J, Weinheimer SP, Stawiski E, Whitcomb JM, Lewis ST, Petropoulos CJ, Huang W. Loss of asparagine-linked glycosylation sites in variable region 5 of human immunodeficiency virus type 1 envelope is associated with resistance to CD4 antibody ibalizumab. J Virol. 2011;85:3872–80.

20. Pace CS, Fordyce MW, Franco D, Kao CY, Seaman MS, Ho DD. Anti-CD4 monoclonal antibody ibalizumab exhibits breadth and potency against HIV-1, with natural resistance mediated by the loss of a V5 glycan in envelope. J Acquir Immune Defic Syndr. 2013;62:1–9.

21. Wagh K, Bhattacharya T, Williamson C, Robles A, Bayne M, Garrity J, Rist M, Rademeyer C, Yoon H, Lapedes A, et al. Optimal combinations of broadly neutralizing antibodies for prevention and treatment of HIV-1 clade C infection. PLoS Pathog. 2016;12:e1005520.

22. Wagh K, Seaman MS, Zingg M, Fitzsimons T, Barouch DH, Burton DR, Connors M, Ho DD, Mascola JR, Nussenzweig MC, et al. Potential of conventional & bispecific broadly neutralizing antibodies for prevention of HIV-1 subtype A, C & D infections. PLoS Pathog. 2018;14:e1006860.

23. Burkly LC, Olson D, Shapiro R, Winkler G, Rosa JJ, Thomas DW, Williams C, Chisholm P. Inhibition of HIV infection by a novel CD4 domain 2-specific monoclonal antibody. Dissecting the basis for its inhibitory effect on HIV-induced cell fusion. J Immunol. 1992;149:1779–87.

24. Trkola A, Ketas TJ, Nagashima KA, Zhao L, Cilliers T, Morris L, Moore JP, Maddon PJ, Olson WC. Potent, broad-spectrum inhibition of human immunodeficiency virus type 1 by the CCR5 monoclonal antibody PRO 140. J Virol. 2001;75:579–88.

25. Huang Y, Yu J, Lanzi A, Yao X, Andrews CD, Tsai L, Gajjar MR, Sun M, Seaman MS, Padte NN, Ho DD. Engineered bispecific antibodies with exquisite HIV-1-neutralizing activity. Cell. 2016;165:1621–31.

26. Emu B, Fessel J, Schrader S, Kumar P, Richmond G, Win S, Weinheimer S, Marsolais C, Lewis S. Phase 3 study of ibalizumab for multidrug-resistant HIV-1. N Engl J Med. 2018;379:645–54.

27. Markham A. Ibalizumab: first global approval. Drugs. 2018;78:781–5.

28. A Randomized, Double-blind, Placebo-controlled Trial, Followed by Single-arm Treatment of PRO 140 in Combination w/Optimized Background Therapy in Treatment-Experienced HIV Subjects (PRO 140). ClinicalTrials.gov. U.S. National Library of Medicine. https://clinicaltrials.gov/ct2/show/NCT02483078?term=PRO140&rank=2. Accessed 11 May 2018.

29. Morris L, Mkhize NN. Prospects for passive immunity to prevent HIV infection. PLoS Med. 2017;14:e1002436.

30. Diskin R, Scheid JF, Marcovecchio PM, West AP Jr, Klein F, Gao H, Gnanapragasam PN, Abadir A, Seaman MS, Nussenzweig MC, Bjorkman PJ. Increasing the potency and breadth of an HIV antibody by using structure-based rational design. Science. 2011;334:1289–93.

31. Kwon YD, Georgiev IS, Ofek G, Zhang B, Asokan M, Bailer RT, Bao A, Caruso W, Chen X, Choe M, et al. Optimization of the solubility of HIV-1-neutralizing antibody 10E8 through somatic variation and structure-based design. J Virol. 2016;90:5899–914.

32. VRC 610: Phase I Safety and Pharmacokinetics Study to Evaluate a Human Monoclonal Antibody (MAB) VRC-HIVMAB095-00-AB (10E8VLS) Administered Alone or Concurrently with MAB VRC- HIVMAB075-00-AB (VRC07-523LS) via Subcutaneous Injection in Healthy Adults. ClinicalTrials.gov. U.S. National Library of Medicine. https://clinicaltrials.gov/ct2/show/NCT03565315. Accessed 03 Aug 2018.

33. Kwon YD, Chuang GY, Zhang B, Bailer RT, Doria-Rose NA, Gindin TS, Lin B, Louder MK, McKee K, O'Dell S, et al. Surface-matrix screening identifies semi-specific interactions that improve potency of a near pan-reactive HIV-1-neutralizing antibody. Cell Rep. 2018;22:1798–809.

34. Freeman MM, Seaman MS, Rits-Volloch S, Hong X, Kao CY, Ho DD, Chen B. Crystal structure of HIV-1 primary receptor CD4 in complex with a potent antiviral antibody. Structure. 2010;18:1632–41.

35. Song R, Franco D, Kao CY, Yu F, Huang Y, Ho DD. Epitope mapping of ibalizumab, a humanized anti-CD4 monoclonal antibody with anti-HIV-1 activity in infected patients. J Virol. 2010;84:6935–42.

36. Song R, Oren DA, Franco D, Seaman MS, Ho DD. Strategic addition of an N-linked glycan to a monoclonal antibody improves its HIV-1-neutralizing activity. Nat Biotechnol. 2013;31:1047–52.

37. Product Pipeline: TMB-360/365. TaiMed Biologics. http://www.taimedbiologics.com/pipeline/36. Accessed 18 May 2018.

38. Karpovsky B, Titus JA, Stephany DA, Segal DM. Production of target-specific effector cells using hetero-cross-linked aggregates containing anti-target cell and anti-Fc gamma receptor antibodies. J Exp Med. 1984;160:1686–701.

39. Perez P, Hoffman RW, Shaw S, Bluestone JA, Segal DM. Specific targeting of cytotoxic T cells by anti-T3 linked to anti-target cell antibody. Nature. 1985;316:354–6.

40. Staerz UD, Kanagawa O, Bevan MJ. Hybrid antibodies can target sites for attack by T cells. Nature. 1985;314:628–31.

41. Chames P, Baty D. Bispecific antibodies for cancer therapy: the light at the end of the tunnel? MAbs. 2009;1:539–47.

42. Brinkmann U, Kontermann RE. The making of bispecific antibodies. MAbs. 2017;9:182–212.

43. Sun M, Pace CS, Yao X, Yu F, Padte NN, Huang Y, Seaman MS, Li Q, Ho DD. Rational design and characterization of the novel, broad and potent bispecific HIV-1 neutralizing antibody iMabm36. J Acquir Immune Defic Syndr. 2014;66:473–83.

44. Song R, Pace C, Seaman MS, Fang Q, Sun M, Andrews CD, Wu A, Padte NN, Ho DD. Distinct HIV-1 neutralization potency profiles of ibalizumab-based bispecific antibodies. J Acquir Immune Defic Syndr. 2016;73:365–73.

45. Zhou T, Georgiev I, Wu X, Yang ZY, Dai K, Finzi A, Kwon YD, Scheid JF, Shi W, Xu L, et al. Structural basis for broad and potent neutralization of HIV-1 by antibody VRC01. Science. 2010;329:811–7.

46. Schaefer W, Regula JT, Bähner M, Schanzer J, Croasdale R, Durr H, Gassner C, Georges G, Kettenberger H, Imhof-Jung S, et al. Immunoglobulin domain crossover as a generic approach for the production of bispecific IgG antibodies. Proc Natl Acad Sci USA. 2011;108:11187–92.

47. Asokan M, Rudicell RS, Louder M, McKee K, O'Dell S, Stewart-Jones G, Wang K, Xu L, Chen X, Choe M, et al. Bispecific antibodies targeting different epitopes on the HIV-1 envelope exhibit broad and potent neutralization. J Virol. 2015;89:12501–12.

48. Ho DD, Neumann AU, Perelson AS, Chen W, Leonard JM, Markowitz M. Rapid turnover of plasma virions and CD4 lymphocytes in HIV-1 infection. Nature. 1995;373:123–6.

49. Perelson AS, Neumann AU, Markowitz M, Leonard JM, Ho DD. HIV-1 dynamics in vivo: virion clearance rate, infected cell life-span, and viral generation time. Science. 1996;271:1582–6.

50. Wei X, Ghosh SK, Taylor ME, Johnson VA, Emini EA, Deutsch P, Lifson JD, Bonhoeffer S, Nowak MA, Hahn BH, et al. Viral dynamics in human immunodeficiency virus type 1 infection. Nature. 1995;373:117–22.

51. Haynes BF, Shaw GM, Korber B, Kelsoe G, Sodroski J, Hahn BH, Borrow P, McMichael AJ. HIV-host interactions: implications for vaccine design. Cell Host Microbe. 2016;19:292–303.

52. Merchant AM, Zhu Z, Yuan JQ, Goddard A, Adams CW, Presta LG, Carter P. An efficient route to human bispecific IgG. Nat Biotechnol. 1998;16:677–81.

53. Steinmetz A, Vallee F, Beil C, Lange C, Baurin N, Beninga J, Capdevila C, Corvey C, Dupuy A, Ferrari P, et al. CODV-Ig, a universal bispecific tetravalent and multifunctional immunoglobulin format for medical applications. MAbs. 2016;8:867–78.

54. Xu L, Pegu A, Rao E, Doria-Rose N, Beninga J, McKee K, Lord DM, Wei RR, Deng G, Louder M, et al. Trispecific broadly neutralizing HIV antibodies mediate potent SHIV protection in macaques. Science. 2017;358:85–90.

55. Klein JS, Gnanapragasam PN, Galimidi RP, Foglesong CP, West AP Jr, Bjorkman PJ. Examination of the contributions of size and avidity to the neutralization mechanisms of the anti-HIV antibodies b12 and 4E10. Proc Natl Acad Sci USA. 2009;106:7385–90.

56. Liu J, Bartesaghi A, Borgnia MJ, Sapiro G, Subramaniam S. Molecular architecture of native HIV-1 gp120 trimers. Nature. 2008;455:109–13.

57. Zhu P, Liu J, Bess J Jr, Chertova E, Lifson JD, Grise H, Ofek GA, Taylor KA, Roux KH. Distribution and three-dimensional structure of AIDS virus envelope spikes. Nature. 2006;441:847–52.

58. Mouquet H, Scheid JF, Zoller MJ, Krogsgaard M, Ott RG, Shukair S, Artyomov MN, Pietzsch J, Connors M, Pereyra F, et al. Polyreactivity increases the apparent affinity of anti-HIV antibodies by heteroligation. Nature. 2010;467:591–5.

59. Galimidi RP, Klein JS, Politzer MS, Bai S, Seaman MS, Nussenzweig MC, West AP Jr, Bjorkman PJ. Intra-spike crosslinking overcomes antibody evasion by HIV-1. Cell. 2015;160:433–46.

60. Roux KH, Strelets L, Brekke OH, Sandlie I, Michaelsen TE. Comparisons of the ability of human IgG3 hinge mutants, IgM, IgE, and IgA2, to form small immune complexes: a role for flexibility and geometry. J Immunol. 1998;161:4083–90.

61. Roux KH, Strelets L, Michaelsen TE. Flexibility of human IgG subclasses. J Immunol. 1997;159:3372–82.

62. Bournazos S, Gazumyan A, Seaman MS, Nussenzweig MC, Ravetch JV. Bispecific anti-HIV antibodies with enhanced breadth and potency. Cell. 2016;165:1609–20.

63. Steinhardt JJ, Guenaga J, Turner HL, McKee K, Louder MK, O'Dell S, Chiang CI, Lei L, Galkin A, Andrianov AK, et al. Rational design of a trispecific antibody targeting the HIV-1 Env with elevated anti-viral activity. Nat Commun. 2018;9:877.

64. Chen W, Bardhi A, Feng Y, Wang Y, Qi Q, Li W, Zhu Z, Dyba MA, Ying T, Jiang S, et al. Improving the CH1-CK heterodimerization and pharmacokinetics of 4Dm2 m, a novel potent CD4-antibody fusion protein against HIV-1. MAbs. 2016;8:761–74.

65. Chen W, Feng Y, Prabakaran P, Ying T, Wang Y, Sun J, Macedo CD, Zhu Z, He Y, Polonis VR, Dimitrov DS. Exceptionally potent and broadly cross-reactive, bispecific multivalent HIV-1 inhibitors based on single human CD4 and antibody domains. J Virol. 2014;88:1125–39.

66. Gardner MR, Kattenhorn LM, Kondur HR, von Schaewen M, Dorfman T, Chiang JJ, Haworth KG, Decker JM, Alpert MD, Bailey CC, et al. AAV-expressed eCD4-Ig provides durable protection from multiple SHIV challenges. Nature. 2015;519:87–91.

67. Fetzer I, Gardner MR, Davis-Gardner ME, Prasad NR, Alfant B, Weber JA, Farzan M. eCD4-Ig variants that more potently neutralize HIV-1. J Virol. 2018;92:e02011–17.

68. Pace CS, Song R, Ochsenbauer C, Andrews CD, Franco D, Yu J, Oren DA, Seaman MS, Ho DD. Bispecific antibodies directed to CD4 domain 2 and HIV envelope exhibit exceptional breadth and picomolar potency against HIV-1. Proc Natl Acad Sci USA. 2013;110:13540–5.

69. Miller LL, Korn EL, Stevens DS, Janik JE, Gause BL, Kopp WC, Holmlund JT, Curti BD, Sznol M, Smith JW 2nd, et al. Abrogation of the hematological and biological activities of the interleukin-3/granulocyte-macrophage colony-stimulating factor fusion protein PIXY321 by neutralizing anti-PIXY321 antibodies in cancer patients receiving high-dose carboplatin. Blood. 1999;93:3250–8.

70. Gokemeijer J, Jawa V, Mitra-Kaushik S. How close are we to profiling immunogenicity risk using in silico algorithms and in vitro methods? An industry perspective. AAPS J. 2017;19:1587–92.

71. Guidance for Industry: Immunogenicity Assessment for Therapeutic Protein Products. U.S. Department of Health and Human Services. Food and Drug Administration. Center for Drug Evaluation and Research (CDER). Center for Biologics Evaluation and Research (CBER). 2014.

72. Bacac M, Fauti T, Sam J, Colombetti S, Weinzierl T, Ouaret D, Bodmer W, Lehmann S, Hofer T, Hosse RJ, et al. A novel carcinoembryonic antigen T-cell bispecific antibody (CEA TCB) for the treatment of solid tumors. Clin Cancer Res. 2016;22:3286–97.

73. Brunker P, Wartha K, Friess T, Grau-Richards S, Waldhauer I, Koller CF, Weiser B, Majety M, Runza V, Niu H, et al. RG7386, a novel tetravalent FAP-DR5 antibody, effectively triggers FAP-dependent, avidity-driven DR5 hyperclustering and tumor cell apoptosis. Mol Cancer Ther. 2016;15:946–57.

74. Chakravarthy U, Bailey C, Brown D, Campochiaro P, Chittum M, Csaky K, Tufail A, Yates P, Cech P, Giraudon M, Delmar P, Szczesny P, Sahni J, Boulay A, Nagel S, Fürst-Recktenwald S, Schwab D. Phase I trial of anti-vascular endothelial growth factor/anti-angiopoietin 2 bispecific antibody RG7716 for neovascular age-related macular degeneration. Ophthalmol Retina. 2017;1:474–85.

75. Regula JT, Lundh von Leithner P, Foxton R, Barathi VA, Cheung CM, Bo Tun SB, Wey YS, Iwata D, Dostalek M, Moelleken J, et al. Targeting key angiogenic pathways with a bispecific CrossMAb optimized for neovascular eye diseases. EMBO Mol Med. 2016;8:1265–88.

76. Tabernero J, Melero I, Ros W, Argiles G, Marabelle A, Rodriguez-Ruiz ME, Albanell J, Calvo E, Moreno V, Cleary JM, Eder JP, Karanikas V, Bouseida S, Sandoval F, Sabanes D, Sreckovic S, Hurwitz H, Paz-Ares LG, Saro Suarez JM, Segal NH. Phase Ia and Ib studies of the novel carcinoembryonic antigen (CEA) T-cell bispecific (CEA CD3 TCB) antibody as a single agent and in combination with atezolizumab: preliminary efficacy and safety in patients with metastatic colorectal cancer (mCRC). J Clin Oncol. 2017;35:3002.

77. Anti-HIV-1 gp41 Monoclonal (10E8), Catalog Number: 12294. NIH AIDS Reagent Program. https://www.aidsreagent.org/reagentdetail.cfm?t=monoclonal_antibodies&id=680. Accessed 27 May 2018.

78. Chennamsetty N, Voynov V, Kayser V, Helk B, Trout BL. Design of therapeutic proteins with enhanced stability. Proc Natl Acad Sci USA. 2009;106:11937–42.

79. Drugs@FDA: FDA approved drug products. U.S. Food and Drug Administration. https://www.accessdata.fda.gov/scripts/cder/daf. Accessed 18 May 2018.

80. Feige MJ, Groscurth S, Marcinowski M, Shimizu Y, Kessler H, Hendershot LM, Buchner J. An unfolded CH1 domain controls the assembly and secretion of IgG antibodies. Mol Cell. 2009;34:569–79.

81. Gilbert PB, Juraska M, deCamp AC, Karuna S, Edupuganti S, Mgodi N, Donnell DJ, Bentley C, Sista N, Andrew P, et al. Basis and statistical design of the passive HIV-1 antibody mediated prevention (AMP) test-of-concept efficacy trials. Stat Commun Infect Dis. 2017;9:20160001.

82. Points to Consider in the Manufacture and Testing of Monoclonal Antibody Products for Human Use. U.S. Department of Health and Human Services. Food and Drug Administration. Center for Biologics Evaluation and Research (CBER). 1997.

83. Guidance for Industry: Assay Development and Validation for Immunogenicity Testing of Therapeutic Protein Products. U.S. Department of Health and Human Services. Food and Drug Administration. Center for Drug Evaluation and Research (CDER). Center for Biologics Evaluation and Research (CBER). Center for Devices and Radiological Health (CDRH). 2016.

84. Chao DT, Ma X, Li O, Park H, Law D. Functional characterization of N297A, a murine surrogate for low-Fc binding anti-human CD3 antibodies. Immunol Invest. 2009;38:76–92.

8

Reticuloendotheliosis virus and avian leukosis virus subgroup J synergistically increase the accumulation of exosomal miRNAs

Defang Zhou[1], Jingwen Xue[1], Shuhai He[1], Xusheng Du[1], Jing Zhou[1], Chengui Li[1], Libo Huang[1], Venugopal Nair[2], Yongxiu Yao[2] and Ziqiang Cheng[1*]

Abstract

Background: Co-infection with avian leukosis virus subgroup J and reticuloendotheliosis virus induces synergistic pathogenic effects and increases mortality. However, the role of exosomal miRNAs in the molecular mechanism of the synergistic infection of the two viruses remains unknown.

Results: In this study, exosomal RNAs from CEF cells infected with ALV-J, REV or both at the optimal synergistic infection time were analysed by Illumina RNA deep sequencing. A total of 54 (23 upregulated and 31 downregulated) and 16 (7 upregulated and 9 downregulated) miRNAs were identified by comparing co-infection with two viruses, single-infected ALV-J and REV, respectively. Moreover, five key miRNAs, including miR-184-3p, miR-146a-3p, miR-146a-5p, miR-3538 and miR-155, were validated in both exosomes and CEF cells by qRT-PCR. GO annotation and KEGG pathway analysis of the miRNA target genes showed that the five differentially expressed miRNAs participated in virus-vector interaction, oxidative phosphorylation, energy metabolism and cell growth.

Conclusions: We demonstrated that REV and ALV-J synergistically increased the accumulation of exosomal miRNAs, which sheds light on the synergistic molecular mechanism of ALV-J and REV.

Keywords: Reticuloendotheliosis virus, Avian leukosis virus subgroup J, Exosomal miRNAs, Synergistic infection

Background

Viral synergism occurs commonly in nature when co-infection of two or more unrelated viruses invades the same host. Both reticuloendotheliosis virus (REV) and avian leukosis virus subgroup J (ALV-J), as two oncogenic retroviruses, consist of a set of retroviral genes, env, pol, gag and LTR, and mainly induce reticuloendotheliosis and myelocytomas, respectively [1, 2]. Due to similar transmission routes, co-infection with ALV-J and REV can readily occur [3, 4] and spreads very rapidly [5–7]. Co-infection of ALV-J and REV induces more serious pathogenic effects, such as immunosuppression, growth retardation, accelerated neoplasia progression, secondary infection in chickens [3, 5], and increased mortality.

Exosomes, intraluminal vesicles ranging approximately 30-100 nm in diameter secreted by live cells, have emerged as important molecules for intercellular communication that are involved in both normal and pathophysiological conditions, such as lactation, immune response and neuronal function, and in the development and progression of diseases, such as liver disease, neurodegenerative diseases and cancer [8–17]. Exosomes contain a wide variety of proteins, lipids, RNAs, non-transcribed RNAs, microRNAs and small RNAs to induce a diverse range of functions from intercellular communication to tumour proliferation [14, 18]. As useful biomarkers, exosomes are also helpful for exploring the synergistic mechanisms of co-infection with ALV-J and REV.

MicroRNAs (miRNAs) constitute a large family of small noncoding RNAs functioning as major regulators of gene expression in cancer development [19–21]. The

*Correspondence: czqsd@126.com
[1] College of Veterinary Medicine, Shandong Agricultural University, Tai'an 271018, China
Full list of author information is available at the end of the article

mature miRNA regulates spatio-temporal gene expression by binding to a seed region in the 3′ untranslated region (UTR) but may also bind to the 5′ UTR of target mRNA to enhance mRNA translation inhibition or degradation, resulting in decreased protein expression [22, 23]. Although miRNAs occupy negligible genomic space, their influence on a myriad of physiological processes, such as growth, differentiation, apoptosis, host–pathogen interactions and energy metabolism, is indubitable and relevant in tumour progression [24–30]. A growing number of studies have certified that miRNAs, including miR-122, miR-29b, miR-34a and miR-155, are key regulators of tumourigenesis, especially in viral synergistic infection [31–33]. However, the role of miRNA-mediated regulation of co-infection with ALV-J and REV remains unknown.

In the present study, to reveal the roles of miRNA profiles in the synergistic infection with ALV-J and REV, exosomal miRNAs were extracted from CEF infected with ALV-J, REV or both at the optimal synergistic infection time to analyse by Illumina RNA deep sequencing. The

key miRNAs obtained from deep sequencing were validated in exosomes and CEFs by qRT-PCR. Furthermore, the affected miRNA–mRNA interactions and associated biological processes were defined by integrated target prediction analyses.

Results

Synergistic infection of ALV-J and REV increases virus replication in CEF

To determine the best synergistic co-infection time of ALV-J and REV in vitro, we built an in vitro model of CEFs co-infected with ALV-J and REV and conducted viral RNA transcription analysis. The qRT-PCR results showed that both ALV-J and REV RNA levels in the co-infection group were increased significantly compared to those in the single infection groups at 48 hpi and 72 hpi and reached the highest peak at 72 hpi (Fig. 1a and 1b). However, the ALV-J RNA levels in the co-infection group were dramatically declined compared to those in the single infection groups at 96 hpi, 122 hpi and 144 hpi (Fig. 1a) while ALV-J still synergized with REV

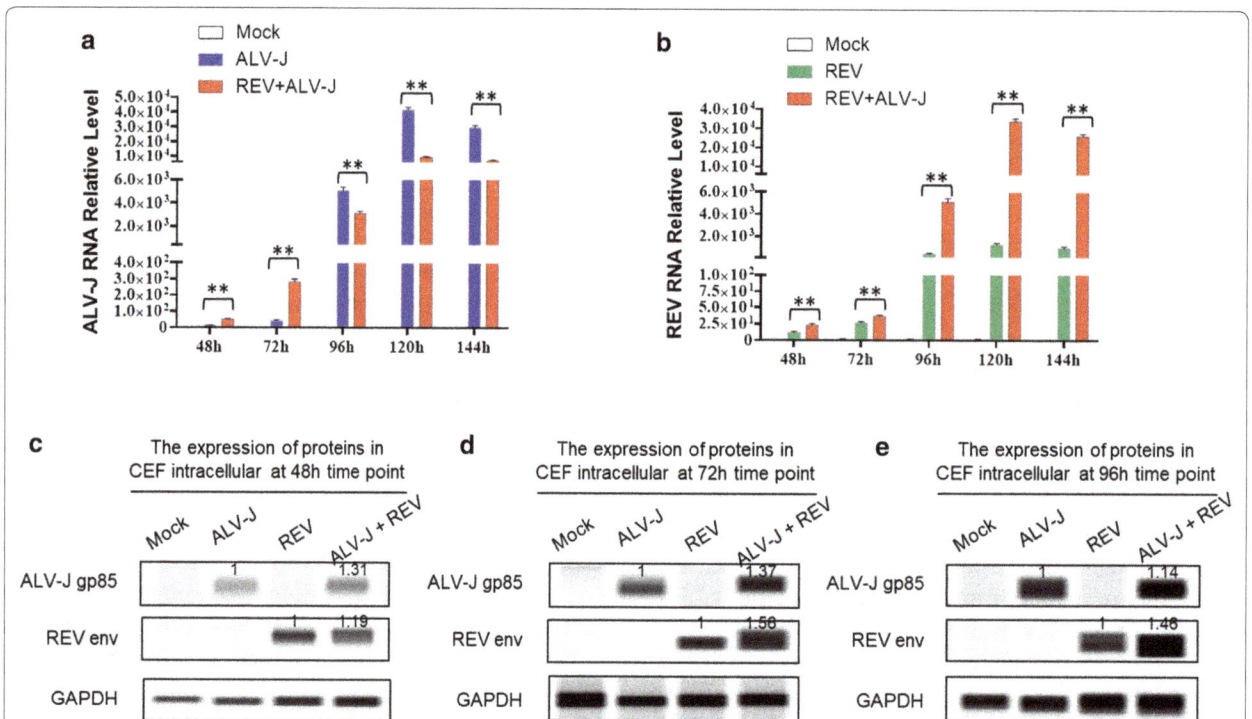

Fig. 1 Co-infection of ALV-J and REV promoted viral replication in CEFs. **a** REV increased the ALV-J RNA level at 48 hpi and 72 hpi while the ALV-J RNA levels in the co-infection group were decreased compared to those in the singly infected ALV-J at 96 hpi, 122 hpi and 144 hpi. The data represent the mean ± SEM determined from three independent experiments (n = 3), with each experiment containing three technical replicates. Compared with the single-infection group: **P < 0.01. **b** ALV-J increased the REV RNA level at 48, 72, 96, 122 and 144 hpi. The data represent the mean ± SEM determined from three independent experiments (n = 3), with each experiment containing three technical replicates. Compared with the single-infection group: **P < 0.01. **c** ALV-J synergized with REV to promote viral protein levels in CEF cells at 48 hpi detected by western blot with an anti-ALV-J gp85 antibody and anti-REV env antibody. **d** ALV-J synergized with REV to promote viral protein levels in CEF cells at 72 hpi detected by western blot with an anti-ALV-J gp85 antibody and anti-REV env antibody. **e** ALV-J synergized with REV to promote viral protein levels in CEF cells at 96 hpi detected by western blot with an anti-ALV-J gp85 antibody and anti-REV env antibody

to promote viral replication at 96 hpi, 120 hpi and 144 hpi (Fig. 1b). The viral protein expression levels were detected by western blot with anti-gp85 of ALV-J or anti-env of REV, and the results showed that the synergistic infection of ALV-J and REV increased each virus protein expression at 48 hpi, 72 hpi and 96 hpi (Fig. 1c, 1d and 1e). Consequently, co-infection of ALV-J and REV leads to the enhancement of viral transcription and protein expression in vitro.

Deep sequence analysis of exosomal miRNAs

To explore the miRNA profile of co-infection with ALV-J and REV, the exosomal miRNA from CEFs infected with ALV-J, REV or both were analysed using miRNA whole-genome sequencing at 72 hpi. We obtained the exosomes successfully and did not have any impurities by transmission electron microscopy. The photo showed that the exosomes had the typical goblet structure, and the size varied between 40 and 150 nm (Fig. 2a). The purities of exosomes were also verified by western blot with

anti-Hsp70, anti-Grp78 and anti-CD81. Western blot analysis showed that both exosomal protein samples were positive for CD81, a known exosomal protein, and negative for Grp78, an endoplasmic reticulum marker (Fig. 2b).

Further, 4 miRNA libraries were generated from exosomes of normal CEFs (ExoN), CEFs infected with ALV-J (ExoJ), REV (ExoR), and both (ExoRJ), and each group had two duplicates. In total, approximately 18,482,128 to 27,087,654 high-quality raw reads were obtained from the exosome libraries (Table 1). The selected reads from these libraries mapped well to the chicken genome, and the perfect match rates were 42.42% and 78.75% of the total reads (Table 1). After filtering the empty adaptors, low-quality sequences and single-read sequences, almost 100% clean reads of 15-35 nt were selected for further analysis. The remainder of the sequences were found to be other types of RNA, including rRNA, snRNA, snoRNA, tRNA, and noncoding RNA. The size distribution of small RNAs is summarized in

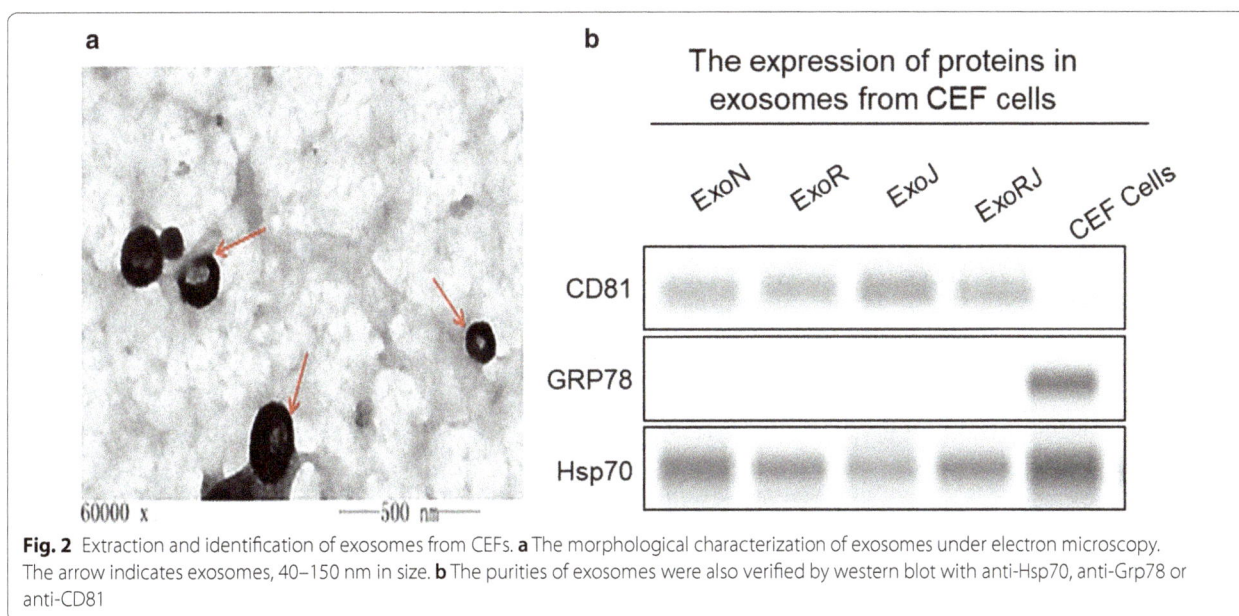

Fig. 2 Extraction and identification of exosomes from CEFs. **a** The morphological characterization of exosomes under electron microscopy. The arrow indicates exosomes, 40–150 nm in size. **b** The purities of exosomes were also verified by western blot with anti-Hsp70, anti-Grp78 or anti-CD81

Table 1 Summary of deep sequencing data for small RNAs in ExoN, ExoJ, ExoR, or ExoRJ

Categories	ExoJ1	ExoJ2	ExoN1	ExoN2	ExoR1	ExoR2	ExoRJ1	ExoRJ2
Raw reads	32,802,706	33,930,695	34,958,139	32,703,162	40,626,293	39,142,674	35,806,903	47,791,565
Clean reads	25,528,138	22,734,959	18,482,128	25,269,659	26,451,518	19,409,373	27,087,654	26,375,518
Map to genome percent (%)	72.43	77.02	67.15	78.75	61.58	58.72	44.3	42.42
Exon-antisense	993,966	1,018,809	418,741	761,889	516,146	323,086	414,847	346,494
Intron-sense	82,595	67,299	67,235	94,664	78,494	59,812	75,956	60,438
Intron-antisense	66,891	66,383	48,160	84,863	56,699	33,887	63,692	54,035
miRNAs	5,564,323	5,391,541	3,120,429	3,314,531	1,154,633	583,363	1,048,558	714,469

Fig. 3. The results showed that the peaks in CEF-uninfected, infected ALV-J, REV, or both were concentrated at 21–23 nt.

Identification of ALV-J and REV synergistic activated exosomal miRNAs in CEFs

To compare the differentially expressed miRNAs between co-infected and the two single virus infected CEFs, the differentially expressed miRNAs were mapped to the miRNA precursors of the reference species in the Sanger miRBase 21.0 database [34]. Using a P-value <

0.05 and $|$log2 (fold change)$| \geq 1$ as the cut-off values, a total of 54 (23 upregulated and 31 downregulated) and 16 (7 upregulated and 9 downregulated) miRNA genes were identified by comparing ExoRJ with ExoJ and ExoR, respectively (Fig. 4, Tables 2, 3).

Validation of miRNA expression using qRT-PCR

To validate the results of deep sequencing, five miRNAs, including miR-184-3p, miR-146a-3p, miR-146a-5p, miR-3538 and miR-155 that changed significantly in the co-infection group compared to each single infection

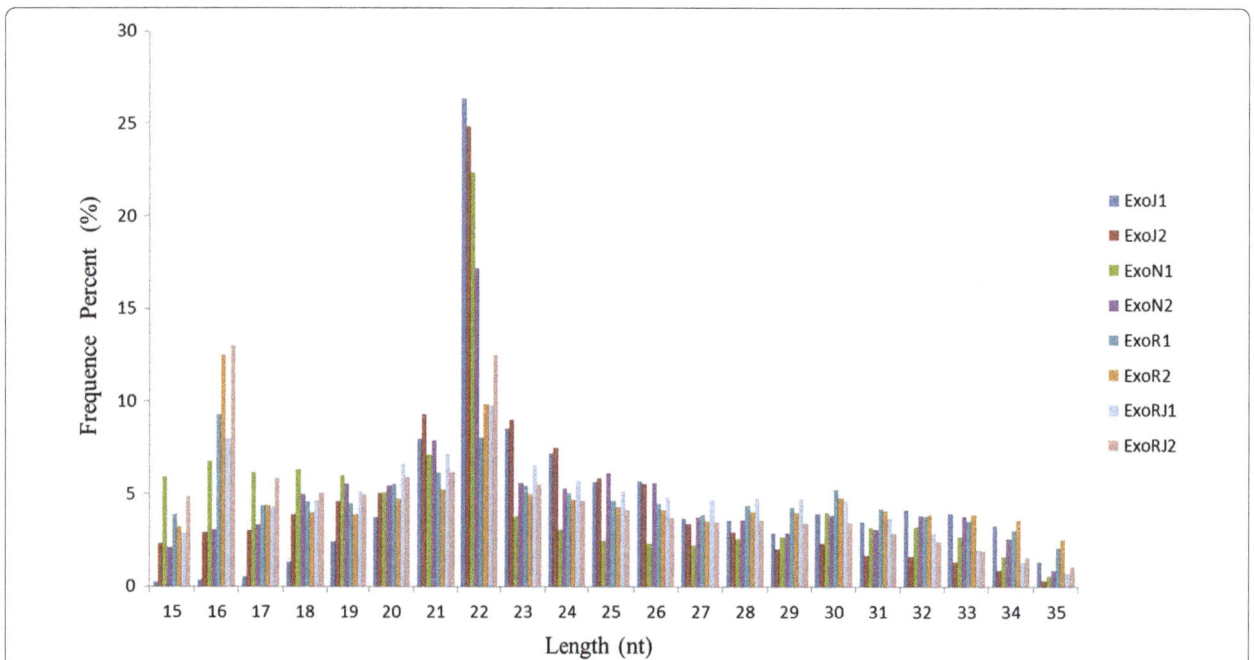

Fig. 3 Length distributions of the clean reads of the sequences. The abundances of the sequences in the peaks are shown. The peaks in CEF-uninfected, infected with ALV-J, REV, or both were at 21–23 nt

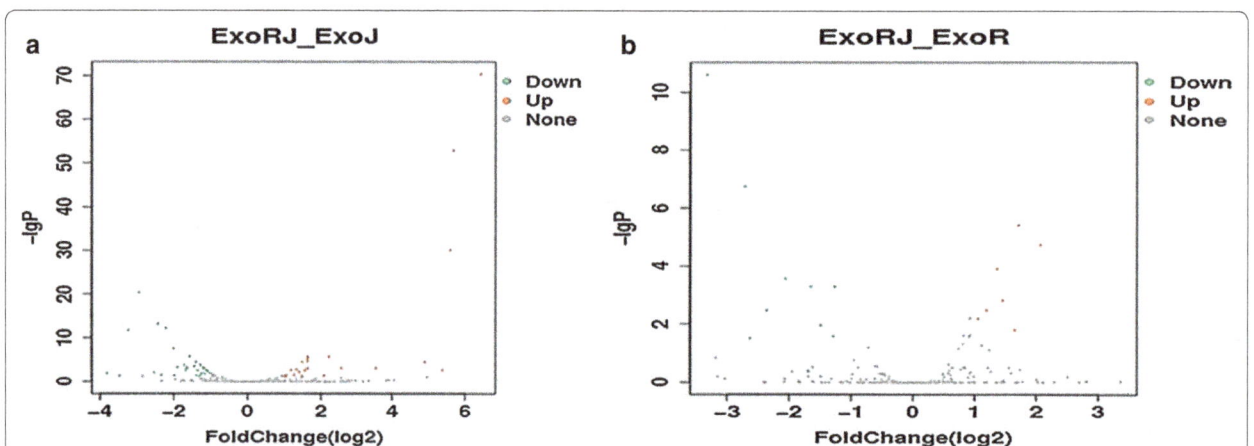

Fig. 4 The volcano plots of miRNAs by comparing co-infection with two viruses with ALV-J-infected (**a**) and REV-infected (**b**) groups. The x and y axes represent the fold change of the relative expression (log2) and the relative expression of the miRNAs, respectively

Table 2 Differentially   expressed   microRNAs between ExoRJ and ExoJ

miRNA name	FC	P value	FDR	Up/down
gga-miR-92-3p	2.77	4.45×10^{-3}	0.04	Up
gga-miR-456-3p	2.8	9.21×10^{-7}	3.18×10^{-5}	Up
gga-miR-429-3p	86	8.65×10^{-74}	4.47×10^{-71}	Up
gga-miR-375	29.1	8.16×10^{-7}	3.02×10^{-5}	Up
gga-miR-3538	3.1	4.48×10^{-7}	1.78×10^{-5}	Up
gga-miR-3529	3.08	5.52×10^{-5}	1.06×10^{-3}	Up
gga-miR-30c-2-3p	2.05	4.18×10^{-3}	0.04	Up
gga-miR-30a-3p	3.1	1.04×10^{-7}	4.47×10^{-6}	Up
gga-miR-223	2.06	3.87×10^{-3}	0.039	Up
gga-miR-222b-3p	11.8	3.48×10^{-5}	7.50×10^{-4}	Up
gga-miR-221-3p	4.65	3.67×10^{-8}	1.89×10^{-6}	Up
gga-miR-2131-3p	2.66	4.54×10^{-4}	6.35×10^{-3}	Up
gga-miR-184-3p	5.94	2.85×10^{-5}	7.01×10^{-4}	Up
gga-miR-1684a-3p	2.51	8.90×10^{-5}	1.64×10^{-3}	Up
gga-miR-155	50.8	5.03×10^{-56}	1.30×10^{-53}	Up
gga-miR-146a-5p	41	1.37×10^{-4}	2.37×10^{-3}	Up
gga-miR-146a-3p	47.7	5.35×10^{-33}	9.22×10^{-31}	Up
gga-miR-144-3p	2.95	1.79×10^{-4}	2.72×10^{-3}	Up
gga-miR-142-5p	2.27	1.33×10^{-4}	2.37×10^{-3}	Up
gga-miR-1416-5p	4.24	3.94×10^{-3}	0.039	Up
gga-miR-1329-5p	2.41	2.72×10^{-3}	0.03	Up
gga-let-7c-5p	2.06	3.45×10^{-3}	0.036	Up
gga-miR-6548-5p	0.071	9.08×10^{-4}	0.011	Down
gga-miR-460a-3p	0.382	3.29×10^{-3}	0.035	Down
gga-miR-455-5p	0.336	3.03×10^{-8}	1.74×10^{-6}	Down
gga-miR-455-3p	0.38	1.13×10^{-6}	3.64×10^{-5}	Down
gga-miR-34a-3p	0.322	3.22×10^{-5}	7.24×10^{-4}	Down
gga-miR-32-3p	0.172	5.48×10^{-4}	7.45×10^{-3}	Down
gga-miR-30e-5p	0.305	4.99×10^{-6}	1.51×10^{-4}	Down
gga-miR-30d	0.45	1.44×10^{-3}	0.017	Down
gga-miR-30b-5p	0.215	6.92×10^{-15}	5.96×10^{-13}	Down
gga-miR-301b-3p	0.434	3.98×10^{-5}	8.02×10^{-4}	Down
gga-miR-301a-3p	0.487	6.54×10^{-4}	8.68×10^{-3}	Down
gga-miR-2954	0.185	6.53×10^{-16}	6.75×10^{-14}	Down
gga-miR-26a-3p	0.199	2.51×10^{-3}	0.028	Down
gga-miR-219b	0.472	2.5×10^{-4}	3.63×10^{-3}	Down
gga-miR-2131-5p	0.412	5.73×10^{-6}	1.65×10^{-4}	Down
gga-miR-20a-3p	0.253	3.68×10^{-3}	0.038	Down
gga-miR-203a	0.09	5.58×10^{-3}	0.049	Down
gga-miR-199-5p	0.313	1.88×10^{-4}	2.78×10^{-3}	Down
gga-miR-193b-3p	0.13	3.44×10^{-23}	4.45×10^{-21}	Down
gga-miR-190a-5p	0.268	2.00×10^{-5}	5.18×10^{-4}	Down
gga-miR-18a-5p	0.465	1.66×10^{-4}	2.69×10^{-3}	Down
gga-miR-181a-3p	0.439	3.01×10^{-5}	7.08×10^{-4}	Down
gga-miR-1729-5p	0.106	$2.66E-14$	1.99×10^{-12}	Down
gga-miR-16-5p	0.414	2.19×10^{-3}	0.025	Down
gga-miR-148a-5p	0.462	1.64×10^{-4}	2.69×10^{-3}	Down
gga-miR-146c-5p	0.317	4.03×10^{-5}	8.02×10^{-4}	Down
gga-miR-146c-3p	0.404	5.18×10^{-3}	0.0461	Down
gga-miR-146b-5p	0.368	1.09×10^{-5}	2.97×10^{-4}	Down

Table 2 (continued)

miRNA name	FC	P value	FDR	Up/down
gga-miR-1451-5p	0.249	3.64×10^{-10}	2.35×10^{-8}	Down
gga-miR-10b-3p	0.426	8.66×10^{-4}	0.011	Down
gga-miR-101-2-5p	0.39	1.76×10^{-4}	2.72×10^{-3}	Down

FC fold change, *FDR* false discovery rate (corrected *P* value)

Table 3 Differentially   expressed   microRNAs between ExoRJ and ExoR

miRNA name	FC	p value	FDR	Up/down
gga-miR-146a-3p	4.18	1.66×10^{-7}	1.84×10^{-5}	Up
gga-miR-155	3.27	2.62×10^{-8}	3.87×10^{-6}	Up
gga-miR-184-3p	3.13	5.41×10^{-4}	1.59×10^{-2}	Up
gga-let-7a-2-3p	2.74	3.08×10^{-5}	1.51×10^{-3}	Up
gga-miR-458a-3p	2.29	8.31×10^{-5}	3.34×10^{-3}	Up
gga-miR-429-3p	2.08	1.89×10^{-4}	6.44×10^{-3}	Up
gga-miR-3538	0.42	9.19×10^{-6}	5.08×10^{-4}	Down
gga-miR-1454	0.41	1.04×10^{-3}	2.56×10^{-2}	Down
gga-miR-460b-5p	0.36	3.45×10^{-4}	1.09×10^{-2}	Down
gga-miR-133c-3p	0.32	8.86×10^{-6}	5.08×10^{-4}	Down
gga-miR-489-3p	0.24	3.68×10^{-6}	2.71×10^{-4}	Down
gga-miR-499-5p	0.19	7.76×10^{-5}	3.34×10^{-3}	Down
gga-miR-1677-3p	0.16	1.36×10^{-3}	3.01×10^{-2}	Down
gga-miR-1563	0.15	7.89×10^{-10}	1.75×10^{-7}	Down
gga-miR-206	0.1	5.71×10^{-14}	2.53×10^{-11}	Down

FC fold change, *FDR* false discovery rate (corrected *P* value)

group, were selected for qRT-PCR analysis with primers in Table 4. After RNA was isolated from ExoN, ExoJ, ExoR and ExoRJ at 72 hpi, all 5 miRNAs showed expression profiles in CEF exosomes that were consistent with the small RNA sequencing data (Fig. 5a). Furthermore, the expressions of these five miRNAs were also verified in CEF cells co-infected with ALV-J and REV 72 hpi. Although the variation trends of miR-184-3p, miR-146a-3p, miR-3538 and miR-155 in both CEF cells and exosomes were consistent, some changes in each miRNA in CEF cells were less than in exosomes, indicating that the exosomes stably maintained these miRNAs (Fig. 5b).

Target prediction

To understand the biological functions of the miRNAs identified in our analysis, miRanda was used to predict targets of the differentially expressed miRNA. Numerous target genes, 19,450 and 6058 for 54 and 16 miRNAs, respectively, were predicted as potential miRNA targets (Additional files 1 and 2). A GO annotation of the predicted target genes revealed that 100 and 35 target genes were significantly annotated for the 54 and 16 miRNAs, respectively, and they were involved in cellular processes,

Table 4 Primers used to detect miRNA expression using qRT-PCR

miRNA name	Mature sequences	Primer (5′–3′)
gga-miR-146a-5p	UGAGAACUGAAUUCCAUGGGUU	GTGAGAACTGAATTCCATGGGTT
gga-miR-146a-3p	ACCCAUGGGCUCAGUUCUUCAG	ACCCATGGGGCTCAGTTCTTC
gga-miR-184-3p	UGGACGGAGAACUGAUAAGGGU	TGGACGGAGAACTGATAAGGGT
gga-miR-3538	GUUCGGUGAUGAAACCAUGGA	GGTTCGGTGATGAAACCATGGA
gga-miR-155	UUAAUGCUAAUCGUGAUAGGG	GGTTAATGCTAATCGTGATAGGG
U6-F		CTCGCTTCGGCAGCACA
U6-R		AACGCTTCACGAATTTGCGT

immune system processes, biology regulation, such as cytoskeleton organization, regulation of Ras protein signal transduction, ATP binding and guanyl-nucleotide exchange factor activity (Fig. 6, Additional files 3 and 4). To further analyse the roles that these miRNAs might play in regulatory networks, the putative miRNA targets were assigned to KEGG pathways using the KEGG GENES Database, PATHWAY Database and LIGAND Database. The results indicated that the most abundant KEGG terms were involved in the Toll-like receptor signalling pathway, oxidative phosphorylation, ribosome and other biological processes (Fig. 7, Additional files 5 and 6). In summary, these findings demonstrated that the differentially expressed miRNAs play important regulatory roles in virus-vector interaction, energy metabolism and cell growth.

Discussion

In this study, an enhancement of viral transcription and protein expression was observed in ALV-J and REV co-infected CEF cells and reached a peak at 72 hpi. After Illumina small RNA deep sequencing of exosomes from CEFs co-infected with ALV-J and REV, a total of 54 (23 upregulated and 31 downregulated) and 16 (7 upregulated and 9 downregulated) miRNAs were identified by comparing the significantly differentially expressed miRNAs of ExoRJ with ExoJ and ExoR, respectively. Further, 5 miRNAs, including miR-184-3p, miR-146a-3p, miR-146a-5p, miR-3538 and miR-155, were verified by qRT-PCR and found to be consistent with the sequencing analysis. The analysis of the target prediction data demonstrated that these differentially expressed miRNAs participated in aspects of virus-vector interaction, oxidative

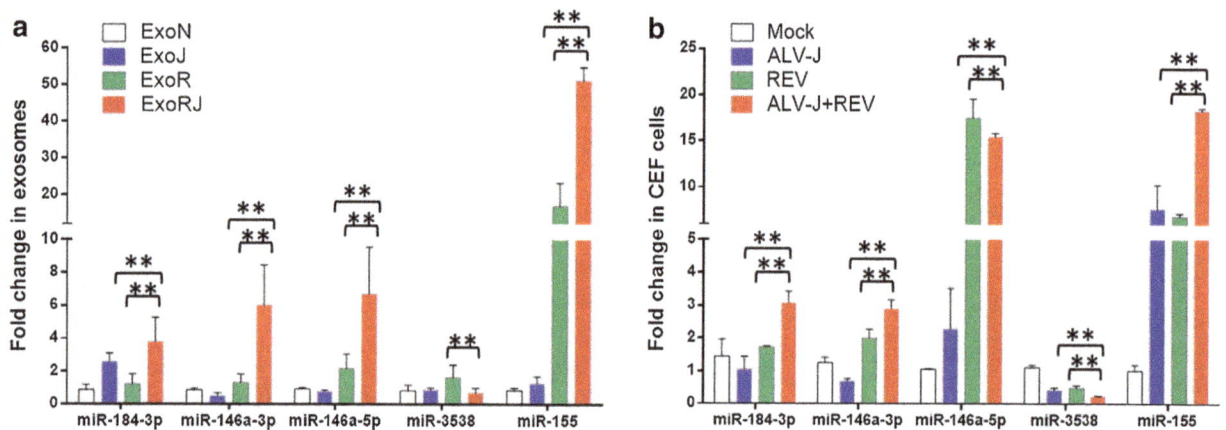

Fig. 5 The qRT-PCR analysis for five miRNAs from exosomes and CEF cells. **a** The qRT-PCR results of the five miRNAs in exosomes were consistent with the sequencing. The data represent the mean ± SEM determined from three independent experiments (n = 3), with each experiment containing three technical replicates. Compared with the single-infection group: **$P < 0.01$. **b** The qRT-PCR results of four miRNAs in CEFs, including miR-184-3p, miR-146a-3p, miR-3538 and miR-155, were consistent with that in exosomes while miR-146a-5p expression in singly infected REV was significantly higher than co-infection with two viruses. The data represent the mean ± SEM determined from three independent experiments (n = 3), with each experiment containing three technical replicates. Compared with the single-infection group: **$P < 0.01$

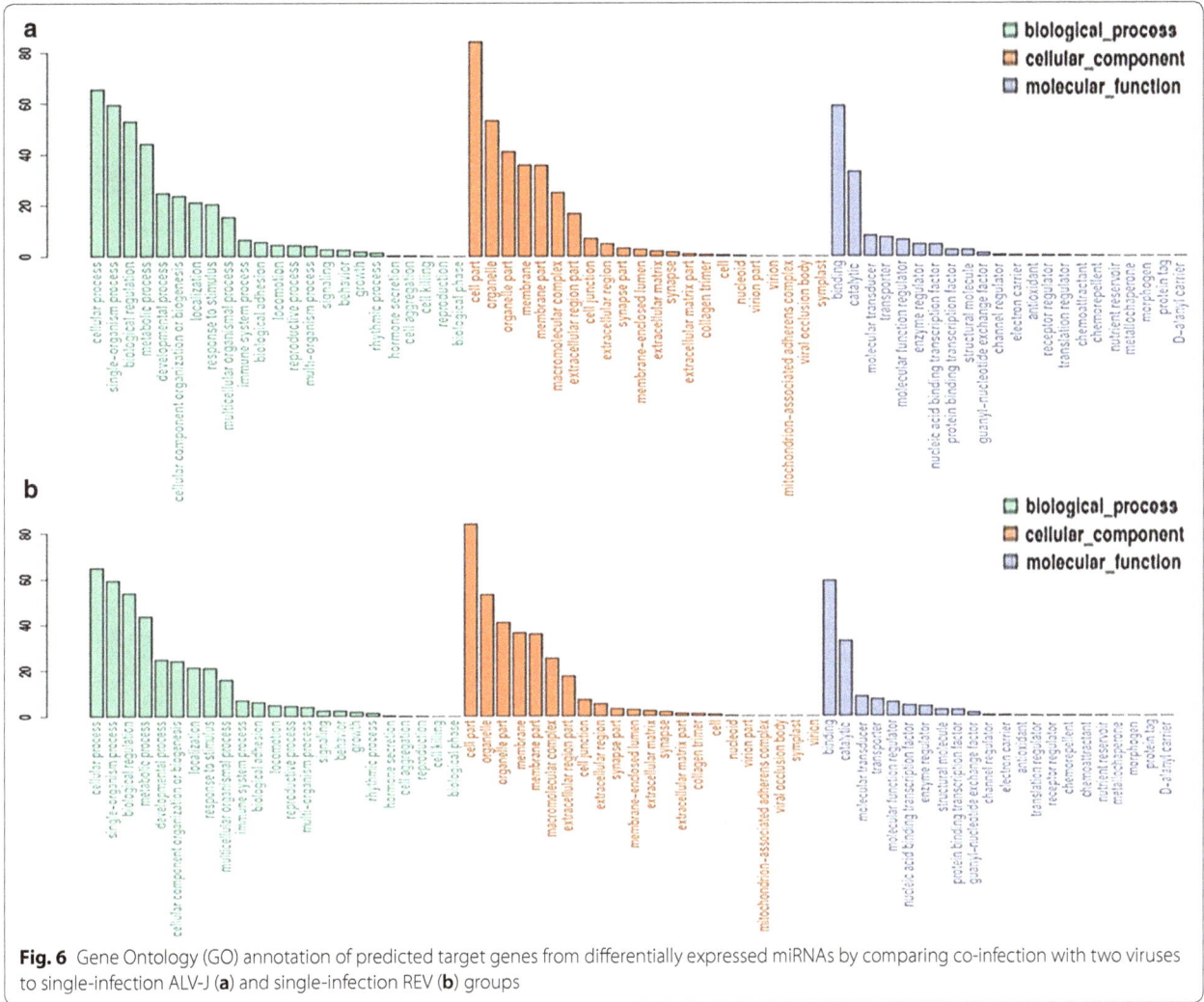

Fig. 6 Gene Ontology (GO) annotation of predicted target genes from differentially expressed miRNAs by comparing co-infection with two viruses to single-infection ALV-J (**a**) and single-infection REV (**b**) groups

phosphorylation, energy metabolism and cell growth in the process of co-infection with ALV-J and REV.

Useful as a biomarker, exosomes are overproduced by most proliferating cell types and contain a wide variety of microRNAs to induce a diverse range of functions, such as antigen presentation, cellular responses to environmental stresses, and propagation of pathogens [35–39]. Some miRNAs, such as let-7, miR-1, miR-15, miR-16, miR-151 and miR-375, which have roles in angiogenesis, haematopoiesis, exocytosis and tumourigenesis, have been reported in exosomes [40–44]. To further understand the relationship between exosomes and the parental CEF cells, miR-184-3p, miR-146a-3p, miR-146a-5p, miR-3538 and miR-155 expression was verified in both exosomes and CEF cells. In addition to miR-146a-5p, the qRT-PCR results in CEF cells of miR-184-3p, miR-146a-3p, miR-3538 and miR-155 were consistent with that in exosomes, suggesting that these miRNAs are key regulators in co-infection with ALV-J and REV.

In tumour progression, especially induced by viral synergistic infection, several studies have verified that miRNAs influence growth, differentiation, apoptosis, host-pathogen interactions, energy metabolism and other physiological processes [31–33]. While infecting cells, viruses integrate into the host genome to ensure viral persistence, which requires certain conditions for virus-vector interaction [45]. Simultaneously, the viral replication also benefits the cell's transcriptional and translational machinery, which may enhance the growth of the host cells. In addition, these regulations are based on energy metabolism [46, 47]. Our data suggested that the significantly differentially expressed miRNAs between co-infected and two single virus infected CEFs participated in energy metabolism, virus-vector interaction and cell growth, suggesting that these miRNAs are key regulators in co-infection with ALV-J and REV. These initial findings will lead to further exploration of the mechanism of ALV-J synergistic infection with REV.

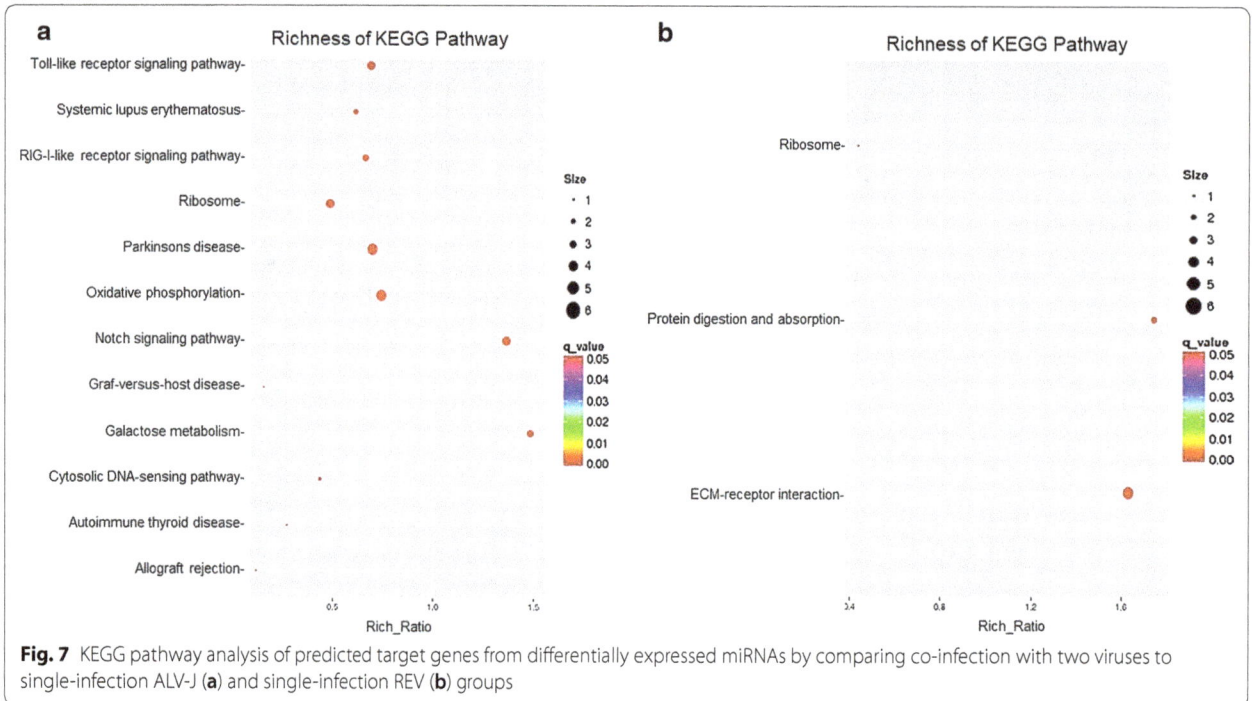

Fig. 7 KEGG pathway analysis of predicted target genes from differentially expressed miRNAs by comparing co-infection with two viruses to single-infection ALV-J (**a**) and single-infection REV (**b**) groups

Conclusion

We demonstrated that REV and ALV-J synergistically increased the accumulation of exosomal miRNAs. We revealed that a total of 54 and 16 miRNA genes were identified by comparing co-infection with two viruses with single-infected ALV-J and REV, respectively. These differentially expressed miRNAs participated in virus-vector interaction, oxidative phosphorylation, energy metabolism and cell growth, indicating potential new avenues to study the mechanism of synergistic infection of ALV-J and REV.

Methods

Cells and virus

DF-1 and chicken embryo fibroblasts (CEFs) cells were maintained in Dulbecco's modified Eagle's medium (DMEM) supplemented with 10% foetal bovine serum (FBS), 1% penicillin/streptomycin, and 1% l-glutamine, in a 5% CO_2 incubator at 37°C. The stock SNV strain of REV at $10^{3.2}$ 50% tissue culture infectious doses ($TCID_{50}$) and NX0101 strain of ALV-J at $10^{3.8}$ $TCID_{50}$ were maintained in our laboratory. The $TCID_{50}$ of the SNV and NX0101 strains were titrated by limiting dilution in DF-1 culture.

Extraction of exosomes from CEF cells

The exosomes from Mock, single infection of ALV-J or REV, or co-infection of both ALV-J and REV CEFs were isolated using Total Exosome Isolation Reagent

(Thermo Fisher Scientific) based on the manufacturer's instructions.

Transmission electron microscopy

The protocol was conducted as described in a previous study [48].

Western blotting

CEF cells were lysed in cell lysis buffer (Beyotime) and incubated on ice for 5 minutes. ALV-J gp85, REV env expression, Hsp70, GRP78 and CD81 were detected by simple western analysis with anti-NX0101 gp85, anti-SNV env antibody, anti-Hsp70 (Bioss), anti-GRP78 (Bioss) antibody and anti-CD81 (Bioss) antibody at a 1:200, 1:200, 1:1000, 1:1000 and 1:1000 dilution, respectively.

Illumina small RNA deep sequencing

Total RNA of the infected CEF exosome samples was separated by 15% agarose gels to extract the small RNA (18-30 nt). After precipitation by ethanol and centrifugal enrichment of the small RNA population, the library was prepared according to the method and process of the Small RNA Sample Preparation Kit (Illumina, RS-200-0048). The RNA concentration of the library was measured using Qubit® RNA Assay Kit in Qubit® 2.0 to preliminarily quantify and then dilute to

1 ng/μl. The insert size was assessed using the Agilent Bioanalyzer 2100 system (Agilent Technologies, CA, USA). The library with the expected insert size was then quantified accurately using TaqMan fluorescence probes of the AB Step One Plus Real-Time PCR system (library valid concentration >2 nM). The qualified libraries were sequenced by an Illumina HiSeq 2500 platform and 50 bp single-end reads were generated.

Real-time quantitative reverse transcription polymerase chain reaction

Total RNA from CEF exosomes of either Mock, single infection of ALV-J or REV, or co-infection of both ALV-J and REV were isolated using the Tiangen RNeasy mini kit according to the manufacturer's instructions, with optional on-column DNase digestion. RNA integrity and concentration were assessed by agarose gel electrophoresis and spectrophotometry. RNA (1 μg per triplicate reaction) was reverse transcribed to cDNA using the TaqMan Gold Reverse Transcription kit (Applied Biosystems). Real-time RT-PCR (qRT-PCR) was carried out using SYBR® Premix Ex TaqTM, and ALV-J or REV specific primers (Table 5). All values were normalized to the endogenous control GAPDH to control for variation. For qRT-PCR of miR-184-3p, miR-146a-3p, miR-146a-5p, miR-3538 and miR-155, we used a miRcute miRNA first-stand cDNA synthesis kit and a miRcute miRNA qPCR detection kit (SYBR Green) (TIANGEN). The reverse primer was provided in the miRcute miRNA qPCR detection kit as a primer complementary to the poly (T) adapter. Data were collected on an ABI PRISM 7500 and analysed via Sequence Detector v1.1 software. All values were normalized to the endogenous control U6 to control for variation. The specific primer for U6 was described in Table 4. Assays were performed in triplicate and average threshold cycle (CT) values were used to determine relative concentration differences based on the ΔΔCT method of relative quantization described in the manufacturer's protocol.

Target prediction

miRanda (http://www.microrna.org/microrna/) was used to predict targets of the differentially expressed miRNA. Gene enrichment and functional annotation analyses were conducted using Gene Ontology (GO; www.geneontology.org), Kyoto Encyclopedia of Genes and Genomes (KEGG, http://www.genome.jp/kegg), PATHWAY Database and LIGAND Database.

Statistical analysis

Results are presented as the mean ± standard deviation(s). The T test and one-way ANOVA test was performed using SPSS 13.0 statistical software. A P value less than 0.05 was considered statistically significant.

Additional files

Additional file 1. The potential miRNA targets of the differentially expressed miRNA between ExoRJ and ExoJ. Numerous target genes, 19,450 for 54 miRNAs, were predicted as potential miRNA targets.

Additional file 2. The potential miRNA targets of the differentially expressed miRNA between ExoRJ and ExoR. Numerous target genes, 6058 for 16 miRNAs, were predicted as potential miRNA targets.

Additional file 3. The GO annotation of the predicted target genes of the differentially expressed miRNA between ExoRJ and ExoJ. A GO annotation of the predicted target genes revealed that 100 target genes were annotated significantly for the 54 differentially expressed miRNAs between ExoRJ and ExoJ.

Additional file 4. The GO annotation of the predicted target genes of the differentially expressed miRNA between ExoRJ and ExoR. A GO annotation of the predicted target genes revealed that 35 target genes were annotated significantly for the 16 miRNAs between ExoRJ and ExoR.

Additional file 5. The KEGG analysis of the predicted target genes of the differentially expressed miRNA between ExoRJ and ExoJ. The KEGG analysis of the predicted target genes revealed that 7 regulatory networks were annotated significantly for the 54 differentially expressed miRNAs between ExoRJ and ExoJ.

Additional file 6. The KEGG analysis of the predicted target genes of the differentially expressed miRNA between ExoRJ and ExoR. The KEGG analysis of the predicted target genes revealed that 3 regulatory networks were annotated significantly for the 16 differentially expressed miRNAs between ExoRJ and ExoR.

Authors' contributions
ZC conceived and designed the research. DZ wrote the manuscript. DZ and JW performed the experiments. SH, XD and JZ contributed reagents and materials. CL, LH, VN, and YY commented on the manuscript. All authors read and approved the final manuscript.

Author details
[1] College of Veterinary Medicine, Shandong Agricultural University, Tai'an 271018, China. [2] The Pirbright Institute & UK-China Centre of Excellence on Avian Disease Research, Pirbright, Ash Road, Guildford, Surrey GU24 0NF, UK.

Acknowledgements
We are grateful to Ms. Pingping Zhuang, Dr. Guihua Wang, Ms. Li Zhang and the Annoroad Gene Technology Company for their technical assistance. We thank Dr. Gen Li and Dr. Mingjun Zhu for their helpful discussion and manuscript revision.

Table 5 Primers used for real-time PCR

Gene	Primer	Primer sequence	Size of PCR product
REV	F	TTGTTGAAGGCAAGCATCAG	105 bp
	R	GAGGATAGCATCTGCCCTTT	
ALV-J	F	TGCGTGCGTGGTTATTATTTC	144 bp
	R	AATGGTGAGGTCGCTGACTGT	
GADPH	F	GAACATCATCCCAGCGTCCA	132 bp
	R	CGGCAGGTCAGGTCAACAAC	

Competing interests

The authors declare no competing financial interests.

Funding

The study was supported by grants from the China-UK Partnership on Global Food Security: Combating tumour diseases for Sustainable Poultry Production (31761133002, BB/R012865/1), the Natural Science Foundation of China (31672521), the Shandong Modern Agricultural Technology & Industry System (SDAIT-11-04) and the Fund of Shandong "Double Tops" Program (2017).

References

1. Payne LN, Brown SR, Bumstead N, Howes K, Frazier JA, Thouless ME. A novel subgroup of exogenous avian leukosis virus in chickens. J Gen Virol. 1991;72(Pt 4):801–7.
2. Bai J, Payne LN, Skinner MA. HPRS-103 (exogenous avian leukosis virus, subgroup J) has an env gene related to those of endogenous elements EAV-0 and E51 and an E element found previously only in sarcoma viruses. J Virol. 1995;69:779–84.
3. Dong X, Ju S, Zhao P, Li Y, Meng F, Sun P, Cui Z. Synergetic effects of subgroup J avian leukosis virus and reticuloendotheliosis virus co-infection on growth retardation and immunosuppression in SPF chickens. Vet Microbiol. 2014;172:425–31.
4. Guo H, Li H, Cheng Z, Liu J, Cui Z. Co-Infection on immunologic function of T lymphocytes and histopathology in broiler chickens. J Integr Agric. 2010;09:1667–76.
5. Cui Z, Sun S, Zhang Z, Meng S. Simultaneous endemic infections with subgroup J avian leukosis virus and reticuloendotheliosis virus in commercial and local breeds of chickens. Avian Pathol. 2009;38:443–8.
6. Davidson I, Borenstein R. Multiple infection of chickens and turkeys with avian oncogenic viruses: prevalence and molecular analysis. Acta Virol. 1999;43:136–42.
7. Cheng Z, Zhang H, Wang G, Liu Q, Liu J, Guo H, Zhou E. Investigations of avian leukosis virus subgroup J and reticuloendotheliosis virus infections in broiler breeders in China. Isr J Vet Med. 2011;66:34–8.
8. Harding C, Heuser J, Stahl P. Receptor-mediated endocytosis of transferrin and recycling of the transferrin receptor in rat reticulocytes. J Cell Biol. 1983;97:329–39.
9. Admyre C, Johansson SM, Qazi KR, Filen JJ, Lahesmaa R, Norman M, Neve EP, Scheynius A, Gabrielsson S. Exosomes with immune modulatory features are present in human breast milk. J Immunol. 2007;179:1969–78.
10. Masyuk AI, Masyuk TV, Larusso NF. Exosomes in the pathogenesis, diagnostics and therapeutics of liver diseases. J Hepatol. 2013;59:621–5.
11. Vella LJ, Sharples RA, Nisbet RM, Cappai R, Hill AF. The role of exosomes in the processing of proteins associated with neurodegenerative diseases. Eur Biophys J. 2008;37:323–32.
12. Bard MP, Hegmans JP, Hemmes A, Luider TM, Willemsen R, Severijnen LA, van Meerbeeck JP, Burgers SA, Hoogsteden HC, Lambrecht BN. Proteomic analysis of exosomes isolated from human malignant pleural effusions. Am J Respir Cell Mol Biol. 2004;31:114–21.
13. Schorey JS, Bhatnagar S. Exosome function: from tumor immunology to pathogen biology. Traffic. 2008;9:871–81.
14. Beach A, Zhang HG, Ratajczak MZ, Kakar SS. Exosomes: an overview of biogenesis, composition and role in ovarian cancer. J Ovarian Res. 2014;7:14.
15. El-Saghir J, Nassar F, Tawil N, El-Sabban M. ATL-derived exosomes modulate mesenchymal stem cells: potential role in leukemia progression. Retrovirology. 2016;13:73.
16. Milane L, Singh A, Mattheolabakis G, Suresh M, Amiji MM. Exosome mediated communication within the tumor microenvironment. J Control Release. 2015;219:278–94.
17. Greening DW, Gopal SK, Xu R, Simpson RJ, Chen W. Exosomes and their roles in immune regulation and cancer. Semin Cell Dev Biol. 2015;40:72–81.
18. Narayanan A, Jaworski E, Duyne RV, Iordanskiy S, Guendel I, Das R, Currer R, Sampey G, Chung M, Kehn-Hall K. Exosomes derived from HTLV-1 infected cells contain the viral protein Tax. Retrovirology. 2014;11:O46.
19. Selbach M, Schwanhausser B, Thierfelder N, Fang Z, Khanin R, Rajewsky N. Widespread changes in protein synthesis induced by microRNAs. Nature. 2008;455:58–63.
20. Baek D, Villen J, Shin C, Camargo FD, Gygi SP, Bartel DP. The impact of microRNAs on protein output. Nature. 2008;455:64–71.
21. Shin VY, Chu KM. MiRNA as potential biomarkers and therapeutic targets for gastric cancer. World J Gastroenterol. 2014;20:10432–9.
22. Lytle JR, Yario TA, Steitz JA. Target mRNAs are repressed as efficiently by microRNA-binding sites in the 5′UTR as in the 3′UTR. Proc Natl Acad Sci USA. 2007;104:9667–72.
23. Towler BP, Jones CI, Newbury SF. Mechanisms of regulation of mature miRNAs. Biochem Soc Trans. 2015;43:1208–14.
24. Ambros V. MicroRNAs and developmental timing. Curr Opin Genet Dev. 2011;21:511–7.
25. Blahna MT, Hata A. Regulation of miRNA biogenesis as an integrated component of growth factor signaling. Curr Opin Cell Biol. 2013;25:233–40.
26. Subramanian S, Steer CJ. MicroRNAs as gatekeepers of apoptosis. J Cell Physiol. 2010;223:289–98.
27. Zhou R, Rana TM. RNA-based mechanisms regulating host-virus interactions. Immunol Rev. 2013;253:97–111.
28. Bhaskaran M, Mohan M. MicroRNAs: history, biogenesis, and their evolving role in animal development and disease. Vet Pathol. 2014;51:759–74.
29. Hartig SM, Hamilton MP, Bader DA, McGuire SE. The miRNA interactome in metabolic homeostasis. Trends Endocrinol Metab. 2015;26:733–45.
30. Rosado J, Alvarez C, Clark D, Gotuzzo E, Talledo M. Differential miRNA expression profiles in Peruvian HTLV-1 carriers. Retrovirology. 2014;11:1.
31. Gupta P, Liu B, Wu JQ, Soriano V, Vispo E, Carroll AP, Goldie BJ, Cairns MJ, Saksena NK. Genome-wide mRNA and miRNA analysis of peripheral blood mononuclear cells (PBMC) reveals different miRNAs regulating HIV/HCV co-infection. Virology. 2014;450–451:336–49.
32. Janssen HL, Reesink HW, Lawitz EJ, Zeuzem S, Rodriguez-Torres M, Patel K, van der Meer AJ, Patick AK, Chen A, Zhou Y, et al. Treatment of HCV infection by targeting microRNA. N Engl J Med. 2013;368:1685–94.
33. Pilotti E, Casoli C, Bianchi MV, Bignami F, Prati F. MiRNA profile in CD4 positive T cells from HTLV-2 and HIV-1 mono- and co-infected subjects. Retrovirology. 2012;9:P2.
34. Quinlan AR, Hall IM. BEDTools: a flexible suite of utilities for comparing genomic features. Bioinformatics. 2010;26:841–2.
35. Cho JA, Yeo DJ, Son HY, Kim HW, Jung DS, Ko JK, Koh JS, Kim YN, Kim CW. Exosomes: a new delivery system for tumor antigens in cancer immunotherapy. Int J Cancer. 2005;114:613–22.
36. Hegmans JP, Bard MP, Hemmes A, Luider TM, Kleijmeer MJ, Prins JB, Zitvogel L, Burgers SA, Hoogsteden HC, Lambrecht BN. Proteomic analysis of exosomes secreted by human mesothelioma cells. Am J Pathol. 1807;2004:164.
37. Lamparski HG, Metha-Damani A, Yao JY, Patel S, Hsu DH, Ruegg C, Le PJ. Production and characterization of clinical grade exosomes derived from dendritic cells. J Immunol Methods. 2002;270:211–26.
38. Schorey JS, Cheng Y, Singh PP, Smith VL. Exosomes and other extracellular vesicles in host-pathogen interactions. EMBO Rep. 2015;16:24–43.
39. Fleming A, Sampey G, Chung MC, Bailey C, van Hoek ML, Kashanchi F, Hakami RM. The carrying pigeons of the cell: exosomes and their role in infectious diseases caused by human pathogens. Pathog Dis. 2014;71:109–20.
40. Taylor DD, Zacharias W, Gerceltaylor C. Exosome isolation for proteomic analyses and RNA profiling. Methods Mol Biol. 2011;728:235.
41. Yang G, Zhang W, Yu C, Ren J, An Z. MicroRNA let-7: regulation, single nucleotide polymorphism, and therapy in lung cancer. J Cancer Res Ther. 2015;11(Suppl 1):C1–6.
42. Minemura H, Takagi K, Miki Y, Shibahara Y, Nakagawa S, Ebata A, Watanabe M, Ishida T, Sasano H, Suzuki T. Abnormal expression of miR-1 in breast carcinoma as a potent prognostic factor. Cancer Sci. 2015;106:1642–50.
43. Porrello ER, Johnson BA, Aurora AB, Simpson E, Nam YJ, Matkovich SJ, Dorn GW 2nd, van Rooij E, Olson EN. MiR-15 family regulates postnatal mitotic arrest of cardiomyocytes. Circ Res. 2011;109:670–9.
44. Pekarsky Y, Croce CM. Role of miR-15/16 in CLL. Cell Death Differ. 2015;22:6–11.
45. Kramer LD. Complexity of virus-vector interactions. Curr Opin Virol. 2016;21:81–6.
46. Hirschey MD, DeBerardinis RJ, Diehl AME, Drew JE, Frezza C, Green MF, Jones LW, Ko YH, Le A, Lea MA, et al. Dysregulated metabolism contributes to oncogenesis. Semin Cancer Biol. 2015;35(Suppl):S129–50.

Selective resistance profiles emerging in patient-derived clinical isolates with cabotegravir, bictegravir, dolutegravir, and elvitegravir

Maureen Oliveira[1], Ruxandra-Ilinca Ibanescu[1], Kaitlin Anstett[1], Thibault Mésplède[1,2], Jean-Pierre Routy[3], Marjorie A. Robbins[4], Bluma G. Brenner[1,2,3]* [ID] and the Montreal Primary HIV (PHI) Cohort Study Group

Abstract

Background: Integrase strand transfer inhibitors (INSTIs) are recommended for first-line HIV therapy based on their relatively high genetic barrier to resistance. Although raltegravir (RAL) and elvitegravir (EVG) resistance profiles are well-characterized, resistance patterns for dolutegravir (DTG), bictegravir (BIC), and cabotegravir (CAB) remain largely unknown. Here, in vitro drug selections compared the development of resistance to DTG, BIC, CAB, EVG and RAL using clinical isolates from treatment-naïve primary HIV infection (PHI) cohort participants (n = 12), and pNL4.3 recombinant strains encoding patient-derived Integrase with (n = 5) and without (n = 5) the E157Q substitution.

Results: Patient-derived viral isolates were serially passaged in PHA-stimulated cord blood mononuclear cells in the presence of escalating concentrations of INSTIs over the course of 36–46 weeks. Drug resistance arose more rapidly in primary clinical isolates with EVG (12/12), followed by CAB (8/12), DTG (8/12) and BIC (6/12). For pNL4.3 recombinant strains encoding patient-derived integrase, the comparative genetic barrier to resistance was RAL > EVG > CAB > DTG and BIC. The E157Q substitution in integrase delayed the advent of resistance to INSTIs. With EVG, T66I/A, E92G/V/Q, T97A or R263K (n = 16, 3, 2 and 1, respectively) arose by weeks 8–16, followed by 1–4 accessory mutations, conferring high-level resistance (> 100-fold) by week 36. With DTG and BIC, solitary R263K (n = 27), S153F/Y (n = 7) H51Y (n = 2), Q146 R (n = 3) or S147G (n = 1) mutations conferred low-level (< 3-fold) resistance at weeks 36–46. Similarly, most CAB selections (n = 18) resulted in R263K, S153Y, S147G, H51Y, or Q146L solitary mutations. However, three CAB selections resulted in Q148R/K followed by secondary mutations conferring high-level cross-resistance to all INSTIs. EVG-resistant viruses (T66I/R263K, T66I/E157Q/R263K, and S153A/R263K) retained residual susceptibility when switched to DTG, BIC or CAB, losing T66I by week 27. Two EVG-resistant variants developed resistance to DTG, BIC and CAB through the additional acquisition of E138A/Q148R and S230N, respectively. One EVG-resistant variant (T66I) acquired L74M/ G140S/S147G, L74M/E138K/S147G and H51Y with DTG CAB and BIC, respectively.

Conclusions: Second generation INSTIs show a higher genetic barrier to resistance than EVG and RAL. The potency of CAB was lower than BIC and DTG. The development of Q148R/K with CAB can result in high-level cross-resistance to all INSTIs.

Keywords: HIV-1, Integrase inhibitors, Antiretroviral drug resistance, Cell culture selections, Primary HIV infection isolates, HIV subtypes

*Correspondence: bluma.brenner@mcgill.ca
[1] McGill University AIDS Centre, Lady Davis Institute for Medical Research, Jewish General Hospital, 3755 Côte Ste-Catherine Road, Montreal, QC H3T 1E2, Canada
Full list of author information is available at the end of the article

Background

Over the past 40 years, remarkable advances in antiretroviral therapy has enabled people living with HIV to enjoy longer life expectancy and an improved quality of life. Despite these advances, ongoing development of more robust and durable drug regimens remain critical to avoid the long-term risk of drug resistance and treatment failure [1, 2]. Presently, integrase strand transfer inhibitors (INSTIs) are the favored class of drugs in first-line combination therapy based on their high potency, improved tolerability, low toxicity and high genetic barrier to resistance [3–5].

Raltegravir (RAL) and elvitegravir (EVG) were the first INSTIs to be approved in 2007 and 2012, respectively [6, 7]. Although highly efficacious in the management of HIV, both RAL and EVG were shown to be prone to the development of resistance when used in salvage therapy without other active antiretroviral drugs [8, 9]. The resistance and cross-resistance profile for RAL and EVG have been well described [8, 10, 11]. Drug resistance is associated with the accumulation of primary resistance substitutions and relevant compensatory substitutions along several pathways including the (1) N155H and G140A/G148R/H/Q pathways conferring high level cross-resistance to RAL and EVG; (2) the T66I or E92Q/G pathways leading to resistance to EVG; or (3) the Y143R/H/C RAL-specific resistance pathway [4, 12].

The emergence of viruses displaying resistance and cross-resistance to RAL and EVG spurred research into the development of "second-generation" INSTIs [4, 12]. These include dolutegravir (DTG) that was approved in 2013, bictegravir (BIC) that was approved in the US in February 2018 and cabotegravir (CAB) that is in phase III clinical development with anticipated release in 2019 [13–15]. Dolutegravir displays a higher genetic barrier to resistance than RAL and EVG, retaining efficacy against many RAL- and EVG-resistant variants [16–18]. In the SAILING clinical study, only 4 of 354 treatment-experienced, INSTI-naïve patients treated with dolutegravir acquired integrase-inhibitor resistance substitutions upon virological failure. Two of these individuals acquired the R263K mutation [19] that had previously been selected in culture by DTG to confer low-level resistance [20]. Interestingly, R263K-containing viruses do not seem able to acquire compensatory substitutions that might increase levels of resistance [21–24]. In cell culture selections with DTG, the emergence of singleton R263K, S153Y or H51Y mutations confers low-level resistance (<3-fold resistance) and contributes to a significant negative impact on viral replicative fitness [4, 20, 25, 26]. DTG has been shown to have a longer binding half-life to the HIV integrase enzyme than either RAL or EVG which may help to explain why it maintains activity against most RAL or EVG resistant variants [27, 28].

The recent phase 3 randomized GS-US-380-1489 and GS-US-380-1490 clinical trials demonstrated bictegravir BIC, co-formulated with tenofovir alafenamide and emtricitabine, to be non-inferior to DTG, when co-formulated with either abacavir and lamivudine or tenofovir alafenamide and emtricitabine at week 48 [13, 15, 29]. No resistance to any drug was observed with either BIC- or DTG-based regimens. BIC and DTG showed high barriers to in vitro resistance in MT-2 cells, with emergent M50I and R263K conferring low-fold resistance in the nM range [30]. BIC, like DTG, appears to show broad-range potency against viruses with primary INSTI mutations conferring resistance to RAL or EVG [31].

CAB, a structural analogue of DTG, displays unique physicochemical and pharmacokinetic properties that permits formulation as a single oral tablet for daily dosing and as a long-acting nanosuspension for monthly to quarterly intramuscular injection. Toxicity profiles for CAB, like that reported for DTG, BIC and RAL, include headache, nausea and diarrhea, [5, 13, 32, 33]. Long-acting CAB showed mild to moderate injection-site reactions that rarely resulted in treatment discontinuation (<1%) [14]. The ability of injectable CAB to achieve and maintain clinically relevant plasma concentrations for 16 weeks may circumvent the need for daily dosing, allowing for long-acting treatment and pre-exposure prophylaxis (PreP) regimens [14]. The LATTE-2 clinical trial showed non-inferiority of the two-drug oral CAB plus rilpivirine (RIL) regimen to the CAB-abacavir-lamivudine drug regimen, with 2/115 experiencing virological failure. One patient acquired virus with the Q148R mutation, conferring phenotypic resistance to RAL, EVG and CAB, in association with the K103N, E138G, and K238T, conferring cross-resistance to non-nucleoside RT inhibitors (NNRTIs) [14]. Similarly, at week 48 in the Phase 2 Latte study, the injectable long-acting formulation of CAB and RIL was non-inferior to efavirenz on a dual nucleoside reverse transcriptase inhibitor (NRTI) backbone with one virological failure in injectable CAB/RIL arm harbouring viruses acquiring the INSTI-associated Q148R mutation with the E138Q NNRTI-resistant mutation [32].

To gain a better understanding of the possibility of resistance to newer INSTIs, we performed in vitro cell culture selections with DTG, BIC, CAB and EVG against primary isolates from newly infected persons harbouring subtype B (n=7) and non-B subtype (n=5) infections. In addition, recombinant strains of HIV-1 with integrase derived from clinical isolates assessed the impact of E157Q substitution on emergent resistance to relevant INSTIs was assessed at weeks 8, 16, 24 and 46.

We observed a higher genetic barrier to DTG and BIC as compared to CAB across the different viral subtypes.

Results

Differential selection of resistance to newer integrase inhibitors

This study was designed to compare the differential ability of a panel of patient-derived clinical isolates (n = 12) and recombinant strains (n = 10) to develop resistance to the integrase inhibitors, DTG, BIC, CAB and EVG. Baseline integrase natural polymorphisms, viral subtype and GenBank accession numbers are summarized in Tables 1 and 2.

Primary viral isolates from PHI cohort participants harbouring subtype B (n = 7) and non-B subtype (n = 5) infections were serially passaged over the course of 46 weeks in the presence of escalating concentrations of DTG, BIC, CAB and EVG (Table 1). Tissue culture selections were performed using PHA-stimulated CBMCs since newly-infected persons typically use the CCR5 receptor and do not grow in MT-2 cells.

Cell culture selections of resistance were conducted in parallel with DTG, BIC, CAB and EVG under the same conditions. DTG, BIC and CAB exhibited high subnanomolar potency against primary HIV-1 isolates grown in CBMCs with baseline inhibitory concentrations (IC50s) of 0.25 ± 0.25 nM, 0.25 ± 0.15 nM and 0.13 ± 0.02 nM, respectively (mean ± SD, n = 10 isolates). The progress of viral outgrowth in the presence of stepwise increasing

concentrations of INSTIs was monitored over the course of 46 weeks. Drug-dose escalations for individual INSTIs were based on weekly RT assays, performed in the presence and absence of drug [34]. Genotyping at weeks 8, 16, 24–27, and 36–46 ascertained the differential acquisition and accumulation of drug-associated mutations.

The drug dose-escalations and viral outgrowth over time for HIV clinical isolates 5326 and 96USSN20 are illustrated in Fig. 1. The drug-dose escalations with DTG and BIC progressed at rates that were considerably slower than CAB or EVG. With DTG and BIC, the acquisitions of solitary mutations, including R263K, H51Y, or S153F, conferred low-level resistance to DTG or BIC. These resistance mutations conferred a negative impact on viral replication reflected in lower RT activity, precluding further escalations of DTG or BIC drug concentrations (Fig. 1).

In contrast, the respective first appearance of R263K or S153F mutations by 96USSN20 and 5326 viral strains with CAB at weeks 8, was followed by the serial accumulation of mutations along the Q148K/R resistance pathway leading to viral escape by week 48 (Fig. 1). The development of resistance to CAB progressed more slowly than EVG. For the 96USSN20 isolate, the acquisition of T66I, S147G, Q146R, and S147G conferred viral escape from EVG at week 25 (Fig. 1). Resistance codons Q146R and Q95R for this CRF002_AG isolate have been hitherto unreported. The Q146P is a reported mutation selected in vitro with EVG, reducing RAL and

Table 1 Baseline natural integrase polymorphisms for the HIV-1 clinical isolates used for the in vitro selections with integrase inhibitors

Isolate ID	GenBank accession number	Subtype	Natural polymorphisms in integrase
14514	KT988124	B	K7R, D10E, S17N, M50I, K111Q, T112V, G123S, T125V, R127K, I220L, Y227F, N232D, D256E
10387	KX7140173	B	D10E, V31I, L45Q, K111E, I113V, G123S, A124T, T125A, R127K, M154I, V201I, D207N, N232D, L234I
10249	KX714014	B	D10E, V31I, L45Q, L101I, K111E, I113V, G123S, A124T, R127K, D207N, N232D, L234I
14624	KX714018	B	D10E, S17N, A23V, L28I, S39C, V72I, L101I, G123S, R127K, N232D
14637	KT988125	B	D10E, E11D, R20K, V31I, S39N, M50I, V72I, S119T, G123S, A124N, R127K, G193E, V201I, D286N
14947	KT988126	B	D10E, E11D, R20K, V31I, S39N, M50I, S119T, G123S, A124N, R127K, G193E, V201I, T218S, D286N
5326	KX714021	B	K7R, D10E, E11D, K14R, V31I, V32I, M50L, V72I, L101I, G123S, A124N, R127K, S195T, I203M, I220L, Y227F, N232D
4742	MG805951	C	D10E, V31I, S39C, V72I, I84M, Q95P, F100Y, L101I, T112V, G123S, A124N, T125A, R127K, D167E, V201I, I203M, K215N, T218L, N232D, L234I, D278A, S283G, R284G
10947	MG805955	C	D6E, D25E, V31I, L45Q, M50I, V72I, P90S, T93S, F100Y, L101I, G106A, T112V, G123S, T125A, R127K, K136Q, V201I, T218I, N232D, L234I, R269K, D278A, S283G, D288N
6343	MG805950	CRF01_AE	D10E, K14R, A21T, V31I, S39N, T112V, G123S, T125A, R127K, G134N, I135V, K136R, D167E, V201I, N232D, L234I, S283G
14515	MG805952	CRF02_AG	D10E, E11D, R20K, A21T, V31I, V72I, L101I, T112V, G123S, T125A, R127K, G134N, K136Q, D167E, V201I, N232D, L234I, V249I, S283G
96USSN20	MG805953	AG	D10E, K14R, V31I, V72I, L101I, T112V, G123S, T125A, R127K, G134N, I135V, K136T, V201I, T206S, N232D, L234I, D256E, R269K, S283G
pNL4.3		B	D10E, I113V, S119R, G123S, A124T, R127K, V151I, L234V

Table 2 Treatment status and baseline natural integrase polymorphisms of the HIV-1 recombinant viruses used for the in vitro selections with integrase inhibitors

Sample ID	GenBank accession number	Treatment status	Integrase baseline polymorphisms
E78001	MH513660	ART-naïve	D10E, V31I, L68LV, V72I, I73IV, T112IT, I113V, G123S, R127K, I162IV, V201I, N232D, R284GR
E78003	MHS13661	ART-naive	D10E, E11D, S24N, V31IV, V32I, L45IL, V72I, L101I, T112A, S119PRST, T122IT, G123S, A124AT, R127K, K136KN, V201IV, N232D
E78004	MHS13662	ART-naïve	D10AE, E11D, V37I, K111A, T112A, S119P, G123S, A124T, T125A, R127K, V201IV, T206S, I208IL, N232D
E78005	MHS13663	ART-naïve	D10E, V72I, L101I, G123S, A124T, R127K, I203M, T206ST, N232D
E78060	MHS13664	ART-naive	L45V, V72I, L74I, L101I, S119G, G123S, A124T, R127K, A128AT, N232D
E78110	MHS13665	ART-naïve	D10E, E11D, V31I, A91AT, L101I, S119T, G123S, A124T, R127K, K156N, *E157Q*, F181L, V201I, K211R, N232D, A265AV, I268IL
E102430[†] (subtype D)	MHS13666	INSTI (DTG)-experienced	D10E, S17K, K34KR, L45I, V72I, L101I, T112V, G123S, T125A, R127K, G134DG, I141IV, *E157Q*, K160E, D167E, G193E, V201I, I220V, N232D, L234I, D270DN, D288N
E102952[†] (subtype D)	MHS13667	INSTI (DTG)-experienced	D10E, S17N, K34KR, L45I, V72I, L101I, T112IV, G123S, T125A, R127K, *E157Q*, K160E, D167E, G193E, V201I, I220V, N232D, L234I, D288N
E103211*	MHS13668	INSTI-naive	D10E, S17N, V31I, V72I, L101I, K111R, T112A, S119RS, T122IT, G123CS, A124N, R127K, *E157Q*, K160Q, V201I, K215N, N232D, D256E, S283GS
E103212*	MHS13669	INSTI-naive	D10E, S17N, V31I, V72I, L101I, K111R, T112A, S119RS, T122IT, G123CS, A124NT, T125AT, R127K, *E157Q*, K160Q, V201I, K215N, N232D, D256E

Italic refers to the presence of the E157Q substitution at baseline

[†] E102430 and E102952 contain integrase from the same patient

* E103211 and E103212 contain integrase from the same patient. Blood samples were drawn a few months apart for each of the patients

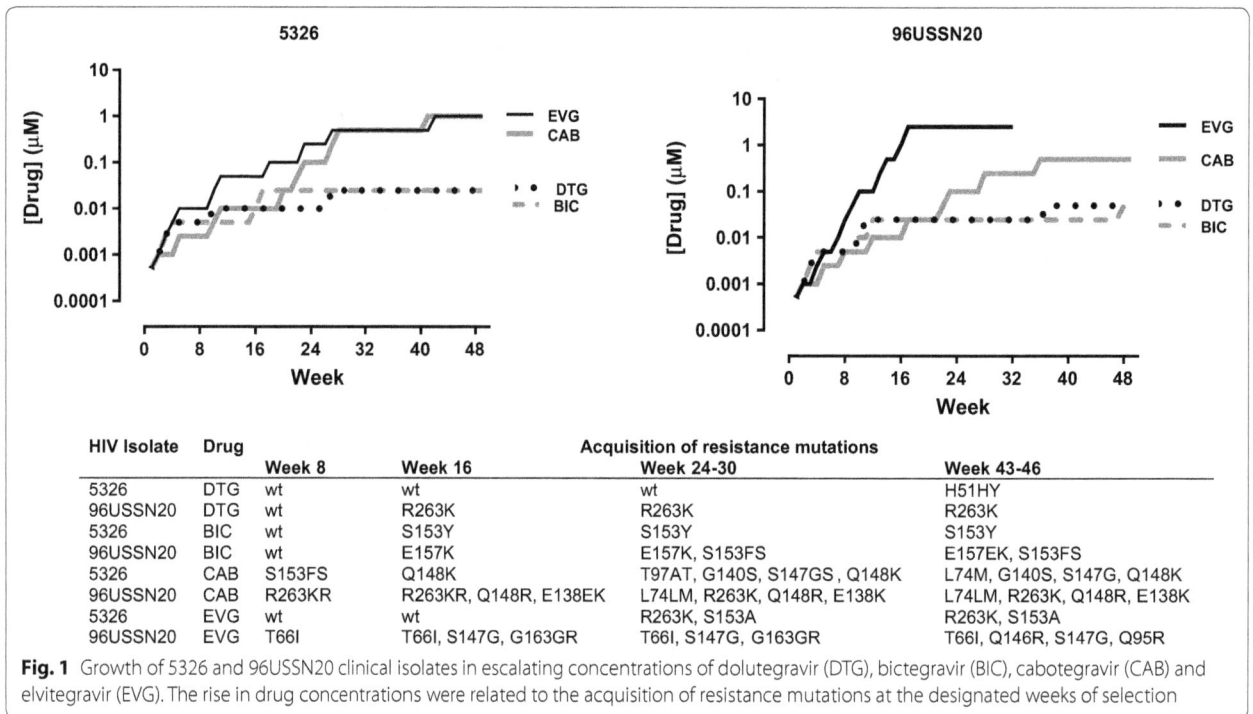

HIV Isolate	Drug	Acquisition of resistance mutations			
		Week 8	Week 16	Week 24-30	Week 43-46
5326	DTG	wt	wt	wt	H51HY
96USSN20	DTG	wt	R263K	R263K	R263K
5326	BIC	wt	S153Y	S153Y	S153Y
96USSN20	BIC	wt	E157K	E157K, S153FS	E157EK, S153FS
5326	CAB	S153FS	Q148K	T97AT, G140S, S147GS, Q148K	L74M, G140S, S147G, Q148K
96USSN20	CAB	R263KR	R263KR, Q148R, E138EK	L74LM, R263K, Q148R, E138K	L74LM, R263K, Q148R, E138K
5326	EVG	wt	wt	R263K, S153A	R263K, S153A
96USSN20	EVG	T66I	T66I, S147G, G163GR	T66I, S147G, G163GR	T66I, Q146R, S147G, Q95R

Fig. 1 Growth of 5326 and 96USSN20 clinical isolates in escalating concentrations of dolutegravir (DTG), bictegravir (BIC), cabotegravir (CAB) and elvitegravir (EVG). The rise in drug concentrations were related to the acquisition of resistance mutations at the designated weeks of selection

EVG susceptibility by 10-fold [7]. The Q95K is rare non-polymorphic accessory resistance mutation conferring little if any effect on drug susceptibility to INSTIs [7]. The

acquisition of R263K with S153A by isolate 5326 conferred > 100-fold resistance to EVG.

Overall, variations in the acquisition of resistance to antiretroviral drugs are multifactorial, dependent on drug efficacy and viral heterogeneity [1]. The genetic barrier to resistance is defined by the number of mutations required to confer resistance, the level of resistance conferred by the acquired specific mutation(s) (ranging from 2 to > 1000 fold) and the resultant costs of resistance substitutions on viral replicative fitness [1]. The patterns of viral outgrowth at the final passage (week 46) for the panel of primary HIV-1 clinical isolates (n = 12) under selective pressure with DTG, BIC, CAB and EVG are shown in Table 3. Collectively, resistance selections proceeded at a considerably slower rate for DTG and BIC than CAB or EVG. By 46 weeks, resistance substitutions were observed in 12/12, 8/12, 8/12 and 7/12 of HIV isolates with EVG, CAB, DTG, or BIC, respectively (Table 3). With BIC or DTG, the acquisition of solitary resistance mutations, including R263K (n = 8), S153Y/F (n = 3) or H51H/Y (n = 1) negatively impacted on viral fitness, precluding drug-dose escalations beyond 0.005–0.025 μM.

Of note, CAB, an analogue of DTG, showed a lower genetic barrier to resistance than DTG and BIC. Although resistance patterns to CAB was like DTG and BIC for 10 of 12 isolates, two isolates showed a lower barrier to CAB resistance. Two viral variants 5326 and 96USSN20 variants acquired complex L74M/G140S/S147G/Q148K and L74M/E138K/Q148R/R263K resistant species allowing

for drug-dose escalations to 1 and 0.5 μM by week 46, respectively (Fig. 1; Table 3). Two other variants, 14947 and 6343, acquired R263K/S153A and S153Y/G163R variants.

In this study, several clinical strains (14514, 10387, 10249, 14624 and 14515) showed a lower propensity to develop resistance to all tested INSTIs. Resistance profiles to DTG, BIC and CAB developed along the R263K or S153F/Y pathway; resistance to EVG was limited to the acquisition of T66I or E92Q at week 46. For the remaining seven isolates, CAB showed a lower barrier to resistance than DTG and BIC, with the acquisition of Q148R/K + 3 mutations in two isolates (Table 3).

EVG showed the lowest genetic barrier with emergent resistance observed in all 12 HIV strains (Table 3). Clinical isolates that failed to develop resistance with DTG, BIC, or CAB, including 14514, 10387, 10249, and 14515, acquired only T66I (n = 3) or E92Q (n = 1) singleton mutations with EVG at weeks 36 or 46. The other isolates accumulated 2–4 secondary drug resistance mutations along the T66I and E92QV pathways, leading to viral escape and EVG dose escalations to 1–5 μM.

Resistance was only observed in a proportion of the primary isolates. We speculate that this viral strain heterogeneity may explain why most primary viral strains rarely develop resistance to DTG and BIC in clinical

Table 3 Selection of drug resistance to dolutegravir (DTG), bictegravir (BIC), cabotegravir (CAB) and elvitegravir at the final week of passage

Virus isolate	Subtype	Acquired mutations at final passage (week 46) of selective drug pressure[a]			Acquired mutations (week 26–40)[b]	
		DTG	BIC	CAB	EVG	RAL
14514	B	R263K	None	None	T66I	–
10387	B	None	None	None	T66I	E92Q
10249	B	R263K	None	None	E92Q	None
14624	B	none	None	H51HY	T66I	T97A, *N155H*
14637	B	R263K	R263K0	R263K	*T66I, E157Q, R263K*	*N155H*
14947	B	R263K	R263K	R263K, S153A	*T66I, E138EK, S147G, Q148R*	*Y143R, L74M, E92V, F121Y, G163GR*
5326	B	H51HY	S153Y	*L74M, G140S, S147G, Q148K*	*R263K, S153A*	*Y143R, L74M, T97A, E157Q*
4742	C	None	None	R263K	*E92EG, R263KR*	T66K
10947	C	R263K	R263K	S147G	*E92V, R263K*	–
6343	AE	R263K	S153Y	S153Y, G163R	*T66I, R263K*	–
14515	AG	None	R263K	None	T66I, H51HY	–
96USSN20	AG	R263K	S153FS, E157EK	*L74M, E138K, Q148R, R263K*	*T66I, Q146R, S147G, Q95R*	L74M, V79I, E138K, *G140A, Q148R*
-pNL4.3	B	R263K, M50I	R263K, M50I	S153F	*T66I, T97A, S147G, S119R, S153A*	*T66I, T97A, G163R, D232N*

Primary patient-derived viruses were passaged in CBMCs in the presence of escalating concentrations of DTG, BIC, CAB, and EVG for 46 weeks

[a] Genotypic analysis was performed of at weeks 0, 16, 24 and 46. The mutations acquired at final week of passage are listed in the order of their first appearance. Mutations highlighted in italics conferred high-level resistance. The acquired R263K, H51Y, S153Y/F mutations conferred low-level resistance with 1–10 nM final drug concentrations as compared to the high-level resistance highlighted in italics where the acquisition of complex resistance mutational motifs with CAB or EVG allowed for viral breakthrough at final drug concentrations of 0.1–2.5 μM

[b] The emerging resistance patterns to RAL determined in previous studies on viral strains are shown for comparative contextual purposes

settings. Our recent studies showed that select HIV-1 viral strains, including 14637 and 14947, associated with large cluster transmission outbreaks may show accelerated escape from integrase in cell culture compared with viral isolates from singleton/small clusters [25]. Large cluster strains can assist in deducing potential pathways implicated in the development of resistance to DTG, BIC and CAB (Table 3).

Different viral subtypes resulted in similar resistance profiles to INSTIs. In our previous studies, drug selections with the subtype C 4742 strain, the G118R resistance pathway arose with DTG and the Merck investigational MK2048 [35]. MK2048, the Merck investigational integrase inhibitors, showed high potency against most RAL/EVG resistant variants but its clinical development was halted due to poor pharmacokinetics [4]. The development of the G118R resistance was ascribed to a signature natural polymorphism at codon 118 in isolate 4742. In this study, 4742 developed no resistance with DTG and BIC, R263K with CAB, and E92V/R263K with EVG (Table 3).

Resistance to integrase inhibitors using patient-derived recombinant strains

The integrase E157Q substitution has been described as a common natural polymorphism present in 2.3%

of HIV-1 viral sequences, including 3.8% and 6.0% of treatment-naïve patients with subtype B and subtype CRF02_AG subtype infections, respectively (Los Alamos database, www.hiv.lanl.gov, accessed June 8, 2018). The E157Q has also been observed in several persons failing INSTI-based regimens, including RAL and DTG [36–39]. To date, very few data are available regarding virological response in patients harbouring E157Q-mutated viruses.

To assess the potential impact of E157Q on emergent resistance to INSTIs, recombinant viruses were constructed where patient-derived integrase were inserted on a pNL4-3Δ integrase background. Viruses included recombinant strains with (n = 5) and without (n = 5) the E157Q substitution (n = 5) in integrase.

The progress of viral selections in CBMCS in stepwise increasing concentrations of DTG, BIC, CAB, EVG, and RAL over time is depicted in Fig. 2. It was noteworthy that strains harbouring the E157Q substitution showed a significantly attenuated development of resistance to RAL and EVG. The hypersensitivity of viruses to E157Q suggests that this mutation is a compensatory mutation, commonly selected with INSTIs with minimal effects on drug susceptibility [4, 40]. The E157Q mutation arose in a EVG and RAL selections in recombinant strains E78004 and E78060, respectively (Table 4).

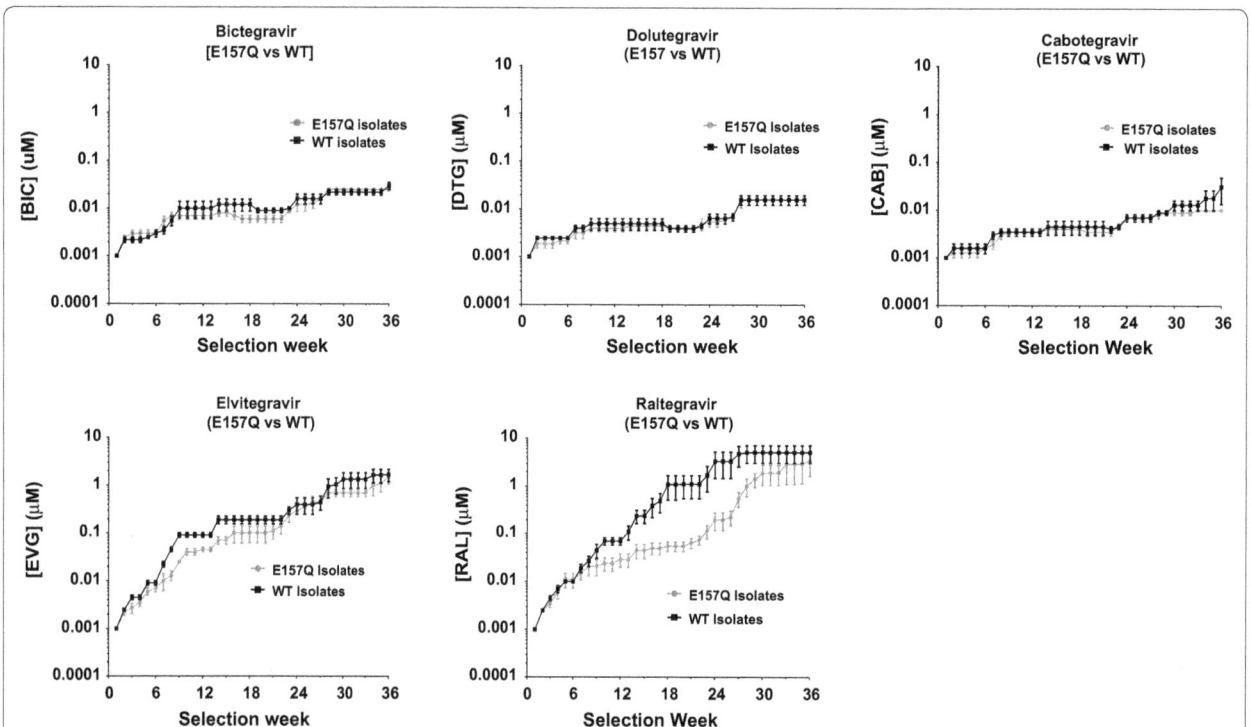

Fig. 2 Drug dose escalations (mean ± SEM) reflect the differential emergence of resistance to integrase inhibitors by recombinant strains encoding patient-derived integrase with (n = 5) and without (n = 5) the E157Q resistance substitution

Table 4 Cell culture selections of viral recombinant strains bearing the integrase from patient samples with and without the E157Q polymorphisms

Virus[a]	Codon 157	Acquired mutations at final passage (week 36–38) of selective drug pressure[b]				
		DTG	BIC	CAB	EVG	RAL
pNLWT	WT	R263K, M50I	R263K, M50I	S153F	T66I, T97A, S147G, S119R, S153A	*ND*
pNL157Q	E157Q	R263K, M50IM	Q146R	R263K, M50I	T66I, S147G, Q95K	E92Q
E78001	WT	S153F	S153Y	R263K, M50I	T66I, Q146R, S230R	*Y143R*, L74M, V151I
E78003	WT	S147G, H51Y	R263K, M50I	N155H	Q95R, *S147G, Q148R*	T97A, G163R, V151I, L74M
E78004	WT	Q146R, Q95KQ	Q146R, Q95KQ	*Q148R, E138K, G140GS, L74I*	T66I, Q95K, E157Q, S230R	T66A, A128T, *Y143G, G163R*, V151I
E78005	WT	R263K	S153Y	S153F	T66A, *Q146I*	T97A, *Y143R*, V151I
E78060	WT	R263K	R263K, M50I	Q146L	T97A Q146R, T66IT	T97A, E157Q, A128AT, V151I
E78110	E157Q	R263K, M50I	R263K	R263K	*T66I, R263K*, M50I	*Y143R*
E102430	E157Q	R263K	R263K	R263K, M50I	*E138K, Q148K*	V151S, L74LM
E102952	E157Q	S153F	R263K, M50I	R263K	T66I, E92Q	*Q148R, E138K, G140A*, V151IV
E103211	E157Q	R263K	R263K	R263K, H51N	S147G, *Q148R, E138K*	*Y143R*
E103212	E157Q	R263K	R263K	R263K, M50I	H51Y, S147G, T97A	T97A

The underline refers to the de novo aquisition of E157Q during selection

[a] Integrase derived from clinical isolates with or without the E157Q substitution were inserted into integrase-depleted pNL4.3 plasmids. Isolated recombinant viruses were serially passaged in escalating concentrations of dolutegravir (DTG), bictegravir (BIC), cabotegravir (CAB), elvitegravir (EVG) or raltegravir (RAL) over the course of 36 weeks

[b] Genotypic analysis was performed of at weeks 0, 16, 24 and 36–38. The mutations acquired at final week of passage are listed in the order of their first appearance. Mutations highlighted in italics conferred high-level resistance

In contrast, patient-derived pNL4-3 recombinant strains showed a high genetic barrier to resistance for DTG, BIC, and CAB, both in the presence or absence of E157Q. All recombinant strains harbouring patient-derived integrase developed resistance to all INSTIs over 36–38 weeks. With DTG, BIC and CAB, the predominant resistance profile included R263K (n = 11), R263K/M50I (n = 7), and S153Y/F (n = 5).

Selection of strain E78004 with CAB resulted in high level resistance along a Q148R/E138K/G140GS/L74I pathway (Table 4). This isolate developed Q146R/Q95KQ with DTG and BIC, a hitherto unreported profile for both drugs. Resistance profiles associated with escape from EVG drug pressure were associated with T66I and the accumulation of major resistance including Q148R/K, E138K, and S147G. Emergent high-level resistance to RAL were associated with the Y143R/G and Q148R pathways.

Phenotypic drug susceptibility of CAB- and EVG-resistant viral variants

Phenotypic drug susceptibility to DTG, BIC, CAB, EVG and RAL was deduced in PHA-stimulated CBMC using select clinical isolates (Table 5) and recombinant strains with patient-derived integrase (Table 6).

Here, we showed two isolates 5326 and 96USSN20 serially accumulated resistance mutations with CAB, leading

to drug dose escalation of 0.5 and 1 μM, respectively. Viruses were amplified at weeks 8, 16, 24 and 46 weeks (Table 5). The first appearance of Q148K as a solitary mutation under CAB pressure in clinical isolate 5326) and recombinant strain E78004 at weeks 18 conferred low-level (< 2–3 fold) resistance to CAB, DTG, BIC and RAL with moderate (12–32-fold) reduced susceptibility to EVG (Tables 5, 6). For isolate 5326, the progressive accumulation of Q148K/G140S/G147GS resulted in increasingly high cross-resistance to CAB, RAL and EVG while retaining susceptibility to DTG and BIC (Table 3). The resistant variant of 5326 amplified at week 48 under selective CAB pressure, harbouring L74M/G140S/S147G/Q148K mutations showed high-level cross-resistance to all INSTIs, including DTG, BIC, CAB, EVG and RAL (Table 5). Similarly, 96USSN20 and E78004 viruses developed resistance along a Q148R pathway leading to L74M/E138K/G148R/R263K and L74I/E138K/G140S/Q148R conferring cross-resistance to all INSTIs.

Phenotypic drug susceptibility assays explored the potential impact of the E157Q substitution drug susceptibility to INSTIs (Table 6). Viral strains E78004 and E78060 acquiring the E157Q under EVG and RAL showed hypersensitivity to DTG, BIC, CAB, consistent with the observed attenuated development of resistance to RAL and EVG of E157Q relative to wild-type recombinant strains.

Table 5 Phenotypic drug susceptibility of viral strains to integrase strand transfer inhibitors (INSTIs) harvested at the designated week of selection with cabotegravir (CAB) or elvitegravir (EVG)

Virus selection week drug[a]	Acquired resistance mutations	EC$_{50}$ (nM) in CBMCs (fold-resistance relative to WT control)				
		DTG	BIC	CAB	EVG	RAL
6343 No drug	WT	0.10	0.17	0.23	0.21	ND
6343 Wk 46 CAB	S153Y, G163R	0.60 (6 ×)	1.33 (8 ×)	0.87 (3.2 ×)	0.53 (2.5 ×)	ND
5326 No drug	WT	0.77	0.41	0.20	0.253	1.12
5326 Wk 45 EVG (1 µM)	S263K, S153A	0.52 (0.7 ×)	0.53 (1.3 ×)	0.19 (1.0 ×)	53 (212 ×)	1.12 (1.0 ×)
5326 Wk 17 CAB (0.01 µM)	Q148K	1.57 (2.0 ×)	0.90 (2.2 ×)	0.61 (3.1 ×)	2.96 (11.8 ×)	3.57 (3.2 ×)
5326 Wk 28 CAB (0.5 µM)	Q148K, G140S, G147GS	3.60 (4.7 ×)	0.72 (1.8 ×)	8.07 (40 ×)	180 (720 ×)	66.5 (60 ×)
5326 Wk 48 CAB (1.0 µM)	Q148K, G140S, S147G, L74M	125 (162 ×)	49.01 (120 ×)	139.7 (700 ×)	3429 (> 1000 ×)	1007 (900 ×)
96USSN20 No drug	WT	0.58	0.77	0.29	0.20	1.60
96USSN20 Wk27 EVG (2.5 µM)	T66I, T97A, Q147G	0.40 (0.7 ×)	0.80 (1 ×)	1.20 (4 ×)	>100 (> 500 ×)	1.7 (1 ×)
96USSN20 Wk 17 CAB (0.025 µM)	Q148R, E138EK, R263KR	8.08 (14 ×)	5.83 (8 ×)	2.40 (8.3 ×)	22.35 (112 ×)	12.01 (7 ×)
96USSN20 Wk 27 CAB (0.25 µM)	Q148R, E138K, R263K, L74LM	10.0 (17 ×)	9.01 (12 ×)	>30 (> 100 ×)	>300 (> 1500 ×)	300 (188 ×)
96USSN20 Wk 45 CAB (0.5 µM)	Q148R, E138K, R263K, L74M	13.93 (24 ×)	13.40 (17 ×)	47.8 (165 ×)	1612 (8060 ×)	568 (355 ×)

[a] Viruses were harvested at the designated week of selection, amplified in PHA-stimulated CBMCs and genotyped. Viruses were co-cultured in PHA-stimulated CBMCs to deduce drug susceptibility against dolutegravir (DTG), bictegravir (BIC), cabotegravir (CAB), elvitegravir (EVG) and raltegravir (RAL). Samples in italics represent greater than 5-fold reduction in drug susceptibility

Table 6 Phenotypic drug susceptibility of viral strains to integrase strand transfer inhibitors (INSTIs) harvested at the designated week of selection with cabotegravir (CAB) or elvitegravir (EVG)

Viral variant-drug selection week (drug)[a]	Acquired resistance mutations	EC$_{50}$ (nM) in CBMCs (fold-resistance relative to WT control)				
		DTG	BIC	CAB	EVG	RAL
pNL4.3	WT	0.71	0.49	0.39	0.13	–
pNL4.3-R263K	R263K	1.56 (2.2 ×)	1.60 (3.3 ×)	0.91 (2.4 ×)	0.79 (6.1 ×)	–
pNL4.3-S153Y	S153Y	3.34 (4.7 ×)	3.40 (7.0 ×)	1.01 (2.6 ×)	<0.3 (2 ×)	–
pNL4.3-S153F	S153F	0.45 (0.63 ×)	0.63 (1.3 ×)	0.56 (1.4 ×)	<0.3	–
E78004 No drug	WT	0.49	1.26	0.27	0.65	1.18
E78004 Wk18 CAB (0.0025 µM)	Q95KQ, Q148R	1.28 (2.6 ×)	1.17 (0.9 ×)	0.67 (2.5 ×)	0.90 (32 ×)	1.64 (1.4 ×)
E78004 Wk26 CAB (0.005 µM)	Q95KQ, Q148R, E138EK	1.60 (3.3 ×)	1.77 (1.4 ×)	3.04 (11.3 ×)	93.57 (144 ×)	20.76 (18 ×)
E78004 Wk36 CAB (0.25 µM)	Q148R, E138K, L74I, G140GS	12.34 (25 ×)	6.08 (5.3 ×)	23.6 (87 ×)	36.16 (57 ×)	3182 (> 100 ×)
E78004 No drug	WT	0.66	0.66	0.43	0.79	1.69
E78004 Wk18 EVG (0.25 µM)	T66I, Q95K, E157EQ	0.59 (0.9 ×)	0.56 (0.9 ×)	0.24 (0.5 ×)	29.10 (37 ×)	14.57 (8.6 ×)
E78004 Wk26 EVG (0.25 µM)	T66I, Q95K, E157Q	0.53 (0.8 ×)	0.38 (0.6 ×)	0.39 (0.9 ×)	69.76 (89 ×)	7.98 (4.7 ×)
E78004 Wk36 EVG (2.5 µM)	T66I, Q95K, E157Q, S230R	0.06 (0.1 ×)	0.01 (0.01 ×)	0.03 (0.1 ×)	123.10 (156 ×)	5.47 (3.2 ×)
E78060 No drug	WT	0.52	0.92	0.45	0.46	2.43
E78060 Wk36 RAL (0.5 µM)	T97A, A128AT, E157Q, V151I	0.31 (0.6 ×)	0.30 (0.3 ×)	0.22 (0.5 ×)	23.79 (52 ×)	49.83 (21 ×)
E102952 No drug	WT (E157Q)	0.09	0.25	0.13	0.33	0.44
E102952 Wk18 RAL (0.025 µM)	Q148R (E157Q)	0.17 (1.8 ×)	0.10 (0.4 ×)	0.14 (1 ×)	0.41 (1.3 ×)	0.75 (1.7 ×)
E102952 Wk38 RAL (20 µM)	Q148R, E138K, G140A, V151IV (E157Q)	5.46 (58 ×)	2.63 (10.6 ×)	2.13 (16.3 ×)	1255 (> 100 ×)	1519 (> 100 ×)

The underline refers to the de novo aquisition of E157Q during selection

[a] Viruses were harvested at the designated week of selection, amplified in PHA-stimulated CBMCs and genotyped. Viruses were co-cultured in PHA-stimulated CBMCs to deduce drug susceptibility against dolutegravir (DTG), bictegravir (BIC), cabotegravir (CAB), elvitegravir (EVG) and raltegravir (RAL). Samples in italics represent greater than 5-fold reduction in drug susceptibility. pNL4.3 recombinant virus are included as controls with R263K and S153Y mutations inserted by site-directed mutagenesis

One recombinant strain, E78004, acquired a Q148R resistance pathway under selective pressure with CAB. The appearance of Q148R/Q95KQ followed by Q148R/ Q95KQ/E138EK resistant strains at weeks 18 and 26 resulted in moderate 2.5- and 11.3-fold resistance to CAB, while retaining susceptibility to DTG and BIC. The outgrowth of the L74I/E138K/G140GS, Q148R showed 25-, 5.3-, 87-, 57- and > 100-fold cross-resistance to DTG, BIC, CAB, EVG, and RAL, respectively.

Switching EVG-resistant strains to DTG, BIC, or CAB

To gain further understanding of the residual efficacies of DTG, BIC, and CAB on EVG-resistant variants, we performed switch experiments. Six EVG-resistant variants and the pNL4.3 recombinant strain showed high-level resistance at week 46, growing in the presence of

Table 7 Viral outgrowth of elvitegravir (EVG) resistant viruses switched to dolutegravir (DTG), bictegravir (BIC) or cabotegravir (CAB)

Virus	Initial EVG selection	Drug switch selection		Resistance mutations at week 27	Lost EVG mutations	Acquired mutations
		2nd drug	Drug (µM)			
6343	EVG Wk 46	Pre-switch	0.25	T66I, R263K		
6343		DTG	0.010	M50MI, R263K	T66I	M50IM
6343		BIC	0.050	R263K	T66I	
6343		CAB	0.050	R263K	T66I	
6343		No drug		R263K	T66I	
14637	EVG Wk 46	Pre-switch	1.0	T66I, E157Q, R263K		
14637		DTG	0.010	E157Q, R263K	T66I	
14637		BIC	0.025	E157Q, R263K	T66I	
14637		CAB	0.050	E157Q, R263K	T66I	
14637		No drug		E157Q, R263K	T66I	
5326	EVG Wk 46	Pre-switch	1	S153A, R263K		
5326		DTG	0.010	S153A, R263K		
5326		BIC	0.010	S153A, R263K		
5326		CAB	0.050	S153A, R263K		
5326		No drug		S153A	R263K	
14624	EVG Wk 46	Pre-switch	1	T66I		
14624		DTG	0.005	T66I, L74M, E138K, S147G, M154IM		L74M, E138K, S147G, M154IM
14624		BIC	0.010	H51HY	T66I	H51HY
14624		CAB	0.10	T66I, L74M, G140GS, S147GS		L74M, G140GS, S147GS
14624		No drug		T66I		
14947	EVG Wk 46	Pre-switch	5	T66I, E138EK, S147G, Q148R		
14947		DTG	0.005	T66I, E138EK, S147G, Q148R, S230N		S230N
14947		BIC	0.025	T66I, E138EK, S147G, Q148R, S230N		S230N
14947		CAB	0.100	T66I, L74M, E138EK, S147G, Q148R, S230N		L74M, S230N
14947		No drug		T66I, S147G, S230NS	E138EK, Q148R	S230NS
96USSN20	EVG Wk 46	Pre-switch	2.5	T66I, Q146R, S147G		
96USSN20		DTG	0.100	T66I, Q146R, S147G, E138E1AEKT, Q148R	Q146R	E138AEKT, Q148R
96USSN20		BIC	0.050	T66I, Q146R, S147G, E138A, T97A	Q146R	T97A, E138A, Q148R
96USSN20		CAB	0.25	T66I, Q146QR, S147G, E138A, Q148QR	Q146QR	E138A, Q148QR
96USSN20		No drug		T66I, S147G	Q146R	
pNL4.3	EVG Wk 46	Pre-switch	2.5	T66I, T97A, S147G, V151I, S153A		
pNL4.3		DTG	0.025	T66I, T97A, S147G, V151I, S153A		
pNL4.3		BIC	0.025	T66I, T97A, S147G, V151I, S153A		
pNL4.3		CAB	0.250	T66I, T97A, S147G, V151I, S153A		
pNL4.3		No drug		T66I, T97A, S147G, V151I, S153A		

Patient-derived viral strains, subjected to EVG selective pressure for 46 weeks, were switched to serially increasing concentrations of DTG, BIC, CAB or no drug for 27 weeks. Genotyping was performed at week 27 and re-genotyped to monitor the loss and acquisition of mutations

1–2.5 μM EVG. These resistant variants were amplified at week 47 and switched to serial drug-dose escalations with DTG, BIC or CAB for a further 27 weeks.

As summarized in Table 7, The EVG-resistant variants retained residual susceptibility to second generation INSTIs. There was however, broader antiviral sensitivity to DTG and BIC than CAB. Drug dose escalations with the latter three drugs were initiated at 0.001 μM. Following passage for 17 weeks, drug-dose escalations reached 0.023 ± 0.012 μM, 0.027 ± 0.006 μM, and 0.121 ± 0.034 at week 27. Drug dose escalations were significantly higher for CAB than DTG or BIC (Bartlett's statistic $= 14.16$, $p = 0.0008$, $p < 0.05$, post hoc Tukey's test).

Genotypic analysis showed the switch of EVG-resistant strains ($n = 6$) to DTG, BIC, CAB or a no drug control for 27 weeks resulted in the loss of the T66I (3/6 selections) or Q146R (1/6) substitutions associated with primary resistance to EVG (Table 7). For isolate 6343, the loss of T66I was accompanied by the acquisition of M50I with DTG (Table 7). The EVG-resistant isolates 6343, 14637 and 5326, harbouring R263K, E157Q/R263K and S153A/R263K, showed residual susceptibility to DTG, BIC and CAB with no further acquisition of resistance mutations at week 27 (Table 7).

The EVG-resistant 14624 T66I variant displayed a higher residual antiviral susceptibility to BIC than DTG and CAB (Table 7). With BIC, T66I was lost and H51HY was acquired. In contrast, the loss of T66I in 14624 was accompanied by the acquisition of L74M/E138K/S147G/M154IM and L74M/G140GS/S147G at week 27 with DTG and CAB, respectively.

The EVG-resistant 14947 variant T66I/E138K/S147G/Q148R variant accumulated S230N with BIC and DTG and L74M/S230N with CAB. The 96USSN20 virus resistant to EVG (T66I, Q146R, and S147G) lost Q146R and acquired E138A and Q148R with DTG, BIC and CAB. The final concentrations at week 27 revealed CAB escape.

Taken together, DTG, BIC and CAB showed broad antiviral efficacies against wild-type and EVG-resistant viruses. BIC and DTG appear to be better able to inhibit viral replication than CAB in several primary HIV-1 isolates and EVG-resistant variants.

Discussion

The findings in this study demonstrated that DTG and BIC showed higher barriers to resistance than EVG. With EVG, resistance was observed in all 12 clinical isolates. In 4/12 and 6/12 selections with DTG and BIC, no resistance mutations arose in long-term passage, respectively. In the remaining selections, the acquisition of singleton R263K, S153Y/F or H51Y substitutions conferred low-level resistance, regardless of viral subtype. Although 4/12 and 6/12 selections with CAB, yielded no resistance

or minor resistance, respectively, two selections with CAB (one subtype B and one CRF02_AG), resulted in the acquisition of Q148R/K with multiple secondary resistance substitutions conferring high-level cross-resistance to all INSTIs.

Although there is a high correlation in the genotypic and phenotypic characteristics associated with resistance to DTG and BIC, CAB may show a lower barrier to resistance. In selections of two clinical isolates and a patient-derived recombinant strain, resistance to CAB arose through a Q148R. The first appearance of Q148R showed < 3-fold resistance to CAB, DTG and BIC. The sequential accumulation of mutations by these three strains resulted in Q148R/E138K/R263K/L74M, Q148K/G140S/S147G/L74M and Q148R/E138K/L74I/G140GS mutational motifs conferring in high-level cross-resistance to all five INSTIs.

BIC and CAB, like DTG displayed antiviral efficacies against viral variants acquiring EVG-resistance mutations. Overall, BIC and DTG were superior to CAB. This is consistent with recent studies modelling the respective binding of CAB, BIC and DTG within the active site of the integrase enzyme [31].

The selection of Q148R in CAB selections is consistent with the observed acquisition of Q148R in two patients in the Latte clinical trials [14, 32]. Molecular models suggest that there is more conformational rigidity with CAB than DTG in metal-chelating scaffold leading to potential steric interactions between CAB and the Q148 locus [41]. The potential steric interactions induced by Q148R at and near the β4–α2 loop may affect binding kinetics of CAB, leading to a decreased dissociative half-life with Q148R between that of DTG and RAL [41].

CAB, an analogue of DTG, has been formulated as an oral tablet (half-life 40 h) and as a long-acting injectable nanosuspension with an intramuscular and subcutaneous half-life of 40 days. CAB/RIL has shown durable viral suppression in patients who are suppressed to less than 50 copies/ml, providing proof of principle for its' use in two-drug maintenance therapy, as well as a potential PreP strategy [14, 32, 42]. The observed emergence of resistance through the Q148R pathway may lead to cross-resistance to the entire class of INSTIs. Although in vitro findings may not arise in the clinic, careful attention may be needed to assure drug adherence and prevent tail periods of declining drug in injectable formulations.

It is noteworthy that HIV-1 viral variants may differ in their replicative fitness and their ability to override resistance bottlenecks. In our previous studies, we showed that viral variants associated with large cluster transmission outbreaks may show a facilitated development of resistance to DTG and EVG than viruses leading to singleton transmission [25]. In this study, isolates 14637 and 14947 were associated with large cluster outbreaks.

This study utilized a panel of clinical isolates reflective of newly-infected treatment-naïve persons harbouring CCR5 viruses. Our analysis also included recombinant CXCR4-tropic pNL4.3 recombinants constructs encoding patient-derived integrase. Most reported studies to date, have limited their performed in vitro analysis of BIC and CAB using pNL4.3 vector constructs or MT-2 or MT-4 cells [31, 43–45].

In previous studies, subtype C variant, 4742, developed the G118R mutation in cell culture selections with DTG and Merck investigation INSTI, MK2048 [46]. The development of G118R was associated with a rare GGA natural polymorphism at codon 118, facilitating a G to A transition leading to G118R (AGA). In this study, the 4742-viral strain gave rise to no resistance with either DTG or BIC, R263KR with CAB, and E92EG/R263K with EVG.

Taken together, our findings show improved resistance profiles for DTG and BIC in all tested viral strains. The CAB, an analogue of DTG with high potency, may be prone to the development of Q148K/R leading to cross-resistance to the entire class of integrase inhibitors. The high potency of DTG and BIC confirms their suitability for use in resource-limited settings dominated by non-B subtypes. A larger panel of viral isolates are needed to address the potential development of the Q148R/K resistance pathway with CAB [43].

Conclusions

The advent of integrase inhibitors has transformed the management of HIV-1 infection. Although treatment failure with RAL and EVG can result in the emergence of INSTI resistance, DTG and BIC have been quite impervious to the development of resistance in the clinical setting [15, 47, 48]. To date, there have been few reports of virological failure and resistance in treatment-naïve persons receiving triple combination DTG-containing regimens [47, 48] and in virologically suppressed patients receiving DTG monotherapy [46, 49]. The present study used in vitro selections using viral isolates from 20 persons to show patterns of resistance to DTG, BIC and CAB that may potentially arise in real-world settings. Our findings indicate that drug resistance monitoring in patients on INSTI-based regiments is essential, despite the high-genetic barriers of thcsc drugs. Although in vitro experiments might not always reflect what, will happen in patients, resistance may be breached when INSTIs are given in monotherapy and in select patients failing INSTI-based regimens [50]. As treatment options coalesce around the use of second-generation integrase

inhibitors in resource-limited settings, more information is needed on emergent resistance to DTG, BIC and CAB and their potential impact on viral response to later-line treatment options [50].

Methods
Cells and antiviral compounds
BIC and EVG were kindly provided by Gilead Sciences Inc. (Foster City, California). CAB was purchased from Toronto Research Chemicals (Toronto, Canada). DTG was kindly provided by ViiV Healthcare (Research Triangle Park, Inc). MT-2 and 96USSN20 cells were obtained from the NIH AIDS Reagent program, Division of AIDS, NAID, NIH with cell line provided by Dr D Richman and Drs D Ellenberger, P Sullivan and RB Lai, respectively [51, 52]. Cord blood mononuclear cells (CBMCs) were isolated as previously described from non-nominative discarded blood obtained through the Department of Obstetrics, Jewish General Hospital [53]. The CEM-GXR cells and HIV-1 pNL4.3 delta integrase plasmid (Δint) were kindly provided by Dr. Mark Brockman (Simon Fraser University, Burnaby, Canada [54].

Isolation of patient-derived HIV-1 primary isolates and recombinant strains encoding patient-derived HIV-1 integrase
The FRQS-Réseau SIDA supports a representative cohort of newly-infected persons with clinical indication of primary infection. In this study, HIV-1 strains were isolated from seven subjects harboring subtype B infections and four subjects harboring non-B subtype infections. HIV-1 isolates were amplified as previously described through co-culture of patient CD8-depleted peripheral blood mononuclear cells (PBMCs) with CD8-depleted phytohemagglutinin-stimulated CBMCs [53, 55]. Amplified cell-free viral supernatants were tittered and stored at − 70 °C until use [53, 55]. In addition, viruses were amplified from the 96USSN20 strain (subtype CRF02_AG) and the pNL4.3 subtype B reference clone obtained from the NIH AIDS Reagent program, Division of AIDS, NIAID, NIH.

Clinical plasma samples were also obtained from treatment-naive persons harboring the WT (n = 5) or E157Q (n = 5) substitution in integrase. Patient-derived amplicons encoding the integrase gene (1064 nucleotides long) were inserted into the pNL4-3 recombinant vector as previously described [54]. Briefly, HIV-1 was RT-PCR amplified from plasma HIV RNA using sequence-specific subtype B primers [56, 57]. Second round PCR was performed using Expand™ High Fidelity Enzyme (Roche Diagnostics, Laval, Quebec) with forward (IN4155F-5′-GTACCAGCACACAAAGGAATTGGAG) and reverse primer (IN5219R-5′-CCTAGTGGGATGTGTACTTCT

GAAC). primers. Recombinant viruses were generated by co-transfecting sequence verified second-round PCR amplicons with linearized Δint-pNL4.3 into CEM-GXR cells via electroporation cells [58]. Transfection cultures were maintained and resulting viruses harvested as described previously [54]. Upon harvest, recombinant viruses were sequence validated.

Amplified infectious clinical isolates and recombinant viral stocks were genotyped and stored at −70 °C. GenBank accession numbers and integrase polymorphisms are indicated in Tables 1 and 2.

Cell culture-based selection of resistance to integrase inhibitors

Selections of HIV-1 variants resistant to INSTIs were performed through serial passage of patient-derived clinical isolates (n = 12) or recombinant strains (n = 10) in CBMCs, in the presence of serially escalating concentrations of DTG, BIC, CAB and EVG over the course of 36–46 weeks, as previously described [53, 59–61]. At each passage, aliquots of cell-free supernatant were stored at −70 °C for further analysis.

Stepwise drug-dose escalations were based on weekly reverse transcriptase (RT) enzymatic assays performed for each isolate in the presence and absence of the relevant INSTI [34]. Briefly, 10 μl clarified culture supernatant were incubated in a 50 μl reaction mixture containing 50 mM Tris (pH 8.0), 5 mM $MgCl_2$, 150 mM KCl, 5 mM dithiothreitol, 0.3 mM glutathione, 0.5 mM EGTA, 0.05% Triton X-100, 50 μg of poly(rA)–oligo(dT)$_{12–18}$ per ml and 0.1 μCi of [^{3}H-TPP]. After a 4 h incubation at 37 °C, 150 μl of ice-cold 10% trichloroacetic acid (TCA) was added for 30 min at 4 °C to precipitate incorporated [3H]-TTP. The precipitated mixture is transferred onto a Millipore multiscreen Glass Fiber FC plates with 10% TCA, vacuum drained. and washed twice with 10% TCA and once with cold ethanol using a Millipore multiscreen manifold. Scintillation cocktail (30 μl) is added to each well. Radioactivity is measured using a Perkin Elmer MicroBeta Trilux microplate counter.

Residual viral efficacy to DTG, BIC and CAB against EVG-resistant viruses was assessed by switch experiments. EVG-resistant viruses isolated at week 46 were grown in escalating concentrations of DTG, BIC, CAB or no drug control for a further 17 and 27 weeks. Genotyping at week 17 and 27 monitored the loss of EVG-associated resistance mutations and acquisition of mutations to second generation INSTIs.

Genotypic analyses were performed at weeks, 8, 16, 27–30 and 46 weeks to evaluate the acquisition and accumulation of amino acid substitutions that could be associated with reduced susceptibility to antiretroviral drugs (i.e., drug resistance mutations). Sanger (population) sequencing of viral RNA extracted from culture supernatants across the integrase coding regions was performed as previously described [60, 62].

Phenotypic susceptibility to DTG, BIC, CAB, EVG and RAL were monitored using a cell-based in vitro assay. Briefly, viruses were amplified from stored cell culture supernatants at designated weeks following in vitro selection. Resistant and wild-type control viruses were infected with serial dilutions of INSTIs. After 7 days, culture supernatants were collected and analyzed for RT activity. The 50% effective concentrations were calculated on the analysis of dose–response curves using GraphPad Prism version 6.07 software.

Authors' contributions

We dedicate this paper in the memory of Mark A. Wainberg, who dedicated his career in the field of HIV/AIDS drug resistance. BB designed and supervised the study and wrote the manuscript. MO and RI performed the drug selections. RI performed the genotyping. TM provided the pNL4.3 with R263K and S153Y introduced by site-directed mutagenesis. J-PR supervised the collection of plasma and cells from persons recruited into the Montreal PHI cohort. All authors read and approved the final manuscript.

Author details

[1] McGill University AIDS Centre, Lady Davis Institute for Medical Research, Jewish General Hospital, 3755 Côte Ste-Catherine Road, Montreal, QC H3T 1E2, Canada. [2] Department of Microbiology and Immunology, McGill University, Montreal, QC, Canada. [3] Faculty of Medicine (Surgery, Experimental Medicine, Infectious Disease), McGill University, Montreal, QC, Canada. [4] BC Children's Hospital Research Institute, Vancouver, BC, Canada.

Acknowledgements

The authors thank all participants of in the Montreal PHI cohort, Mario Legault, coordinator of the cohort and all participating physicians from Clinique médicale L'Actuel, Clinique médicale Quartier Latin, Centre hospitalier Université de Montréal, Clinique Roger Leblanc/Opus, Centre hospitalier Université McGill, including Jean-Guy Baril, Louise Charest, Marc-André Charron, Pierre Côté, Alexandra de Pokomandy, Serge Dufresne, Claude Fortin, Jason Friedman, Norbert Gilmore, Emmanuelle Huchet, Marina Klein, Louise Labreque, Richard Lalonde, Roger Leblanc, Bernard Lessard, Catherine Milne, Marie Munoz, Martin Potter, Danielle Rouleau, Jean-Pierre Routy, Jason Szabo, Réjean Thomas, Cecile Tremblay, Benoît Trottier, and Sylvie Vézina.

Competing interests

The authors declare that they have no competing interests.

Funding

This study was sponsored in part, by grants from Gilead Sciences (Grant No. 9883), the Fonds de Recherche du Québec (FRQ, 202685), Genome Canada and Quebec (142HIV). The funders had no role in data collection and interpretation, or the decision to submit the work for publication.

References

1. Brenner BG, Ibanescu RI, Hardy I, Roger M. Genotypic and phylogenetic insights on prevention of the spread of HIV-1 and drug resistance in "real-world" settings. Viruses. 2017;10:10.

2. Wainberg MA, Zaharatos GJ, Brenner BG. Development of antiretroviral drug resistance. N Engl J Med. 2011;365:637–46.

3. Brenner BG, Wainberg MA. Clinical benefit of dolutegravir in HIV-1 management related to the high genetic barrier to drug resistance. Virus Res. 2017;239:1–9.

4. Anstett K, Brenner B, Mesplede T, Wainberg MA. HIV drug resistance against strand transfer integrase inhibitors. Retrovirology. 2017;14:36.

5. Elzi L, Erb S, Furrer H, Cavassini M, Calmy A, Vernazza P, Gunthard H, Bernasconi E, Battegay M. Swiss HIVCSG: adverse events of raltegravir and dolutegravir. AIDS. 2017;31:1853–8.

6. Grinsztejn B, Nguyen BY, Katlama C, Gatell JM, Lazzarin A, Vittecoq D, Gonzalez CJ, Chen J, Harvey CM, Isaacs RD. Safety and efficacy of the HIV-1 integrase inhibitor raltegravir (MK-0518) in treatment-experienced patients with multidrug-resistant virus: a phase II randomised controlled trial. Lancet. 2007;369:1261–9.

7. Shimura K, Kodama E, Sakagami Y, Matsuzaki Y, Watanabe W, Yamataka K, Watanabe Y, Ohata Y, S Y, Sato M, et al. Broad antiretroviral activity and resistance profile of the novel human immunodeficiency virus integrase inhibitor elvitegravir (JTK-303/GS-9137). J Virol. 2008;82:764–74.

8. Delelis O, Thierry S, Subra F, Simon F, Malet I, Alloui C, Sayon S, Calvez V, Deprez E, Marcelin AG, et al. Impact of Y143 HIV-1 integrase mutations on resistance to raltegravir in vitro and in vivo. Antimicrob Agents Chemother. 2010;54:491–501.

9. Maiga AI, Malet I, Soulie C, Derache A, Koita V, Amellal B, Tchertanov L, Delelis O, Morand-Joubert L, Mouscadet JF, et al. Genetic barriers for integrase inhibitor drug resistance in HIV type-1 B and CRF02_AG subtypes. Antivir Ther. 2009;14:123–9.

10. Bar-Magen T, Donahue DA, McDonough EI, Kuhl BD, Faltenbacher VH, Xu H, Michaud V, Sloan RD, Wainberg MA. HIV-1 subtype B and C integrase enzymes exhibit differential patterns of resistance to integrase inhibitors in biochemical assays. AIDS. 2010;24:2171–9.

11. Malet I, Delelis O, Soulie C, Wirden M, Tchertanov L, Mottaz P, Peytavin G, Katlama C, Mouscadet JF, Calvez V, Marcelin AG. Quasispecies variant dynamics during emergence of resistance to raltegravir in HIV-1-infected patients. J Antimicrob Chemother. 2009;63:795–804.

12. Mesplede T, Quashie PK, Zanichelli V, Wainberg MA. Integrase strand transfer inhibitors in the management of HIV-positive individuals. Ann Med. 2014;46:123–9.

13. Gallant J, Lazzarin A, Mills A, Orkin C, Podzamczer D, Tebas P, Girard PM, Brar I, Daar ES, Wohl D, et al. Bictegravir, emtricitabine, and tenofovir alafenamide versus dolutegravir, abacavir, and lamivudine for initial treatment of HIV-1 infection (GS-US-380-1489): a double-blind, multicentre, phase 3, randomised controlled non-inferiority trial. Lancet. 2017;390:2063–72.

14. Margolis DA, Gonzalez-Garcia J, Stellbrink HJ, Eron JJ, Yazdanpanah Y, Podzamczer D, Lutz T, Angel JB, Richmond GJ, Clotet B, et al. Long-acting intramuscular cabotegravir and rilpivirine in adults with HIV-1 infection (LATTE-2): 96-week results of a randomised, open-label, phase 2b, non-inferiority trial. Lancet. 2017;390:1499–510.

15. Sax PE, DeJesus E, Crofoot G, Ward D, Benson P, Dretler R, Mills A, Brinson C, Peloquin J, Wei X, et al. Bictegravir versus dolutegravir, each with emtricitabine and tenofovir alafenamide, for initial treatment of HIV-1 infection: a randomised, double-blind, phase 2 trial. Lancet HIV. 2017;4:e154–60.

16. Kobayashi M, Yoshinaga T, Seki T, Wakasa-Morimoto C, Brown KW, Ferris R, Foster SA, Hazen RJ, Miki S, Suyama-Kagitani A, et al. In Vitro antiretroviral properties of S/GSK1349572, a next-generation HIV integrase inhibitor. Antimicrob Agents Chemother. 2011;55:813–21.

17. Lenz JC, Rockstroh JK. S/GSK1349572, a new integrase inhibitor for the treatment of HIV: promises and challenges. Expert Opin Investig Drugs. 2011;20:537–48.

18. Prada N, Markowitz M. Novel integrase inhibitors for HIV. Expert Opin Investig Drugs. 2010;19:1087–98.

19. Cahn P, Pozniak AL, Mingrone H, Shuldyakov A, Brites C, Andrade-Villanueva JF, Richmond G, Buendia CB, Fourie J, Ramgopal M, et al. Dolutegravir versus raltegravir in antiretroviral-experienced, integrase-inhibitor-naive adults with HIV: week 48 results from the randomised, double-blind, non-inferiority SAILING study. Lancet. 2013;382:700–8.

20. Quashie PK, Mesplede T, Han YS, Oliveira M, Singhroy DN, Fujiwara T, Underwood MR, Wainberg MA. Characterization of the R263K mutation in HIV-1 integrase that confers low-level resistance to the second-generation integrase strand transfer inhibitor dolutegravir. J Virol. 2012;86:2696–705.

21. Mesplede T, Quashie PK, Osman N, Han Y, Singhroy DN, Lie Y, Petropoulos CJ, Huang W, Wainberg MA. Viral fitness cost prevents HIV-1 from evading dolutegravir drug pressure. Retrovirology. 2013;10:22.

22. Mesplede T, Osman N, Wares M, Quashie PK, Hassounah S, Anstett K, Han Y, Singhroy DN, Wainberg MA. Addition of E138K to R263K in HIV integrase increases resistance to dolutegravir, but fails to restore activity of the HIV integrase enzyme and viral replication capacity. J Antimicrob Chemother. 2014;69:2733–40.

23. Wares M, Mesplede T, Quashie PK, Osman N, Han Y, Wainberg MA. The M50I polymorphic substitution in association with the R263K mutation in HIV-1 subtype B integrase increases drug resistance but does not restore viral replicative fitness. Retrovirology. 2014;11:7.

24. Mesplede T, Quashie PK, Hassounah S, Osman N, Han Y, Liang J, Singhroy DN, Wainberg MA. The R263K substitution in HIV-1 subtype C is more deleterious for integrase enzymatic function and viral replication than in subtype B. AIDS. 2015;29:1459–66.

25. Brenner BG, Ibanescu RI, Oliveira M, Roger M, Hardy I, Routy JP, Kyeyune F, Quinones-Mateu ME, Wainberg MA. Montreal PHICSG: HIV-1 strains belonging to large phylogenetic clusters show accelerated escape from integrase inhibitors in cell culture compared with viral isolates from singleton/small clusters. J Antimicrob Chemother. 2017;72:2171–83.

26. Quashie PK, Oliviera M, Veres T, Osman N, Han YS, Hassounah S, Lie Y, Huang W, Mesplede T, Wainberg MA. Differential effects of the G118R, H51Y, and E138K resistance substitutions in different subtypes of HIV integrase. J Virol. 2015;89:3163–75.

27. Hightower KE, Wang R, Deanda F, Johns BA, Weaver K, Shen Y, Tomberlin GH, Carter HL 3rd, Broderick T, Sigethy S, et al. Dolutegravir (S/GSK1349572) exhibits significantly slower dissociation than raltegravir and elvitegravir from wild-type and integrase inhibitor-resistant HIV-1 integrase-DNA complexes. Antimicrob Agents Chemother. 2011;55:4552–9.

28. Osman N, Mesplede T, Quashie PK, Oliveira M, Zanichelli V, Wainberg MA. Dolutegravir maintains a durable effect against HIV replication in tissue culture even after drug washout. J Antimicrob Chemother. 2015;70:2810–5.

29. Sax PE, Pozniak A, Montes ML, Koenig E, DeJesus E, Stellbrink HJ, Antinori A, Workowski K, Slim J, Reynes J, et al. Coformulated bictegravir, emtricitabine, and tenofovir alafenamide versus dolutegravir with emtricitabine and tenofovir alafenamide, for initial treatment of HIV-1 infection (GS-US-380-1490): a randomised, double-blind, multicentre, phase 3, non-inferiority trial. Lancet. 2017;390:2073–82.

30. Tsiang M, Jones GS, Goldsmith J, Mulato A, Hansen D, Kan E, Tsai L, Bam RA, Stepan G, Stray KM, et al. Antiviral activity of bictegravir (GS-9883), a novel potent HIV-1 integrase strand transfer inhibitor with an improved resistance profile. Antimicrob Agents Chemother. 2016;60:7086–97.

31. Smith SJ, Zhao XZ, Burke TR Jr, Hughes SH. Efficacies of cabotegravir and bictegravir against drug-resistant HIV-1 integrase mutants. Retrovirology. 2018;15:37.

32. Margolis DA, Brinson CC, Smith GHR, de Vente J, Hagins DP, Eron JJ, Griffith SK, Clair MHS, Stevens MC, Williams PE, et al. Cabotegravir plus rilpivirine, once a day, after induction with cabotegravir plus nucleoside reverse transcriptase inhibitors in antiretroviral-naive adults with HIV-1 infection (LATTE): a randomised, phase 2b, dose-ranging trial. Lancet Infect Dis. 2015;15:1145–55.

33. Sax PE, DeJesus E, Crofoot G, Ward D, Benson P, Dretler R, Mills A, Brinson C, Peloquin J, Wei X, et al. Bictegravir versus dolutegravir, each with emtricitabine and tenofovir alafenamide, for initial treatment of HIV-1 infection: a randomised, double-blind, phase 2 trial. Lancet HIV. 2017;4:e154–60.

34. Boulerice F, Bour S, Geleziunas R, Lvovich A, Wainberg MA. High frequency of isolation of defective human immunodeficiency virus type 1 and heterogeneity of viral gene expression in clones of infected U-937 cells. J Virol. 1990;64:1745–55.

35. Brenner BG, Thomas R, Blanco JL, Ibanescu RI, Oliveira M, Mesplede T, Golubkov O, Roger M, Garcia F, Martinez E, Wainberg MA. Development of a G118R mutation in HIV-1 integrase following a switch to dolutegravir monotherapy leading to cross-resistance to integrase inhibitors. J Antimicrob Chemother. 2016;71:1948–53.

36. Ghosn J, Mazet AA, Avettand-Fenoel V, Peytavin G, Wirden M, Delfraissy JF, Chaix ML. Rapid selection and archiving of mutation E157Q in HIV-1 DNA during short-term low-level replication on a raltegravir-containing regimen. J Antimicrob Chemother. 2009;64:433–4.

37. Malet I, Delelis O, Valantin MA, Montes B, Soulie C, Wirden M, Tchertanov L, Peytavin G, Reynes J, Mouscadet JF, et al. Mutations associated with failure of raltegravir treatment affect integrase sensitivity to the inhibitor in vitro. Antimicrob Agents Chemother. 2008;52:1351–8.

38. Danion F, Belissa E, Peytavin G, Thierry E, Lanternier F, Scemla A, Lortholary O, Delelis O, Avettand-Fenoel V, Duvivier C. Non-virological response to a dolutegravir-containing regimen in a patient harbouring a E157Q-mutated virus in the integrase region. J Antimicrob Chemother. 2015;70:1921–3.

39. Charpentier C, Descamps D. Resistance to HIV integrase inhibitors: about R263K and E157Q mutations. Viruses. 2018;10:41.

40. Charpentier C, Malet I, Andre-Garnier E, Storto A, Bocket L, Amiel C, Morand-Joubert L, Tumiotto C, Nguyen T, Maillard A, et al. Phenotypic analysis of HIV-1 E157Q integrase polymorphism and impact on virological outcome in patients initiating an integrase inhibitor-based regimen. J Antimicrob Chemother. 2018;73:1039–44.

41. Dudas K DF, Wang R, Margolis D, Demarest J, Griffith S, St Clair MH. Characterization of NRTI and INI resistance mutations observed in a study subject on ral two-drug therapy with 10 mg cabotegravir and 25 mg rilpivirine. In: International workshop on antiretroviral drug resistance, 21–22 Feb 2015, Seattle, WA.

42. Margolis DA, Boffito M. Long-acting antiviral agents for HIV treatment. Curr Opin HIV AIDS. 2015;10:246–52.

43. Neogi U, Singh K, Aralaguppe SG, Rogers LC, Njenda DT, Sarafianos SG, Hejdeman B, Sonnerborg A. Ex-vivo antiretroviral potency of newer integrase strand transfer inhibitors cabotegravir and bictegravir in HIV type 1 non-B subtypes. AIDS. 2018;32:469–76.

44. Yoshinaga T, Kobayashi M, Seki T, Miki S, Wakasa-Morimoto C, Suyama-Kagitani A, Kawauchi-Miki S, Taishi T, Kawasuji T, Johns BA, et al. Antiviral characteristics of GSK1265744, an HIV integrase inhibitor dosed orally or by long-acting injection. Antimicrob Agents Chemother. 2015;59:397–406.

45. Yoshinaga T, Seki T, Miki S, Miyamoto T, Suyama-Kagitani A, Kawauchi-Miki S, Kobayashi M, Sato A, Stewart E, Underwood M, Fujiwara T. Novel secondary mutations C56S and G149A confer resistance to HIV-1 integrase strand transfer inhibitors. Antiviral Res. 2018;152:1–9.

46. Brenner BG, Thomas R, Blanco JL, Ibanescu RI, Oliveira M, Mesplede T, Golubkov O, Roger M, Garcia F, Martinez E, Wainberg MA. Development of a G118R mutation in HIV-1 integrase following a switch to dolutegravir monotherapy leading to cross-resistance to integrase inhibitors. J Antimicrob Chemother. 2016;71:1948–53.

47. Cahn P, Pozniak AL, Mingrone H, Shuldyakov A, Brites C, Andrade-Villanueva JF, Richmond G, Buendia CB, Fourie J, Ramgopal M, et al. Dolutegravir versus raltegravir in antiretroviral-experienced, integrase-inhibitor-naive adults with HIV: week 48 results from the randomised, double-blind, non-inferiority SAILING study. Lancet. 2013;382:700–8.

48. Lepik KJ, Harrigan PR, Yip B, Wang L, Robbins MA, Zhang WW, Toy J, Akagi L, Lima VD, Guillemi S, et al. Emergent drug resistance with integrase strand transfer inhibitor-based regimens. AIDS. 2017;31:1425–34.

49. Wijting IEA, Lungu C, Rijnders BJA, van der Ende ME, Pham HT, Mesplede T, Pas SD, Voermans JJC, Schuurman R, van de Vijver D, et al. HIV-1 resistance dynamics in patients failing dolutegravir maintenance monotherapy. J Infect Dis. 2018;218(5):688–97.

50. Kuritzkes DR. Resistance to dolutegravir—a chink in the armor? J Infect Dis. 2018;218:673–5.

51. Sullivan PS, Do AN, Ellenberger D, Pau CP, Paul S, Robbins K, Kalish M, Storck C, Schable CA, Wise H, et al. Human immunodeficiency virus (HIV) subtype surveillance of African-born persons at risk for group O and group N HIV infections in the United States. J Infect Dis. 2000;181:463–9.

52. Haertle T, Carrera CJ, Wasson DB, Sowers LC, Richman DD, Carson DA. Metabolism and anti-human immunodeficiency virus-1 activity of 2-halo-2′,3′-dideoxyadenosine derivatives. J Biol Chem. 1988;263:5870–5.

53. Oliveira M, Brenner BG, Wainberg MA. Isolation of drug-resistant mutant HIV variants using tissue culture drug selection. Methods Mol Biol. 2009;485:427–33.

54. Brockman MA, Chopera DR, Olvera A, Brumme CJ, Sela J, Markle TJ, Martin E, Carlson JM, Le AQ, McGovern R, et al. Uncommon pathways of immune escape attenuate HIV-1 integrase replication capacity. J Virol. 2012;86:6913–23.

55. Gonzalez N, Perez-Olmeda M, Mateos E, Cascajero A, Alvarez A, Spijkers S, Garcia-Perez J, Sanchez-Palomino S, Ruiz-Mateos E, Leal M, Alcami J. A sensitive phenotypic assay for the determination of human immunodeficiency virus type 1 tropism. J Antimicrob Chemother. 2010;65:2493–501.

56. Gonzalez-Serna A, Min JE, Woods C, Chan D, Lima VD, Montaner JS, Harrigan PR, Swenson LC. Performance of HIV-1 drug resistance testing at low-level viremia and its ability to predict future virologic outcomes and viral evolution in treatment-naive individuals. Clin Infect Dis. 2014;58:1165–73.

57. Lapointe HR, Dong W, Lee GQ, Bangsberg DR, Martin JN, Mocello AR, Boum Y, Karakas A, Kirkby D, Poon AF, et al. HIV drug resistance testing by high-multiplex "wide" sequencing on the MiSeq instrument. Antimicrob Agents Chemother. 2015;59:6824–33.

58. Reuman EC, Bachmann MH, Varghese V, Fessel WJ, Shafer RW. Panel of prototypical raltegravir-resistant infectious molecular clones in a novel integrase-deleted cloning vector. Antimicrob Agents Chemother. 2010;54:934–6.

59. Brenner BG, Oliveira M, Doualla-Bell F, Moisi DD, Ntemgwa M, Frankel F, Essex M, Wainberg MA. HIV-1 subtype C viruses rapidly develop K65R resistance to tenofovir in cell culture. AIDS. 2006;20:F9–13.

60. Brenner B, Turner D, Oliveira M, Moisi D, Detorio M, Carobene M, Marlink RG, Schapiro J, Roger M, Wainberg MA. A V106M mutation in HIV-1 clade C viruses exposed to efavirenz confers cross-resistance to non-nucleoside reverse transcriptase inhibitors. AIDS. 2003;17:F1–5.

61. Asahchop EL, Wainberg MA, Oliveira M, Xu H, Brenner BG, Moisi D, Ibanescu IR, Tremblay C. Distinct resistance patterns to etravirine and rilpivirine in viruses containing nonnucleoside reverse transcriptase inhibitor mutations at baseline. AIDS. 2013;27:879–87.

62. Brenner BG, Lowe M, Moisi D, Hardy I, Gagnon S, Charest H, Baril JG, Wainberg MA, Roger M. Subtype diversity associated with the development of HIV-1 resistance to integrase inhibitors. J Med Virol. 2011;83:751–9.

63. Routy JP, Machouf N, Edwardes MD, Brenner BG, Thomas R, Trottier B, Rouleau D, Tremblay CL, Cote P, Baril JG, et al. Factors associated with a decrease in the prevalence of drug resistance in newly HIV-1 infected individuals in Montreal. AIDS. 2004;18:2305–12.

10

Pre-exposure prophylaxis (PrEP) in an era of stalled HIV prevention: Can it change the game?

Robyn Eakle[1,2]* ⓘ, Francois Venter[1] and Helen Rees[1]

Abstract

Pre-exposure prophylaxis (PrEP) for HIV prevention has evolved significantly over the years where clinical trials have now demonstrated the efficacy of oral PrEP, and the field is scaling-up implementation. The WHO and UNAIDS have made PrEP implementation a priority for populations at highest risk, and several countries have developed guidelines and national plans accordingly, largely based on evidence generated by demonstration projects. PrEP presents the opportunity to change the face of HIV prevention by offering a new option for protection against HIV and disrupting current HIV prevention systems. Nevertheless, as with all new technologies, both practical and social requirements for implementation must be taken into account if there is to be sustained and widespread adoption, which will also apply to forthcoming prevention technologies. Defining and building success for PrEP within the scope of scale-up requires careful consideration. This review summarises where the PrEP field is today, lessons learned from the past, the philosophy and practicalities of how successful programming may be defined, and provides perspectives of costs and affordability. We argue that a successful PrEP programme is about effective intervention integration and ultimately keeping people HIV negative.

Keywords: HIV prevention, Biomedical prevention products, Pre-exposure prophylaxis (PrEP)

Introduction

Pre-exposure prophylaxis (PrEP) for HIV prevention has evolved significantly since the early conceptualization of protection tested in animal models [1] following evidence of prevention using antiretrovirals for occupational and non-occupational post-exposure prophylaxis [2, 3]. Since then, clinical trials have demonstrated the efficacy of oral PrEP, with evidence from 18 studies showing that "PrEP significantly reduced the risk of HIV acquisition" [4]. However, the level of efficacy varied according to differences in adherence within and across the study populations, with MSM showing higher levels of efficacy than found in the women-only studies [4]. Adherence is a central component for consideration of programme planning, budget, and PrEP effectiveness.

*Correspondence: reakle@wrhi.ac.za; robyn.eakle@lshtm.ac.uk
[1] Wits Reproductive Health and HIV Institute, Faculty of Health Sciences, University of the Witwatersrand, Hillbrow Health Precinct, 22 Esselen Street, Hillbrow, Johannesburg 2001, South Africa
Full list of author information is available at the end of the article

The primacy of a combined effort including early antiretroviral treatment (ART) for HIV-positive people, rendering them non-infectious, and efficient prevention interventions for HIV-negative people including condom distribution, treatment of sexually transmitted infections (STIs), post-exposure prophylaxis, and oral PrEP, voluntary medical male circumcision (VMMC), as well as continued outreach and education programming, is necessary if the goal of controlling the epidemic by 2030 is to be realized [5]. The World Health Organization (WHO) and UNAIDS have made PrEP implementation a priority for populations at "substantial risk" [6, 7], and several countries have developed guidelines and national plans integrating PrEP into programming, with the United States, South Africa, and Kenya among the first with official government-supported guidance [8–12]. These guidelines have been developed based on evidence emerging from demonstration projects [13].

Developing relevant and successful PrEP interventions, as well as defining what success is for those programmes is a challenge that the HIV prevention world is currently evaluating and debating. Since PrEP will not be a standalone intervention and rather integrated into existing programming and systems, measures of success should take into account combination prevention and programming as a whole. In addition, data suggest that while men can achieve good protection with PrEP even if doses are missed, women need to take PrEP every day to achieve high levels of efficacy [14, 15]. Evaluating effectiveness in a female population is thus strongly influenced by adherence, making its performance in the field harder to predict.

Mathematical modelling has suggested that PrEP could be part of changing the HIV prevention game, with the potential to enhance conventional prevention efforts, depending on the ability of programmes to prioritise those at risk and manage costs [16–19]. There is a desperate need for improved prevention efforts, so understanding how to strategically focus PrEP interventions to achieve optimal outcomes and to reinvigorate prevention programmes, is of critical importance. Coupled with strategic planning is the need for demand and support for the intervention. In the United Kingdom (UK), grass-roots advocacy and support largely from the men who have sex with men (MSM) community has pushed for expanded availability of PrEP beyond those able and willing to pay out of their own pockets [20]. In Swaziland, a national pilot is underway to capitalize the success of the implementation of test and treat for HIV-positive people by adding PrEP as an option for those at higher risk of HIV in the general community [21]. These are just two separate examples of where ground up and top down support have pushed the availability of PrEP into a position to make a difference as a prevention system disrupter.

This review summarises the literature on where the PrEP field is today, discusses lessons learned thus far from intervention and service delivery integration salient to the introduction of PrEP, discusses the philosophy and practicalities of how successful PrEP programming may be defined, explores how the newness of PrEP may be leveraged as a system disrupter to encourage demand, and provides perspectives of prevention costs and cost effectiveness. We argue that developing and measuring a successful PrEP programme is about effective prevention intervention integration aimed at keeping people HIV negative.

PrEP: Where are we now?

Oral PrEP is now included as part of the recommended standard of prevention by the World Health Organization (WHO) for people defined as being at "substantial risk" of HIV infection [6]. Substantial risk was defined in the 2016 Consolidated Guidelines on the Use of Antiretroviral drugs for Treating and Preventing HIV as geographical incidence of 3% or higher. However, the recommendation also suggests that 2% is sufficient, and considerations of population context, as well as demand should be taken into account, thereby effectively allowing countries to interpret this definition as it is relevant to their particular settings. Oral PrEP has been registered for use by sexually active men and women, by several national drug regulatory authorities including the United States Food and Drug Administration (US FDA) and the South African Medicines Control Council (MCC). Implementation studies for different target populations have been completed or are in various stages across the globe [13].

The current oral PrEP strategy itself requires a daily commitment to pill taking, in particular for heterosexual women who appear to require higher concentrations of antiretrovirals in the genital tract to confer protection [14]. This is supported by preliminary evidence which suggests that in order to reach adequate drug levels in tissues exposed to potential HIV infection (e.g. vaginal and/or anal), women require near perfect adherence to a seven day regimen, where MSM may reach adequate levels in anal tissues with only 4 days of pill taking in a week which can be non consecutive [14, 15]. Because of the significant behaviour requirements to maintain consistent daily pill taking, additional options for PrEP delivery, including long-acting injectables, vaginal rings and films, are being developed to increase the selection of PrEP products and allow people to make choices about which technology best fits their lifestyles [22–24]. This scope of development is comparable to contraception where increasing the number of contraceptive options has been shown to significantly increase the overall uptake of contraception [25]. This seems to also be the case with the female condom where expanding the choice of product has improved access and use [26]. A vaginal ring containing the HIV drug dapivirine was recently tested in clinical trials and showed modest efficacy in preventing HIV, and an open label trial is now ongoing [27, 28]. Other products are in development, and it may take a few years to complete clinical efficacy studies, secure licensure and assess needs for implementation and cost [29]. In the meantime, noting the persistently high HIV incidence particularly among adolescent girls and young women (AGYW), and other vulnerable populations, it is critical to rollout oral PrEP as an expansion of prevention technology options and learn from the experiences of scaling it up which can later ease the way for new products.

Figure 1 shows a timeline for the last 20 years of ARV-based prevention development and demonstrates the rapid increase in development activities over the last

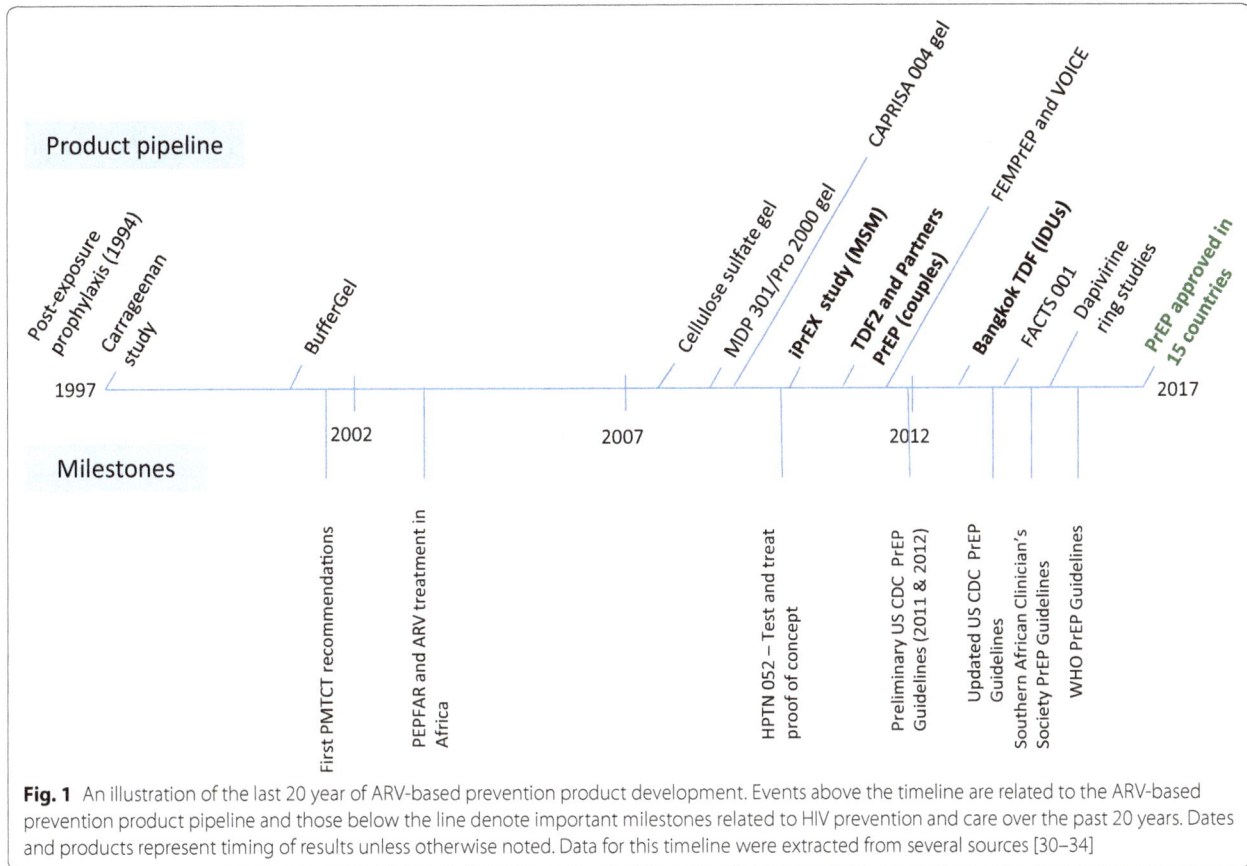

Fig. 1 An illustration of the last 20 year of ARV-based prevention product development. Events above the timeline are related to the ARV-based prevention product pipeline and those below the line denote important milestones related to HIV prevention and care over the past 20 years. Dates and products represent timing of results unless otherwise noted. Data for this timeline were extracted from several sources [30–34]

10 years compared with the previous decade. This timeline depicts the 'scale-up' in knowledge which happened over a period of time, gaining momentum with the results of each product. Although not all of the products or stepping stones illustrated here are of equal impact, each step in the development process contributed to the evolution of thinking and decisions in the development of ARV-based prevention technologies. Now, as the oral PrEP intervention is scaled-up in countries and new products come online, a similar escalation in learning from and accelerating implementation will ideally occur. Additional graphics and details of development can be accessed on the AVAC website [30].

Per recommendations from mathematical modelling studies [16, 18, 35] as well as the WHO [36], first wave implementation studies have focused on delivering PrEP to populations at higher risk of HIV, in particular MSM and sex workers, as well as people who use drugs (PWUD) and AGYW to a lesser extent. This approach was aimed at optimising impact and cost effectiveness. In practice, these projects have mostly focused on MSM and sex workers where programmes have already been established as a sort of "low hanging fruit" [13]. Beyond these first waves in defined programmes, however, identifying

those at highest risk and prioritising risk groups brings significant challenges. Most populations at highest risk experience structural vulnerabilities such as lack of access to services, lack of information and/or criminalization making them harder to reach [37]. Others have pursued studies for the harder to reach such as such as the SAPPH-IRe trial in Zimbabwe which combined provision of PrEP and test and treat through mobile clinics in rural areas throughout the country [38]. Second wave projects have been focusing on AGYW, which, while comprising only 11% of the population, are estimated to make up 20% of new HIV infections globally and are in great need of additional HIV prevention options [7, 39]. However, beyond sexual and reproductive health services, to varying degrees depending on settings, AGYW are more difficult to engage in care or interventions such as PrEP because they are not necessarily grouping together in particular clinics or geographical/contextual areas (as opposed to MSM or sex workers) and therefore require a whole different approach to communication, education, and support for PrEP use.

From the few results reported thus far from demonstration projects, it appears that people at high risk are self-identifying and taking up PrEP [40, 41], but it may be that these people represent "early adopters" as the numbers are relatively small. These early adopters sit at the front of the bell curve that represents the Diffusion of Innovations theory [42]. This theory states that uptake of any new technology or behaviour starts with a small proportion of people adopting and promoting it to their communities. Perhaps one of the greatest challenges in PrEP delivery will be to engage the next level of adopters who are at high risk, but may not initially be highly motivated to take it up. Promoting uptake, or generating demand in more sceptical communities, may involve a combination of strategies including social marketing and creative adherence support driven by lessons learned from outside the public health arena such as behavioural economics [43, 44]. Approaches will also have to be tailored according to each population and geography. In this regard, viewing PrEP itself as a system "disrupter", where the newness and promise of the product is a motivator in and of itself, will both require new strategies to engage PrEP-sceptical potential end-users as well as those who may have become impervious to prevention messaging and disinterested in available technologies. This element of capitalizing on the introduction of a new prevention option could be an important component of generating demand among the next set of adopters.

New prevention interventions: integration, programming, and lessons learned

The implementation of oral PrEP comprises a few critical logistical components. These include initial HIV testing to confirm an HIV-negative status, continued testing to ensure no change in HIV status, and monitoring of kidney health. These are the basic clinical requirements as recommended in several guidelines [6, 8, 11, 12]. Additionally, these guidelines highlight the need to monitor for potential hepatitis B infection, which does not exclude but could complicate PrEP use, other potential co-infections, and especially women who may be pregnant or breastfeeding where guidance on PrEP use is mixed. These components as currently stipulated require informed healthcare providers who can support their clients with information when they are making the decision as to whether to start PrEP, as well as support them during their time using PrEP with tailored adherence strategies.

With these requirements in mind, it is clear that new prevention technologies or interventions may be challenging to integrate into existing services if the specific requirements of introduction are different from what exists in the established system. Male condoms are the commonest and most successful prevention technology so far introduced. Overall they are inexpensive and widely utilised [45, 46], however, no intervention is perfect and

male condoms have suffered from challenges like any other. Programmatic challenges have included issues with reliable distribution and access, as well as negative social connotations around trust and sex, and some reported problems with breakage [47–53]. Female condom programmes have been more challenging to introduce and sustain because of higher unit costs, limited distribution outlets, negative health care worker attitudes, and user acceptability [54, 55]. Similar challenges should be anticipated in the introduction of oral PrEP programme, as many female condom programmes floundered because of these obstacles. As with male and female condoms, consideration of where PrEP can and should be delivered will be critical so as not to limit access or stigmatise the product. Potential outlets could be specialised key population clinics, general public health clinics, school health programmes, and sexual and reproductive health clinics, as well as mobile versions of all of these.

Another example is VMMC, a relatively simple, one-time surgical, typically outpatient procedure, and once done offers lifelong partial protection against HIV. However, it took time to build VMMC into a viable service from both the provider and the client perspectives. From the service delivery side, factors including "country ownership; sustained political will; service delivery efficiencies, such as task shifting and task sharing; use of outreach and mobile services; disposable, pre-packaged VMMC kits; external funding; and a standardized set of indicators for VMMC" were found to be the ingredients required for successful implementation and scale-up, while continual failures in supply chain management and unreliable funding sources caused issues in maintaining consistent service provision [56]. PrEP will need some of these same components to be successfully implemented and scaled-up, and in addition will have challenges such as repeat HIV testing, blood draws, and regular client follow up. These ingredients for implementation speak to the required ownership, accountability, and pragmatism of integrating a new prevention intervention into systems already burdened with heavy patient volumes and logistical management issues.

Implementation of VMMC taught important lessons which could also inform PrEP rollout. Issues such as task shifting, the need for specific, easy to use kits for VMMC and the negative response of some men to compulsory HIV testing, had not been anticipated as challenges [57]. To address these issues, more resources were needed to develop strong community-based social marketing campaigns as well as mechanisms to support men. Resources were aimed at messaging for men and women to promote the intervention, and in some cases, providing cancer screening services for women to promote a holistic health programme [58]. The observation that adjustments to the

VMMC programmes were required once implementation had begun, demonstrates the importance of continuous, iterative programme review once a new technology is introduced. As with VMMC, developing supportive partner services, or options for partner engagement, could strengthen overall PrEP services and help to mitigate stigma and rumours arising from misunderstanding of the intervention.

Additionally, for PrEP to become normalized as an intervention, communities will need to become familiar and accepting of the concept. This will be challenging if only certain key populations are prioritised for rollout [59]. Messaging around the intervention will need to consider social aspects of delivery which were also barriers in VMMC implementation. These include the potential for loss of income when at the clinic, fear of the procedure or of side effects in the case of PrEP, lack of HIV risk perception, and lack of partner support [60–62].

Finally, and perhaps most unique to PrEP, is that it will be aimed at maintaining an HIV negative status in those at risk for HIV and will be used during periods of high risk rather than for a person's entire life. The social and risk element is especially complex with the potential difficulties of identifying the high-risk groups, maintaining engagement with them while mitigating stigma (and criminalization for some marginalised groups), providing tailored services that are acceptable, and having the individuals who are identified as being at risk, self-assess sufficiently to ensure adequate adherence. Getting these pieces right will also depend on how the larger community understands the product (e.g. not as a "sex worker or MSM product"), and accepts and supports its implementation. The use of PrEP for limited portions of time will also add to the complexity of maintaining use during the time of need in these high-risk populations and conveying appropriate messaging to that extent.

The focus on adherence

Like oral contraception, PrEP is a highly effective prevention technology if taken consistently, notwithstanding the different efficacy requirements for women and men mentioned above. Adherence to PrEP is therefore key to the method's success, yet there have been many challenges in ensuring adherence in clinical trials. Adherence to PrEP (or lack thereof) was why parts of one study [63], and another entire study [64] were not able to adequately measure efficacy among women, where at least 70% of participants in the VOICE trial and 60% in FEM-PrEP did not use PrEP properly. The qualitative research published following the VOICE [65] and FEMPrEP [66] studies revealed highly nuanced reasons for lack of use, including misconceptions about personal risk, logistical issues attending the clinic, apathy towards research, and

general lack of interest in the product but intense interest in the high quality health services provided by the clinical trial clinics [65, 66]. This presented a challenge in the trials where women would tell clinical staff that they were adhering to their assigned regimens in order to keep coming to the clinic. Some observers questioned whether oral PrEP would ever be a viable product for women who, in large numbers in these studies, demonstrated little interest in consistent PrEP use. However it was generally agreed that in the absence of many prevention choices, that the product should be made available following additional research into the nuanced feedback received from the trials and previous prevention efforts [43, 67–70].

These insights are important as they point towards a need to conceptualize oral PrEP differently from other prevention methods and from the provision of ART, as well as build PrEP interventions into care valued by the community. Importantly, the duration of use will be determined by the needs of the individual. Taking PrEP over a period of time has been likened to "seasons of risk", where someone may choose to take PrEP for a time, and then switch to another method [43, 71], as happens with contraception. As with contraception, as long as this engagement with products results in the desired outcome (maintaining a negative HIV status), then the programming will be successful—e.g. PrEP does not have to be implemented in place of or to the detriment of male and female condoms, or other prevention strategies.

The provision of ART, especially as it expands into test and treat programming worldwide, has focused on uptake and consistent use of HIV treatment for life. This cannot be the mind set for PrEP, which must be delivered by providers with a message of flexibility thus promoting honest feedback from clients who will need to engage with the best product available to stay negative. Presenting PrEP to health care workers as being analogous to contraception is likely to be better understood rather than locating PrEP alongside HIV treatment. In addition, the early experiences of ART and its side effects persist in the memories of communities, which could be off putting for clients considering PrEP. With these issues in mind, supportive adherence counselling will be imperative for PrEP success [72].

Defining and building success

The primary measure of success for any HIV prevention technology is the number of HIV infections averted over a period of time and in a prescribed population. However, this retrospective analysis can take a significant effort and time to produce. To more accurately assess progress in shorter periods of time (quarterly or even annually), measurement of success is often limited to programmatic counting. For instance, the number of condoms distributed to a given population in a given year is usually taken as whether a condom campaign has been successful. This metric, however, does not shed light as to whether people used the condoms.

Overall, for evaluating PrEP success, numbers of HIV infections averted will need to be modelled based on a range of composite programmatic measures. One important metric will be uptake among those eligible for PrEP. However, eligibility will have to be well-defined and is currently different in some countries. There is clinical eligibility of being HIV-negative with healthy kidney function which is universal in guidelines, however the question of risk is where countries currently differ. Kenya is prioritising people at higher risk in certain geographical areas [73], while South Africa is focusing only on key populations and has excluded pregnant and breastfeeding women for the time being [10, 12]. Therefore, any comparisons of uptake across countries will need to keep these differences in mind. In addition, the denominator for who is actually eligible may be difficult to calculate depending on the validity of population demographics in a given setting.

Measuring uptake should also go a step further in determining the number of people newly engaging in or returning to care because of interest in PrEP. Since PrEP may actually act as a catalyst to reignite interest in HIV prevention services overall then accounting for increases in numbers of people coming to the clinic because of PrEP, whether they end up using it or not, is also an important measure of success for the larger prevention goal of staying HIV-negative. This will depend, however, on programmes having reliable data from before PrEP is introduced to be able to assess increases in numbers, as well as ideally recording in a standardized manner the purpose for engagement in care as well as date of previous HIV test and/or visit. In addition, it will be important to then analyse who is coming to the clinic in terms of (on a basic level) age, sexual behaviour, and gender.

Retention is a critical metric, but is also not so straight forward as there is the question of whether it is retention with use of PrEP, or rather maintaining consistent retention in care. Arguably, the latter could pose a better metric provided individuals remain HIV-negative given that is the primary purpose of PrEP and engagement in prevention services in the larger picture. Potentially both should be included, but in either case, the number of people returning for services will be important to capture. This brings a whole host of issues around how to track health service clients which are being tackled and tested through multiple creative efforts such as health cards, biometrics, and/or national electronic databases. The retention aspect should also take into account the notion that some people may fall out of PrEP use and so

should be able to track whether they maintain consistent engagement with the system while they are in periods of lesser HIV risk [72, 74].

For the metric of retention including PrEP, there has been evidence to show that recording repeat refills can be useful as a composite measure for use and one that is far more sustainably collected as compared with MEMS or pill counting [72]. As with condoms, just counting the number of people taking up PrEP or pills distributed will not account for whether people actually used the product. Adherence was a common metric in the PrEP efficacy studies, but the measurement required drug level analyses, pill counting and some more advanced technologies such as medical event monitoring systems (MEMS) on pill bottles to electronically record when bottles are opened. These strategies were also used to determine how reliable participants' self-reports were. Adherence measured in these relatively sophisticated fashions is not likely to be sustainable in a real-world environment due to labour burden, facility and budget capacities. In addition, measurement of adherence needs to be nuanced considering the cycles of risk, and differing levels of efficacy between men and women.

Seroconversions to HIV-positive status can also be tracked to assess programme success in promoting and supporting PrEP use, or at the very least, success in engaging people in effective HIV prevention. Additionally, if PrEP cycling is not managed well, there will be a risk for generating ARV resistance, although the PrEP efficacy and implementation studies, as well as pharmacovigiliance research to date have shown the probability of resistance generated by PrEP to be very low [4, 75].

These indicators will inherently depend, however, on ongoing successful personal and provider assessment of risk which also does not negatively stigmatize those at higher risk. Many pilot studies are investigating the use of risk assessment tools with varying degrees of depth. Results over the coming months from these studies will provide insight as to whether these tools have been useful and to what degree they should be used in scale-up.

Finally, for there to be PrEP interventions to assess, there must be a market and therefore demand and support for them. Testing implementation in the field and paths to guidelines in the few countries which have already taken it on board have varied greatly according to context. In the UK, the PROUD study definitively demonstrated the HIV protection potential of PrEP even before the end of the trial [76] and sparked grassroots demand from the MSM population for it to be offered through the National Health System (NHS). Negotiations are still ongoing due to the cost of integrating the drug into the NHS, however analyses have shown that existing PrEP provision through private clinics has likely contributed to the significant decrease in new infections in the UK [20, 77], further motivating continuous calls for PrEP availability. In Swaziland, where the test and treat strategy for ART was taken on board and had significant effects on reduction of community viral load, the government seized the opportunity to adopt PrEP through a national pilot in order to test the most effective way to utilize this new tool to further drive down the epidemic [21, 78]. These are two examples of how PrEP is making its way into systems from the bottom up and top down, where people have seen a need and seek to implement PrEP in a strategic way. This support is instrumental in paving the way for successful programming.

Cost-effectiveness and affordability

Since before the clinical trials reported results of PrEP efficacy, there were significant modelling efforts to estimate impact and cost-effectiveness of PrEP [79–81]. These studies relied heavily on estimated service costs as well as cost of the PrEP drugs themselves as there were no practical data from implementation. Since then, commodity costs have evolved, with tiered pricing which allow low and middle income countries to pay less for drugs than richer countries. The markets are now with opening further the availability of generic options [82].

Models have also evolved, updated and informed by efficacy estimates and service delivery costing demonstrated in rollout studies [41, 83]. Cost-effectiveness, however, will depend on the ability of programmes to efficiently integrate PrEP into existing services, and generate demand appropriately and relevantly among people at highest risk to take it up. To add to the complexity, it will also be important to consider whether PrEP become less cost-effective over time due to saturation and decreasing burden of new HIV infections necessitating the addition or increase of scale of other interventions.

In light of these complexities, an on-going challenge for many countries is how to incorporate PrEP into national plans with tight budget already allocated to existing services, such as South Africa where PrEP is being considered within the context of an ever-growing national health budget and one of the largest ART programmes in the world [83]. In Kenya, a framework for PrEP implementation was developed highlighting a projected 5-year cost for PrEP sitting at just over at $328 million, and a funding gap of about $314 million. This is based on mathematical modelling of sub-county incidence rates with population estimates aiming to geographically prioritize those at highest risk. The majority of the budget is devoted to commodity costs, knowing that the intervention is being integrated into existing services. With time, these services should adjust to make PrEP delivery more efficient and leverage the cyclical nature of individual PrEP use.

For now, no global funding programmes are providing country-level support specifically for PrEP. The United States Agency for International Development (USAID) provides some funding for PrEP through special large programme grants with specific aims. As yet, the Global Fund has only recently included PrEP in its country in its 2017–2022 strategy, but as stated it will be for select countries and it is not clear yet when this will be effected. For now, countries are making due with leveraging anything available in their existing budgets as well as special programming to get PrEP provision off the ground.

In the meantime, the recent FDA approval [82], as well as approvals in other countries such as India and South Africa, of generic PrEP drugs should help to promote the availability of lower cost drugs especially in developing country settings. Additionally, the Medicines Patent Pool, an United Nations initiative launched in 2010 with a public health business model aimed at lowering prices for essential medicines, has played an important role in the license for the PrEP combination of TDF/FTC [84]. Following an update in 2017, the MPP license for PrEP now includes 116 countries. These efforts should help to alleviate pressure on many national budgets, as well as expand PrEP markets where it is currently not included in national health plans. The HIV epidemic in developing countries, and in particular sub-Saharan Africa, are in great need of new options such as PrEP and reduction in commodity costs is imperative to making new options available a reality. Additionally, there are also people in developed countries who do not have access to PrEP and want it, such as in the UK, Canada, and much of Europe [85, 86]. In 2015, the average cost of brand name Truvada-based PrEP in the United States was $1700 per month [87], and has been reported to be between 500 and 850 euros per month in Europe [88], thus placing high hopes on lowering costs and promoting better uptake among key populations. Advocacy to push for reducing the cost of PrEP to be offered through national health plans or insurance will be key to increasing availability in both developing and developed settings.

Conclusions

Oral PrEP is an effective HIV prevention intervention when taken consistently, and should be made easily available to those at high risk of HIV who are self-aware and able to make the commitment to be sufficiently adherent. Oral PrEP can pave the way for these new technologies, and the lessons learned in its implementation can be used to build stronger, more adaptable programmes. PrEP will not change the game on its own, but as a component of HIV programming has the ability to disrupt current systems and reinvigorate the HIV prevention field. The measurement of PrEP success should be reflected in the numbers of people coming for prevention services that include targeted PrEP, and ultimately in demonstrated reductions in new HIV infections. Nevertheless, as with all new technologies, there needs to be a social shift at a population level if there is to be sustained and widespread adoption, which will also apply to prevention technologies in the development pipeline.

What is the cost of not implementing PrEP, or other new prevention options? Research has shown that ART will not reduce the epidemic enough to move towards elimination, or even control [5]. For many populations, the reliance on old prevention interventions means that the risk of acquiring HIV remains unacceptably high [89]. If the goal of PrEP and other prevention programming is to prevent new HIV infections, also reducing the escalating costs of ART as a lifelong public health intervention, then offering PrEP in the spirit of promoting choice, accessibility, flexibility, and efficiency should be the first step in paving the way for new HIV prevention interventions.

Authors' contributions
RE drafted the main manuscript, FV and HR contributed content. All authors read and approved the final manuscript.

Author details
[1] Wits Reproductive Health and HIV Institute, Faculty of Health Sciences, University of the Witwatersrand, Hillbrow Health Precinct, 22 Esselen Street, Hillbrow, Johannesburg 2001, South Africa. [2] Faculty of Public Health and Policy, London School of Hygiene and Tropical Medicine, London, United Kingdom.

Acknowledgements
Not applicable.

Competing interests
The authors declare that they have no competing interests in relation to this manuscript.

Funding
Not applicable.

References
1. Garcia-Lerma JG, Heneine W. Animal models of antiretroviral prophylaxis for HIV prevention. Curr Opin HIV AIDS. 2012;7:505–13.
2. Rey D, Bendiane MK, Moatti JP, Wellings K, Danziger R, MacDowall W, et al. Post-exposure prophylaxis after occupational and non-occupational exposures to HIV: an overview of the policies implemented in 27 European countries. AIDS Care. 2000;12(6):695–701.
3. Bryant J, Baxter L, Hird S. Non-occupational postexposure prophylaxis for HIV: a systematic review. Health Technol Assess Winch Engl. 2009;13(14):iii–ix.
4. Fonner VA, Dalglish SL, Kennedy CE, Baggaley R, O'Reilly KR, Koechlin FM, et al. Effectiveness and safety of oral HIV preexposure prophylaxis for all populations. AIDS Lond Engl. 2016;30(12):1973–83.
5. Stover J, Bollinger L, Izazola JA, Loures L, DeLay P, Ghys PD, et al. What is required to end the AIDS epidemic as a public health threat by 2030? The cost and impact of the fast-track approach. PLoS ONE. 2016;11(5):e0154893.
6. World Health Organization. Consolidated guidelines on the use of antiretroviral drugs for treating and preventing HIV infection | Recommendations for a public health approach—Second edition [Internet]. 2016 [cited 2016 Jun 28]. http://www.who.int/hiv/pub/arv/arv-2016/en/.
7. UNAIDS. Prevention Gap Report [Internet]. 2016. http://www.unaids.org/sites/default/files/media_asset/2016-prevention-gap-report_en.pdf.
8. CDC. Pre-exposure prophylaxis (PrEP) | HIV risk and prevention [Internet]. [cited 2017 Aug 8]. https://www.cdc.gov/hiv/risk/prep/index.html.
9. NASCOP. Pre exposure prophylaxis for HIV (Oral PrEP) [Internet]. NASCOP. [cited 2017 Aug 8]. http://www.nascop.or.ke/index.php/nascop-pre-exposure-prophylaxis-for-hiv-oral-prep/.
10. South African National AIDS Programme. South Africa's National Strategic Plan for HIV, TB, and STIs 2017–2022 [Internet]. 2017. http://sanac.org.za/wp-content/uploads/2017/05/NSP_FullDocument_FINAL.pdf.
11. Bekker L-G, Rebe K, Venter F, Maartens G, Moorhouse M, Conradie F, et al. Southern African guidelines on the safe use of pre-exposure prophylaxis in persons at risk of acquiring HIV-1 infection. South Afr J HIV Med [Internet]. 2016 [cited 2017 Apr 4]. http://www.sahivsoc.org/Files/Guidelines%20on%20the%20safe%20use%20of%20PrEP%20(March%202016).pdf.
12. Department of Health, South Africa. Oral pre-exposure prophylaxis (PrEP) and test and treat national guidelines for sex workers. Pretoria, South Africa; 2016.
13. AVAC. Ongoing and planned PrEP demonstration and implementation studies [Internet]. AVAC. 2016 [cited 2017 Feb 22]. http://www.avac.org/resource/ongoing-and-planned-prep-demonstration-and-implementation-studies.
14. Cottrell ML, Yang KH, Prince HMA, Sykes C, White N, Malone S, et al. A translational pharmacology approach to predicting outcomes of preexposure prophylaxis against HIV in men and women using tenofovir disoproxil fumarate with or without emtricitabine. J Infect Dis. 2016;214(1):55–64.
15. Kashuba AD, Gengiah TN, Werner L, Yang K-H, White NR, Karim QA, et al. Genital tenofovir concentrations correlate with protection against HIV infection in the CAPRISA 004 trial: importance of adherence for microbicide effectiveness. J Acquir Immune Defic Syndr 1999. 2015;69(3):264–9.
16. Cremin I, Alsallaq R, Dybul M, Piot P, Garnett G, Hallett TB. The new role of antiretrovirals in combination HIV prevention: a mathematical modelling analysis. AIDS. 2013;27(3):447–58.
17. Cremin I, McKinnon L, Kimani J, Cherutich P, Gakii G, Muriuki F, et al. PrEP for key populations in combination HIV prevention in Nairobi: a mathematical modelling study. Lancet HIV. 2017;4(5):e214–22.
18. Gomez GB, Borquez A, Case KK, Wheelock A, Vassall A, Hankins C. The cost and impact of scaling up pre-exposure prophylaxis for HIV prevention: a systematic review of cost-effectiveness modelling studies. PLoS Med. 2013;10(3):e1001401.
19. Smith JA, Anderson S-J, Harris KL, McGillen JB, Lee E, Garnett GP, et al. Maximising HIV prevention by balancing the opportunities of today with the promises of tomorrow: a modelling study. Lancet HIV. 2016;3(7):e289–96.
20. Brady M. Pre-exposure prophylaxis as HIV prevention in the UK. Ther Adv Chronic Dis. 2016;7(3):150–2.
21. Nkambule R. Substantial progress in confronting the HIV epidemic in Swaziland: first evidence of national impact. In 2017 [cited 2017 Aug 24]. http://programme.ias2017.org/Abstract/Abstract/5837.
22. Delany-Moretlwe S, Mullick S, Eakle R, Rees H. Planning for HIV preexposure prophylaxis introduction: lessons learned from contraception. Curr Opin HIV AIDS. 2016;11(1):87–93.

23. Abdool Karim S, Baxter C, Frohlich J, Abdool Karim Q. The need for multipurpose prevention technologies in sub-Saharan Africa. BJOG Int J Obstet Gynaecol. 2014;1(121):27–34.

24. Boonstra H, Barot S, Lusti-Narasimhan M. Making the case for multipurpose prevention technologies: the socio-epidemiological rationale. BJOG Int J Obstet Gynaecol. 2014;1(121):23–6.

25. WHO. WHO | Expanding contraceptive choice [Internet]. WHO. [cited 2017 Aug 10]. http://www.who.int/reproductivehealth/publications/family_planning/expanding-contraceptive-choice/en/.

26. Match Research. Evaluation of the South African female condom programme: parallel programming of female condoms [Internet]. 2016 [cited 2017 Aug 19]. http://www.femalecondoms4all.org/wp-content/uploads/2016/06/Parallel-Programming-of-Female-Condoms-Evaluation-of-the-South-African-Female-Condom-Programme.pdf.

27. Baeten JM, Palanee-Phillips T, Brown ER, Schwartz K, Soto-Torres LE, Govender V, et al. Use of a vaginal ring containing dapivirine for HIV-1 prevention in women. N Engl J Med. 2016;375(22):2121–32.

28. Nel A, van Niekerk N, Kapiga S, Bekker L-G, Gama C, Gill K, et al. Safety and efficacy of a dapivirine vaginal ring for HIV prevention in women. N Engl J Med. 2016;375(22):2133–43.

29. AVAC. MPT products in the pipeline: selected highlights [Internet]. AVAC. [cited 2017 Aug 9]. http://www.avac.org/infographic/mpt-products-pipeline.

30. AVAC. Infographics [Internet]. AVAC: global advocacy for HIV Prevention. [cited 2017 Sep 11]. http://www.avac.org/resources/infographics.

31. Centers for Disease Control and Prevention. Case-control study of HIV seroconversion in health-care workers after percutaneous exposure to HIV-infected blood—France, United Kingdom, and United States, January 1988–August 1994. Morb Mortal Wkly Rep. 1995;44(50):929–33.

32. Mayer KH, Peipert J, Fleming T, Fullem A, Moench T, Cu-Uvin S, et al. Safety and tolerability of BufferGel, a novel vaginal microbicide, in women in the United States. Clin Infect Dis Off Publ Infect Dis Soc Am. 2001;32(3):476–82.

33. Van Damme L, Govinden R, Mirembe FM, Guédou F, Solomon S, Becker ML, et al. Lack of effectiveness of cellulose sulfate gel for the prevention of vaginal HIV transmission. N Engl J Med. 2008;359(5):463–72.

34. McCormack S, Ramjee G, Kamali A, Rees H, Crook AM, Gafos M, et al. PRO2000 vaginal gel for prevention of HIV-1 infection (Microbicides Development Programme 301): a phase 3, randomised, double-blind, parallel-group trial. Lancet. 2010;376(9749):1329–37.

35. Hallett TB. Priorities across the continuum of care: modelling the impact of interventions on mortality and HIV transmission. Vancouver, Canada; 2015.

36. World Health Organization. Guidance on oral pre-exposure prophylaxis (PrEP) for serodiscordant couples, men and transgender women who have sex with men at high risk of HIV. 2012. http://www.who.int/hiv/pub/guidance_prep/en/index.html.

37. UNAIDS. HIV prevention among key populations [Internet]. 2016 [cited 2017 Aug 9]. http://www.unaids.org/en/resources/presscentre/featurestories/2016/november/20161121_keypops.

38. Cowan F. Results of the SAPPH-IRe Trial: a cluster randomised trial of a combination intervention to empower female sex workers in Zimbabwe to link and adhere to antiretrovirals for treatment and prevention. In 2016 [cited 2017 Aug 9]. http://programme.aids2016.org/Abstract/Abstract/10619.

39. World Health Organization. Global consultation on lessons from sexual and reproductive health programming to catalyse HIV prevention for adolescent girls and young women [Internet]. 2016 [cited 2018 Jan 31]. http://www.who.int/reproductivehealth/topics/linkages/WHO_Meeting_Rpt_HIV_Prevention_AGYW.pdf.

40. PrEP: demonstration for implementation. In: TUAC02 [Internet]. Vancouver, Canada; 2015. http://pag.ias2015.org/Roadmap/Index.

41. Eakle R, Gomez GB, Naicker N, Mbogua J, Bothma R, Moorhouse M, et al. Treatment and prevention for female sex workers in South Africa: first-year results for the TAPS demonstration project. In: Prepping for PrEP. Chicago, IL, USA; 2016. (PD04.02LB).

42. Rogers EM. Diffusion of innovations. 4th ed. New York: Simon and Schuster; 2010.

43. Celum CL, Delaney-Moretlwe S, McConnell M, van Rooyen H, Bekker L-G, Kurth A, et al. Rethinking HIV prevention to prepare for oral PrEP implementation for young African women. J Int AIDS Soc [Internet]. 2015 Jul 20

[cited 2017 Aug 9];18(4). http://www.jiasociety.org/index.php/jias/article/view/20227.

44. Pettifor A, Nguyen NL, Celum C, Cowan FM, Go V, Hightow-Weidman L. Tailored combination prevention packages and PrEP for young key populations. J Int AIDS Soc [Internet]. 2015 Feb 26;18(2Suppl 1). http://www.ncbi.nlm.nih.gov/pmc/articles/PMC4344537/.

45. Davis KR, Weller SC. The effectiveness of condoms in reducing heterosexual transmission of HIV. Fam Plan Perspect. 1999;31(6):272–9.

46. Giannou FK, Tsiara CG, Nikolopoulos GK, Talias M, Benetou V, Kantzanou M, et al. Condom effectiveness in reducing heterosexual HIV transmission: a systematic review and meta-analysis of studies on HIV serodiscordant couples. Expert Rev Pharmacoecon Outcomes Res. 2016;16(4):489–99.

47. Bradley J, Rajaram S, Alary M, Isac S, Washington R, Moses S, et al. Determinants of condom breakage among female sex workers in Karnataka, India. BMC Public Health. 2011;11(Suppl 6):S14.

48. Wee S, Barrett ME, Lian WM, Jayabaskar T, Chan KWR. Determinants of inconsistent condom use with female sex workers among men attending the STD clinic in Singapore. Sex Transm Infect. 2004;80(4):310–4.

49. Abdool Karim S, Abdool Karim Q, Preston-Whyte E, Sankar N. Reasons for lack of condom use among high school students. South Afr Med J Suid-Afr Tydskr Vir Geneeskd. 1992;82(2):107–10.

50. Carvalho FT, Gonçalves TR, Faria ER, Shoveller JA, Piccinini CA, Ramos MC, et al. Behavioral interventions to promote condom use among women living with HIV. In: Cochrane database of systematic reviews [Internet]. Wiley; 1996 [cited 2013 Jan 24]. http://onlinelibrary.wiley.com/doi/10.1002/14651858.CD007844.pub2/abstract.

51. Agha S. Factors associated with HIV testing and condom use in Mozambique: implications for programs. Reprod Health. 2012;9:20.

52. Bergmann JN, Stockman JK. How does intimate partner violence affect condom and oral contraceptive use in the United States? A systematic review of the literature. Contraception. 2015;91(6):438–55.

53. Maharaj P, Cleland J. Risk perception and condom use among married or cohabiting couples in KwaZulu-Natal, South Africa. Int Fam Plan Perspect. 2005;31(1):24–9.

54. Hoffman S, Mantell J, Exner T, Stein Z. The future of the female condom. Int Fam Plan Perspect [Internet]. 2004 Sep [cited 2013 Jun 24];30(3). https://www.guttmacher.org/pubs/journals/3013904.html.

55. Kaler A. The future of female-controlled barrier methods for HIV prevention: female condoms and lessons learned. Cult Health Sex. 2004;6(6):501–16.

56. Ledikwe JH, Nyanga RO, Hagon J, Grignon JS, Mpofu M, Semo B. Scaling-up voluntary medical male circumcision—what have we learned? HIVAIDS Auckl NZ. 2014;8(6):139–46.

57. Skolnik L, Tsui S, Ashengo TA, Kikaya V, Lukobo-Durrell M. A cross-sectional study describing motivations and barriers to voluntary medical male circumcision in Lesotho. BMC Public Health. 2014;30(14):1119.

58. Kitara DL, Ocero A, Lanyero J, Ocom F. Roll-out of Medical Male circumcision (MMC) for HIV prevention in non-circumcising communities of Northern Uganda. Pan Afr Med J [Internet]. 2013 Jul 15;15. http://www.ncbi.nlm.nih.gov/pmc/articles/PMC3810160/.

59. May C, Finch T, Mair F, Ballini L, Dowrick C, Eccles M, et al. Understanding the implementation of complex interventions in health care: the normalization process model. BMC Health Serv Res. 2007;7:148.

60. Evens E, Lanham M, Hart C, Loolpapit M, Oguma I, Obiero W. Identifying and addressing barriers to uptake of voluntary medical male circumcision in Nyanza, Kenya among men 18–35: a qualitative study. PLoS ONE. 2014;9(6):e98221.

61. Hatzold K, Mavhu W, Jasi P, Chatora K, Cowan FM, Taruberekera N, et al. Barriers and motivators to voluntary medical male circumcision uptake among different age groups of men in Zimbabwe: results from a mixed methods study. PLoS ONE [Internet]. 2014 May 6;9(5). http://www.ncbi.nlm.nih.gov/pmc/articles/PMC4011705/.

62. Mah T. Systematic review of the barriers and facilitators to voluntary male medical circumcision (VMMC) uptake in priority countries and recommendations. In Durban, South Africa; 2016 [cited 2017 Aug 17]. http://programme.aids2016.org/Abstract/Abstract/10420.

63. Marrazzo J, Ramjee G, Palanee T, Mkhize B, Nakabiito C, Taljaard M, et al. Pre-exposure Prophylaxis for HIV in Women: Daily Oral Tenofovir, Oral Tenofovir/Emtricitabine, or Vaginal Tenofovir Gel in the VOICE Study (MTN 003). In: HIV Prevention: ARV, Counseling, Contraception, and Condoms

[Internet]. Atlanta, Georgia; 2013 [cited 2013 Mar 28]. http://www.retro-conference.org/2013b/Abstracts/47951.htm.

64. Van Damme L, Corneli A, Ahmed K, Agot K, Lombaard J, Kapiga S, et al. Preexposure prophylaxis for HIV infection among African women. N Engl J Med. 2012;367:411–22.

65. van der Straten A, Stadler J, Montgomery E, Hartmann M, Magazi B, Mathebula F, et al. Women's experiences with oral and vaginal pre-exposure prophylaxis: the VOICE-C qualitative study in Johannesburg, South Africa. PLoS ONE. 2014;9(2):e89118.

66. Corneli AL, McKenna K, Headley J, Ahmed K, Odhiambo J, Skhosana J, et al. A descriptive analysis of perceptions of HIV risk and worry about acquiring HIV among FEM-PrEP participants who seroconverted in Bondo, Kenya, and Pretoria, South Africa. J Int AIDS Soc [Internet]. 2014 Sep 8 [cited 2015 Aug 7];17(3Suppl 2). http://www.ncbi.nlm.nih.gov/pmc/articles/PMC4164016/.

67. Sheth AN, Rolle CP, Gandhi M. HIV pre-exposure prophylaxis for women. J Virus Erad. 2016;2(3):149–55.

68. Amico KR, Stirratt MJ. Adherence to preexposure prophylaxis: current, emerging, and anticipated bases of evidence. Clin Infect Dis. 2014;59(suppl 1):S55–60.

69. Kirby T. Targeting HIV prevention to young women in Africa. Lancet. 2016;388(10060):2579.

70. Mathur S, Pilgrim N, Pulerwitz J. PrEP introduction for adolescent girls and young women. Lancet HIV. 2016;3(9):e406–8.

71. Namey E, Agot K, Ahmed K, Odhiambo J, Skhosana J, Guest G, et al. When and why women might suspend PrEP use according to perceived seasons of risk: implications for PrEP-specific risk-reduction counselling. Cult Health Sex. 2016;18(9):1081–91.

72. Haberer JE. Current concepts for PrEP adherence. Curr Opin HIV AIDS. 2016;11(1):10–7.

73. National AIDS & STI Control Programme (NASCOP), Ministry of Health. Framework for the implementation of pre-exposure prophylaxis of HIV in Kenya [Internet]. Nairobi, Kenya; 2017 [cited 2017 Aug 18]. http://www.prepwatch.org/wp-content/uploads/2017/05/Kenya_PrEP_Implementation_Framework-1.pdf.

74. Marcus JL, Hurley LB, Nguyen DP, Silverberg MJ, Volk JE. Redefining human immunodeficiency virus (HIV) preexposure prophylaxis failures. Clin Infect Dis. 2017;65(10):1768–9.

75. Abbas UL, Hood G, Wetzel AW, Mellors JW. Factors influencing the emergence and spread of HIV drug resistance arising from rollout of antiretroviral pre-exposure prophylaxis (PrEP). PLoS ONE. 2011;6:e18165.

76. McCormack S, Dunn D. Pragmatic open-label randomised trial of preexposure prophylaxis: the PROUD study. In 2015 [cited 2015 Oct 28]. http://www.croiconference.org/sessions/pragmatic-open-label-randomised-trial-preexposure-prophylaxis-proud-study.

77. Gallagher J. HIV "game-changer" to arrive next month. BBC News [Internet]. 2017 Aug 3 [cited 2018 Feb 1]. http://www.bbc.com/news/health-40814242.

78. Richardson ET. Scale-up of antiretroviral therapy and pre-exposure prophylaxis in Swaziland. In 2016 [cited 2017 Aug 24]. http://www.croiconference.org/sessions/scale-antiretroviral-therapy-and-preexposure-prophylaxis-swaziland.

79. Gomez GB, Borquez A, Caceres CF, Segura ER, Grant RM, Garnett GP, et al. The potential impact of pre-exposure prophylaxis for HIV prevention among men who have sex with men and transwomen in Lima, Peru: a mathematical modelling study. PLoS Med. 2012;9:e1001323.

80. Hallett TB, Baeten JM, Heffron R, Barnabas R, de Bruyn G, Cremin Í, et al. optimal uses of antiretrovirals for prevention in HIV-1 serodiscordant heterosexual couples in South Africa: a modelling study. PLoS Med. 2011;8:e1001123.

81. Alsallaq R, Baeten J, Hughes J, Abu-Raddad L, Celum C, Hallett T. Modelling the effectiveness of combination prevention from a house-to-house HIV testing platform in KwaZulu Natal, South Africa. Sex Transm Infect. 2011;87(Suppl 1):A36.

82. U.S. Food & Drug Administration. First-time generic drug approvals 2017 (ANDA number: 090894) [Internet]. 2017 [cited 2017 Sep 1]. https://www.fda.gov/Drugs/DevelopmentApprovalProcess/HowDrugsareDevelopedandApproved/DrugandBiologicApprovalReports/ANDAGenericDrugApprovals/.

83. Chiu C. Optimising South Africas HIV response: results of the HIV and TB investment case. In Boston, Massachusetts; 2016 [cited 2017 Aug 24]. http://www.croiconference.org/sessions/optimising-south-africa%C2%92s-hiv-response-results-hiv-and-tb-investment-case.

84. Medicines Patent Pool. MPP-TENOFOVIR DISOPROXIL FUMARATE (TDF) [Internet]. [cited 2017 Nov 11]. https://medicinespatentpool.org/licence-post/tenofovir-disoproxil-fumarate-tdf/.

85. AVAC. Country Updates [Internet]. PrEPWatch. [cited 2017 Apr 26]. http://www.prepwatch.org/scaling-up/country-updates/.

86. Bell N. PrEP is now approved in Canada. What happens now? [Internet]. Xtra. 2016 [cited 2017 Sep 5]. https://www.dailyxtra.com/prep-is-now-approved-in-canada-what-happens-now-70344.

87. Project Inform. The FDA has approved generic PrEP—but access may remain difficult [Internet]. [cited 2017 Sep 5]. https://www.projectinform.org/hiv-news/the-fda-has-approved-generic-prep-but-access-may-remain-difficult/.

88. PrEP in Europe Initiative (PEI). PrEP access in Europe [Internet]. 2017 [cited 2017 Nov 15]. https://www.avac.org/sites/default/files/u3/PEI_Report_May2017.pdf.

89. Eakle R, Bourne A, Mbogua J, Mutanha N, Rees H. Exploring acceptability of oral PrEP prior to implementation among female sex workers in South Africa. J Int AIDS Soc. 2018;21(2). https://doi.org/10.1002/jia2.25081.

11

The HIV-1 accessory proteins Nef and Vpu downregulate total and cell surface CD28 in CD4$^+$ T cells

Emily N. Pawlak, Brennan S. Dirk, Rajesh Abraham Jacob, Aaron L. Johnson and Jimmy D. Dikeakos[*]

Abstract

Background: The HIV-1 accessory proteins Nef and Vpu alter cell surface levels of multiple host proteins to modify the immune response and increase viral persistence. Nef and Vpu can downregulate cell surface levels of the co-stimulatory molecule CD28, however the mechanism of this function has not been completely elucidated.

Results: Here, we provide evidence that Nef and Vpu decrease cell surface and total cellular levels of CD28. Moreover, using inhibitors we implicate the cellular degradation machinery in the downregulation of CD28. We shed light on the mechanisms of CD28 downregulation by implicating the Nef LL$_{165}$ and DD$_{175}$ motifs in decreasing cell surface CD28 and Nef DD$_{175}$ in decreasing total cellular CD28. Moreover, the Vpu LV$_{64}$ and S$_{52/56}$ motifs were required for cell surface CD28 downregulation, while, unlike for CD4 downregulation, Vpu W$_{22}$ was dispensable. The Vpu S$_{52/56}$ motif was also critical for Vpu-mediated decreases in total CD28 protein level. Finally, the ability of Vpu to downregulate CD28 is conserved between multiple group M Vpu proteins and infection with viruses encoding or lacking Nef and Vpu have differential effects on activation upon stimulation.

Conclusions: We report that Nef and Vpu downregulate cell surface and total cellular CD28 levels. We identified inhibitors and mutations within Nef and Vpu that disrupt downregulation, shedding light on the mechanisms utilized to downregulate CD28. The conservation and redundancy between the abilities of two HIV-1 proteins to downregulate CD28 highlight the importance of this function, which may contribute to the development of latently infected cells.

Keywords: HIV-1 Nef, HIV-1 Vpu, CD28 downregulation, T cell activation

Background

Adaptive immune responses are primarily driven by B and T lymphocytes, which mediate humoral and cell-mediated immunity (reviewed in [1]). Thymus derived lymphocytes, or T cells, can be classified as CD8$^+$ cytotoxic T-lymphocytes (CTLs) or CD4$^+$ T helper cells, and these cells play key roles in anti-viral responses. Naïve T cells require signaling from antigen presenting cells (APCs) to become competent effector cells. According to the two-signal model of T cell activation, APCs provide two signals to enable these cells to become productive effector cells. The first signal is established during MHC-restricted binding of the T cell receptor (TCR): antigen complex, while signal 2 consists of co-stimulatory signaling (reviewed in [2, 3]). A lack of co-stimulatory signaling results in cells becoming unresponsive or anergic. Key co-stimulatory signaling is provided by binding of CD28, a transmembrane receptor expressed on the surface of T cells, to B7.1/B7.2 (CD80/CD86) on the surface of APCs. Indeed, CD28 receptor ligation initiates downstream signaling, which in conjunction with TCR signaling, results in cell activation and proliferation essential for mounting an immune response [4, 5].

The importance of the TCR and co-stimulatory signaling to the development of an effective immune response makes them prime targets of intracellular pathogens.

*Correspondence: Jimmy.Dikeakos@uwo.ca
Department of Microbiology and Immunology, Schulich School
of Medicine and Dentistry, University of Western Ontario, Dental Sciences
Building, Room 3007J, London, ON N6A 5C1, Canada

Indeed, many viruses have evolved the capabilities to intricately modulate these T cell activation cues to optimize their replication and persistence. For instance, lymphotropic viruses, including the Human Immunodeficiency Virus Type 1 (HIV-1), Human T-lymphotropic virus (HTLV), and Epstein–Barr virus (EBV), inhibit T cell activation by downregulating components of the TCR and TCR-associated kinases essential for TCR signaling [6–11], as well as re-organizing the TCR and immunological synapse [12]. Moreover, viruses inhibit signaling downstream of co-stimulatory receptors, or alter the levels of cell surface co-stimulatory or inhibitory molecules [13–16]. Ultimately, virus-induced changes in T cell activation can result in immune evasion, enhanced replication, and increased persistence. The importance of viral alterations to immune cell activation are evidenced by the specific HIV-1 proteins that play key roles in T cell activation.

HIV-1 encodes four accessory proteins that lack any known enzymatic or structural functions: Vif, Vpr, Nef and Vpu (reviewed in [17–19]). Collectively, these viral proteins play critical roles in increasing infectivity, persistence and pathogenesis. While Nef and Vpu are arguably the most extensively studied accessory proteins, their roles in T cell activation are not fully understood. The ability of Nef and Vpu to downregulate various host cell receptors is a key function mediating their effects. Indeed, both Nef and Vpu downregulated multiple receptors in a screen to identify cell surface proteins that are altered by these viral proteins [20]. Specifically, Nef and Vpu facilitate degradation or intracellular sequestration of host receptors, including restriction factors and immune cell receptors, to thwart their cell surface expression [17]. By hijacking membrane trafficking proteins, such as the adaptor proteins adaptor protein 1 (AP-1) or adaptor protein 2 (AP-2), Nef and Vpu connect multiple cellular receptors to additional cellular trafficking machinery which alters the receptors' subcellular localization. For example, Nef hijacks AP-1 to facilitate the endocytosis and sequestration of major histocompatibility complex type I (MHC-I) molecules [18, 21–23], limiting recognition of infected cells by the immune system [24]. In parallel, the ability of Nef to hijack AP-2 results in the endocytosis and degradation of CD4, which limits superinfection and antibody-dependent cell-mediated cytotoxicity [25–32]. Similarly, Vpu hijacks bone marrow stromal antigen 2 (BST-2) trafficking by associating with adaptor proteins to facilitate its sequestration and degradation [33–37]. Vpu also enables the degradation of CD4 by targeting newly synthesized CD4 to the endoplasmic-reticulum-associated protein degradation (ERAD) pathway [38]. Interestingly, Nef expression leads to endocytosis of CD28 from the cell surface, in a manner

dependent on both AP-1 and AP-2 [39, 40]. However, the fate of CD28 after Nef-mediated endocytosis remains poorly understood and the effects of Vpu on CD28 are unexplored.

In this article, we report that Nef and Vpu decrease cell surface and total cellular CD28 levels within infected $CD4^+$ T cells. Moreover, we can inhibit the observed decreases in total CD28 using inhibitors of the cellular degradation machinery, consistent with Nef and Vpu facilitating trafficking of CD28 to an acidic compartment. Additionally, a mutant Nef protein associated with impaired binding to the vacuolar ATPase was compromised in its ability to reduce cell surface and total CD28 levels, while an non-phosphorylatable Vpu protein that is unable to recruit the protein degradation machinery was impaired in its ability to reduce cell surface and total CD28 levels. Finally, the ability of Vpu to downregulate CD28 is not limited to the lab adapted HIV-1 strain NL4.3 Vpu, and infection of cells with viruses encoding Nef or Vpu have differential effects on activation upon stimulation of CD3 and CD28.

Results

The HIV-1 accessory proteins Nef and Vpu downregulate cell surface and total CD28 protein levels

The co-stimulatory molecule CD28 is essential for immune cell activation and proliferation of naïve and memory T cells [2]. To investigate the effects of the HIV-1 accessory proteins Nef and Vpu on endogenous CD28 levels, $CD4^+$ Sup-T1 T cells were infected with Gag-Pol truncated, VSV-G pseudotyped and eGFP expressing HIV-1 NL4.3 viruses encoding both Nef and Vpu (NL4.3), Vpu alone (dNef), Nef alone (dVpu), or neither accessory protein (dVpu dNef). Infected Sup-T1 cells were analyzed by flow cytometry after staining for cell surface CD28 (Fig. 1). Upon gating on live (Zombie Red^{TM-}), infected (GFP^+) single cells (Additional file 1), significantly greater cell surface levels of CD28 were present on cells infected with viruses lacking Nef (dNef), Vpu (dVpu) or both Nef and Vpu (dVpu dNef), compared to cells infected with virus encoding both Nef and Vpu (NL4.3; Fig. 1a–c). Accordingly, Western blot analysis confirmed the presence or absence of Nef and Vpu in infected Sup-T1 cells (Fig. 1d). Moreover, we examined the ability of Nef and Vpu expressed from replication competent NL4.3 provirus to downregulate cell surface CD28 in infected $CD4^+$ T cells purified from peripheral blood mononuclear cells (PBMCs) (Fig. 1e, f; Additional file 2). In line with our observations in Sup-T1 cells, in the absence of Nef (dNef), Vpu (dVpu) or both Nef and Vpu (dVpu dNef) greater levels of cell surface CD28 were present on infected ($p24^+$) cells compared to cells infected with NL4.3, indicating that Nef and Vpu independently

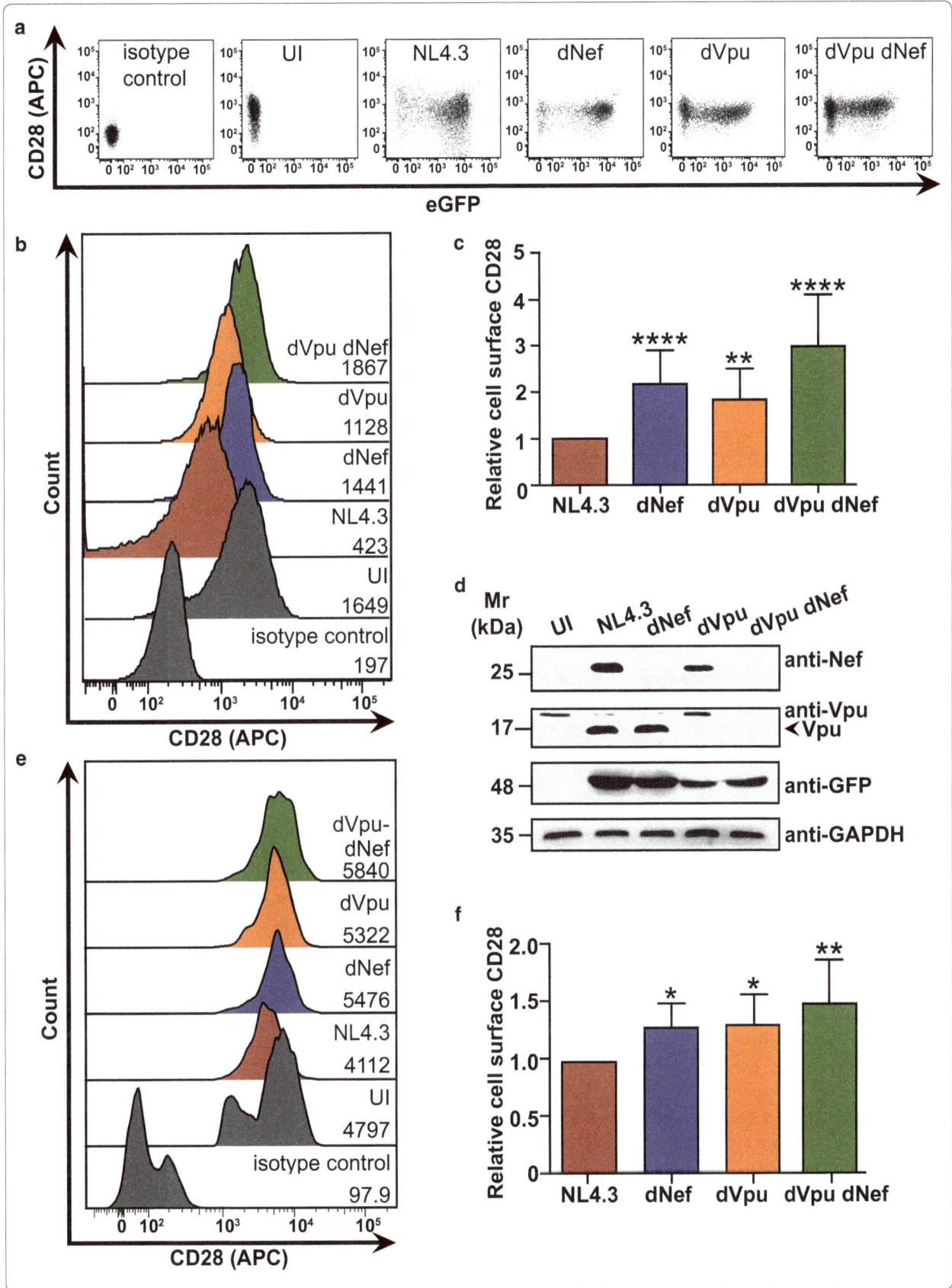

(See figure on previous page.)
Fig. 1 HIV-1 Nef and Vpu downregulate cell surface CD28 protein levels. CD4+ Sup-T1 and primary CD4+ T cells were infected with either VSV-G pseudotyped or replication competent NL4.3, respectively. Viruses encoded Nef and Vpu (NL4.3, red), lacked Nef (dNef, blue) or Vpu (dVpu, orange), or lacked both Nef and Vpu (dVpu dNef, green). Infected cells were stained for CD28 and analyzed by flow cytometry. Live infected Sup-T1 cells were analyzed by gating on Zombie Red™⁻ and GFP+ cells, and infected primary CD4+ T cells were analyzed by gating on p24+ cells. **a** Representative dot plots illustrating cell surface CD28 (APC) and infection (GFP+) of live (Zombie Red™⁻) Sup-T1 cells. **b** Representative histograms illustrating cell surface levels of CD28 or the appropriate isotype control on Sup-T1 cells after gating on live (Zombie Red™⁻) and infected (GFP+) cells. CD28 (APC) geometric mean fluorescence intensities (MFI) are indicated. **c** Summary of the relative mean (± SE) cell surface CD28 levels on infected (GFP+) Sup-T1 cells based on MFIs (n = 17). **d** Western blot illustrating expression of Nef and Vpu in infected Sup-T1 cells. **e** Representative histograms illustrating cell surface levels of CD28 or the appropriate isotype control on uninfected (UI) or infected (p24+) CD4+ PBMCs. MFIs are indicated. **f** Summary of the relative mean (± SE) cell surface CD28 levels on infected CD4+ T cells based on MFIs obtained from infection of CD4+ T cells from two healthy donors (n ≥ 3). (UI: uninfected; SE: standard error; Mr: molecular weight; GAPDH: glyceraldehyde 3-phosphate dehydrogenase; GFP: green fluorescent protein; MFI: geometric mean fluorescent intensity; SE: standard error; *p ≤ 0.05; **p ≤ 0.01; ****p ≤ 0.0001)

downregulate cell surface CD28 in both primary CD4+ T cells and Sup-T1 cells.

We next sought to examine the effects of Nef and Vpu on total CD28 protein levels. Sup-T1 cells or CD4+ T cells purified from healthy donor PBMCs were infected with VSV-G pseudotyped HIV-1 NL4.3 viruses, as in Fig. 1. Infected cells were permeabilized and stained for total CD28, and subsequently analyzed by flow cytometry (Fig. 2). As with cell surface CD28, in Sup-T1 cells the total CD28 levels were significantly higher in cells infected with viruses lacking Nef (dNef) or Vpu (dVpu), relative to cells infected with viruses encoding both viral proteins (NL4.3; Fig. 2a–c). The highest total CD28 levels were observed in cells infected with virus lacking functional *nef* and *vpu* genes (dVpu dNef; Fig. 2a–c). Furthermore, the ability of Nef and Vpu to downregulate total CD28 protein was consistent in primary cells. Indeed, infection of CD4+ T cells purified from PBMCs with VSV-G pseudotyped NL4.3 demonstrated that cells infected with virus lacking either (dNef, dVpu) or both (dVpu dNef) viral proteins had significantly higher mean levels of CD28, compared to cells infected with virus encoding both Nef and Vpu (NL4.3) (Fig. 2d, e). This data suggests that similar to the cell surface receptor CD4 [32, 38], both Nef and Vpu downregulate total cellular CD28 protein levels.

To confirm that the HIV-1 accessory proteins Nef and Vpu altered endogenous CD28, we infected Sup-T1 cells with VSV-G pseudotyped NL4.3 viruses encoding or lacking the viral proteins and examined CD28 localization using widefield microscopy (Fig. 3). Specifically, due to our observed decreases in total CD28 protein levels (Fig. 2), we stained cells for endogenous CD28 and lysosomal-associated membrane protein 1 (LAMP-1), a marker of the degradative lysosomal compartment. Interestingly, we observed that in the presence of Nef and Vpu (NL4.3) CD28 localized away from the cell surface, inconsistent with the plasma membrane localization observed in uninfected cells (Fig. 3a). Moreover, upon elimination of the viral proteins (dVpu dNef) we observed a rescue

in CD28's localization to the cell surface (Fig. 3a). Upon quantification of CD28: LAMP-1 co-localization, we found that in the presence of both viral proteins (NL4.3) the co-localization of CD28 with LAMP-1 was significantly greater than in the absence of either (dNef, dVpu) or both (dVpu dNef) viral proteins (Fig. 3b). This microscopy analysis confirms that Nef and Vpu downregulate endogenous CD28 and suggests this downregulation results in transport of CD28 to the degradative lysosome.

Nef and Vpu-mediated effects on CD28 are dependent on the cellular degradation machinery

Cellular protein levels can be reduced via degradation by acidic hydrolases within acidified endosomal compartments [41]. Since we observed the co-localization of CD28 and LAMP-1 in infected cells (Fig. 3), we sought to determine if the Nef- and Vpu-mediated reduction in total CD28 could be blocked by inhibition of endosomal acidification. To test this, we treated infected Sup-T1 cells with the base ammonium chloride to increase intravesicular pH [42]. We specifically measured total CD28 within Sup-T1 cells infected with pseudotyped NL4.3 and treated with ammonium chloride prior to staining. Interestingly, upon ammonium chloride treatment, total CD28 detected by flow cytometry increased relative to untreated cells (Fig. 4a). Moreover, the fold increase, or recovery, of total CD28 protein levels upon ammonium chloride treatment was significantly lower when cells were infected with viruses lacking either (dNef, dVpu) or both Nef and Vpu (dVpu dNef), compared to Nef- and Vpu-encoding virus (NL4.3; Fig. 4a). In addition, we examined the effects of ammonium chloride on the CD4 receptor (Additional file 3). Similar to CD28, the recovery of CD4 levels upon ammonium chloride treatment was significantly less in cells infected with virus lacking one or both of the accessory proteins (dNef, dVpu, dVpu dNef; Additional file 3). Therefore, in the presence of the viral accessory proteins Nef and Vpu, a decrease in total CD28 occurs and this effect is mitigated by inhibition of endosomal acidification.

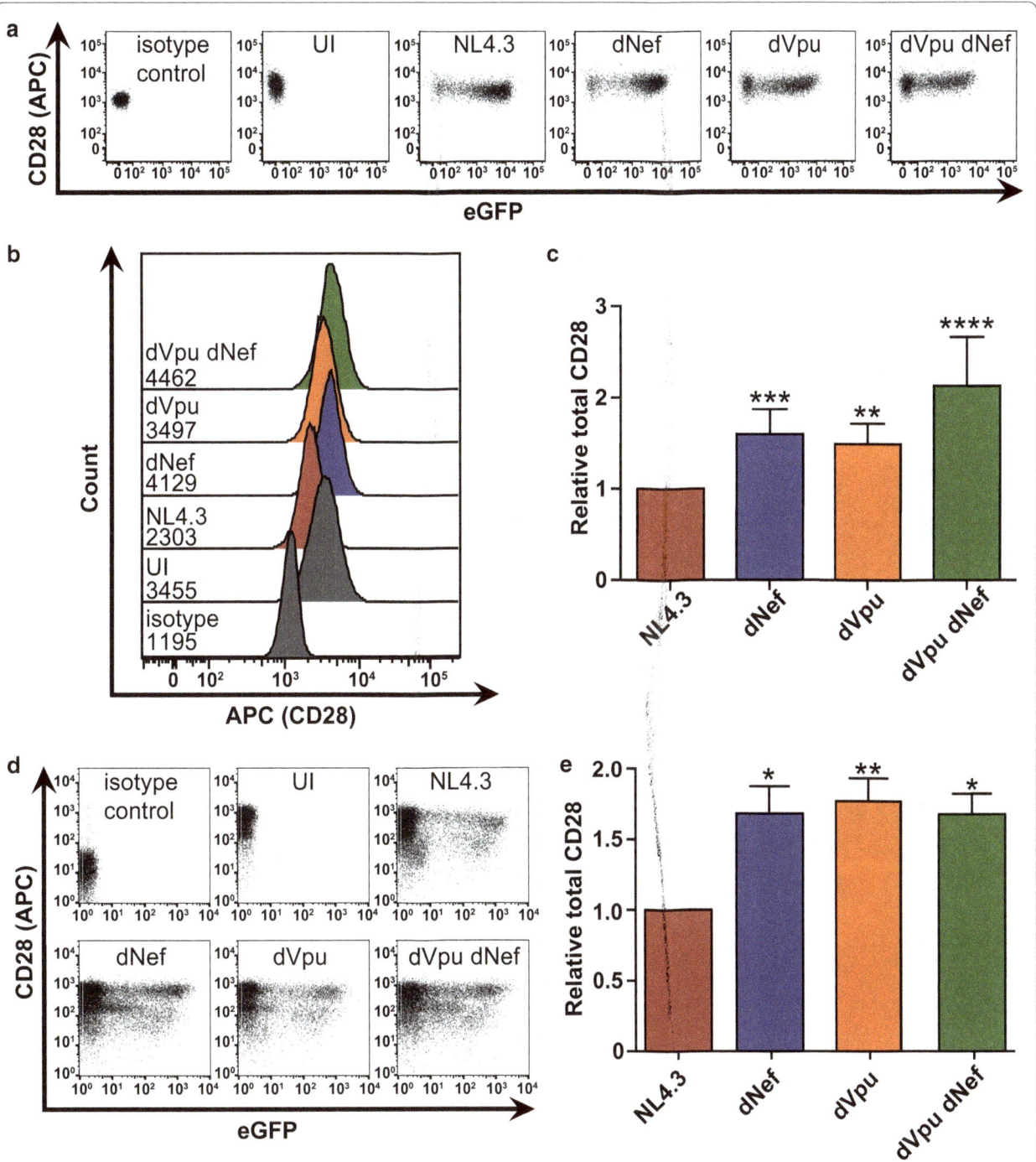

Fig. 2 HIV-1 Nef and Vpu downregulate total CD28 protein levels. CD4[+] Sup-T1 cells or primary CD4[+] T cells were infected with VSV-G pseudotyped NL4.3. Viruses encoded Nef and Vpu (NL4.3, red), lacked Nef (dNef, blue), lacked Vpu (dVpu, orange) or lacked both Nef and Vpu (dNef dVpu, green). Forty-eight hours post-infection, cells were permeabilized, stained for CD28 and analyzed by flow cytometry. **a** Representative dot plots illustrating total CD28 (APC) and infection (GFP) levels of live (Zombie Red[TM−]) Sup-T1 cells. **b** Representative histograms illustrating total levels of CD28 (APC) after gating on live (Zombie Red[TM−]) infected (GFP[+]) cells. Geometric mean fluorescence intensities (MFI) are indicated. **c** Summary of mean (± SE) relative total CD28 based on MFI (n = 12). **d** Representative dot plots illustrating purified CD4[+] T cell infection (GFP) and total CD28 (APC) levels. **e** Summary of mean (± SE) total CD28 levels on Infected (GFP[+]) CD4[+] T cells (n = 5). Data were obtained from infection of cells obtained from two healthy donors. (UI: uninfected; MFI: geometric mean fluorescent intensity; SE: standard error; *p ≤ 0.05; **p ≤ 0.01; ***p ≤ 0.001; ****p ≤ 0.0001)

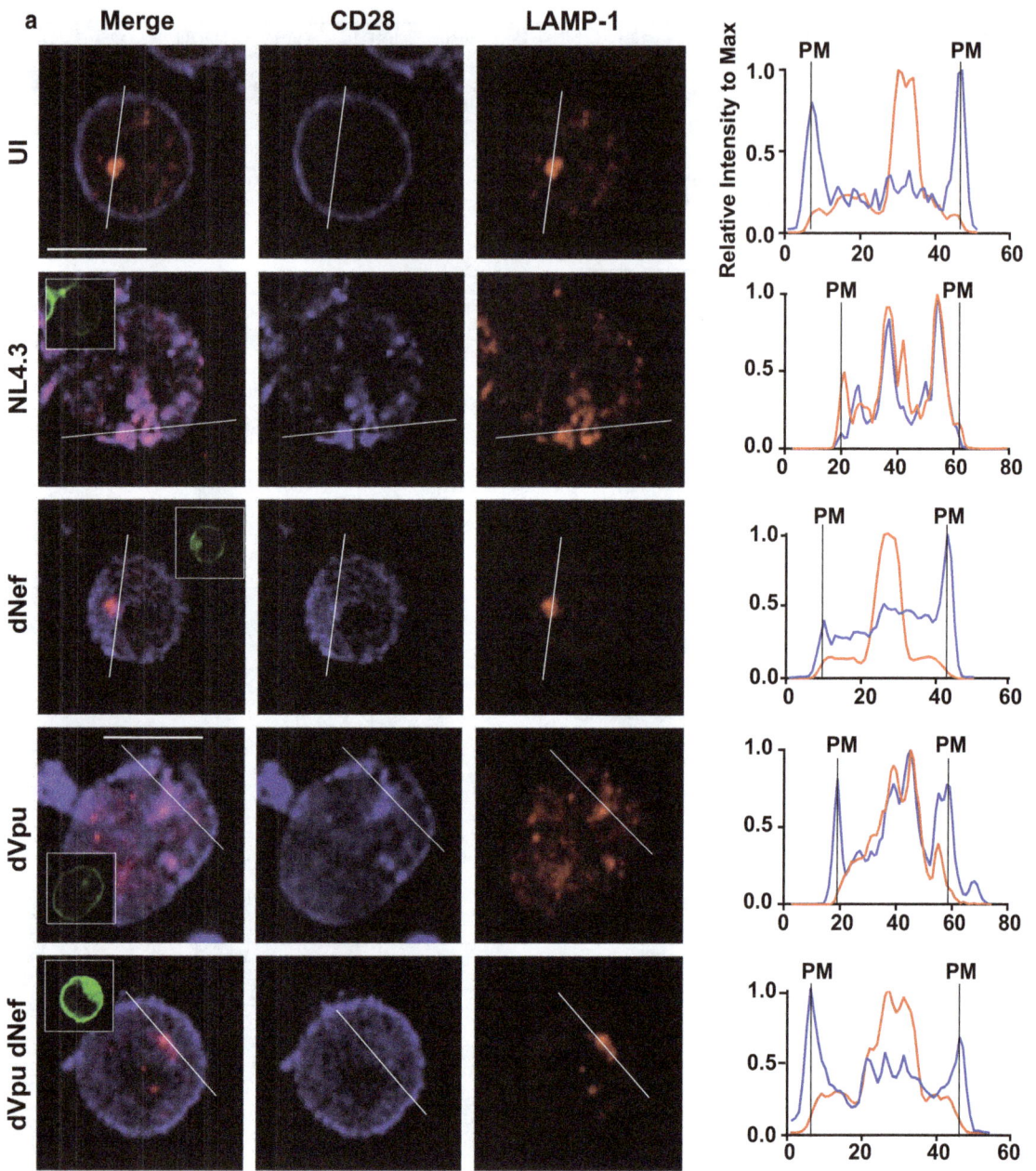

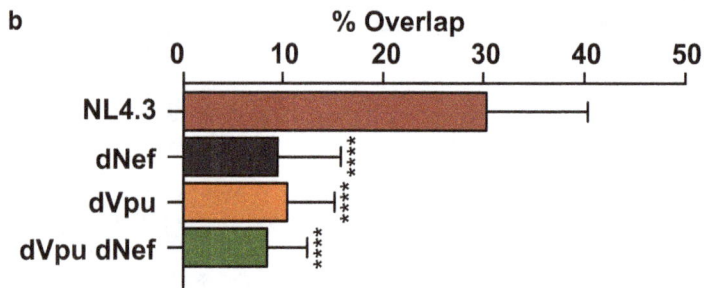

Fig. 3 The subcellular localization of CD28 is altered in the presence of Nef or Vpu. CD4$^+$ Sup-T1 cells were infected with VSV-G pseudotyped NL4.3 viruses encoding or lacking Nef and/or Vpu. Infected cells were stained for CD28 and the lysosomal marker LAMP-1 and visualized by widefield microscopy. **a** Shown are representative infected (GFP$^+$) cells (left) and a graphical representation of CD28 (blue) and LAMP-1 (red) fluorescence intensity relative to the maximum along the illustrated line (right). The scale bar indicates 10 μm and the vertical lines labelled PM indicate where the illustrated line meets the plasma membrane (PM). Insets in the merged panel illustrate the GFP channel. **b** The percentage overlap between CD28 and LAMP-1 is calculated based on the mean ($\pm$ SD) Manders' overlap coefficients from at least 30 cells and 3 independent experiments. (UI: uninfected; LAMP-1: Lysosomal-associated membrane protein 1; SD: standard deviation; ****p $\leq$ 0.0001)

To further confirm these findings, we used widefield microscopy to visualize CD28 within Sup-T1 cells infected with VSV-G pseudotyped NL4.3. Specifically, we examined the subcellular localization of CD28 within infected cells treated with the general endosome acidification inhibitor ammonium chloride or treated with Bafilomycin A1 or Concanamycin A, specific inhibitors of the endosome acidifying proton pump, the vacuolar ATPase [43, 44]. We observed that upon treatment with ammonium chloride, Bafilomycin A1, or Concanamycin A, the distribution of CD28 within VSV-G pseudotyped NL4.3 infected cells was altered relative to vehicle (Dimethyl sulfoxide (DMSO)) treated cells (Fig. 4b). Indeed, inhibitor treatment resulted in the increased localization of CD28 to the cell surface when compared to cells treated with vehicle. Moreover, quantification of the co-localization of CD28 and LAMP-1 in Bafilomycin A1 or Concanamycin A treated cells indicated that upon inhibitor treatment CD28 co-localizes significantly less with the lysosomal marker LAMP-1 (Fig. 4c). These results suggest that the ability of Nef and Vpu to downregulate CD28 is dependent on endolysosomal acidification.

Motifs ascribed to specific Nef:host cell protein interactions are critical for Nef-mediated CD28 downregulation

To further elucidate the mechanisms used by Nef to downregulate CD28, we sought to determine if this function is dependent on motifs within Nef that have been previously implicated in interacting with membrane trafficking regulators that act to downregulate other cell surface receptors. Accordingly, Sup-T1 cells were infected with isogenic Gag-Pol truncated VSV-G pseudotyped NL4.3 viruses that only differed at the following Nef motifs: the myristoylation site (G$_2$; [45]), the methionine residue critical for Nef:AP-1:MHC-I complex formation (M$_{20}$; [22]), the dileucine motif implicated in adaptor protein-complex formation (LL$_{165}$; [46]) and the diacidic motif implicated in vacuolar ATPase binding (DD$_{175}$; [47]). Specifically, Sup-T1 cells were infected with pseudotyped NL4.3 encoding a non-functional Vpu protein and the various Nef mutants. Subsequently, live and infected single cells were analyzed (Additional file 1). In addition, cells were infected with pseudotyped NL4.3 encoding a functional Vpu protein and the various Nef mutants (Additional files 4, 5). As

expected, cells infected with virus encoding Nef G$_2$A [45], which disrupts most known Nef functions, exhibited significantly higher cell surface levels of CD28 compared to cells infected with virus encoding wild-type Nef (Fig. 5a, b; Additional file 5). Interestingly, cells infected with viruses encoding the LL$_{165}$AA and DD$_{175}$GA Nef mutations also showed significantly higher cell surface levels of CD28, suggesting that the LL$_{165}$ and DD$_{175}$ motifs are critical for cell surface CD28 downregulation (Fig. 5a, b; Additional file 5). Conversely, mutation of M$_{20}$ (M$_{20}$A), a residue essential for the downregulation of MHC-I via the interaction with AP-1 [22, 48], did not affect CD28 cell surface downregulation (Fig. 5a, b; Additional file 5). Importantly, the dileucine (LL$_{165}$AA) and diacidic (DD$_{175}$GA) motif mutations did not inhibit other Nef functions, as these mutated Nef proteins retained the ability to downregulate cell surface MHC-I (Additional file 5), demonstrating that the dileucine and diacidic motifs function in downregulating CD28.

In parallel, Sup-T1 cells were infected with the equivalent viruses from Fig. 5b and total CD28 levels were measured by flow cytometry. The observed decrease in total CD28 in the presence of Nef (Fig. 2) was abolished by mutation of the myristoylation site (G$_2$A) and the diacidic motif (DD$_{175}$GA), as cells infected with viruses encoding these mutated Nef proteins exhibited significantly higher total levels of CD28 compared to those infected with virus encoding wild-type Nef (Fig. 5c; Additional file 5). However, unlike cell surface CD28, the total CD28 levels did not differ significantly between cells infected with virus encoding wild-type Nef versus Nef LL$_{165}$AA in cells infected with viruses also encoding Vpu (Additional file 5). Contrastingly, in cells infected with virus lacking Vpu and encoding the Nef LL$_{165}$AA mutation, we observed significantly greater levels of total CD28 (Fig. 5c). Finally, expression of all mutated Nef proteins was confirmed by Western blot (Fig. 5d). Taken together, these findings implicate the Nef diacidic motif (DD$_{175}$) in the downregulation of total and cell surface CD28.

Motifs in Vpu implicated in interactions with specific host cellular proteins are critical for CD28 downregulation

Next, we sought to gain insight into the mechanism used by Vpu to downregulate CD28 by examining the

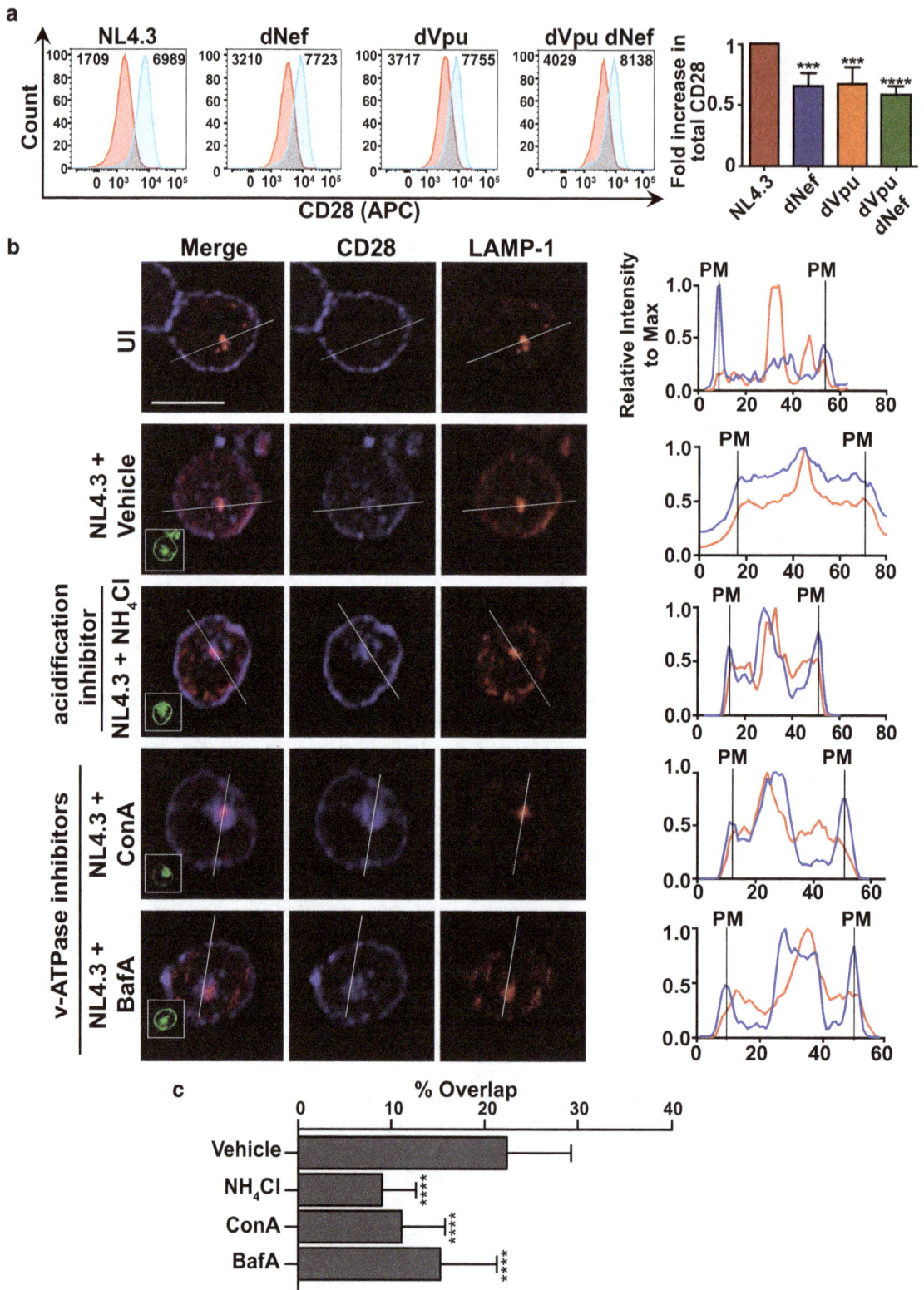

(See figure on previous page.)

Fig. 4 Inhibition of the degradation machinery increases CD28 protein levels in infected cells. CD4$^+$ Sup-T1 cells were infected with VSV-G pseudotyped NL4.3 encoding or lacking Nef and/or Vpu. Infected cells were analyzed 48 h post-infection after treatment for 24 h with 40 mM ammonium chloride or treatment for 5 h with 100 nM Bafilomycin A1 or 100 nM Concanamycin A. Cells were stained for CD28 and the lysosomal marker LAMP-1 and analyzed by widefield microscopy or stained for CD28 and analyzed by flow cytometry. **a** Representative histograms illustrating total CD28 levels of infected cells treated with complete RPMI with (blue) or without (red) 40 mM ammonium chloride. Geometric mean fluorescence intensities (MFIs) are indicated. MFIs of infected cells were determined after gating on live (Zombie Red^{TM-}), infected (GFP$^+$) cells and the relative fold increase ($\pm$ SE) in total CD28 upon ammonium chloride (n $\geq$ 5) treatment is illustrated (right). **b** Representative infected (GFP$^+$) Sup-T1 cells subjected to treatment with vehicle (DMSO), ammonium chloride (NH$_4$Cl), Concanamycin A (ConA) or Bafilomycin A1 (BafA) and visualized by widefield microscopy (left). The scale bar indicates 10 µm and insets in merged panel illustrate GFP channel. A graphical representation of CD28 and LAMP-1 fluorescence intensity relative to max along the illustrated line is shown (right). The vertical lines labelled PM indicate where the illustrated line meets the plasma membrane (PM). **c** The percentage of overlap between CD28 and LAMP-1 is based on the mean ($\pm$ SD) Manders' overlap coefficients measured on at least 30 cells from 3 independent experiments (UI: uninfected; SD: standard deviation; LAMP-1: Lysosomal-associated membrane protein; MFI: geometric mean fluorescent intensity; ***p $\leq$ 0.001; ****p $\leq$ 0.0001)

ability of mutant Vpu proteins to modulate cell surface and total CD28 levels. Mutated motifs within the NL4.3 *vpu* gene which have been previously implicated in the ability of Vpu to downregulate CD4 [49–51] or the restriction factor BST-2 [52–54] were inserted into a NL4.3 viral backbone encoding eGFP, but lacking a functional *nef* gene (pNL4.3 dG/P eGFP dNef). Sup-T1 cells were infected with these VSV-G pseudotyped isogenic NL4.3 viruses, which only differ in the specific *vpu*

mutations. Relative to cells infected with virus encoding wild-type Vpu (dNef), significantly greater levels of cell surface CD28 were present on cells infected with viruses encoding Vpu mutations at the adaptor protein interaction interface (LV$_{64}$AA Vpu dNef) and serine residues (S$_{52/56}$N Vpu dNef) which are phosphorylated by casein kinase II to facilitate recruitment of E3 ubiquitin ligase complex components (Fig. 6a, b) [38]. In contrast, relative to cells infected with virus encoding wild-type Vpu

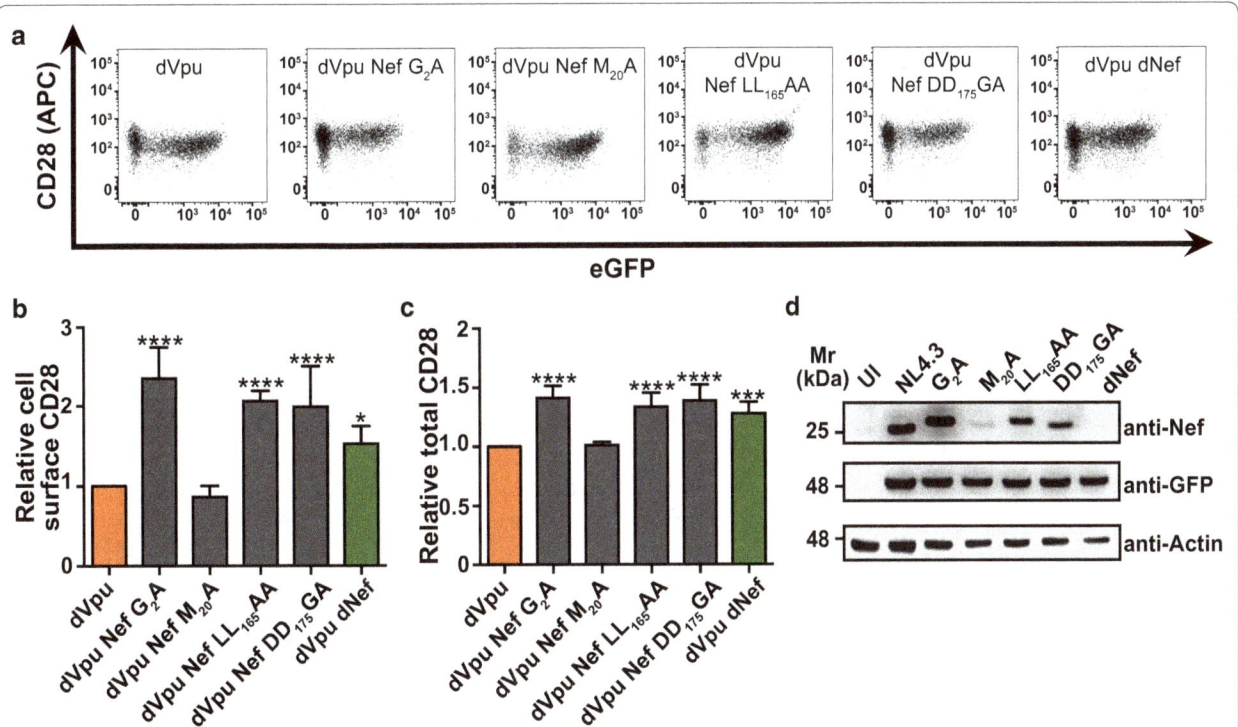

Fig. 5 Nef:host cell protein interaction motifs are critical for Nef-mediated CD28 downregulation. Infected CD4$^+$ Sup-T1 cells were stained for CD28 and analyzed by flow cytometry. Cells infected with VSV-G pseudotyped NL4.3 lacking Vpu (dVpu, orange) or Vpu and Nef (dVpu dNef, green) were used as controls. **a** Representative dot plots illustrating CD28 (APC) and infection (GFP) in live (Zombie Red^{TM-}) cells. **b** Mean ($\pm$ SE) relative cell surface CD28 MFIs of cells infected with NL4.3 lacking Vpu and encoding the indicated mutations in *nef* (n $\geq$ 4). **c** Relative mean ($\pm$ SE) total CD28 within live cells infected with NL4.3 encoding various Nef mutations (n $\geq$ 5). **d** Western blot illustrating expression of the mutated Nef proteins. (Mr: molecular weight; UI: uninfected; SE: standard error; MFI: geometric mean fluorescent intensity; *p $\leq$ 0.05; ***p $\leq$ 0.001; ****p $\leq$ 0.0001)

Fig. 6 Motifs in Vpu are critical for downregulation of CD28. Infected CD4$^+$ Sup-T1 cells were stained for CD28 and analyzed by flow cytometry. Mean geometric fluorescence intensities (MFI) of cells were determined after gating on live and infected (Zombie Red^{TM-} and GFP$^+$) cells. Cells infected with VSV-G pseudotyped NL4.3 lacking Nef (dNef, blue) and both Nef and Vpu (dNef dVpu, green) were used as controls. **a** Representative histograms illustrating cell surface CD28 on live (Zombie Red^{TM-}) infected (GFP$^+$) cells. MFIs are indicated. **b** Mean (± SE) relative cell surface CD28 on cells infected with viruses encoding mutations in *vpu* (n ≥ 9). **c** Relative mean (± SE) total CD28 within cells infected with viruses encoding the indicated *vpu* mutations (n ≥ 7). **d** Western blot illustrating expression of mutated Vpu proteins. (Mr: molecular weight; UI: uninfected; SE: standard error; GAPDH: glyceraldehyde 3-phosphate dehydrogenase; MFI: geometric mean fluorescent intensity; GFP: green fluorescent protein; *p ≤ 0.05; **p ≤ 0.01; ****p ≤ 0.0001)

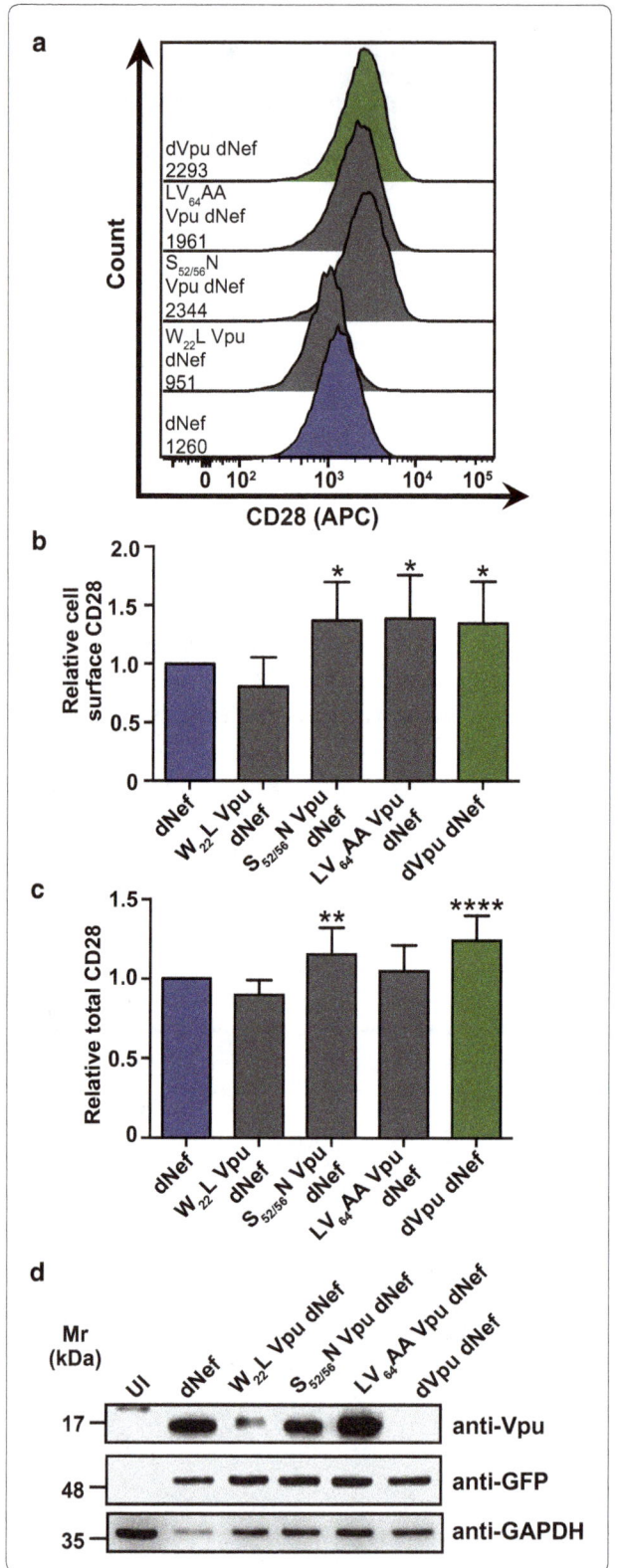

(dNef), cell surface CD28 levels were not significantly different on cells infected with virus encoding a mutation within a Vpu transmembrane domain residue implicated in the downregulation of CD4 and BST-2 (W$_{22}$A Vpu dNef [50, 53]; Fig. 6a, b). The functionality of the mutant Vpu proteins was tested by examining the effects of the mutations on Vpu-mediated CD4 downregulation in Sup-T1 cells (Additional file 6). Indeed, upon infection with viruses encoding the W$_{22}$L, S$_{52/56}$N or LV$_{64}$AA mutations, significantly greater cell surface levels of CD4 were present relative to cells infected with virus encoding wild-type Vpu (dNef) (Additional file 6), suggesting that the W$_{22}$ motif is critical for CD4, but not cell surface CD28 downregulation.

In parallel, viruses encoding mutated Vpu proteins were also tested for their effects on the downregulation of total CD28. Total CD28 levels were not significantly different when comparing cells infected with virus encoding wild-type Vpu or the W$_{22}$L or LV$_{64}$AA mutations (Fig. 6c). In contrast, there was significantly greater total CD28 in the absence of Vpu (dVpu dNef) and in the presence of Vpu encoding the S$_{52/56}$N mutation (S$_{52/56}$N dNef) relative to virus encoding wild-type Vpu (dNef) (Fig. 6c). As an additional control, we demonstrated that cells infected with virus encoding the W$_{22}$L, S$_{52/56}$N or LV$_{64}$AA mutations exhibited significantly greater total levels of CD4 relative to cells infected with virus encoding wild-type Vpu (Additional file 6). Expression of all mutated Vpu proteins was confirmed by Western blot (Fig. 6d). As with our findings for cell surface CD28 downregulation, our results suggest that the molecular determinants of CD28 downregulation by Vpu are distinct from those utilized to downregulate CD4.

Patient-derived Vpu proteins mediate CD28 downregulation

Our findings suggest that HIV-1 NL4.3 can downregulate CD28 by both Nef and Vpu. However, as HIV-1 is genetically diverse, functions observed in the laboratory strain NL4.3 may not necessarily play a prominent role in the epidemic at large. We therefore wanted to determine if Vpu-mediated CD28 downregulation is a conserved function. Thus, we tested the ability of multiple group M Vpu proteins to downregulate cell surface and total CD28. To test this, the NL4.3 *vpu* gene from a Gag-Pol truncated NL4.3 virus lacking Nef (NL4.3 dG/P eGFP dNef) was replaced with *vpu* genes from an HIV-1 subtype B reference strain (B.US.86.JRFL), a subtype C reference strain (C.BR.92.92BR025; [55]), or a gene encoding a subtype C consensus protein (CC). Sup-T1 cells were infected with these VSV-G pseudotyped isogenic viruses which differed only in the encoded Vpu proteins, and cell surface and total CD28 levels were measured by flow cytometry (Additional file 1). Cells infected with virus encoding a subtype C consensus (CC) Vpu protein or a subtype B reference strain (B.US.86.JRFL) Vpu protein did not significantly differ in cell surface levels of CD28 relative to cells infected with virus encoding NL4.3 Vpu (Fig. 7a, b), suggesting that these additional Vpu proteins were capable of downregulating cell surface CD28. In contrast, cells infected with virus encoding a subtype C reference strain (C.BR.92.92BR025) *vpu* gene had significantly greater cell surface levels of CD28, as with virus lacking a functional *vpu* gene (dVpu dNef) (Fig. 7a, b). Moreover, staining for total cellular CD28 revealed that cells infected with virus encoding the B.US.86.JRFL and consensuses C *vpu* genes did not differ in total cellular CD28 levels relative to cells infected with virus encoding NL4.3 *vpu*, while the C.BR.92.92BR025 Vpu protein did not downregulate total CD28 (Fig. 7c). Expression of these proteins in a heterologous system revealed equivalent protein levels for all Vpu proteins except for Vpu from C.BR.92.92BR025, which is weakly expressed (Fig. 7d). To confirm that these findings were not unique to the Sup-T1 cell line, PBMCs

were infected with the same pseudotyped NL4.3 viruses (Fig. 7a) and cell surface CD28 levels on infected (GFP$^+$) CD4$^+$ cells was measured (Additional file 7). A similar trend to that observed in Sup-T1 cells was noted, as the mean levels of CD28 expression were significantly greater on cells infected with virus lacking the *vpu* gene, than in cells infected with virus encoding the NL4.3 and B.US.86. JRFL *vpu* genes (Fig. 7e–g). However, unlike Sup-T1 cells, cell surface levels of CD28 were significantly higher on cells infected with virus encoding the consensus C (CC) Vpu protein, than the NL4.3 Vpu protein. Overall, this suggests that Vpu-mediated cell surface and total CD28 downregulation is not limited to the laboratory adapted HIV-1 strain NL4.3.

Nef and Vpu expression alters the cellular response to external CD28 stimulation

Given that HIV-1 decreases cell surface levels of CD28 (Fig. 1), a key immune cell stimulatory receptor, we postulated that decreased cell surface levels of CD28 on infected cells leads to a decreased ability of cells to become activated by CD28/CD3 stimulation. Thus, we tested what effects Nef and Vpu may have on activation in CD4$^+$ T cells stimulated by CD28/CD3. We therefore infected primary CD4$^+$ T cells with VSV-G pseudotyped NL4.3 encoding both Nef and Vpu (NL4.3), Nef alone (dVpu), Vpu alone (dNef) or lacking both Nef and Vpu (dVpu dNef). Infected cells were stimulated with soluble anti-CD28 and plate bound anti-CD3, and activation was determined by measuring intracytoplasmic production of IL-2, an event that occurs downstream from CD28 activation [56] (Fig. 8). Upon infection with virus lacking Nef (dNef), the percentage of infected cells that produced IL-2 after stimulation was significantly lower than in cells infected with virus encoding Nef and Vpu (NL4.3) (Fig. 8a, b), suggesting that the presence of Nef leads to increased activation, consistent with Nef's previously reported role in T cell activation upon anti-CD3 and anti-CD28 treatment of Jurkat cells [57]. In contrast, in primary cells infected with a virus lacking Vpu

(See figure on next page.)

Fig. 7 Non-NL4.3 Vpu proteins downregulate cell surface CD28. CD4$^+$ Sup-T1 and peripheral blood mononuclear cells (PBMCs) were infected with VSV-G pseudotyped NL4.3 viruses lacking Nef and encoding wild-type Vpu (dNef, blue), no Vpu (dNef dVpu, green) or three non-NL4.3 Vpu proteins (grey). Cells were analyzed by flow cytometry and mean geometric fluorescence intensities (MFI) of infected (GFP$^+$) cells were determined. **a** Representative histograms illustrating cell surface CD28 on live infected (GFP$^+$) Sup-T1 cells. MFIs are indicated. **b** Mean (± SE) relative cell surface CD28 on Sup-T1 cells infected with NL4.3 lacking a functional Nef protein (dNef), but encoding various Vpu proteins (n = 5). **c** Mean (± SE) relative total cellular CD28 of Sup-T1 cells infected with NL4.3 encoding various Vpu proteins (n ≥ 8). **d** Western blot illustrating expression of eGFP-tagged versions of the analyzed Vpu proteins from transfected HEK293T cells. **e** Representative dot plots illustrating infection level (GFP) and cell surface CD28 (APC) on primary CD4$^+$ cells. **f** Representative histograms illustrating cell surface CD28 on either uninfected (isotype control, uninfected) or CD4$^+$ infected (GFP$^+$) cells. MFIs are indicated. **g** Mean (± SE) relative cell surface CD28 on CD4$^+$ cells infected with viruses encoding various *vpu* genes (n = 8). Data were obtained from infection of PBMCs from two healthy donors. (Mr: molecular weight; GAPDH: glyceraldehyde 3-phosphate dehydrogenase; GFP: green fluorescent protein; SE: standard error; UI: uninfected; *p ≤ 0.05; **p ≤ 0.01; ****p ≤ 0.0001)

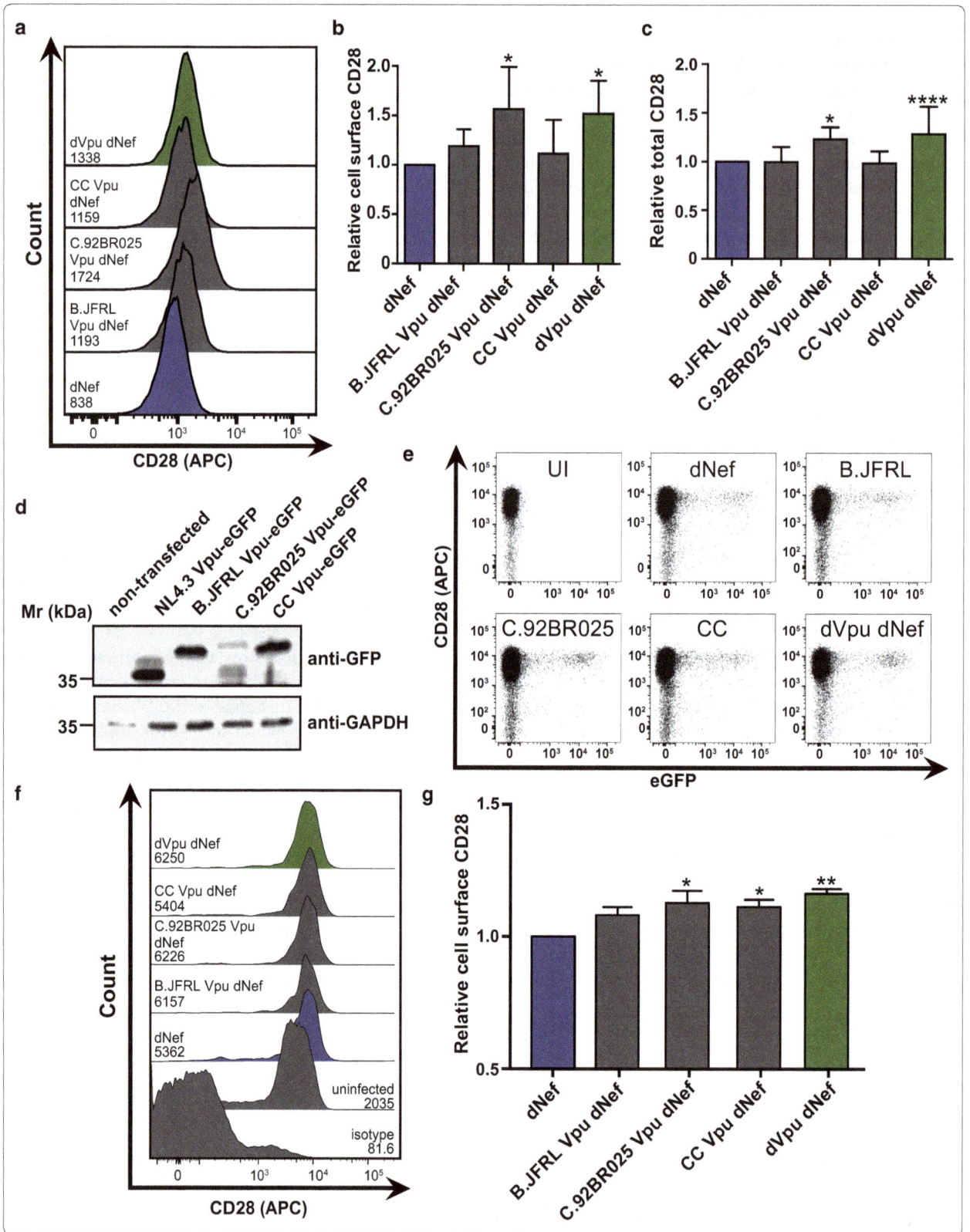

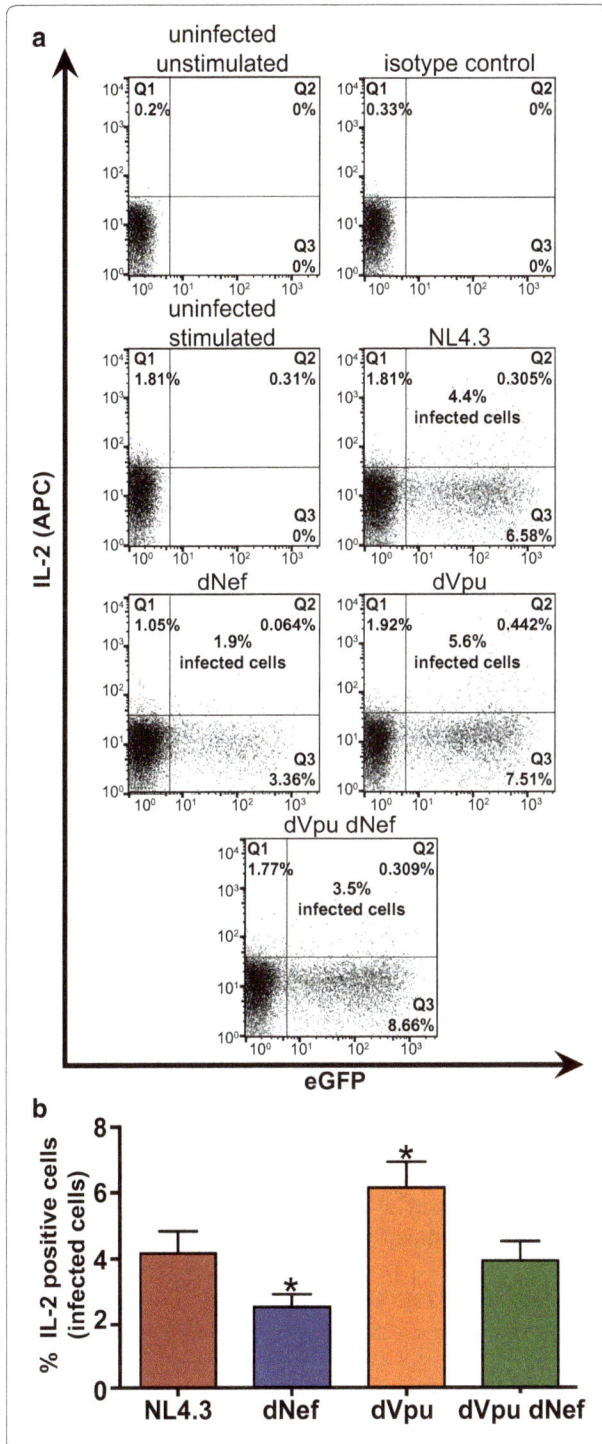

Fig. 8 Response of infected cells to CD28-stimulation is altered in the presence of Nef or Vpu. Purified CD4$^+$ T cells were infected with VSV-G pseudotyped NL4.3 encoding Nef and Vpu (NL4.3, red), lacking Nef (dNef, blue) or Vpu (dVpu, orange), or lacking both Nef and Vpu (dVpu dNef, green). Twenty-four hours post-infection cells were activated with anti-CD3/anti-CD28 for 24 h. Cells were then incubated with Brefeldin A for 12 h and stained for intracellular IL-2 prior to analysis by flow cytometry. **a** Representative dot plots illustrating intracellular IL-2 (APC) and infection (GFP) levels. Quadrants were selected based on the IL-2 isotype antibody control and uninfected controls. The percentage of infected cells that are IL-2 positive is indicated (red). The percentage of cells making up the uninfected and IL-2 negative population (Q4) are as follows: uninfected unstimulated: 99.8%, isotype control: 99.7%, uninfected stimulated: 93.8%, NL4.3: 91.3, dNef: 95.5%, dVpu: 90.1, dVpu dNef: 89.3%. **b** Mean (± SE) percentage of infected cells that are IL-2 positive ($n \geq 6$). The means were obtained by analysis of infected cells from two healthy donors. (SE: standard error; *$p \leq 0.05$)

(dVpu dNef), as the proportion of activated cells did not differ from cells infected with wild-type virus (NL4.3; Fig. 8a, b). Overall, this suggests that Nef and Vpu, which influence cell surface and total CD28 levels, differentially regulate responsiveness to CD28 stimulation.

Discussion

In the current report, we describe the distinct ability of both HIV-1 Nef and Vpu to decrease cell surface and total levels of CD28 in CD4$^+$ T cells. Specifically, we have shown cell surface CD28 downregulation with VSV-G pseudotyped NL4.3 in Sup-T1 cells and primary cells, as well as downregulation in primary CD4$^+$ T cells infected with replication competent NL4.3 (Figs. 1, 7). These results are consistent with observations made in cell lines transiently transfected with Nef and/or Vpu expression vectors. Downregulation of endogenous CD28 was previously illustrated in Jurkat cells transiently expressing Nef [40]. Moreover, Haller et al. completed a large screen for receptors downregulated by Nef and Vpu through transient expression of the viral proteins in A3.01 T lymphocytes, and observed downregulation of CD28 by both HIV-1 Nef and Vpu [20]. Interestingly, the latter study demonstrated varying degrees of downregulation by HIV-1 Nef and Vpu, as well as SIV$_{mac239}$ Nef, with respect to the multiple tested receptors [20]. Accordingly, we observed that the effects of Nef and Vpu on CD28 are subtler than the effects of Nef and Vpu on other receptors, namely MHC-I and CD4 (Additional file 5, 6), but nevertheless Nef and Vpu traffic this receptor to a degradative lysosomal compartment and decrease total CD28 protein levels (Figs. 2, 3, 4). Moreover, it has been shown that there are varying degrees of CD28 downregulation by various Nef proteins, with HIV-2 and certain SIV derived Nef proteins exhibiting more efficient downregulation than HIV-1

(dVpu), the proportion of IL-2 positive infected cells was significantly increased, suggesting that Vpu decreases anti-CD3/CD28 dependent cell activation. This increased activation in the presence of Nef and decreased activation in the presence of Vpu was also evident in experiments conducted with virus lacking both Nef and Vpu

Nef proteins [20, 58]. However, this does not limit the potential physiological relevance of CD28 downregulation by HIV-1 and our current report demonstrates the mechanistic details of Nef and Vpu-mediated CD28 downregulation.

Our results demonstrate that slight increases in cell surface CD28 levels can be observed in cells infected with viruses lacking Nef and Vpu (dVpu dNef) in comparison to uninfected cells (Fig. 1b, e). This suggests that HIV-1 proteins other than Nef and Vpu may also be contributing to changes in cell surface CD28 levels upon infection. The latter effects may be due to events independent of membrane trafficking and could be the consequence of changes at the level of CD28 transcription. Notably, CD28 expression levels may be affected at the transcriptional level via the HIV-1 tat protein, as it interacts with the Sp1 transcription factor which positively affects CD28 transcription [59, 60].

Given that Nef and Vpu collaborate to mediate the downregulation and degradation of cellular receptors, specifically CD4 [28, 61–63], we hypothesized that the observed decreases in total CD28 levels in the presence of Nef and Vpu were due to CD28 degradation. This is supported by our observation that CD28 co-localizes with the lysosome marker LAMP-1 in the presence of the viral proteins (Fig. 3). Moreover, we found that we could limit Nef- and Vpu-mediated decreases in total CD28 and CD4 protein levels upon treatment with ammonium chloride (Fig. 4; Additional file 3). The effects of ammonium chloride on CD4 downregulation are of interest given the previously reported Vpu-dependent proteasomal degradation of CD4 [64]. In our experiments, ammonium chloride may be playing a broader role and impacting cellular physiology by affecting general cell acidification. Importantly, we have used the specific endosomal acidification inhibitors Bafilomycin A1 and Concanamycin A to provide a more specific mechanistic explanation of Nef- and Vpu-dependent effects on CD28 (Fig. 4), thereby bypassing the more general effects of using ammonium chloride. The specific inhibition of the vacuolar ATPase with these molecules limits the co-localization of CD28 with LAMP-1 in Nef and Vpu-expressing cells (Fig. 4).

We also report how CD28 depletion involves the distinct ability of Nef and Vpu to interact with host cellular proteins. Indeed, cell surface CD28 downregulation was inhibited by mutation of Nef LL_{165} and DD_{175}, while maintaining the ability to downregulate MHC-I (Fig. 5; Additional file 5). The findings that Nef LL_{165} and DD_{175} are critical for cell surface CD28 downregulation is in accordance with previously published reports [40, 65], and suggests that AP-2 [46] and the vacuolar ATPase [47] are critical for cell surface downregulation by Nef. Interestingly, mutation of the G_2, LL_{165} and DD_{175} motifs

abolished Nef-dependent decreases in total levels of cellular CD28 in the absence of Vpu (Fig. 5), while mutation of the LL_{165} motif did not significantly alter total CD28 levels in the presence of Vpu (Additional file 5). This may be due to Vpu's ability to compensate for specific Nef mutations. Our observed increases in total cellular CD28 when the ability of Nef to interact with the vacuolar ATPase is inhibited further supports the idea that Nef mediates degradation of CD28 ($DD_{175}GA$; Fig. 5c). The Nef DD_{175} motif is also critical for Nef-mediated lysosomal degradation of the co-inhibitory receptor Cytotoxic T-Lymphocyte-Associated protein 4 (CTLA-4) [66], which interestingly, competes with CD28 for binding the same receptors, B7.1/B7.2 [67]. Overall, this suggests that as with cell surface downregulation, the downregulation of total CD28 levels is dependent on specific Nef:host cell protein interaction motifs.

We have also provided mechanistic details on how Vpu modulates CD28 expression and localization within HIV-1 infected cells. Intriguingly, the mutations exhibited different effects on CD28 and CD4 downregulation (Fig. 6; Additional file 6), indicating that CD28 downregulation by Vpu may have evolved independently. Specifically, mutation of the Vpu W_{22}, $S_{52/56}$ and LV_{64} motifs inhibited the ability of Vpu to downregulate cell surface CD4 (Additional file 6), in agreement with previous reports [49–51]. In contrast, mutation of the highly conserved W_{22} did not inhibit cell surface downregulation of CD28 (Fig. 6a, b), suggesting that this residue is dispensable for CD28 downregulation despite being implicated in the downregulation of CD4 and BST-2 [50, 53, 68, 69].

Similar to CD4 downregulation, mutation of Vpu S_{52}/S_{56} and LV_{64} inhibited cell surface downregulation of CD28 (Fig. 6a, b). Interestingly, these Vpu motifs play distinct roles with AP-1 and AP-2, in addition to contributing to mechanisms that promote the degradation of cellular proteins. Indeed, the non-phosphorylatable mutants of Vpu (Vpu $S_{52/56}N$) do not recruit AP-1 and AP-2 and subsequently fail to downregulate BST-2 [37], whereas Vpu LV_{64} promotes the degradation of BST-2 via autophagy [70]. Thus, the ability of Vpu to downregulate CD28 from the cell surface may require AP-1 or AP-2 binding to the LV_{64} motif in a Vpu S_{52}/S_{56} dependent manner to exclude CD28 from the cell surface post-endocytosis or prior to anterograde transport.

Interestingly, only the $S_{52/56}N$ mutations in Vpu inhibited Vpu-mediated decreases in total CD28, whereas the W_{22}, $S_{52/56}$ and LV_{64} motifs were all imperative to decreasing total CD4 (Fig. 6c; Additional file 6). The adaptor protein-binding motif in Vpu (LV_{64}) was critical for cell surface downregulation, but dispensable for decreasing total CD28 (Fig. 6b, c). This motif may be unnecessary for reducing total CD28 levels as additional host cell binding factors, either known or currently unidentified, may compensate for mutation of the LV_{64} motif. Overall, the mechanism of Vpu-mediated CD28 cell surface downregulation is discrete from that which mediates total decreases in cellular CD28, and this mechanism is distinct from Vpu-mediated downregulation of total CD4.

We demonstrated that the ability of Vpu to downregulate cell surface and total CD28 is not specific to the laboratory adapted NL4.3 strain Vpu protein. Specifically, a subtype C consensus Vpu protein and a subtype B reference strain (B.US.86.JRFL) protein downregulated cell surface and total CD28 in infected Sup-T1 cells (Fig. 7). Contrastingly, the Vpu protein derived from a subtype C reference strain (C.BR.92.92BR025) did not downregulate CD28 (Fig. 7), which may be attributable in part to decreased expression (Fig. 7d). Interestingly, in a separate study we found that this subtype C reference strain encodes a non-functional Nef protein and has previously been shown to have lower fitness when compared to other well described subtype reference strains [71, 72]. Moreover, we found that in infected CD4$^+$ PBMCs both the NL4.3 and B.US.86.JRFL derived Vpu proteins were capable of downregulating cell surface CD28 (Fig. 7e–g). However, unlike in Sup-T1 cells, PBMCs infected with virus encoding the consensus C Vpu protein did not exhibit downregulation (Fig. 7g). The observed difference between Sup-T1 cells and CD4$^+$ PBMCs may be due to intrinsic differences between Sup-T1 and primary cells and potential differences in the expression pattern of the various Vpu proteins in different cell types. None the less, the ability of distinct Vpu proteins to downregulate cell surface and total CD28 suggests that this function is conserved to some extent, despite high HIV-1 diversity [73].

HIV-1 has evolved multiple means of downregulating CD28, which are in part genetically separable from CD4 and MHC-I downregulation, implying that CD28 downregulation is critical during infection. Moreover, we hypothesized that the function of CD28 downregulation is relevant during infection and that CD28 downregulation by Nef and Vpu may alter cell activation through CD28 receptor stimulation. Indeed, we observed that in primary CD4$^+$ T cells infected with pseudotyped virus encoding Vpu alone (dNef), a significantly smaller proportion of infected cells secreted IL-2 upon CD3/CD28 stimulation, relative to cells infected with virus encoding Nef and Vpu (NL4.3; Fig. 8b). In contrast, cells infected with virus lacking Vpu (dVpu) displayed an increase in cell activation (Fig. 8), indicating that Nef alone increases CD28 stimulation responsiveness.

The observed differences in cell activation in the presence or absence of Nef and Vpu may be partially attributable to other reported functions of these viral proteins.

Namely, Nef alters the subcellular localization of the T cell receptor and immunological synapse associated kinase Lck, leading to a physical separation of the T cell receptor from the immunological synapse [6, 74]. Nef also binds and activates the serine/threonine kinase p21 activated kinase 2 (PAK2), which induces T cell activation [57]. Nef thus alters the activation status of cells, perhaps inducing the correct balance between activating and inhibitory signaling, thereby enabling optimal viral replication without inducing anergy or activation induced cell death [75]. However, when compared to Nef, little is known regarding how Vpu alters T cell activation. Nonetheless, Vpu may interfere with T cell activation and IL-2 production through its ability to inhibit nuclear factor kappa-light-chain-enhancer of activated B cells (NF- κB) [76]. Ultimately, the evolution of CD28 downregulation may be one component of the multitude of alterations within infected cells that act to attain optimal levels of cell activation.

The role or function of CD28 downregulation in vivo remains elusive, however we speculate it may play a role in cell activation. CD28 is critical for T cell activation, providing co-stimulatory signalling necessary for activation upon binding to CD80:CD86 [4, 5] and in the absence of CD28, T cell receptor ligation can lead to an unresponsive, anergic state [78]. The importance of CD28 in vivo has been demonstrated through the use of anti-CD28 therapies to induce immunosuppression following transplantation, in patients with autoimmune diseases (reviewed in [79]) and during cancer immunotherapies via CD28 activation [80]. In addition, reductions in IL-2 levels, as observed in the presence of Vpu (Fig. 8), may lead to impairments in T cell survival, proliferation and function (reviewed in [81]). Interestingly, decreases in IL-2 levels are observed in HIV infected individuals [82, 83], and clinical trials have examined the benefit of administering recombinant IL-2 in combination with anti-retroviral therapy [84]. IL-2 has also been associated with reactivation of latently infected cells [85, 86]. Therefore, it is conceivable that CD28 downregulation alters responsiveness and activation of infected T cells.

Alterations in activation status of infected cells, which may in part be achieved through CD28 downregulation, could have effects in vivo during HIV-1 infection. Upon HIV-1 infection, a transcriptionally silent latent reservoir of cells is formed, which currently present the largest obstacle for achieving a HIV-1 cure [87]. A decrease in cell activation as a result of alterations in cell surface CD28 levels may allow an infected cell to enter a transcriptionally silent, latent state. Indeed, CD28 activation is capable of inducing HIV-1 transcription and replication, even in the absence of TCR activation [88]. Moreover, viral microRNA-mediated silencing of genes that contribute to cellular activation, which may include CD28 [77], have been suggested to be important for the development of latency [89]. Furthermore, CD28 activation is utilized to reactivate latent cells, as mTOR, a kinase activated downstream of CD28 signaling [90], was identified as a critical controller of HIV-1 latency [91].

Conclusions

We illustrate that the HIV-1 Nef and Vpu accessory proteins downregulate CD28 from the cell surface and at the cellular level. This effect is observed with more than just the laboratory adapted NL4.3 strain, indicating this function is conserved. We propose that the decreases in total cellular CD28 may be potentiated by lysosomal degradation of CD28. Moreover, our analysis of Nef and Vpu mutants suggest that the Nef:vacuolar ATPase interaction and phosphorylation of Vpu $S_{52/56}$ are both critical for downregulation of cell surface and total protein levels of this key co-stimulatory molecule. Finally, the presence or absence of Nef and Vpu modulates the ability of cells to respond to CD28-mediated stimulation.

Methods
DNA constructs

Viral infection plasmids used for VSV-G pseudotyped lentivirus production were engineered from the previously described pNL4.3 dG/P eGFP or pNL4.3 dG/P eGFP dNef backbones [92, 93]. To make viral constructs lacking Vpu, HIV-1$_{NL4-3}$ *vpu/nef/UD* Deletion Mutant (p230-11; NIH-AIDS reagents catalog number 2535) was digested with EcoRI and BamHI and the fragment encoding the *vpu* gene was sub-cloned into pNL4.3 dG/P eGFP or pNL4.3 dG/P eGFP dNef. Mutations in the NL4.3 *nef* gene were produced by site directed mutagenesis within a pN1 expression vector (Clontech, Mountain View, CA) encoding NL4.3 Nef. Mutagenesis primers were created with the Agilent Technologies QuickChange Primer Design program (Agilent Technologies, Santa Clara, CA). The *nef* genes containing mutations were subsequently PCR amplified with primers encoding XmaI and NotI cut sites, and were inserted into a previously described vector encoding XmaI and NotI cut sites flanking the *nef* gene [94]. Mutations in the NL4.3 *vpu* gene were produced by site directed mutagenesis in a pN1 Vpu-FLAG expression vector. *Vpu* genes encoding mutations were subsequently PCR amplified and inserted into pRECnfl HIV-1 dVpu/URA3 (obtained from Eric Arts, University of Western Ontario), using a previously described yeast recombination system [95]. The *vpu*-encoding fragment was then sub-cloned into a NL4.3 backbone lacking a functional *nef* gene (pNL4.3 dG/P eGFP dNef) using the EcoRI and BamHI restriction sites. *Vpu* genes derived from a subtype C reference strain (C.BR.92.92BR025),

subtype B reference strain (B.US.86.JRFL) or a consensus C protein synthesized using Invitrogen GeneArt Synthesis (Thermo Fisher Scientific, Mississauga, ON) were inserted into the pRECnfl HIV-1 dVpu/URA3 vector followed by sub-cloning into pNL4.3 dG/P eGFP dNef, as described above. To test the expression of the non-NL4.3 Vpu proteins the *vpu* encoding fragments were PCR amplified and sub-cloned into the peGFP-N1 expression vector (Clontech).

Viral infection plasmids utilized to make replication competent NL4.3 were engineered from the previously described pNL4.3 vector [93]. A Nef deficient plasmid (pNL4.3 dNef) was obtained from Gary Thomas (University of Pittsburgh) and Vpu (dVpu) and Nef and Vpu (dVpu dNef) deficient plasmids were produced by sub-cloning the *vpu* encoding portion of HIV-1$_{NL4-3}$ *vpu/nef/UD* Deletion Mutant into pNL4.3 or pNL4.3 dNef, as described above.

Cell culture

HEK293T (ATCC) and U87 CD4$^+$ CXCR4$^+$ (NIH-AIDS Research and Reference Reagent program; catalog number 4036) cells were maintained in Dulbecco's modified Eagle's medium (DMEM) containing 4 mM L-glutamine, 4500 mg/L glucose and sodium pyruvate (HyClone, Logan, UT) and supplemented with 1% Penicillin–Streptomycin (Hyclone) and 10% fetal bovine serum (FBS; Wisent, St-Bruno, QC). Sup-T1 cells were maintained in Roswell Park Memorial Institute media (RPMI) 1640 media with L-glutamine supplemented with 100 µg/ml penicillin–streptomycin, 1% sodium pyruvate, 1% nonessential amino acids, 2 mM L-glutamine (Hyclone) and 10% FBS. All cell lines were grown at 37 °C in the presence of 5% CO_2 and sub-cultured in accordance with supplier's recommendations.

Primary peripheral blood mononuclear cells were isolated from four healthy donors by density centrifugation using Histopaque (Sigma-Aldrich, Oakville, ON) and cryopreserved. Upon revival, cells were maintained in RPMI with L-glutamine supplemented with 100 µg/ml penicillin–streptomycin, 1% sodium pyruvate, 1% nonessential amino acids, 2 mM L-glutamine (Hyclone) and 10% FBS at 37 °C and 5% CO_2 in the presence or absence of IL-2 and phytohemagglutinin (PHA) stimulation, as indicated. CD4$^+$ T cells were purified from PBMCs using the MojoSort^{TM} human CD4 T cell isolation kit (BioLegend, San Diego, CA) and MACS cell separation columns (Miltenyi Biotec, Auburn, CA), according to the manufacturer's protocol.

For ammonium chloride treatment, cells were pelleted and culture medium was replaced with complete RPMI containing or lacking 40 mM ammonium chloride (Sigma-Aldrich) in phosphate buffered saline (PBS)

24 h prior to analysis. For vacuolar ATPase inhibitor treatment, cells were pelleted and culture medium was replaced with complete RPMI containing vehicle, 100 nM Concanamycin A (Santa Cruz Biotechnology, Dallas, TX) or 100 nM Bafilomycin A1 (Sigma-Aldrich) in DMSO 5 h prior to analysis.

Transfections and infections

For VSV-G pseudotyped lentivirus production, HEK293T cells were triply transfected with the pNL4.3 dG/P eGFP vector of interest, the VSV-G envelope-encoding pMD2.G plasmid (Addgene; catalog number 12259) and pCMV-DR8.2 (Addgene; catalog number 12263) using PolyJet (FroggaBio, North York, ON) as per the manufacturer's protocol. Forty-eight hours post transfection, lentivirus was harvested via cell culture supernatant clarification by spinning at $1500 \times g$, followed by 20 µm filtration. For production of NL4.3 provirus, viral vectors were transfected into HEK293T cells using PolyJet. Forty-eight hours post-transfection, cell supernatant was applied to U87 CD4$^+$ CXCR4$^+$ cells to propagate the virus. Cell supernatant was harvested 4–6 days post infection as described above. Viruses were stored in 20% FBS at − 80 °C.

For infection of Sup-T1 cells with VSV-G pseudotyped viruses, 8×10^5 Sup-T1 cells were pelleted and re-suspended in the appropriate volume of pseudovirus in 20% FBS, 8 µg/mL polybrene and brought to 1 mL with 10% complete RPMI. Forty-eight hours post infection, cells were analyzed via flow cytometry, microscopy or Western blotting. For infection of peripheral blood mononuclear cells with VSV-G pseudotyped viruses, cells were cultured for 3 days in 10 ng/mL IL-2 (PeproTech, Rocky Hill, NJ) and 5 µg/mL PHA (Sigma-Aldrich). Cells were then pelleted and re-suspended in the appropriate volume of pseudovirus containing 8 µg/mL polybrene. Cells were subsequently spinoculated for 4 h at $2880 \times g$ at room temperature, re-suspended in fresh RPMI and incubated for 2 days prior to analysis. For infection of primary CD4$^+$ T cells with replication competent NL4.3 viruses, cells were cultured for 3 days in 10 ng/mL IL-2 and 5 µg/mL PHA-L. CD4$^+$ T cells were then purified as described above and re-suspended in the appropriate volume of virus in 20% FBS and 8 µg/mL polybrene. Subsequently, cells were spinoculated for 4 h at $2880 \times g$ at room temperature, re-suspended in fresh complete RPMI containing 5 ng/mL IL-2 and 5 µg/mL PHA-L. Two days post-infection, cells were pelleted and re-suspended in fresh media containing PHA and IL-2 and 4 days post-infection cells were fixed and stained. For infection of purified CD4$^+$ T cells with VSV-G pseudotyped virus, cells were cultured for 3 days in 10 ng/mL IL-2 and 5 µg/ mL PHA-L. CD4$^+$ T cells were then purified as described

above and re-suspended in the appropriate volume of virus in 20% FBS and 8 µg/mL polybrene. Subsequently, cells were spinoculated for 4 h at $2880 \times g$ at room temperature, re-suspended in fresh complete 10% RPMI and analyzed 48 h post-infection.

Flow cytometry analysis of cell surface receptors

For cell surface staining of Sup-T1 cells, 48 h post infection, cells were washed twice with PBS, followed by staining for 20 min at room temperature with 1:6000 Zombie Red^{TM} (BioLegend) in PBS, where appropriate. Cells were then washed in FACS buffer (1% FBS, 50 mM ethylenediaminetetraacetic acid (EDTA) in PBS) and fixed in 1% paraformaldehyde (PFA) for 20 min at room temperature. Cells were subsequently washed twice with FACS buffer and stained with the appropriate antibodies by rocking for 40 min at room temperature. Cells were then washed twice with FACS buffer and re-suspended in PBS. For staining of CD28 and CD4, 1:25 APC-conjugated mouse-anti-CD28 (clone CD28.2, BioLegend) and 1:25 APC-conjugated mouse-anti-CD4 (clone OKT4, BioLegend) were utilized, respectively. For cell surface MHC-I staining, cells were stained with W6/32 (anti-MHC-I, pan-selective for HLA-A, B and C, provided by D. Johnson, Oregon Health and Science University), washed twice with FACS buffer, incubated with an APC-conjugated species specific secondary antibody, followed by washing with FACS buffer and re-suspending in PBS. For analysis of total CD28 or CD4 levels, cells were prepared as above, but were permeabilized and blocked prior to staining. Specifically, after fixation, cells were permeabilized by incubation with 0.5% saponin for 15 min at room temperature. Cells were then washed with 1% FBS, 0.1% saponin, 5 mM EDTA and blocked for 30 min with blocking buffer (10% FBS, 0.1% saponin, 5 mM EDTA in PBS). Cells were incubated with primary antibody diluted in blocking buffer followed by washing with 1% FBS, 0.1% saponin, 5 mM EDTA and re-suspending in PBS.

For cell surface staining of peripheral blood mononuclear cells infected with VSV-G pseudotyped NL4.3 encoding eGFP, cells were fixed in 2% PFA for 20 min at room temperature, followed by washing twice with cell staining buffer (BioLegend). Cells were then incubated for 40 min at room temperature with the appropriate fluorescently labeled primary antibodies (1:50 APC-Cy7 conjugated anti-CD4 (Clone OKT4, BioLegend), 1:25 APC conjugated anti-CD28 (clone CD28.2, BioLegend)). Cells were then washed twice with cell staining buffer and re-suspended in PBS prior to analysis.

For analysis of total CD28 in primary CD4$^+$ T cells infected with VSV-G pseudotyped NL4.3 provirus, cells were washed twice with cell staining buffer (BioLegend) and fixed and permeabilized in BD Cytofix/Cytoperm solution (BD Biosciences, San Jose, CA). Cells were subsequently washed twice with Perm/Wash buffer (BD Biosciences) and stained for 30 min at 4 °C for CD28 level analysis [1:25 APC conjugated anti-CD28 (clone CD28.2, BioLegend)]. Cells were then washed, re-suspended in PBS and analyzed.

For analysis of cell surface CD28 on primary CD4$^+$ T cells infected with replication competent NL4.3 provirus, cells were washed twice with cell staining buffer (BioLegend) and incubated for 30 min at 4 °C with fluorophore conjugated primary antibodies against the appropriate cell surface antigen [1:25 APC conjugated anti-CD28 (clone CD28.2, BioLegend)]. Cells were then washed twice with cell staining buffer and then fixed and permeabilized in BD Cytofix/Cytoperm solution (BD Biosciences, San Jose, CA). Cells were subsequently washed twice with Perm/Wash buffer (BD Biosciences) and stained for 30 min at 4 °C for p24 level analysis (1:50 anti-p24; clone KC57, Beckman Coulter). Cells were then washed, re-suspended in PBS and analyzed. The following isotype control antibodies were used in lieu of primary antibody as required: APC-Cy7 conjugated mouse IgG2b, κ isotype (clone MOPC-21, BioLegend), APC mouse IgG1 κ isotype control (clone MOPC-21, BioLegend), PE mouse IgG1κ (clone: MOPC-21, BioLegend).

Cells were analyzed using a BD Biosciences FACS-Canto SORP (BD Biosciences). Data analysis was performed using FlowJo software (version 9.6.4, FlowJo LLC, Ashland, OR).

Protein analysis

Infected Sup-T1 cells or HEK293T cells transfected using PolyJet (FroggaBio) were lysed 48 h post transduction or transfection for protein expression analysis. Briefly, cells were pelleted and lysed by rocking in lysis buffer [0.5 M HEPES, 1.25 M NaCl, 1 M MgCl$_2$, 0.25 M EDTA, 0.1% Triton X-100 and 1× complete Protease Inhibitor Tablets (Roche, Indianapolis, IN)] for 1 h at 4 °C. The supernatant was then clarified by spinning at 16,100×g for 30 min at 4 °C, mixed with SDS-PAGE sample buffer (0.312 M Tris pH 6.8, 3.6 M 2-Mercaptoethanol, 50% glycerol, 10% SDS) and boiled at 95 °C for 10 min. Samples were run on 12 or 14% SDS-PAGE gels followed by transferring to nitrocellulose. Membranes were blocked with 5% milk in TBST (50 mM Tris, 150 mM NaCl, 0.1% Tween 20) for 1 h at room temperature, followed by incubation overnight at 4 °C with the appropriate primary antibody in 5% milk in TBST. The following primary antibodies were used: 1:1000 rabbit anti-Nef polyclonal antibody (NIH-AIDS Research and Reference Reagent program, catalog number 2949), 1:2000 rabbit anti-GFP polyclonal antibody (Clontech), 1:5000 rabbit anti-Vpu polyclonal antibody (NIH-AIDS Research and Reference Reagent

program, catalog number 969), 1:2000 mouse anti-Actin monoclonal antibody (Thermo Fisher Scientific, 1:1000 rabbit anti-GAPDH polyclonal antibody (Thermo Fisher Scientific). The next day, membranes were washed three times with TBST and incubated for 2 h at room temperature with the appropriate species specific HRP-conjugated secondary antibodies (1:2000, Thermo Fisher Scientific) in 5% milk in TBST. Blots were subsequently washed and developed using ECL substrates (Millipore, Etobicoke, ON) and a C-DiGit chemiluminescence Western blot scanner (LI-COR Biosciences, Lincoln, NE).

Microscopy

For microscopy experiments, cells were infected and treated with inhibitors as described above. Cells were then adhered to poly-L-lysine (Sigma-Aldrich) coated coverslips and fixed in 2% PFA for 10 min at room temperature. Cells were subsequently washed twice with PBS and permeabilized with methanol for 20 min. Cells were then washed twice with PBS and blocked in 2% bovine serum albumin (BSA) in PBS for 1 h at room temperature. Cells were subsequently stained for 2 h with mouse anti-CD28 (Thermo Fisher Scientific) and rabbit anti-LAMP-1 (Developmental Studies Hybridoma Bank, University of Iowa) diluted at 1:200 in 0.2% BSA in PBS, washed twice with 0.2% BSA in PBS and incubated for one and a half hours with the appropriate fluorophore conjugated secondary antibodies (Alexa-Fluor-647 conjugated anti-mouse and Cy3-conjugated anti-rabbit; Jackson ImmunoResearch, West Grove, PA) at 1:400 in 0.2% BSA in PBS. Finally, cells were washed twice with PBS and mounted on coverslips with DAPI Fluoromount-G (SouthernBiotech, Birmingham, AL). Cells were imaged on a Leica DMI6000 B at 63× or 100× magnification using the FITC, Cy3, Cy5 and DAPI filter settings and imaged with a Hamamatsu Photometrics Delta Evolve camera. Images were subsequently deconvolved using the Advanced Fluorescence Deconvolution application (Lecia, Wetzlar, Germany) on the Leica Application Suite software. Co-localization analysis was conducted using Mander's Coefficent from the ImageJ plugin JACoP, as described previously [96].

Cell activation analysis

To examine activation in infected cells, cryopreserved PBMCs were revived and rested for 6 h in complete RPMI media (without PHA/IL-2) at 37 °C and 5% CO$_2$. CD4$^+$ T cells were then purified as described above and spinoculated with the appropriate VSV-G pseudotyped NL4.3 virus encoding both Nef and Vpu (NL4.3 dG/P eGFP), encoding Vpu alone (NL4.3 dG/P eGFP dNef), encoding Nef alone (NL4.3 dG/P eGFP dNef), or lacking both Nef and Vpu (NL4.3 dG/P eGFP dVpu dNef). After spinoculation, cells were incubated in complete 10%

RPMI for 24 h prior to incubating with anti-CD3 (10 µg/ml, clone OKT3, BioLegend) immobilized on a plate and soluble anti-CD28 (5 µg/ml, clone CD28.2, BioLegend). After 24 h of activation, cells were treated with Brefeldin A (1:1000 dilution, BD Biosciences) for 12 h before proceeding for intracellular IL-2 staining.

For intracellular staining of IL-2, infected CD4$^+$ T cells were fixed using Cytofix/Cytoperm solution (BD Biosciences) for 20 min at 4 °C, washed twice with Perm/Wash buffer (BD Biosciences) and stained for intracellular IL-2 with an APC-conjugated anti-IL-2 antibody (clone MQ1-17H12, BD Biosciences), or the appropriate isotype control (APC Rat IgG2a, κ isotype control, clone R35-95, BD Biosciences), for 1 h at 4 °C (1:20 dilution in Perm/Wash buffer). Cells were then washed twice using Perm/Wash buffer prior to analysis by flow cytometry. In order to determine the percentage of the infected cells that were IL-2 positive, the percentage of GFP$^+$ IL-2$^+$ cells (Q_2, Fig. 8) was divided by the total percentage of infected cells (sum of GFP$^+$ IL-2$^+$ (Q_2, Fig. 8) and GFP$^+$ IL-2$^-$ (Q_3, Fig. 8)) and multiplied by 100.

Data and statistical analysis

For analyses of flow cytometry data obtained for Sup-T1 cells infected with VSV-G pseudotyped NL4.3 encoding Vpu and various Nef mutations, relative levels of receptors were determined by normalizing geometric mean fluorescence intensity after gating on infected (GFP$^+$) cells (Additional file 4). For all other analysis of cell surface receptors on Sup-T1 cells infected with VSV-G pseudotyped NL4.3, relative levels of receptors were determined by normalizing geometric mean fluorescence intensity after gating on single, live (Zombie Red^{TM-}), infected (GFP$^+$) cells (Additional file 1). Relative levels of CD28 on primary CD4$^+$ T cells infected with replication competent NL4.3 were determined by normalizing geometric mean fluorescence intensity after gating on single, p24 high and CD28$^+$ cells (Additional file 2). Relative levels of CD28 on VSV-G pseudotyped NL4.3 infected PBMCs, were determined by normalizing geometric mean fluorescence intensity after gating on CD4$^+$ and infected (GFP$^+$) lymphocytes (Additional file 7). For all cell surface or total receptor analysis by flow cytometry, the geometric mean fluorescence intensity of the control in each experiment (left-most sample on each graph) was set to 1 and the other sample MFIs were calculated relative to the control having an MFI of 1. To calculate the relative increase in intracellular staining upon ammonium chloride treatment, the geometric mean fluorescence intensity of the live and infected cells treated with ammonium chloride was divided by the geometric mean fluorescence intensity of cells that were untreated. This ratio was then normalized such that the fold increase in

MFI for cells infected with NL4.3 was equal to one. All statistics for analysis of receptor levels were conducted using a one-way analysis of variance with Bonferroni's multiple comparison test. For analysis of CD28: LAMP-1 co-localization, the mean Manders' overlap coefficients were compared using a one-way analysis of variance with Bonferroni's multiple comparison test to compare wild-type infected cells to cells infected with viruses encoding or lacking Nef and/or Vpu (Fig. 3) or wild-type infected cells treated with vehicle to cells treated with various inhibitors (Fig. 4). Alternatively, for analysis of the percentage of IL-2 positive infected cells, a paired two-tailed t test was used. All statistical tests were completed using Graph Pad Prism (Graph Pad Software Inc., La Jolla, CA).

Additional files

Additional file 1. Gating of live infected Sup-T1 cells infected with Gag-Pol truncated VSV-G pseudotyped NL4.3. To examine live and infected cells, dead cells were excluded by gating on Zombie Red^{TM-} cells, doublets were excluded and subsequently infected (GFP$^+$) cells were gated on. In a representative experiment, 80.3% of cells were live (Zombie Red^{TM-}) and 83.1% of live single cells were infected (GFP$^+$). Gates were set based on FMO (fluorescence minus one) controls stained for all fluorophores except that which is being gated on.

Additional file 2. Analysis of primary CD4$^+$ T cells infected with replication competent virus. Primary CD4$^+$ T cells were purified and infected with replication competent NL4.3 viruses and stained for cell surface CD28 and intracellular p24. (A) To examine the cells surface CD28 levels on infected cells, single cells were gated on followed by gating on the p24 (PE) and CD28 (APC) high population. In a representative experiment, 5.22% of cells were p24 high. (B) Representative dot plots illustrating p24 (PE) and CD28 (APC) on the following groups: uninfected and unstained, stained with the appropriate APC isotype control, infected and stained with the appropriate PE isotype control, or infected with the indicated viruses and stained with both anti-CD28 (APC) and anti-p24 (PE).

Additional file 3. Ammonium chloride treatment increases total CD4 levels in infected cells. CD4$^+$ Sup-T1 cells were infected with Gag-Pol truncated VSV-G pseudotyped NL4.3 encoding or lacking Nef and/or Vpu. Infected cells were treated with 40 mM ammonium chloride for 48 h prior to staining for CD4 and analyzed by flow cytometry. (A) Representative histograms illustrating CD4 (APC) levels on live, infected cells. Mean geometric fluorescence intensities (MFIs) are indicated. (B) MFIs of infected cells were determined after gating on live, infected (Zombie Red^{TM-} and GFP$^+$) cells and the relative fold increase (± SE) in total CD4 (n ≥ 5) upon ammonium chloride treatment is illustrated. (SE: standard error; ****p ≤ 0.0001).

Additional file 4. Gating of Sup-T1 cells infected with VSV-G pseudotyped NL4.3 encoding various Nef mutants. To examine the population of interest, cells were gated on, followed by gating on infected (GFP$^+$) cells. In a representative experiment 97.9% of cells were infected (GFP$^+$).

Additional file 5. Nef: host protein interaction motifs are critical for Nef-mediated CD28 downregulation in the presence of Vpu. Infected CD4$^+$ Sup-T1 cells were stained for CD28 or MHC-I and analyzed by flow cytometry. Cells infected with VSV-G pseudotyped wild-type NL4.3 (NL4.3, red) or NL4.3 lacking Nef (dNef, blue) were used as controls. (A) Mean (± SE) relative cell surface CD28 of cells infected with NL4.3 encoding various mutations in the *nef* gene (n ≥ 5). (B) Mean (± SE) relative cell surface MHC-I on cells infected with NL4.3 encoding various *nef* mutations (n ≥ 4). (C) Relative mean (± SE) total CD28 within live cells infected with NL4.3 encoding various *nef* mutations (n ≥ 6). (SE: standard error; *p ≤ 0.05; **p ≤ 0.01; ****p ≤ 0.0001).

Additional file 6. Specific motifs in Vpu are critical for downregulation of CD4. Infected CD4+ Sup-T1 cells were stained for CD4 and analyzed by flow cytometry. Mean geometric fluorescence intensities of cells (MFI) were determined after gating on live and infected (Zombie Red™− and GFP+) cells. Cells infected with VSV-G pseudotyped NL4.3 lacking Nef (dNef, blue) and both Nef and Vpu (dNef dVpu, green) were used as controls. (A) Mean (± SE) relative cell surface CD4 on cells infected with NL4.3 encoding various mutations *in vpu* (n ≥ 4). (B) Relative mean (± SE) total CD4 within cells infected with NL4.3 encoding various Vpu mutations (n ≥ 5). (SE: standard error; *p ≤ 0.05; **p ≤ 0.01; ***p ≤ 0.001; ****p ≤ 0.0001).

Additional file 7. Gating of CD4+ peripheral blood mononuclear cells infected with VSV-G pseudotyped NL4.3. To examine the population of interest, lymphocytes were gated on, followed by gating on CD4+ (APC-Cy7) positive and infected (GFP+) cells. In a representative experiment 35.9% of lymphocytes were CD4+ and 1.3% of these were infected (GFP+). Gates were set based on isotype stained (APC-Cy7) and uninfected controls.

Authors' contributions

ENP, BSD and RAJ conducted experiments. ENP, BSD, RAJ and JDD conceived and designed experiments. ENP, BSD, RAJ, ALJ analyzed data. ENP, BSD, RAJ, ALJ, JDD aided in writing the manuscript. All authors read and approved the final manuscript.

Acknowledgements

We acknowledge the NIH AIDS Research and Reference Reagent Program, David Johnson, Eric Arts and Gary Thomas for providing antibodies and reagents for this project. This work was supported by an operating grant from the Canadian Institutes of Health Research (CIHR) to JDD (CIHR-MOP 286719) and by infrastructure grants from the Canadian Foundation for Innovation and The University of Western Ontario. ENP is supported by an Alexander Graham Bell Doctoral Canada Graduate Scholarship from NSERC. BSD is supported by a Frederick Banting and Charles Best Canada Graduate Scholarship from CIHR and ALJ is partially supported by an Ontario Graduate Studentship.

Competing interests

The authors declare they have no competing interests.

References

1. Warrington R, Watson W, Kim HL, Antonetti FR. An introduction to immunology and immunopathology. Allergy Asthma Clin Immunol. 2011;7(Suppl 1):S1.
2. Chen L, Flies DB. Molecular mechanisms of T cell co-stimulation and co-inhibition. Nat Rev Immunol. 2013;13(4):227–42.
3. Smith-Garvin JE, Koretzky GA, Jordan MS. T cell activation. Annu Rev Immunol. 2009;27:591–619.
4. Weiss A, Manger B, Imboden J. Synergy between the T3/antigen receptor complex and Tp44 in the activation of human T cells. J Immunol. 1986;137(3):819–25.
5. Jenkins MK, Taylor PS, Norton SD, Urdahl KB. CD28 delivers a costimulatory signal involved in antigen-specific IL-2 production by human T cells. J Immunol. 1991;147(8):2461–6.

6. Thoulouze MI, Sol-Foulon N, Blanchet F, Dautry-Varsat A, Schwartz O, Alcover A. Human immunodeficiency virus type-1 infection impairs the formation of the immunological synapse. Immunity. 2006;24(5):547–61.
7. Simmons A, Gangadharan B, Hodges A, Sharrocks K, Prabhakar S, Garcia A, et al. Nef-mediated lipid raft exclusion of UbcH7 inhibits Cbl activity in T cells to positively regulate signaling. Immunity. 2005;23(6):621–34.
8. Haller C, Rauch S, Michel N, Hannemann S, Lehmann MJ, Keppler OT, et al. The HIV-1 pathogenicity factor Nef interferes with maturation of stimulatory T-lymphocyte contacts by modulation of N-Wasp activity. J Biol Chem. 2006;281(28):19618–30.
9. de Waal Malefyt R, Yssel H, Spits H, de Vries JE, Sancho J, Terhorst C, et al. Human T cell leukemia virus type I prevents cell surface expression of the T cell receptor through down-regulation of the CD3-gamma, -delta, -epsilon, and -zeta genes. J Immunol. 1990;145(7):2297–303.
10. Koga Y, Oh-Hori N, Sato H, Yamamoto N, Kimura G, Nomoto K. Absence of transcription of lck (lymphocyte specific protein tyrosine kinase) message in IL-2-independent, HTLV-I-transformed T cell lines. J Immunol. 1989;142(12):4493–9.
11. Ingham RJ, Raaijmakers J, Lim CS, Mbamalu G, Gish G, Chen F, et al. The Epstein–Barr virus protein, latent membrane protein 2A, co-opts tyrosine kinases used by the T cell receptor. J Biol Chem. 2005;280(40):34133–42.
12. Silva JG, Martins NP, Henriques R, Soares H. HIV-1 Nef impairs the formation of calcium membrane territories controlling the signaling nanoarchitecture at the immunological synapse. J Immunol. 2016;197(10):4042–52.
13. Barber DL, Wherry EJ, Masopust D, Zhu B, Allison JP, Sharpe AH, et al. Restoring function in exhausted CD8 T cells during chronic viral infection. Nature. 2006;439(7077):682–7.
14. Muthumani K, Choo AY, Shedlock DJ, Laddy DJ, Sundaram SG, Hirao L, et al. Human immunodeficiency virus type 1 Nef induces programmed death 1 expression through a p38 mitogen-activated protein kinase-dependent mechanism. J Virol. 2008;82(23):11536–44.
15. El-Far M, Ancuta P, Routy JP, Zhang Y, Bakeman W, Bordi R, et al. Nef promotes evasion of human immunodeficiency virus type 1-infected cells from the CTLA-4-mediated inhibition of T-cell activation. J Gen Virol. 2015;96(Pt 6):1463–77.
16. Chaudhry A, Das SR, Jameel S, George A, Bal V, Mayor S, et al. A two-pronged mechanism for HIV-1 Nef-mediated endocytosis of immune costimulatory molecules CD80 and CD86. Cell Host Microbe. 2007;1(1):37–49.
17. Sugden SM, Bego MG, Pham TN, Cohen EA. Remodeling of the host cell plasma membrane by HIV-1 Nef and Vpu: a strategy to ensure viral fitness and persistence. Viruses. 2016;8(3):67.
18. Pawlak EN, Dikeakos JD. HIV-1 Nef: a master manipulator of the membrane trafficking machinery mediating immune evasion. Biochim Biophys Acta. 2015;1850(4):733–41.
19. Guenzel CA, Herate C, Benichou S. HIV-1 Vpr-a still "enigmatic multitasker". Front Microbiol. 2014;5:127.
20. Haller C, Muller B, Fritz JV, Lamas-Murua M, Stolp B, Pujol FM, et al. HIV-1 Nef and Vpu are functionally redundant broad-spectrum modulators of cell surface receptors, including tetraspanins. J Virol. 2014;88(24):14241–57.
21. Roeth JF, Williams M, Kasper MR, Filzen TM, Collins KL. HIV-1 Nef disrupts MHC-I trafficking by recruiting AP-1 to the MHC-I cytoplasmic tail. J Cell Biol. 2004;167(5):903–13.
22. Jia X, Singh R, Homann S, Yang H, Guatelli J, Xiong Y. Structural basis of evasion of cellular adaptive immunity by HIV-1 Nef. Nat Struct Mol Biol. 2012;19(7):701–6.
23. Dirk BS, Pawlak EN, Johnson AL, Van Nynatten LR, Jacob RA, Heit B, et al. HIV-1 Nef sequesters MHC-I intracellularly by targeting early stages of endocytosis and recycling. Sci Rep. 2016;6:37021.
24. Collins KL, Chen BK, Kalams SA, Walker BD, Baltimore D. HIV-1 Nef protein protects infected primary cells against killing by cytotoxic T lymphocytes. Nature. 1998;391(6665):397–401.
25. Ren X, Park SY, Bonifacino JS, Hurley JH. How HIV-1 Nef hijacks the AP-2 clathrin adaptor to downregulate CD4. Elife. 2014;3:e01754.
26. Chaudhuri R, Lindwasser OW, Smith WJ, Hurley JH, Bonifacino JS. Downregulation of CD4 by human immunodeficiency virus type 1 Nef is

dependent on clathrin and involves direct interaction of Nef with the AP2 clathrin adaptor. J Virol. 2007;81(8):3877–90.

27. Ross TM, Oran AE, Cullen BR. Inhibition of HIV-1 progeny virion release by cell-surface CD4 is relieved by expression of the viral Nef protein. Curr Biol. 1999;9(12):613–21.

28. Wildum S, Schindler M, Munch J, Kirchhoff F. Contribution of Vpu, Env, and Nef to CD4 down-modulation and resistance of human immunodeficiency virus type 1-infected T cells to superinfection. J Virol. 2006;80(16):8047–59.

29. Michel N, Allespach I, Venzke S, Fackler OT, Keppler OT. The Nef protein of human immunodeficiency virus establishes superinfection immunity by a dual strategy to downregulate cell-surface CCR5 and CD4. Curr Biol. 2005;15(8):714–23.

30. Pham TN, Lukhele S, Hajjar F, Routy JP, Cohen EA. HIV Nef and Vpu protect HIV-infected CD4+ T cells from antibody-mediated cell lysis through down-modulation of CD4 and BST2. Retrovirology. 2014;11:15.

31. Veillette M, Desormeaux A, Medjahed H, Gharsallah NE, Coutu M, Baalwa J, et al. Interaction with cellular CD4 exposes HIV-1 envelope epitopes targeted by antibody-dependent cell-mediated cytotoxicity. J Virol. 2014;88(5):2633–44.

32. Piguet V, Gu F, Foti M, Demaurex N, Gruenberg J, Carpentier JL, et al. Nef-induced CD4 degradation: a diacidic-based motif in Nef functions as a lysosomal targeting signal through the binding of beta-COP in endosomes. Cell. 1999;97(1):63–73.

33. Jia X, Weber E, Tokarev A, Lewinski M, Rizk M, Suarez M, et al. Structural basis of HIV-1 Vpu-mediated BST2 antagonism via hijacking of the clathrin adaptor protein complex 1. Elife. 2014;3:e02362.

34. Van Damme N, Goff D, Katsura C, Jorgenson RL, Mitchell R, Johnson MC, et al. The interferon-induced protein BST-2 restricts HIV-1 release and is downregulated from the cell surface by the viral Vpu protein. Cell Host Microbe. 2008;3(4):245–52.

35. Mitchell RS, Katsura C, Skasko MA, Fitzpatrick K, Lau D, Ruiz A, et al. Vpu antagonizes BST-2-mediated restriction of HIV-1 release via beta-TrCP and endo-lysosomal trafficking. PLoS Pathog. 2009;5(5):e1000450.

36. Mangeat B, Gers-Huber G, Lehmann M, Zufferey M, Luban J, Piguet V. HIV-1 Vpu neutralizes the antiviral factor Tetherin/BST-2 by binding it and directing its beta-TrCP2-dependent degradation. PLoS Pathog. 2009;5(9):e1000574.

37. Kueck T, Foster TL, Weinelt J, Sumner JC, Pickering S, Neil SJ. Serine phosphorylation of HIV-1 Vpu and its binding to tetherin regulates interaction with clathrin adaptors. PLoS Pathog. 2015;11(8):e1005141.

38. Margottin F, Bour SP, Durand H, Selig L, Benichou S, Richard V, et al. A novel human WD protein, h-beta TrCp, that interacts with HIV-1 Vpu connects CD4 to the ER degradation pathway through an F-box motif. Mol Cell. 1998;1(4):565–74.

39. Leonard JA, Filzen T, Carter CC, Schaefer M, Collins KL. HIV-1 Nef disrupts intracellular trafficking of major histocompatibility complex class I, CD4, CD8, and CD28 by distinct pathways that share common elements. J Virol. 2011;85(14):6867–81.

40. Swigut T, Shohdy N, Skowronski J. Mechanism for down-regulation of CD28 by Nef. EMBO J. 2001;20(7):1593–604.

41. Mindell JA. Lysosomal acidification mechanisms. Annu Rev Physiol. 2012;74:69–86.

42. Cardelli JA, Richardson J, Miears D. Role of acidic intracellular compartments in the biosynthesis of Dictyostelium lysosomal enzymes. The weak bases ammonium chloride and chloroquine differentially affect proteolytic processing and sorting. J Biol Chem. 1989;264(6):3454–63.

43. Yoshimori T, Yamamoto A, Moriyama Y, Futai M, Tashiro Y. Bafilomycin A1, a specific inhibitor of vacuolar-type H(+)-ATPase, inhibits acidification and protein degradation in lysosomes of cultured cells. J Biol Chem. 1991;266(26):17707–12.

44. Drose S, Bindseil KU, Bowman EJ, Siebers A, Zeeck A, Altendorf K. Inhibitory effect of modified bafilomycins and concanamycins on P- and V-type adenosinetriphosphatases. Biochemistry. 1993;32(15):3902–6.

45. Kaminchik J, Bashan N, Pinchasi D, Amit B, Sarver N, Johnston MI, et al. Expression and biochemical characterization of human immunodeficiency virus type 1 nef gene product. J Virol. 1990;64(7):3447–54.

46. Bresnahan PA, Yonemoto W, Ferrell S, Williams-Herman D, Geleziunas R, Greene WC. A dileucine motif in HIV-1 Nef acts as an internalization signal for CD4 downregulation and binds the AP-1 clathrin adaptor. Curr Biol. 1998;8(22):1235–8.

47. Geyer M, Yu H, Mandic R, Linnemann T, Zheng YH, Fackler OT, et al. Subunit H of the V-ATPase binds to the medium chain of adaptor protein complex 2 and connects Nef to the endocytic machinery. J Biol Chem. 2002;277(32):28521–9.

48. Noviello CM, Benichou S, Guatelli JC. Cooperative binding of the class I major histocompatibility complex cytoplasmic domain and human immunodeficiency virus type 1 Nef to the endosomal AP-1 complex via its mu subunit. J Virol. 2008;82(3):1249–58.

49. Hill MS, Ruiz A, Schmitt K, Stephens EB. Identification of amino acids within the second alpha helical domain of the human immunodeficiency virus type 1 Vpu that are critical for preventing CD4 cell surface expression. Virology. 2010;397(1):104–12.

50. Tiganos E, Friborg J, Allain B, Daniel NG, Yao XJ, Cohen EA. Structural and functional analysis of the membrane-spanning domain of the human immunodeficiency virus type 1 Vpu protein. Virology. 1998;251(1):96–107.

51. Margottin F, Benichou S, Durand H, Richard V, Liu LX, Gomas E, et al. Interaction between the cytoplasmic domains of HIV-1 Vpu and CD4: role of Vpu residues involved in CD4 interaction and in vitro CD4 degradation. Virology. 1996;223(2):381–6.

52. Tervo HM, Homann S, Ambiel I, Fritz JV, Fackler OT, Keppler OT. beta-TrCP is dispensable for Vpu's ability to overcome the CD317/Tetherin-imposed restriction to HIV-1 release. Retrovirology. 2011;8:9.

53. Pang X, Hu S, Li J, Xu F, Mei S, Zhou J, et al. Identification of novel key amino acids at the interface of the transmembrane domains of human BST-2 and HIV-1 Vpu. Retrovirology. 2013;10:84.

54. Kueck T, Neil SJ. A cytoplasmic tail determinant in HIV-1 Vpu mediates targeting of tetherin for endosomal degradation and counteracts interferon-induced restriction. PLoS Pathog. 2012;8(3):e1002609.

55. Osmanov S. HIV type 1 variation in World Health Organization-sponsored vaccine evaluation sites: genetic screening, sequence analysis, and preliminary biological characterization of selected viral strains. WHO Network for HIV Isolation and Characterization. AIDS Res Hum Retroviruses. 1994;10(11):1327–43.

56. June CH, Ledbetter JA, Gillespie MM, Lindsten T, Thompson CB. T-cell proliferation involving the CD28 pathway is associated with cyclosporine-resistant interleukin 2 gene expression. Mol Cell Biol. 1987;7(12):4472–81.

57. Olivieri KC, Mukerji J, Gabuzda D. Nef-mediated enhancement of cellular activation and human immunodeficiency virus type 1 replication in primary T cells is dependent on association with p21-activated kinase 2. Retrovirology. 2011;8:64.

58. Yu H, Khalid M, Heigele A, Schmokel J, Usmani SM, van der Merwe J, et al. Lentiviral Nef proteins manipulate T cells in a subset-specific manner. J Virol. 2015;89(4):1986–2001.

59. Lin CJ, Tam RC. Transcriptional regulation of CD28 expression by CD28GR, a novel promoter element located in exon 1 of the CD28 gene. J Immunol. 2001;166(10):6134–43.

60. Seve M, Favier A, Osman M, Hernandez D, Vaitaitis G, Flores NC, et al. The human immunodeficiency virus-1 Tat protein increases cell proliferation, alters sensitivity to zinc chelator-induced apoptosis, and changes Sp1 DNA binding in HeLa cells. Arch Biochem Biophys. 1999;361(2):165–72.

61. Geleziunas R, Bour S, Wainberg MA. Cell surface down-modulation of CD4 after infection by HIV-1. FASEB J. 1994;8(9):593–600.

62. Rhee SS, Marsh JW. Human immunodeficiency virus type 1 Nef-induced down-modulation of CD4 is due to rapid internalization and degradation of surface CD4. J Virol. 1994;68(8):5156–61.

63. Willey RL, Maldarelli F, Martin MA, Strebel K. Human immunodeficiency virus type 1 Vpu protein induces rapid degradation of CD4. J Virol. 1992;66(12):7193–200.

64. Magadan JG, Perez-Victoria FJ, Sougrat R, Ye Y, Strebel K, Bonifacino JS. Multilayered mechanism of CD4 downregulation by HIV-1 Vpu involving distinct ER retention and ERAD targeting steps. PLoS Pathog. 2010;6(4):e1000869.

65. Heigele A, Schindler M, Gnanadurai CW, Leonard JA, Collins KL, Kirch-hoff F. Down-modulation of CD8alphabeta is a fundamental activity of primate lentiviral Nef proteins. J Virol. 2012;86(1):36–48.

66. El-Far M, Isabelle C, Chomont N, Bourbonniere M, Fonseca S, Ancuta P, et al. Down-regulation of CTLA-4 by HIV-1 Nef protein. PLoS ONE. 2013;8(1):e54295.

67. Alegre ML, Frauwirth KA, Thompson CB. T-cell regulation by CD28 and CTLA-4. Nat Rev Immunol. 2001;1(3):220–8.

68. Vigan R, Neil SJ. Determinants of tetherin antagonism in the transmem-brane domain of the human immunodeficiency virus type 1 Vpu protein. J Virol. 2010;84(24):12958–70.

69. Magadan JG, Bonifacino JS. Transmembrane domain determinants of CD4 Downregulation by HIV-1 Vpu. J Virol. 2012;86(2):757–72.

70. Madjo U, Leymarie O, Fremont S, Kuster A, Nehlich M, Gallois-Montbrun S, et al. LC3C contributes to Vpu-mediated antagonism of BST2/tetherin restriction on HIV-1 release through a Non-canonical autophagy path-way. Cell Rep. 2016;17(9):2221–33.

71. Johnson AL, Dirk BS, Coutu M, Haeryfar SM, Arts EJ, Finzi A, et al. A highly conserved residue in HIV-1 Nef alpha helix 2 modulates protein expres-sion. mSphere. 2016;1(6):e00288-16.

72. Quinones-Mateu ME, Ball SC, Marozsan AJ, Torre VS, Albright JL, Vanham G, et al. A dual infection/competition assay shows a correlation between ex vivo human immunodeficiency virus type 1 fitness and disease pro-gression. J Virol. 2000;74(19):9222–33.

73. Schindler M, Munch J, Kutsch O, Li H, Santiago ML, Bibollet-Ruche F, et al. Nef-mediated suppression of T cell activation was lost in a lentiviral line-age that gave rise to HIV-1. Cell. 2006;125(6):1055–67.

74. Pan X, Rudolph JM, Abraham L, Habermann A, Haller C, Krijnse-Locker J, et al. HIV-1 Nef compensates for disorganization of the immunological synapse by inducing trans-Golgi network-associated Lck signaling. Blood. 2012;119(3):786–97.

75. Jacob RA, Johnson AL, Pawlak EN, Dirk BS, Van Nynatten LR, Haeryfar SMM, et al. The interaction between HIV-1 Nef and adaptor protein-2 reduces Nef-mediated CD4+ T cell apoptosis. Virology. 2017;509:1–10.

76. Bour S, Perrin C, Akari H, Strebel K. The human immunodeficiency virus type 1 Vpu protein inhibits NF-kappa B activation by interfer-ing with beta TrCP-mediated degradation of Ikappa B. J Biol Chem. 2001;276(19):15920–8.

77. Couturier JP, Root-Bernstein RS. HIV may produce inhibitory microRNAs (miRNAs) that block production of CD28, CD4 and some interleukins. J Theor Biol. 2005;235(2):169–84.

78. Harding FA, McArthur JG, Gross JA, Raulet DH, Allison JP. CD28-mediated signalling co-stimulates murine T cells and prevents induction of anergy in T-cell clones. Nature. 1992;356(6370):607–9.

79. Esensten JH, Helou YA, Chopra G, Weiss A, Bluestone JA. CD28 costimula-tion: from mechanism to therapy. Immunity. 2016;44(5):973–88.

80. Kamphorst AO, Wieland A, Nasti T, Yang S, Zhang R, Barber DL, et al. Rescue of exhausted CD8 T cells by PD-1-targeted therapies is CD28-dependent. Science. 2017;55(6332):1423–7.

81. Gaffen SL, Liu KD. Overview of interleukin-2 function, production and clinical applications. Cytokine. 2004;28(3):109–23.

82. Clerici M, Hakim FT, Venzon DJ, Blatt S, Hendrix CW, Wynn TA, et al. Changes in interleukin-2 and interleukin-4 production in asymptomatic, human immunodeficiency virus-seropositive individuals. J Clin Invest. 1993;91(3):759–65.

83. Orsilles MA, Pieri E, Cooke P, Caula C. IL-2 and IL-10 serum levels in HIV-1-infected patients with or without active antiretroviral therapy. APMIS. 2006;114(1):55–60.

84. INSIGHT-ESPRIT Study Group, SILCAAT Scientific Committee, Abrams D, Levy Y, Losso MH, Babiker A, et al. Interleukin-2 therapy in patients with HIV infection. N Engl J Med. 2009;361(16):1548–59.

85. Chun TW, Engel D, Mizell SB, Ehler LA, Fauci AS. Induction of HIV-1 replica-tion in latently infected CD4+ T cells using a combination of cytokines. J Exp Med. 1998;188(1):83–91.

86. Wang FX, Xu Y, Sullivan J, Souder E, Argyris EG, Acheampong EA, et al. IL-7 is a potent and proviral strain-specific inducer of latent HIV-1 cellular res-ervoirs of infected individuals on virally suppressive HAART. J Clin Invest. 2005;115(1):128–37.

87. Margolis DM, Garcia JV, Hazuda DJ, Haynes BF. Latency reversal and viral clearance to cure HIV-1. Science. 2016;353(6297):aaf6517.

88. Asjo B, Cefai D, Debre P, Dudoit Y, Autran B. A novel mode of human immunodeficiency virus type 1 (HIV-1) activation: ligation of CD28 alone induces HIV-1 replication in naturally infected lymphocytes. J Virol. 1993;67(7):4395–8.

89. Weinberg MS, Morris KV. Are viral-encoded microRNAs mediating latent HIV-1 infection? DNA Cell Biol. 2006;25(4):223–31.

90. Mondino A, Mueller DL. mTOR at the crossroads of T cell proliferation and tolerance. Semin Immunol. 2007;19(3):162–72.

91. Besnard E, Hakre S, Kampmann M, Lim HW, Hosmane NN, Martin A, et al. The mTOR complex controls HIV latency. Cell Host Microbe. 2016;20(6):785–97.

92. Husain M, Gusella GL, Klotman ME, Gelman IH, Ross MD, Schwartz EJ, et al. HIV-1 Nef induces proliferation and anchorage-independent growth in podocytes. J Am Soc Nephrol. 2002;13(7):1806–15.

93. Adachi A, Gendelman HE, Koenig S, Folks T, Willey R, Rabson A, et al. Pro-duction of acquired immunodeficiency syndrome-associated retrovirus in human and nonhuman cells transfected with an infectious molecular clone. J Virol. 1986;59(2):284–91.

94. Dirk BS, Jacob RA, Johnson AL, Pawlak EN, Cavanagh PC, Van Nynat-ten L, et al. Viral bimolecular fluorescence complementation: a novel tool to study intracellular vesicular trafficking pathways. PLoS ONE. 2015;10(4):e0125619.

95. Dudley DM, Gao Y, Nelson KN, Henry KR, Nankya I, Gibson RM, et al. A novel yeast-based recombination method to clone and propagate diverse HIV-1 isolates. Biotechniques. 2009;46(6):458–67.

96. Bolte S, Cordelieres FP. A guided tour into subcellular colocalization analy-sis in light microscopy. J Microsc. 2006;224(Pt 3):213–32.

Promoter expression of HERV-K (HML-2) provirus-derived sequences is related to LTR sequence variation and polymorphic transcription factor binding sites

Meagan Montesion[1,4] , Zachary H. Williams[1], Ravi P. Subramanian[1,5], Charlotte Kuperwasser[2,3] and John M. Coffin[1*]

Abstract

Background: Increased transcription of the human endogenous retrovirus group HERV-K (HML-2) is often seen during disease. Although the mechanism of its tissue-specific activation is unclear, research shows that LTR CpG hypomethylation alone is not sufficient to induce its promoter activity and that the transcriptional milieu of a malignant cell contributes, at least partly, to differential HML-2 expression.

Results: We analyzed the relationship between LTR sequence variation and promoter expression patterns in human breast cancer cell lines, finding them to be positively correlated. In particular, two proviruses (3q12.3 and 11p15.4) displayed increased activity in almost all tumorigenic cell lines sampled. Using a transcription factor binding site prediction algorithm, we identified two unique binding sites in each 5′ LTR that appeared to be associated with inducing promoter activity during neoplasia. Genomic analysis of the homologous proviruses in several non-human primates indicated post-integration genetic drift in two transcription factor binding sites, away from the ancestral sequence and towards the active form. Based on the sequences of 2504 individuals from the 1000 Genomes Project, the active form of the 11p15.4 site was found to be polymorphic within the human population, with an allele frequency of 51%, whereas the activating mutation in the 3q12.3 provirus was fixed in humans but not present in the orthologous provirus in chimpanzees or gorillas.

Conclusions: These data suggest that stage-specific transcription factors at least partly contribute to LTR promoter activity during transformation and that, in some cases, transcription factor binding site polymorphisms may be responsible for the differential HML-2 expression often seen between individuals.

Keywords: Endogenous retrovirus, HERV-K, HML-2, LTR, Transcription, Tumorigenesis

Background

Retroviruses are unique in that they are the only virus family known to exist in both endogenous and exogenous forms [1, 2]. Their integrated DNA sequences, known as proviruses, include at least four genes (*gag, pro, pol,* and *env*) flanked by long terminal repeats (LTRs), which contain all elements necessary to initiate and terminate viral transcription [2, 3]. Genetic transmission of these sequences occurs with germline integration, producing endogenous retroviruses (ERVs). ERVs are inherited in a Mendelian fashion and are subject to natural selection; those with deleterious effects are generally either lost from the population or inactivated by mutation, whereas those with neutral or advantageous effects remain [2, 4]. As a consequence of the accumulation of these elements over time, nearly 8% of the human genome is derived from such viral sequences [5–7].

*Correspondence: john.coffin@tufts.edu
[1] Department of Molecular Biology and Microbiology, Tufts University School of Medicine, Boston, MA, USA
Full list of author information is available at the end of the article

Once classified with other "junk DNA", ERVs are now credited with providing genomic plasticity through the use of viral proteins for host functions and alternative regulation of host gene transcription. For example, proviruses contain numerous promoters, splice sites, transcription factor binding sites, and polyadenylation signals, all of which can have significant effects on neighboring host gene expression [2, 8, 9]. Syncytins, fusogenic proteins derived from ERV *env* sequences, are essential for placenta development and mediate cell fusion to form the syncytiotrophoblast layer [10, 11]. Although ERV expression is usually silenced through epigenetic and chromatin modification, primarily via CpG methylation [8, 12–14], there are a few known instances of host cell co-option of ERV expression. Recent studies show human endogenous retrovirus (HERV) expression to be increased in human embryonic stem cells (hESCs) and human preimplantation embryos and to play a critical role during embryogenesis through the maintenance of pluripotency and hESC identity [15–19]. Increased expression of HERV proteins was found to be correlated with increased IFITM1 expression, resulting in viral immunoprotection during human embryogenesis [19, 20].

Despite these exceptions, increased HERV activity is largely associated with malignancy, especially cancer. Activation of stem cell-associated retroviruses (SCARs) in human cancer is hypothesized to be associated with increased likelihood of metastasis, immune evasion of cancer cells, and a predictive marker of poor prognosis [21, 22]. Increased cancer-related expression is attributable in part to global hypomethylation, a common consequence of tumorigenesis, and LTR hypomethylation is widely documented to result in promoter activation [11, 13, 23]. However, in vitro treatment with 5-aza-2'-deoxycytidine, a DNA methyltransferase inhibitor, shows that LTR hypomethylation alone is not always sufficient to induce promoter activity, suggesting that the proper transcriptional milieu of a cell may also be required [24–26]. Ubiquitous transcription factors, such as Sp1, Sp3, and YY1, are linked with LTR activity but do not explain the cell-specific expression that is often seen [8, 25, 27].

Expression from HERV-K (HML-2), the most recently integrated and biologically active HERV group, is upregulated in up to 85% of breast cancer samples, although the mechanism of activation is still unclear [28–31]. RNA sequence analysis of cells in an in vitro mammary carcinogenesis model shows that LTR-driven transcription of HML-2 proviruses is restricted to tumorigenic human mammary epithelial cells (HMECs), suggesting that stage-specific transcription factors appearing during malignant transformation play a role in LTR activation [32]. The goal of this study was to investigate how

LTR sequence variation among the various HML-2 proviruses affects activation of its promoter during HMEC transformation.

Overall, we found the most widespread increase in promoter activity during transformation in two proviruses (located at 3q12.3 and 11p15.4). Through a combination of reporter construct assays and RNA-Seq analyses, we identified two transcription factor binding sites on each 5' LTR that were associated with promoter activity in transformed cells. Further genomic analysis of these proviruses, using data from the 1000 Genomes Project as well as comparison with homologous proviruses in several other hominoid species, showed that both of these sites had been created by mutations in the 5' LTR that occurred post viral integration. The 3q12.3 site has become fixed in the human population whereas that at 11p15.4 is polymorphic, with the active form having an allele frequency of 51%. In both cases, these sites have evolved away from the inactive ancestral sequence and towards an active form. These results emphasize the importance of studying HERV transcription at the single provirus and single nucleotide level, as polymorphisms in critical binding sites may be responsible for the differential HML-2 expression often seen between individuals.

Results

Differential HML-2 promoter expression is correlated with 5' LTR sequence similarity

The HML-2 5' LTR contains all elements necessary for driving transcription. Removal of core promoter elements results in reduced promoter activity, suggesting that these sequences are critical for proper LTR-driven expression [9, 25, 33]. Each provirus has accumulated numerous unique mutations over time, suggesting that LTR sequence variation could contribute to differential HML-2 expression, particularly through the alteration of transcription factor binding sites. Through a series of dual-luciferase assays, we sought to evaluate whether LTR sequence identity is correlated with similar promoter expression patterns during breast cancer tumorigenesis.

The proviruses of interest for this study were chosen based on a preliminary investigation in which we used single-genome sequencing to detect provirus-specific transcripts from eight human breast cancer cell lines. From this analysis, we produced a list of the top ten highest expressing HML-2 proviruses within these cell lines tested (Additional file 1). 16p11.2 and K105 were excluded from our study since 16p11.2 has no 5' LTR and the unmapped K105 exhibited cloning inconsistencies caused by its location within the unassembled centromeric region Un_g1000219 [4, 34]. The remaining eight proviruses, plus 8p23.1c, a segmental duplication of 11p15.4 [4], were chosen as our loci of interest. The alternative names and chromosomal locations of these proviruses are listed in Table 1.

Phylogenetic analysis of the LTRs from these nine proviruses shows that most of them are classified as LTR-HS, the LTR group that contains the youngest proviruses, including ~90% of the human-specific integrations (Fig. 1a) [4, 9, 35]. The 5′ LTR sequences from each provirus were cloned into pGL4.17[luc2/Neo], a promoterless firefly luciferase vector, directly upstream of the luc2 gene. The relative promoter activity of these sequences was determined based on luc2 expression and normalized against that of an internal control vector, containing a Renilla luciferase gene (Rluc) driven by an SV40 promoter (Fig. 1b). A panel of eighteen human cell lines was transiently co-transfected with these vectors. The panel comprised of two immortalized HMEC cell lines, fifteen tumorigenic breast cancer cell lines (representing all three molecular subtypes), and one teratocarcinoma cell line known to produce HML-2 transcripts and retroviral-like particles (RVLPs) at high levels [9, 36]. Characterization of the cell lines used is shown in Table 2.

Although minimal promoter activity was detected in immortalized HMECs transfected with any of the HML-2 LTR reporter constructs, significant upregulation of expression driven by one or more LTRs was seen in 73% (11/15) of the tumorigenic breast cancer cell lines (Fig. 1c). This expression pattern is consistent with previous reports that suggest up to 85% of breast cancer samples have a significant increase in HML-2 activity [29, 31, 37]. Overall, each LTR was significantly expressed in at least one cell line tested but showed differential expression across the panel. Two proviruses (3q12.3 and 11p15.4) were significantly upregulated in nearly all neoplastic cell lines investigated, whereas others were only upregulated in a select few (Fig. 1d). The highest level

of combined HML-2 expression in a breast cell line was exhibited by T47D (Fig. 1c), a tumorigenic breast cancer cell line known to produce RVLPs under hormonally-stimulated conditions [3, 38, 39]. However, this activity level was only about half that seen in the Tera-1 cells, consistent with our previous report that Tera-1 cells produce markedly higher numbers of HML-2 transcripts than breast cancer cell lines [32].

We next sought to determine if LTRs of similar sequence share similar patterns of promoter activity. For this purpose, we created a percent sequence identity matrix, by multiple sequence alignment using Clustal Omega [40], and an HML-2 percent expression similarity matrix, determined through pairwise comparisons of significant promoter activity within each cell line tested (Additional file 2). We found the two values to be correlated, suggesting that LTRs with high sequence similarity are more likely to exhibit significant promoter activity under the transcriptional environment of the same cell line (Fig. 2a). Overall, LTRs with ~70% sequence similarity shared promoter expression patterns ~60% of the time, whereas LTRs with ~95% sequence identity shared promoter expression patterns ~90% of the time (Fig. 2b). With the exception of the 5′ LTR of 3q12.3 (Fig. 2, red), the sequences clustered into two observable groups. The expression pattern of the 3q12.3 5′ LTR was not similar to any other LTR and instead exhibited unusually high promoter activity levels, with significant promoter expression seen in almost every transformed cell line investigated (Fig. 1d).

Identification of transcription factor binding sites critical for HML-2 promoter activity during neoplasia

The association between LTR sequence and cell line-specific expression suggests that certain sequence-specific elements, such as transcription factor binding sites, play a large role in determining differential promoter activity. Increased HML-2 expression is largely seen during tumorigenesis and our recent results indicate that LTR-driven transcription does not occur until post-transformation [32]. The following experiments were performed to further investigate the relationship between malignant transformation and expression and to elucidate the specific LTR sequences required.

For this purpose, we focused on three cell lines: HME, HMLE-Her2, and HMLE-Ras. These cells were all derived from the same HMEC population and are therefore isogenic, differing only by oncogene overexpression. HME cells are non-transformed but immortalized through hTERT (human telomerase reverse transcriptase) overexpression. The HMLE cells, in addition to being hTERT-immortalized, are transformed through the introduction of SV40 large and small T antigens. HMLE-Her2 and

Table 1 HML-2 proviruses with alternative names and genomic coordinates

Provirus	Alternative names	Chromosomal location (hg19)
1q22	K102, K(C1b), K50a, ERVK-7	chr1:155,596,457–155,605,636
3q12.3	KII, ERVK-5	chr3:101,410,737–101,419,859
3q21.2	KI, ERVK-4	chr3:125,609,302–125,618,439
5p13.3	K104, K50d	chr5:30,486,760–30,496,205
7p22.1b	K108R, ERVK-6	chr7:4,630,561–4,640,031
8p23.1c		chr8:12,073,970–12,083,497
11p15.4	K7	chr11:3,468,656–3,478,209
21q21.1	K60, ERVK-23	chr21:19,933,659–19,941,962
22q11.21	K101, K(C22), ERVK-24	chr22:18,926,187–18,935,361

From Subramanian et al. [4] and Montesion et al. [32]

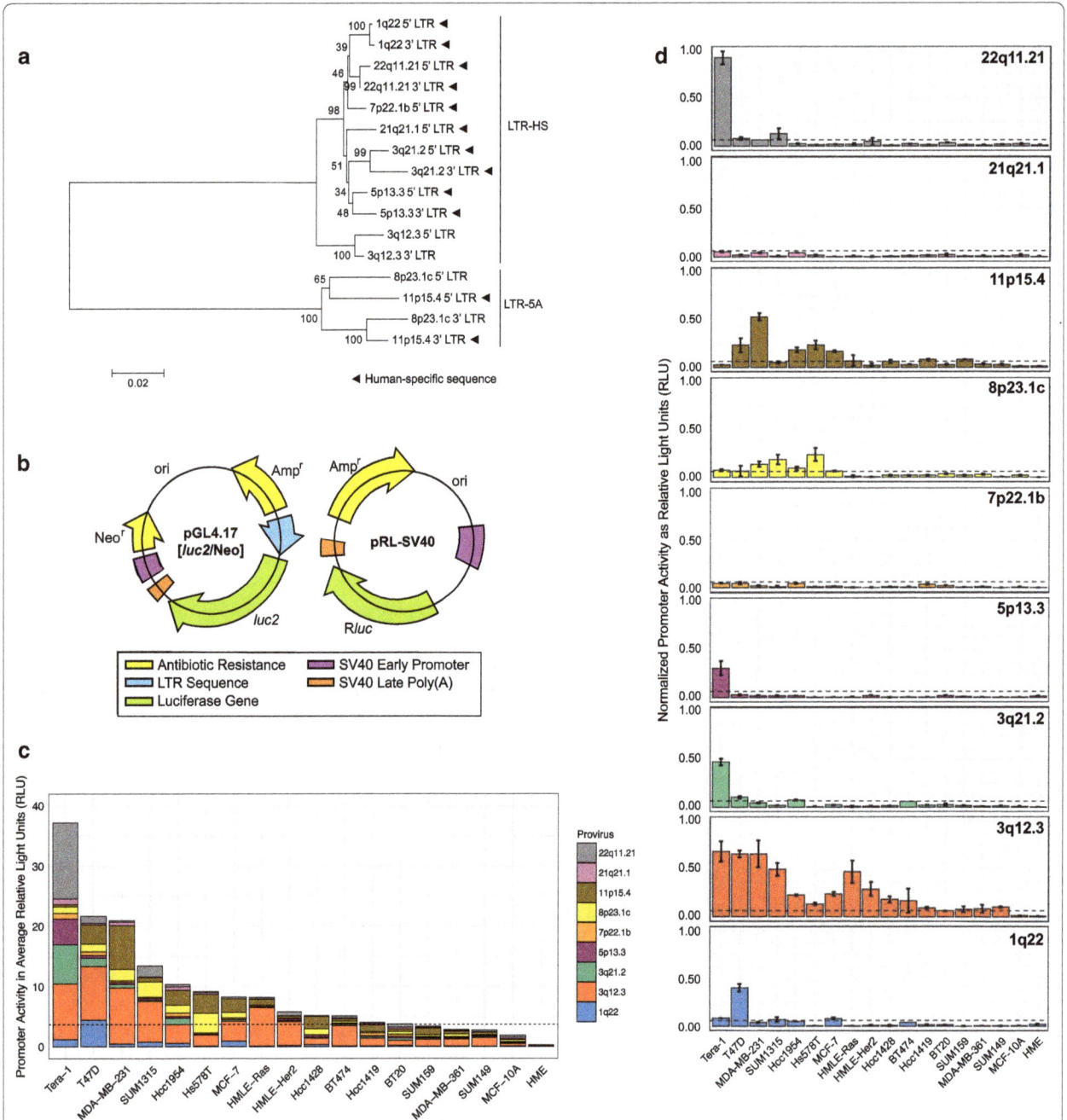

Fig. 1 HML-2 proviruses exhibit differential promoter activity in tumorigenic cells and negligible activity in immortalized HMEs. **a** Neighbor-joining tree displaying 5′ and 3′ LTR sequence relationship of the nine HML-2 proviruses used in this study. Bootstrap values are shown to the left of each node and scale is substitutions/site. LTR type (LTR-HS or LTR-5A) is shown to the right of the tree. Human-specific sequences are designated with a black triangle. **b** Schematic of the reporter constructs used in the dual-luciferase assay. Left, promoter-less firefly luciferase vector (pGL4.17[luc2/Neo]). Right, control *Renilla* luciferase vector (pRL-SV40). Direction of gene transcription is shown by arrows. Important gene regions are differentiated by colors and the names associated with those colors are displayed underneath. **c, d** Relative 5′ LTR promoter activity determined by dual luciferase assay in eighteen human cell lines. Data are organized by cell line in (**c**) and by provirus in (**d**). Promoter activity is displayed as relative light units (RLU) normalized against the internal control *Renilla* expression. Data in (**d**) are normalized against the highest expression value in the dataset. Statistical significance (dashed line, $p < 0.05$) was generated by ANOVA with Bonferroni's multiple comparisons test and is based on comparisons to HME expression. All experiments were conducted in triplicate and data displayed as mean (**c**) or mean ± standard deviation (**d**)

Table 2 Characterization of cell lines used for transfection

Breast cancer molecular subtype	Hormone receptor status	Cell lines
Luminal	ER+ and/or PR + HER2 ±	T47D, MCF-7, Hcc1428, BT474, MDA-MB-361
HER2/*neu*	ER− PR− HER2 +	SUM1315, Hcc1954, Hcc1419
Basal	ER− PR− HER2 −	MDA-MB-231, Hs578T, BT20, SUM159, SUM149

Additional cell types		Cell lines
Immortalized human mammary epithelial cells		HME, MCF-10A
Transformed human mammary epithelial cells		HMLE-Her2, HMLE-Ras
Human teratocarcinoma cells		Tera-1

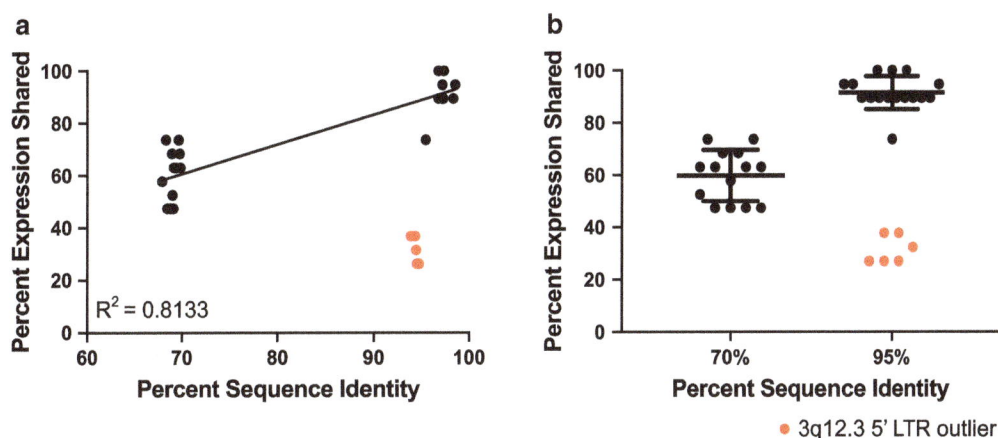

Fig. 2 LTR sequence identity is correlated with promoter expression patterns, with the exception of 3q12.3. Scatter plots displaying the correlation between percent sequence identity and shared percent expression. Raw values are shown in Additional file 2 and are based on pairwise comparisons. Best fit line and its R^2 value are shown for (**a**) (black values only). Error bars depict the mean ± standard deviation in (**b**) (black values only). Outlying 3q12.3 5′ LTR data points are shown in red for both plots

HMLE-Ras differ from one another by their oncogene overexpression, *ERBB2* (also known as HER2/*neu*) and *HRAS*, respectively. These cell lines provided the opportunity to investigate how specific differences in the transcriptional environment of the cell can affect LTR expression.

We detected increased promoter activity from 3q12.3 and 11p15.4 in HMLE-Ras cells as well as increased activity from 3q12.3 in HMLE-Her2 cells. The significance of this expression was determined as compared to the HME cell line (Fig. 3a). In effort to explain this pattern, we sought to identify transcription factor binding sites that are unique to each LTR and therefore may be responsible for the selective activation seen of one LTR over another. Using MatInspector, a transcription factor binding site prediction software by Genomatix [41], we found a total of 63 unique sites among the nine LTRs in this study. Of those, 13 were unique to 3q12.3 and 20 were unique to 11p15.4 (Table 3).

The same software was used to create a list of transcription factors predicted to bind to the unique sites on the 5′ LTRs of 3q12.3 and 11p15.4. In a previous study [32] the expressed RNAs of the HMLE-Ras, HMLE-Her2, and HME cell lines were sequenced, alongside the established human breast cancer cell line Hcc1954, using Illumina MiSeq sequencing. The transcript abundance levels, measured as FPKM, of these transcription factors were compared to assess upregulation of their expression in the tumorigenic cell lines as compared to the non-transformed HME control, and related to levels of expression of the proviruses at 3q12.3 and 11p15.4. Overall, we saw a significant increase in expression of transcription factors known to bind to the HOX-PBX and RFX3 sites on the 3q12.3 5′ LTR as well as a significant increase in those known to bind to the ATF and RORA sites on the 11p15.4 5′ LTR (Fig. 3b), implicating these sites and one or more of the upregulated factors in LTR activation during neoplasia.

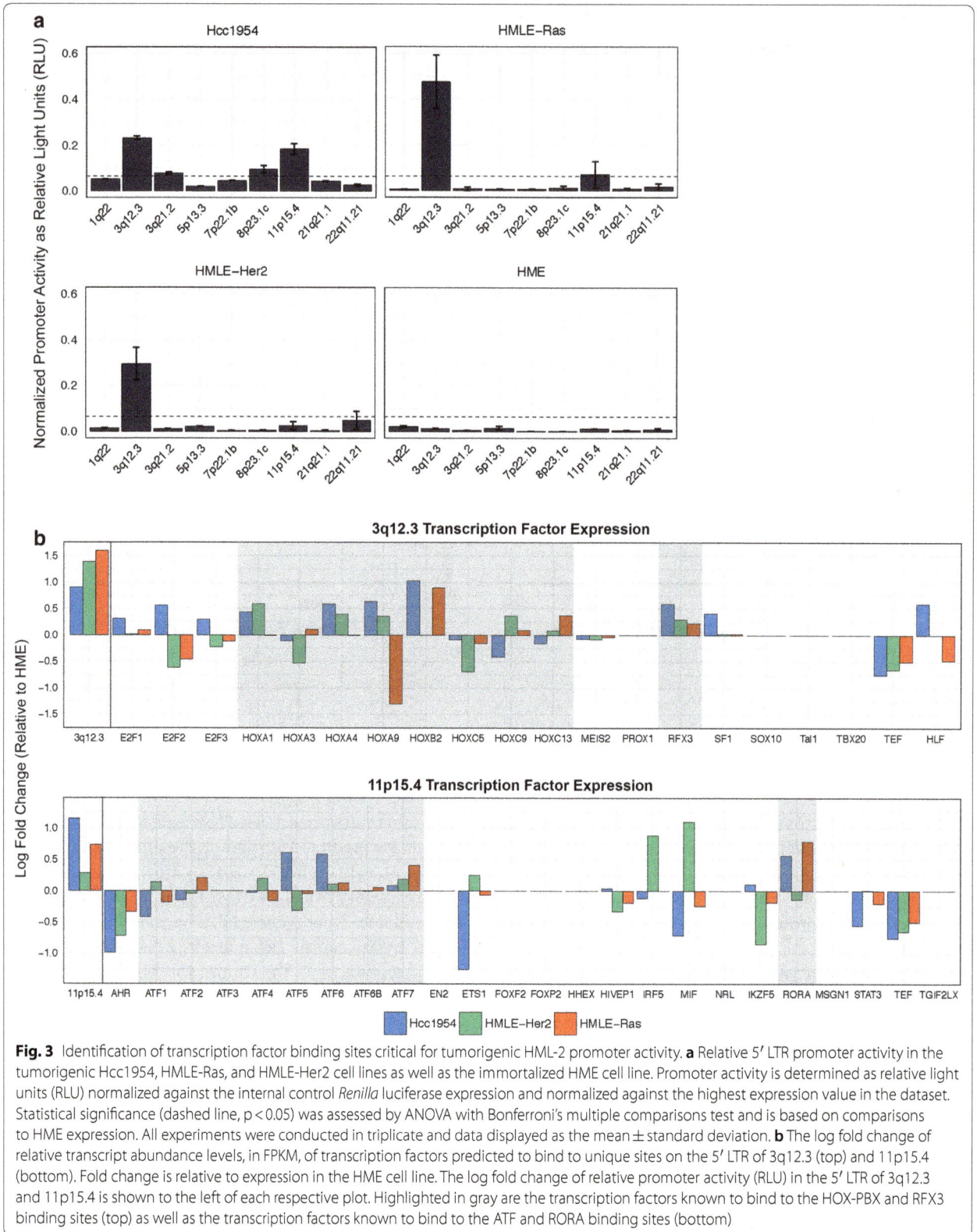

Fig. 3 Identification of transcription factor binding sites critical for tumorigenic HML-2 promoter activity. **a** Relative 5′ LTR promoter activity in the tumorigenic Hcc1954, HMLE-Ras, and HMLE-Her2 cell lines as well as the immortalized HME cell line. Promoter activity is determined as relative light units (RLU) normalized against the internal control *Renilla* luciferase expression and normalized against the highest expression value in the dataset. Statistical significance (dashed line, $p < 0.05$) was assessed by ANOVA with Bonferroni's multiple comparisons test and is based on comparisons to HME expression. All experiments were conducted in triplicate and data displayed as the mean ± standard deviation. **b** The log fold change of relative transcript abundance levels, in FPKM, of transcription factors predicted to bind to unique sites on the 5′ LTR of 3q12.3 (top) and 11p15.4 (bottom). Fold change is relative to expression in the HME cell line. The log fold change of relative promoter activity (RLU) in the 5′ LTR of 3q12.3 and 11p15.4 is shown to the left of each respective plot. Highlighted in gray are the transcription factors known to bind to the HOX-PBX and RFX3 binding sites (top) as well as the transcription factors known to bind to the ATF and RORA binding sites (bottom)

Table 3 Unique transcription factor binding sites found in HML-2 5′ LTRs of interest

Provirus	Unique binding site
1q22	NBRE[‡]
3q12.3	CDE, E2F, HOX-PBX, MRG1[‡], PROX1, RFX3[†], SF1[†], SOX10, TAL1-E2A, TBX20, TEF-HLF[‡], TGIF[†], TR2[‡]
3q21.2	GLI1[†], IK3, NFY[‡], NKX29[†], SIX2[†], STAT5
5p13.3	CARF[‡], MYBL1[‡]
7p22.1b	EKLF[‡], GAGA[‡], GLI3[‡]
8p23.1c	AML1[‡], BHLHB2[‡], DMRT7[‡], HMGA[‡], HOX1-3[‡], MAFF[‡], MEF2[‡], NRF1[†], PAX1[‡], SOX17[‡], STAT5A[‡]
11p15.4	AHRARNT[‡], ATF, ATF6, CETS1P54, EN2[‡], ETS1, FOXP2[†], FREAC2[†], HDBP1-2, HHEX, HIVEP1[†], IRF5, MIF1[†], NRL, PEGASUS, RORA, SGN1, STAT3, TEF[†], TGIF2LX
21q21.1	CHOP[†], NFKAPPAB50[†], USF[†], ZNF300[†]
22q11.21	GRHL1[‡], MASH1[†], TAL1BETAHEB[†]

Only sites unique to each 5′ LTR, as compared to the other eight 5′ LTRs, are shown

[†] Present only in other HML-2 solo LTR(s)

[‡] Present in other HML-2 full length provirus(es) and solo LTR(s)

Removal of critical binding sites decreases HML-2 promoter activity in neoplastic cell lines

The functionality of these sites was assessed by mutating each one individually. A multiple sequence alignment was performed using the sequences of all nine 5′ LTRs. From this analysis, we created a consensus sequence for each critical binding site, which we deemed to be the "non-active" version of each site. The full binding site sequence in each 5′ and 3′ LTR of the nine proviruses of interest in this study are provided in Additional file 3, Additional file 4, Additional file 5 and Additional file 6. The 3q12.3 HOX-PBX binding site differed from the consensus non-active sequence by a five base pairs, including a duplication of four nucleotides (Fig. 4a). Reversion of these sites significantly decreased LTR promoter activity in both neoplastic cell lines, with activity decreasing by twofold in HMLE-Ras cells (Fig. 4c, left) and by sevenfold in HMLE-Her2 cells (Fig. 4c, middle). The 3q12.3 RFX3 binding site only differed from the consensus sequence by one nucleotide, an A to C transversion (Fig. 4b), and yet removal of this site decreased LTR activity by fivefold in both HMLE-Ras cells (Fig. 4c, left) and HMLE-Her2 cells (Fig. 4c, middle). Activity was decreased to levels comparable to that of 1q22, a proviral LTR with no significant promoter activity in these cell lines (Fig. 4c). Mutating these sites did not significantly decrease LTR promoter activity in Hcc1954 cells (Fig. 4c, right), which also showed elevated expression of transcription factors known to bind to five unique 3q12.3 sites (E2F, HOX-PBX, RFX3, SF1, TEF-HLF) (Fig. 3b), suggesting that the other active binding sites can compensate for promoter activity when only some of them are removed.

Similar results were seen with the 11p15.4 5′ LTR. The consensus sequence differed from the ATF binding site by nine nucleotides (Fig. 5a) and back mutating the

binding site to match the consensus sequenced decreased promoter activity by sixfold in HMLE-Ras cells (Fig. 5c, left). The RORA binding site differed by eleven nucleotides from the consensus sequence (Fig. 5b) and mutating all of these to the consensus bases decreased promoter activity by fivefold in HMLE-Ras cells (Fig. 5c, left). Again, these changes decreased activity to levels comparable with 1q22 (Fig. 5c, left). As in the case of 3q12.3, no decrease in promoter activity was seen in the Hcc1954 cell line (Fig. 5c, right), which had elevated expression of transcription factors known to bind to four unique 11p15.4 sites (ATF, HIVEP1, PEGASUS, RORA) (Fig. 3b, bottom).

Most unique HML-2 transcription factor binding sites were acquired over time following integration and are fixed in the human population

At the time of integration, the 5′ and 3′ LTRs of a provirus are almost always identical. Over time, as mutations are accumulated, sequence variation between the two LTRs increases. By aligning the 5′ and 3′ LTRs of 3q12.3 and 11p15.4, we were able to determine whether these critical transcription factor binding sites were present at the time of insertion (as evidenced by its presence in both LTRs) or were acquired over time (and found in only one LTR). We determined that one of the sites, RFX3 found in 3q12.3, was present at the time of insertion, but that three of the binding sites were acquired over time (Table 4). We analyzed the remaining unique binding sites in this same manner, with the exception of sites found on 7p22.1b and 21q21.1, which do not have full 3′ LTRs. Overall, only 21% (12/56) of the unique sites were present at the time of insertion (Fig. 6a, left), the majority of which (58%, 7/12) were found in the 3q12.3 5′ LTR (Fig. 6b).

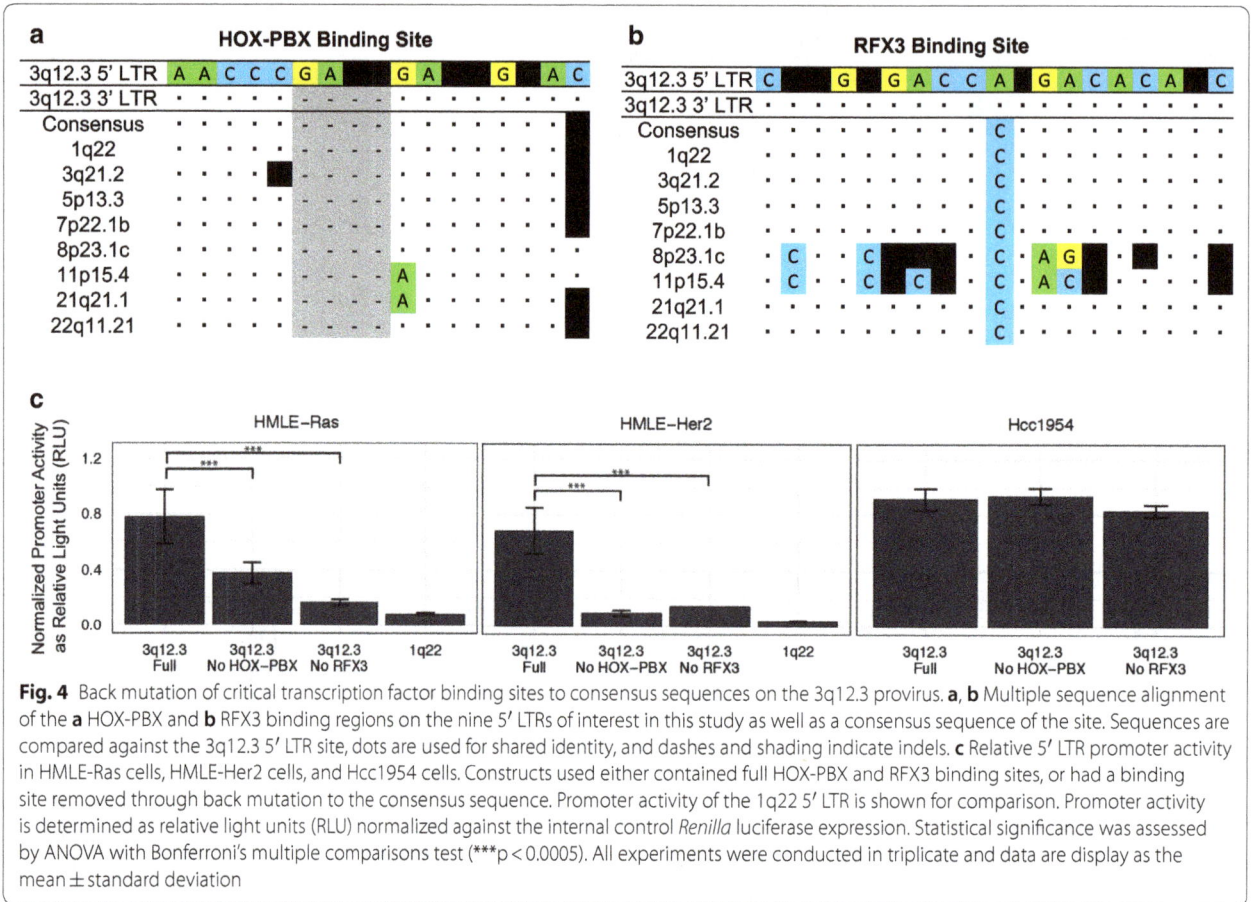

Fig. 4 Back mutation of critical transcription factor binding sites to consensus sequences on the 3q12.3 provirus. **a, b** Multiple sequence alignment of the **a** HOX-PBX and **b** RFX3 binding regions on the nine 5′ LTRs of interest in this study as well as a consensus sequence of the site. Sequences are compared against the 3q12.3 5′ LTR site, dots are used for shared identity, and dashes and shading indicate indels. **c** Relative 5′ LTR promoter activity in HMLE-Ras cells, HMLE-Her2 cells, and Hcc1954 cells. Constructs used either contained full HOX-PBX and RFX3 binding sites, or had a binding site removed through back mutation to the consensus sequence. Promoter activity of the 1q22 5′ LTR is shown for comparison. Promoter activity is determined as relative light units (RLU) normalized against the internal control *Renilla* luciferase expression. Statistical significance was assessed by ANOVA with Bonferroni's multiple comparisons test (***p < 0.0005). All experiments were conducted in triplicate and data are display as the mean ± standard deviation

To determine the distribution of these sites within the human population, we analyzed the VCF (Variant Call Format) files of 2504 individuals, as supplied by phase 3 of the 1000 Genomes Project [42]. Of the four binding sites that we found to be critical for HML-2 promoter expression during neoplasia, three had allele frequencies > 99% and are therefore fixed in the population. The RORA binding site, found in the 11p15.4 5′ LTR, was found to be polymorphic with an allele frequency of 50.76% (Table 4). Overall, only 8% (5/63) of the unique sites that we identified were polymorphic in the human population (Fig. 6a, right).

Evolution of the HML-2 HOX-PBX and RORA binding sites

Alignment of the 5′ and 3′ LTRs of the 3q12.3 provirus revealed a 4 bp insertion, found in the middle of the HOX-PBX site, resulting from duplication of a GATT sequence (Fig. 4a). This provirus is estimated to have integrated ~10 million years ago and is present in gorillas, chimpanzees, and bonobos, as well as humans [4]. Using the UCSC Genome Browser, we examined this LTR in several non-human primate reference genomes. We found that despite the conservation of the 3q12.3

provirus across multiple hominoid species, the 4 bp insertion, and consequently the HOX-PBX binding site, is only present in humans and Denisovans (Fig. 6c). These results suggest that this binding site was acquired sometime after the human-chimpanzee evolutionary split and has been stably integrated in the human genome ever since.

The RORA binding site on 11p15.4 was one of the only polymorphic unique binding sites that we identified. This polymorphism is due to a single nucleotide change, where 51% of alleles in the human population contains an A at the 23rd base pair in the site (and therefore an intact RORA site) and 49% of the population contains a T. This provirus is of particular interest because 11p15.4 is a segmental duplication of 8p23.1c, which is estimated to have integrated ~20 million years ago. Although the proviral sequence is quite old, the duplication occurred after the human-chimpanzee split, and the 11p15.4 sequence is human-specific [4]. We aligned the 5′ and 3′ LTRs of these two proviruses and compared their sequences at the RORA binding site. We found that although both of the 3′ LTRs at this site are identical, the 5′ LTRs differ by one nucleotide,

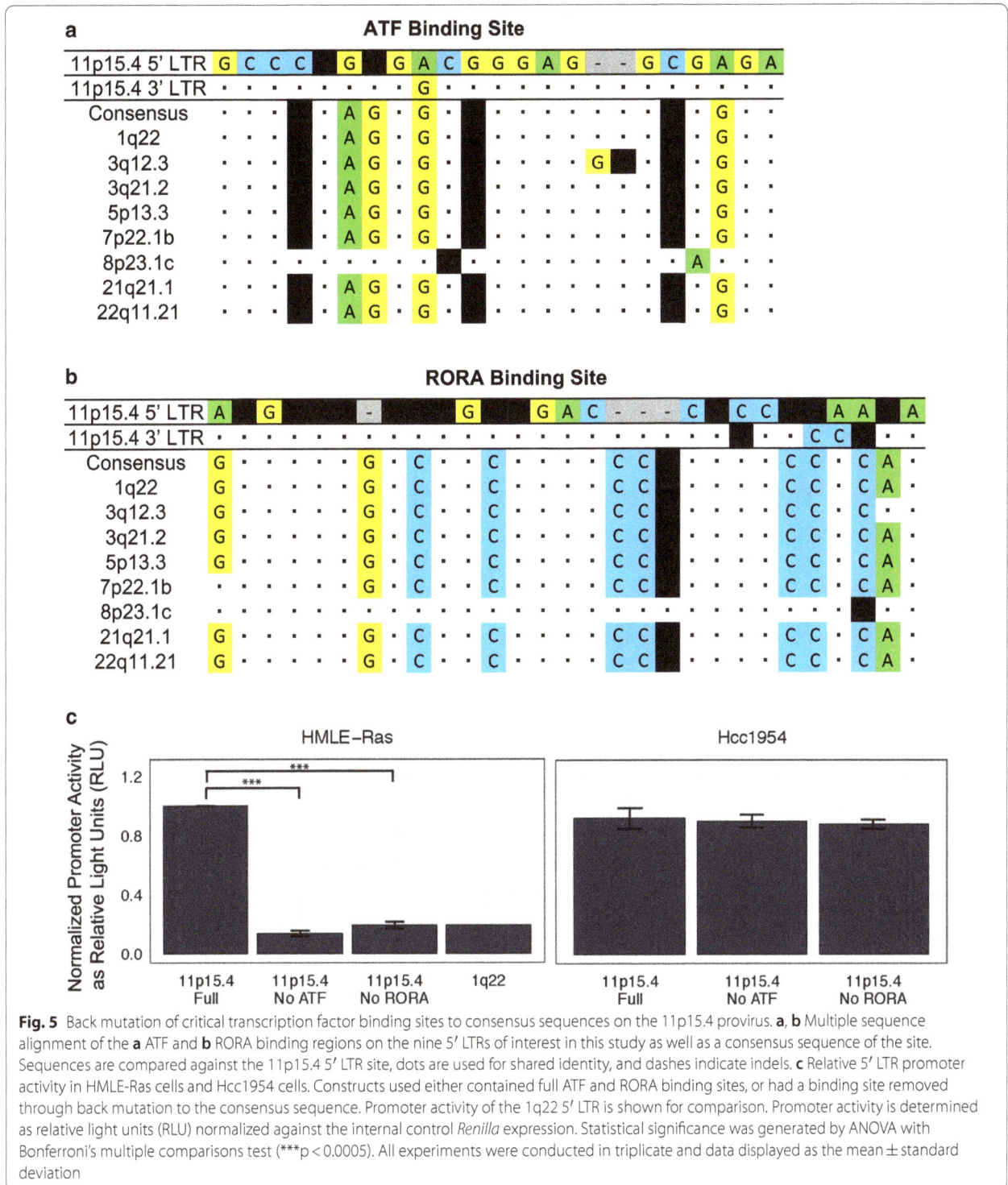

Fig. 5 Back mutation of critical transcription factor binding sites to consensus sequences on the 11p15.4 provirus. **a, b** Multiple sequence alignment of the **a** ATF and **b** RORA binding regions on the nine 5′ LTRs of interest in this study as well as a consensus sequence of the site. Sequences are compared against the 11p15.4 5′ LTR site, dots are used for shared identity, and dashes indicate indels. **c** Relative 5′ LTR promoter activity in HMLE-Ras cells and Hcc1954 cells. Constructs used either contained full ATF and RORA binding sites, or had a binding site removed through back mutation to the consensus sequence. Promoter activity of the 1q22 5′ LTR is shown for comparison. Promoter activity is determined as relative light units (RLU) normalized against the internal control *Renilla* expression. Statistical significance was generated by ANOVA with Bonferroni's multiple comparisons test (***p < 0.0005). All experiments were conducted in triplicate and data displayed as the mean ± standard deviation

the same 23rd nucleotide that is responsible for the RORA polymorphism (Fig. 6d). The 5′ LTR also differed from the 3′ by deletion of 3 bp, which must have predated the segmental duplication of this provirus, as it was also found in the 8p23.1c 5′ LTR. Based on

these observations, it appears as though the provirus at 11p15.4 in half of the human population has evolved away from the ancestral 8p23.1c sequence, resulting in a functional RORA binding site.

Table 4 Characterization of LTR binding sites critical for 3q12.3 and 11p15.4 promoter activity in tumorigenic cells

Provirus	Binding site	LTR	Binding site allele frequency	Binding site evolution
3q12.3	HOX-PBX	5′ LTR	99.68% (fixed)	Acquired
	RFX3	5′ and 3′ LTR	99.96% (fixed)	Present at the time of insertion
11p15.4	ATF	5′ LTR	99.88% (fixed)	Acquired
	RORA	5′ LTR	50.76% (polymorphic)	Acquired

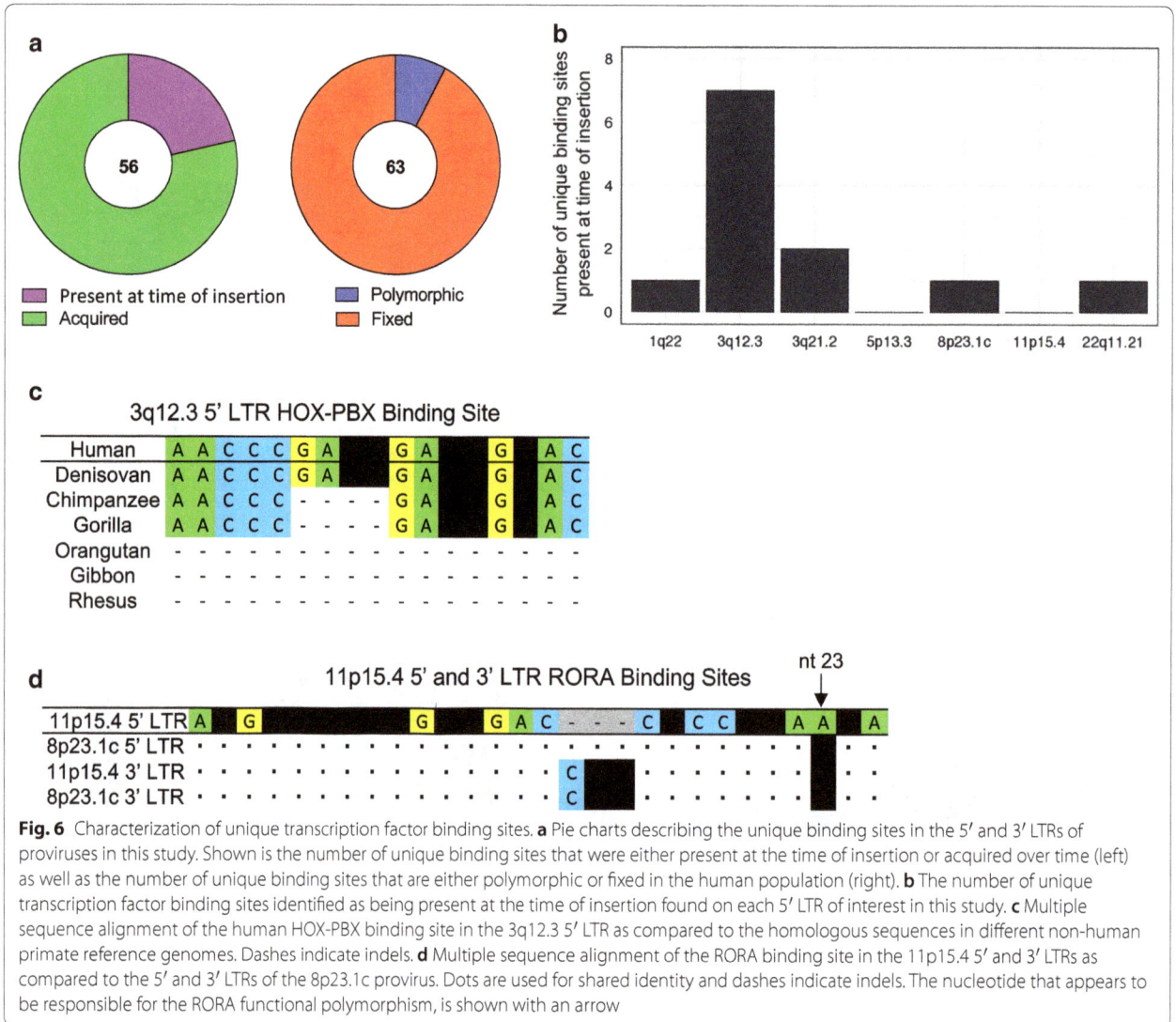

Fig. 6 Characterization of unique transcription factor binding sites. **a** Pie charts describing the unique binding sites in the 5′ and 3′ LTRs of proviruses in this study. Shown is the number of unique binding sites that were either present at the time of insertion or acquired over time (left) as well as the number of unique binding sites that are either polymorphic or fixed in the human population (right). **b** The number of unique transcription factor binding sites identified as being present at the time of insertion found on each 5′ LTR of interest in this study. **c** Multiple sequence alignment of the human HOX-PBX binding site in the 3q12.3 5′ LTR as compared to the homologous sequences in different non-human primate reference genomes. Dashes indicate indels. **d** Multiple sequence alignment of the RORA binding site in the 11p15.4 5′ and 3′ LTRs as compared to the 5′ and 3′ LTRs of the 8p23.1c provirus. Dots are used for shared identity and dashes indicate indels. The nucleotide that appears to be responsible for the RORA functional polymorphism, is shown with an arrow

Discussion

Post-integration, retroviral sequences are transcribed and translated like any other cellular gene and are subject to the same selective pressures. Germline sequences with neutral or advantageous effects can become fixed in the population, resulting in endogenization [2, 25, 43]. These sequences provide unique opportunities to study the evolutionary relationship between host and pathogen, including adaptations for assimilation within the host genome.

The full biological significance of HERVs remains to be uncovered. Repetitive mobile sequences are often credited with contributing to genome plasticity and HERVs, equipped with multiple splice junctions, promoter/

enhancer sites, and polyadenylation signals, are abundantly capable of altering host gene expression [2, 8, 43]. A number of endogenous retroviruses, including the mouse mammary tumor virus, murine leukemia virus, and Jaagsiekte sheep retrovirus, exhibit both endogenous and exogenous transmission and are capable of inducing carcinogenesis. Since the pathogenicity of these viruses is generally due to LTR activity and integration site, which can result in the alteration of expression of nearby proto-oncogenes [43, 44], endogenous viral sequences are often silenced through epigenetic and chromatin modifications such as CpG methylation [12–14].

Our group recently characterized the HML-2 transcriptome during HMEC transformation and found that the site of proviral integration is often crucial for expression, with the majority of expressed proviruses being transcribed by non-LTR-driven mechanisms such as read-through from adjacent promoters. When it was present, LTR-driven transcription was detected only in tumorigenic cells, suggesting that the altered transcriptional milieu of a transformed cell is critical for LTR promoter activation [32]. The goal of this study was to investigate the interplay between LTR sequence variation and cellular environment and to look for evidence of evolutionary adaptations that could result in increased activity during neoplasia.

LTR hypomethylation, commonly seen in malignant cells, is well documented to result in increased ERV expression [13, 29, 45]. To eliminate this issue, we decided to investigate the relationship between LTR sequence similarity and differential expression patterns using reporter construct assays, where methylation status is not a factor. We chose to study nine HML-2 proviruses, shown by single-genome sequencing to be highly transcribed across a number of breast cancer cell lines (Additional file 1). Phylogenetic analysis of these 5′ LTRs classified most of them as LTR-HS, the LTR group that includes the youngest proviruses and most human-specific integrations [4, 9]. Of these, only one provirus (3q12.3) is known to not be human-specific, as it is present in gorillas and chimpanzees as well (Fig. 1a). All proviruses in this study are fixed in the human population, although one provirus (7p22.1b) is considered to be allelically polymorphic. It is present as either a solo LTR, formed through the recombination of the 5′ and 3′ LTRs and excision of the internal proviral sequence, or a full ("2-LTR") provirus [4, 7]. However, in either case, the 5′ LTR of interest is fixed and as such, for the purpose of this study, we do not consider any of these LTRs to be insertionally polymorphic.

Overall, we found significant HML-2 promoter activity in 73% (11/15) of tumorigenic HME cell lines (Fig. 1c), consistent with previous reports of increased HML-2

expression in up to 85% of breast cancer samples [30, 31, 37]. Molecular subtype, as denoted by hormone receptor status, of the cell lines was noted (Table 2), but no significant correlation with HML-2 promoter expression was observed (Additional file 7). Pairwise comparisons of 5′ LTR sequence identity and promoter expression in our luciferase panel revealed a positive correlation between the results of the two assays (Fig. 2). These results suggest that LTRs with similar sequences share similar promoter expression patterns, most likely due to conservation of the same transcription factor binding sites and core promoter elements.

To further investigate the importance of sequence variation on LTR promoter activity, we used MatInspector, a transcription factor binding site prediction software, to generate a list of all binding sites unique to each of the nine LTRs used in this study (Table 3). We considered unique sites to be candidates for sequence variation that may explain why one LTR would be activated under a certain cellular condition instead of another. Two proviruses, 3q12.3 and 11p15.4, exhibited the highest levels of promoter activity across our luciferase panel (Fig. 1d). We used the MatInspector data, alongside RNA-Seq results from a previously published experiment by our group [32], to identify upregulated transcription factors known to bind to the unique binding sites on these two LTRs. These results provided us with two candidate sites per 5′ LTR for the promoter activation we saw during neoplasia: the HOX-PBX and RFX3 sites on 3q12.3 and the ATF and RORA sites on 11p15.4 (Fig. 3b). Removal of these sites individually decreased LTR promoter activity in HMLE-Ras and HMLE-Her2 cells by two to sevenfold (Figs. 4c, 5c).

All four of these binding sites are known to be involved with transcriptional activation, particularly during the regulation of human embryogenesis [46–49]. Interestingly, this observation is consistent with previous literature suggesting that HERVs are regulated in manners similar to stem cell genes, relying on cell-specific transcription factors and epigenetic modifications rather than TATA boxes or other canonical promoter elements [25, 33]. The evolution of the HOX-PBX and RORA binding sites were of most interest. Although the 3q12.3 provirus can be traced back through the primate lineage to gorillas, the HOX-PBX binding site is only found in the 5′ LTR in Denisovan and human genomes (Fig. 6c). Due to lack of coverage of the Neandertal reference genome at this location, it's unclear if this binding site is present in that species. This site, created by duplication of a GATT sequence, appears to have been acquired after the evolutionary split between humans and chimpanzees and has been fixed in the human population ever since. This analysis suggests that although the 3q12.3 provirus is evolutionarily conserved amongst several non-human primate species, the HOX-PBX binding site is human-specific. Although HOX proteins are widely expressed during development, aberrant expression has been documented during malignancy and increased HOX gene expression is being investigated as a potential breast cancer biomarker [50].

Alignments between the 5′ and 3′ LTR of proviruses shed light on the evolution of unique transcription factor binding sites. We were able to determine if sites were present at the time of insertion (present in both LTRs) or acquired over time (present in only one LTR). Only 21% of the unique binding sites that we identified were present at the time of insertion (Fig. 6a, left), implying that the expression patterns observed for these proviruses would not have reflected those of the ancestral virus that gave rise to them. Furthermore, the majority of unique sites were in the 3q12.3 5′ LTR (Fig. 6b). This distribution is consistent with the greater genetic distance and greater age of this provirus from the rest of the LTR-HS group (Fig. 1a). The high degree of unique sites present at the time of insertion may also explain why this particular provirus had an expression pattern widely different from the other LTRs in this study (Fig. 2).

Due to their possible role in pathogenicity, it is essential to study the genetic differences of HML-2 elements among individuals. Most often, such studies focus on whole proviruses, studying insertional polymorphism and its possible contribution to disease. Thus far, however, no polymorphic proviruses have been found to play a role in the genesis of cancer [34, 51]. To our knowledge, ours is the first study to investigate genetic differences at the single nucleotide level, by examining SNPs within LTRs. Of the 63 binding sites unique to one of the expressed LTRs that we identified, only five of them were found to be polymorphic within the 2504 genomes mined (Fig. 6a, right). These allele frequencies were further broken down by super-population, showing only slightly higher prevalence of these binding sites in the African population (Additional file 8).

The RORA binding site, harbored on the 5′ LTR of the 11p15.4 provirus, was the only site critical for HML-2 activation during neoplasia that was also polymorphic (Table 4). This provirus is of particular interest because it is a segmental duplication of 8p23.1c [4], which showed no LTR activity during tumorigenesis. After examining the RORA binding sites on both of these LTRs, we found that 51% of the population contains an active RORA site whereas the other half of the population contains an inactive RORA site, identical to the ancestral 8p23.1c 5′ LTR. Thus, more than half of the human population has evolved away from the ancestral sequence and towards a more active LTR version (Fig. 6d).

Conclusions

The role, if any, of HERV activity during tumorigenesis is unknown. It is currently unclear if HML-2 expression is an ancillary consequence of transformation or if it somehow aids in the event; although recent work shows that Env protein expression may increase the ability of tumor cells to evade immune surveillance during some cancers [52] or even participate directly in the transformation process by interacting with cellular proto-oncogenes [53]. Although no provirus of interest in our study is believed to have a viable open reading frame for any viral gene, protein production in these cell lines as well as any sample used in future investigations, should be examined. Our results show that HML-2 promoter activity is present in the majority (73%) of breast cancer cell lines tested and that LTR sequence similarity is correlated with promoter expression patterns. From there, we were able to map binding sites seemingly crucial for HML-2 promoter expression during neoplasia, many of which were acquired over evolutionary time. The polymorphism of certain sites provides another dimension in regards to what causes differential expression of ERVs between individuals. These data may shed light on adaptive co-evolution of ERVs within their host cells.

In recent years, there have been numerous reports of co-option of endogenous proviral sequences to disparate features of normal human and vertebrate biology, including protection against infection by related exogenous viruses [54], formation of the placental syncytiotrophoblast layer [10], expression of salivary amylase [55], stimulation of innate immunity [56], stimulation of neurological synapses promoting long-term memory [57], among others. It is particularly noteworthy that transcription of the two most highly expressed proviruses in our panel of ex vivo transformed cancer cell lines was facilitated through binding sites that were created by mutations in the 5′ LTRs that arose and spread in the human population following integration, implying that the expression patterns observed do not reflect those of the ancestral virus. It is tempting to speculate that responsiveness of the mutant proviruses to common, development-specific transcription factors might have given them some beneficial property along the lines of the ones listed above, thereby providing a selective advantage to the individuals carrying them and promoting their rapid fixation in the population.

Methods
Cell culture
The HME, HMLE-Her2, HMLE-Ras, MCF-10A, SUM149, SUM159, MDA-MB-361, Hcc1419, Hcc1428, and SUM1315 cell lines were grown in the Kuperwasser lab at Tufts University as previously described [32] and

all other cell lines were obtained from ATCC (Manassas, VA, USA). All cell lines were grown as per ATCC's recommendations and detailed information regarding their origin and culture conditions can be found in Additional file 9.

Single-genome sequencing

ZR-75-1, MCF-7, T47D, SK-BR-3, Hcc1954, BT20, Hs578T, and MDA-MB-231 breast cancer cells were grown to 90% confluency. RNA was extracted and purified using the RNeasy Mini Kit (Qiagen, Valencia, CA, USA, Cat. No. 74104) and all DNA contamination was removed through DNase treatment (Turbo DNA-*free* Kit, Ambion, Foster City, CA, USA, Cat. No. AM1907). RT reactions were set up as recommended by the manufacturer's protocol using an oligo(dT) primer (SuperScript III One-Step RT-PCR System, Invitrogen, Carlsbad, CA, USA, Cat. No. 12574-018). The resulting cDNA was serially diluted down to an average of 1/3 genome per sample and amplified using Taq DNA polymerase (Invitrogen, Cat. No. 10342-020). Two forward primers (5′-TTCCTT TACAAAGTTGCGTAAAGC-3′, 5′-GTTGCGTAAAGC CCCCTTAT-3′) and one reverse primer (5′-CACAGA CACAGTAACAATCTG-3′), all targeting the HML-2 *env* region, were used in the reaction. The amplified products were gel extracted with the QIAquick Gel Extraction Kit (Qiagen, Cat. No. 28704) and purified samples were sent out for sequencing. The primers used for sequencing were 5′-GACTCCCAGACTATAACCTGTC-3′ and 5′-CGAAGCATCAAAAGCCCA-3′. Sequencing results were BLAT searched in the UCSC Genome Browser [58] to identify expressed proviruses.

Phylogenetic analysis

The 5′ and 3′ LTR sequence of each provirus of interest was obtained from the UCSC Genome Browser's Repeat-Masker Track [58, 59] and imported as FASTA files into the Molecular Evolutionary Genetics Analysis (MEGA, v6.06) program for alignment using Multiple Sequence Comparison by Log-Expectation (MUSCLE) [60, 61]. Phylogeny of aligned sequences was determined by sequence dissimilarity and a neighbor-joining tree was constructed using a p-distance algorithm. Bootstrap values were determined using 1000 replicate tests.

Dual-luciferase assay

Primers for LTR amplification were selected using the Primer3 program [62]. Restriction enzyme cleavage sites were appended to the 5′ end of the primer sequences for proper vector ligation. The primers created are listed in Additional file 10. The LTR sequences were PCR-amplified using Taq DNA polymerase. Template DNA

was purified from Tera-1 cells using the DNeasy Blood and Tissue Kit (Qiagen, Cat. No. 69504). The amplified sequences were cloned using basic molecular biology techniques and ligated into the multiple cloning region of the pGL4.17[*luc2*/Neo] promoter-less firefly luciferase vector (Promega, Madison, WI, USA, Cat. No. E6721). All constructs were sequenced to check for PCR-induced mutations before transfection. All cell cultures were seeded in triplicate at 100,000 cells/well in a 24-well plate for transfection. Cultures were co-transfected with the pGL4 vector alongside a pRL-SV40 internal control *Renilla* luciferase vector (Promega, Cat. No. E2231) at a 30:1 ratio using Opti-MEM reduced serum media (Gibco, Cat. No. 31985-070) and Lipofectamine 2000 (Thermo Fisher Technologies, Cat. No. 11668-019), as recommended by the manufacturer's protocol. Post-transfection, cells were incubated at 37 °C for 48 h before lysis and analysis. Luminescence was measured via the dual-luciferase assay system (Promega, Cat. No. E1910) and quantified as relative light units (RLU) on a BioTek Synergy HT plate reader using Gen5 Data Analysis Software (BioTek Instruments, Winooski, VT, USA). Empty vectors as well as non-transfected cells were measured as a control to determine any cell-specific background signal. LTR promoter activity was calculated as *luc2* activity normalized against that of the internal *Renilla* luciferase control signal.

HML-2 similarity matrices

The sequence of each "full length" (i.e., not solo LTR) HML-2 provirus annotated within the human reference genome (hg19 build) was obtained from the UCSC Genome Browser [58]. These sequences were input into the Clustal Omega program (The European Bioinformatics Institute (EMBL-EBI), Hinxton, Cambridge, UK) [40] to create a multiple sequence alignment using the HHalign algorithm [63] and to create a percent sequence identity matrix. The HML-2 percent expression similarity matrix was created by making pairwise comparisons of significant promoter expression in each of the eighteen cell lines used in our dual-luciferase analysis.

Transcription factor binding site analysis

The full sequence of each 5′ LTR of interest was imported into MatInspector, a transcription factor binding site prediction software provided by Genomatix [41]. Any site that was identified in more than one provirus was removed from the analysis to produce a list containing all predicted binding sites unique to each LTR. This program also provided information regarding transcription factors that are known to bind to these sites. Transcript abundance levels of these transcription factors in the Hcc1954, HMLE-Ras, HMLE-Her2, and HME cell lines were determined by Cuffdiff analysis of our previous RNA-Seq results. A full description of the study used to obtain these values is detailed in our previous publication [32] and the RNA-Seq data are deposited in the NCBI Gene Expression Omnibus database under Accession Number GSE84275.

Consensus sequences of the HOX-PBX, RFX3, ATF, and RORA binding sites were determined through a separate MEGA alignment. New reporter constructs containing the consensus (non-active) sites were created through IDT's gBlocks® Gene Fragments synthesis service (Integrated DNA Technologies, Inc., Coralville, IA, USA). These fragments were directly cloned into the pGL4[*luc2*/Neo] firefly luciferase vector and transfected into cell lines as previously described in the Dual-Luciferase Assay section of the Materials and Methods.

The 5′ and 3′ LTRs of each of the nine proviruses of interest were analyzed in an additional MEGA alignment. All unique transcription factor binding sites found in only one LTR were regarded as being "acquired" and any unique binding sites found in both LTRs were characterized as "present at time of insertion". Sites located in the 7p22.1b and 21q21.1 proviruses were excluded from the analysis since they no longer possess intact 3′ LTRs [4].

The allele frequencies of each unique binding site were calculated from the VCF (Variant Call Format) files of 2504 individuals, as supplied by phase 3 of the 1000 Genomes Project [42]. VCF files were analyzed computationally using VCFtools, by specifying the genomic coordinates (hg19 build) of each site of interest. All sites with an allele frequency of at least 89% were considered to be fixed in the human population. All sites that were classified as polymorphic within the population had allele frequencies of 52% or less. No binding site that we identified had an allele frequency intermediate of those two thresholds, i.e. calculated to be greater than 52% but less than 89%.

The HOX-PBX binding site was further analyzed in several non-human primate reference genomes as supplied by the UCSC Genome Browser [58]. The Denisovan reference genome sequence was obtained from the Denisova High-Coverage Sequence Reads of the Denisova Seq Track. The chimpanzee, gorilla, orangutan, gibbon, and rhesus reference genome sequences were obtained from the Vertebrate Multiz Alignment & Conservation Track.

Additional files

Additional file 1: Table S1. HML-2 transcript levels detected through single-genome sequencing in breast cancer cell lines of varying molecular subtype.

Additional file 2: Table S2. HML-2 similarity matrices.

Additional file 3: Table S3. HOX-PBX binding site sequences and genomic coordinates (hg19).

Additional file 4: Table S4. RFX3 binding site sequences and genomic coordinates (hg19).

Additional file 5: Table S5. ATF binding site sequences and genomic coordinates (hg19).

Additional file 6: Table S6. RORA binding site sequences and genomic coordinates (hg19).

Additional file 7: Figure S1. HML-2 promoter activity is not breast cancer subtype-specific. Total relative 5′ LTR promoter activity levels of fifteen tumorigenic breast cancer cell lines broken down by molecular subtype (luminal, HER2+, and basal-like) as compared to two immortalized HME cell lines. Hormone receptor status and cell lines identified as being each molecular subtype are shown in detail in Table 2. All experiments were conducted in triplicate and data display the mean ± standard deviation.

Additional file 8: Figure S2. Allele frequencies of polymorphic HML-2 5′ LTR transcription factor binding sites within each superpopulation. Allele frequencies were determined for the proviruses shown from 2504 individuals from the 1000 Genomes Project and broken down by superpopulation (EAS = East Asian; AMR = Ad Mixed American; AFR = African; EUR = European; SAS = South Asian). The name of the transcription factor binding site as well as the provirus of interest are shown at the top of each graph.

Additional file 9: Table S7. Culture methods for cell lines used.

Additional file 10: Table S8. Primers used to amplify 5′ LTRs of transfected HML-2 proviruses.

Authors' contributions

MM, CK, and JMC conceived and designed the experiments. MM and RPS performed the experiments. MM, ZHW, RPS, and JMC analyzed the data. MM and JMC wrote the paper and all authors read and approved the final manuscript.

Author details

[1] Department of Molecular Biology and Microbiology, Tufts University School of Medicine, Boston, MA, USA. [2] Department of Developmental, Chemical, and Molecular Biology, Tufts University School of Medicine, Boston, MA, USA. [3] Raymond and Beverly Sackler Convergence Laboratory, Tufts University School of Medicine, Boston, MA, USA. [4] Present Address: Foundation Medicine, Inc., Cambridge, MA, USA. [5] Present Address: Excerpta Medica, New York, NY, USA.

Acknowledgements

We thank the Tufts University Genomics core facility for their RNA-Seq advice and as John Yoon for helpful discussion and editorial advice.

Competing interests

The authors declare that they have no competing interests.

Funding
This project was supported by research Grants R37 CA 089441 and R35 CA 200421 from the National Cancer Institute.

References

1. Lower R, Lower J, Tondera-Koch C, Kurth R. A general method for the identification of transcribed retrovirus sequences (R-U5 PCR) reveals the expression of the human endogenous retrovirus loci HERV-H and HERV-K in teratocarcinoma cells. Virology. 1993;192:501–11. https://doi.org/10.1006/viro.1993.1066.

2. Jern P, Coffin JM. Effects of retroviruses on host genome function. Annu Rev Genet. 2008;42:709–32. https://doi.org/10.1146/annurev.genet.42.110807.091501.

3. Ono M, Yasunaga T, Miyata T, Ushikubo H. Nucleotide sequence of human endogenous retrovirus genome related to the mouse mammary tumor virus genome. J Virol. 1986;60:589–98.

4. Subramanian RP, Wildschutte JH, Russo C, Coffin JM. Identification, characterization, and comparative genomic distribution of the HERV-K (HML-2) group of human endogenous retroviruses. Retrovirology. 2011;8:90. https://doi.org/10.1186/1742-4690-8-90.

5. Armbruester V, Sauter M, Krautkraemer E, Meese E, Kleiman A, Best B, et al. A novel gene from the human endogenous retrovirus K expressed in transformed cells. Clin Cancer Res. 2002;8:1800–7.

6. Gonzalez-Hernandez MJ, Cavalcoli JD, Sartor MA, Contreras-Galindo R, Meng F, Dai M, et al. Regulation of the human endogenous retrovirus K (HML-2) transcriptome by the HIV-1 Tat protein. J Virol. 2014;88:8924–35. https://doi.org/10.1128/JVI.00556-14.

7. Wildschutte JH, Williams ZH, Montesion M, Subramanian RP, Kidd JM, Coffin JM. Discovery of unfixed endogenous retrovirus insertions in diverse human populations. Proc Natl Acad Sci U S A. 2016. https://doi.org/10.1073/pnas.1602336113.

8. Schmitt K, Reichrath J, Roesch A, Meese E, Mayer J. Transcriptional profiling of human endogenous retrovirus group HERV-K(HML-2) loci in melanoma. Genome Biol Evol. 2013;5:307–28. https://doi.org/10.1093/gbe/evt010.

9. Bhardwaj N, Montesion M, Roy F, Coffin JM. Differential expression of HERV-K (HML-2) proviruses in cells and virions of the teratocarcinoma cell line Tera-1. Viruses. 2015;7:939–68. https://doi.org/10.3390/v7030939.

10. Mi S, Lee X, Li X, Veldman GM, Finnerty H, Racie L, et al. Syncytin is a captive retroviral envelope protein involved in human placental morphogenesis. Nature. 2000;403:785–9. https://doi.org/10.1038/35001608.

11. Reiss D, Zhang Y, Mager DL. Widely variable endogenous retroviral methylation levels in human placenta. Nucleic Acids Res. 2007;35:4743–54. https://doi.org/10.1093/nar/gkm455.

12. Gotzinger N, Sauter M, Roemer K, Mueller-Lantzsch N. Regulation of human endogenous retrovirus-K Gag expression in teratocarcinoma cell lines and human tumours. J Gen Virol. 1996;77(Pt 12):2983–90. https://doi.org/10.1099/0022-1317-77-12-2983.

13. Florl AR, Lower R, Schmitz-Drager BJ, Schulz WA. DNA methylation and expression of LINE-1 and HERV-K provirus sequences in urothelial and renal cell carcinomas. Br J Cancer. 1999;80:1312–21. https://doi.org/10.1038/sj.bjc.6690524.

14. Conklin KF, Coffin JM, Robinson HL, Groudine M, Eisenman R. Role of methylation in the induced and spontaneous expression of the avian endogenous virus ev-1: DNA structure and gene products. Mol Cell Biol. 1982;2:638–52.

15. Santoni FA, Guerra J, Luban J. HERV-H RNA is abundant in human embryonic stem cells and a precise marker for pluripotency. Retrovirology. 2012;9:111. https://doi.org/10.1186/1742-4690-9-111.

16. Xie W, Schultz MD, Lister R, Hou Z, Rajagopal N, Ray P, et al. Epigenomic analysis of multilineage differentiation of human embryonic stem cells. Cell. 2013;153:1134–48. https://doi.org/10.1016/j.cell.2013.04.022.

17. Smith ZD, Chan MM, Humm KC, Karnik R, Mekhoubad S, Regev A, et al. DNA methylation dynamics of the human preimplantation embryo. Nature. 2014;511:611–5. https://doi.org/10.1038/nature13581

18. Ohnuki M, Tanabe K, Sutou K, Teramoto I, Sawamura Y, Narita M, et al. Dynamic regulation of human endogenous retroviruses mediates factor-induced reprogramming and differentiation potential. Proc Natl Acad Sci U S A. 2014;111:12426–31. https://doi.org/10.1073/pnas.1413299111.

19. Grow EJ, Flynn RA, Chavez SL, Bayless NL, Wossidlo M, Wesche DJ, et al. Intrinsic retroviral reactivation in human preimplantation embryos and pluripotent cells. Nature. 2015. https://doi.org/10.1038/nature14308.

20. Frank JA, Feschotte C. Co-option of endogenous viral sequences for host cell function. Curr Opin Virol. 2017;25:81–9. https://doi.org/10.1016/j.coviro.2017.07.021.

21. Glinsky GV. Activation of endogenous human stem cell-associated retroviruses (SCARs) and therapy-resistant phenotypes of malignant tumors. Cancer Lett. 2016;376:347–59. https://doi.org/10.1016/j.canlet.2016.04.014.

22. Kudo-Saito C, Yura M, Yamamoto R, Kawakami Y. Induction of immunoregulatory CD271+ cells by metastatic tumor cells that express human endogenous retrovirus H. Cancer Res. 2014;74:1361–70. https://doi.org/10.1158/0008-5472.CAN-13-1349.

23. Kreimer U, Schulz WA, Koch A, Niegisch G, Goering W. HERV-K and LINE-1 DNA methylation and reexpression in urothelial carcinoma. Front Oncol. 2013;3:255. https://doi.org/10.3389/fonc.2013.00255.

24. Lavie L, Kitova M, Maldener E, Meese E, Mayer J. CpG methylation directly regulates transcriptional activity of the human endogenous retrovirus family HERV-K(HML-2). J Virol. 2005;79:876–83. https://doi.org/10.1128/JVI.79.2.876-883.2005.

25. Fuchs NV, Kraft M, Tondera C, Hanschmann KM, Lower J, Lower R. Expression of the human endogenous retrovirus (HERV) group HML-2/HERV-K does not depend on canonical promoter elements but is regulated by transcription factors Sp1 and Sp3. J Virol. 2011;85:3436–48. https://doi.org/10.1128/JVI.02539-10.

26. Stengel S, Fiebig U, Kurth R, Denner J. Regulation of human endogenous retrovirus-K expression in melanomas by CpG methylation. Genes Chromosomes Cancer. 2010;49:401–11. https://doi.org/10.1002/gcc.20751.

27. Knossl M, Lower R, Lower J. Expression of the human endogenous retrovirus HTDV/HERV-K is enhanced by cellular transcription factor YY1. J Virol. 1999;73:1254–61.

28. Ono M, Kawakami M, Ushikubo H. Stimulation of expression of the human endogenous retrovirus genome by female steroid hormones in human breast cancer cell line T47D. J Virol. 1987;61:2059–62.

29. Wang-Johanning F, Frost AR, Johanning GL, Khazaeli MB, LoBuglio AF, Shaw DR, et al. Expression of human endogenous retrovirus k envelope transcripts in human breast cancer. Clin Cancer Res. 2001;7:1553–60.

30. Wang-Johanning F, Frost AR, Jian B, Epp L, Lu DW, Johanning GL. Quantitation of HERV-K env gene expression and splicing in human breast cancer. Oncogene. 2003;22:1528–35. https://doi.org/10.1038/sj.onc.1206241.

31. Zhao J, Rycaj K, Geng S, Li M, Plummer JB, Yin B, et al. Expression of human endogenous retrovirus type K envelope protein is a novel candidate prognostic marker for human breast cancer. Genes Cancer. 2011;2:914–22. https://doi.org/10.1177/1947601911431841.

32. Montesion M, Bhardwaj N, Williams ZH, Kuperwasser C, Coffin JM. Mechanisms of HERV-K (HML-2) Transcription during human mammary epithelial cell transformation. J Virol. 2018. https://doi.org/10.1128/jvi.01258-17.

33. Manghera M, Douville RN. Endogenous retrovirus-K promoter: a landing strip for inflammatory transcription factors? Retrovirology. 2013;10:16. https://doi.org/10.1186/1742-4690-10-16.

34. Wildschutte JH, Ram D, Subramanian R, Stevens VL, Coffin JM. The distribution of insertionally polymorphic endogenous retroviruses in breast cancer patients and cancer-free controls. Retrovirology. 2014;11:62. https://doi.org/10.1186/PREACCEPT-1720768941312026.

35. Buzdin A, Ustyugova S, Khodosevich K, Mamedov I, Lebedev Y, Hunsmann G, et al. Human-specific subfamilies of HERV-K (HML-2) long terminal repeats: three master genes were active simultaneously during branching of hominoid lineages. Genomics. 2003;81:149–56.

36. Ruprecht K, Ferreira H, Flockerzi A, Wahl S, Sauter M, Mayer J, et al. Human endogenous retrovirus family HERV-K(HML-2) RNA transcripts are selectively packaged into retroviral particles produced by the human germ

cell tumor line Tera-1 and originate mainly from a provirus on chromosome 22q11.21. J Virol. 2008;82:10008–16. https://doi.org/10.1128/JVI.01016-08.

37. Wang-Johanning F, Radvanyi L, Rycaj K, Plummer JB, Yan P, Sastry KJ, et al. Human endogenous retrovirus K triggers an antigen-specific immune response in breast cancer patients. Cancer Res. 2008;68:5869–77. https://doi.org/10.1158/0008-5472.CAN-07-6838.

38. Seifarth W, Baust C, Murr A, Skladny H, Krieg-Schneider F, Blusch J, et al. Proviral structure, chromosomal location, and expression of HERV-K-T47D, a novel human endogenous retrovirus derived from T47D particles. J Virol. 1998;72:8384–91.

39. Keydar I, Ohno T, Nayak R, Sweet R, Simoni F, Weiss F, et al. Properties of retrovirus-like particles produced by a human breast carcinoma cell line: immunological relationship with mouse mammary tumor virus proteins. Proc Natl Acad Sci U S A. 1984;81:4188–92.

40. McWilliam H, Li W, Uludag M, Squizzato S, Park YM, Buso N, et al. Analysis Tool Web Services from the EMBL-EBI. Nucleic Acids Res. 2013;41:W597–600. https://doi.org/10.1093/nar/gkt376.

41. Cartharius K, Frech K, Grote K, Klocke B, Haltmeier M, Klingenhoff A, et al. MatInspector and beyond: promoter analysis based on transcription factor binding sites. Bioinformatics. 2005;21:2933–42. https://doi.org/10.1093/bioinformatics/bti473.

42. Genomes Project C, Auton A, Brooks LD, Durbin RM, Garrison EP, Kang HM, et al. A global reference for human genetic variation. Nature. 2015;526:68–74. https://doi.org/10.1038/nature15393.

43. Lower R, Lower J, Kurth R. The viruses in all of us: characteristics and biological significance of human endogenous retrovirus sequences. Proc Natl Acad Sci U S A. 1996;93:5177–84.

44. Wang-Johanning F, Liu J, Rycaj K, Huang M, Tsai K, Rosen DG, et al. Expression of multiple human endogenous retrovirus surface envelope proteins in ovarian cancer. Int J Cancer. 2007;120:81–90. https://doi.org/10.1002/ijc.22256.

45. Fanning T, Alves G. A family of repetitive DNA sequences in Old World primates. Gene. 1997;199:279–82.

46. Shah N, Sukumar S. The Hox genes and their roles in oncogenesis. Nat Rev Cancer. 2010;10:361–71. https://doi.org/10.1038/nrc2826.

47. Tammimies K, Bieder A, Lauter G, Sugiaman-Trapman D, Torchet R, Hokkanen ME, et al. Ciliary dyslexia candidate genes DYX1C1 and DCDC2 are regulated by regulatory factor (RF) X transcription factors through X-box promoter motifs. FASEB J. 2016. https://doi.org/10.1096/fj.201500124RR.

48. Jiang S, Zhang E, Zhang R, Li X. Altered activity patterns of transcription factors induced by endoplasmic reticulum stress. BMC Biochem. 2016;17:8. https://doi.org/10.1186/s12858-016-0060-2.

49. Cook DN, Kang HS, Jetten AM. Retinoic acid-related orphan receptors (RORs): regulatory functions in immunity, development, circadian rhythm, and metabolism. Nucl Recept Res. 2015. https://doi.org/10.11131/2015/101185.

50. Morgan R, Boxall A, Harrington KJ, Simpson GR, Gillett C, Michael A, et al. Targeting the HOX/PBX dimer in breast cancer. Breast Cancer Res Treat. 2012;136:389–98. https://doi.org/10.1007/s10549-012-2259-2.

51. Burmeister T, Ebert AD, Pritze W, Loddenkemper C, Schwartz S, Thiel E. Insertional polymorphisms of endogenous HERV-K113 and HERV-K115 retroviruses in breast cancer patients and age-matched controls. AIDS Res Hum Retrovir. 2004;20:1223–9. https://doi.org/10.1089/0889222042545081.

52. Serafino A, Balestrieri E, Pierimarchi P, Matteucci C, Moroni G, Oricchio E, et al. The activation of human endogenous retrovirus K (HERV-K) is implicated in melanoma cell malignant transformation. Exp Cell Res. 2009;315:849–62. https://doi.org/10.1016/j.yexcr.2008.12.023.

53. Lemaitre C, Tsang J, Bireau C, Heidmann T, Dewannieux M. A human endogenous retrovirus-derived gene that can contribute to oncogenesis by activating the ERK pathway and inducing migration and invasion. PLoS Pathog. 2017;13:e1006451. https://doi.org/10.1371/journal.ppat.1006451.

54. Blanco-Melo D, Gifford RJ, Bieniasz PD. Co-option of an endogenous retrovirus envelope for host defense in hominid ancestors. Elife. 2017. https://doi.org/10.7554/elife.22519.

55. Samuelson LC, Wiebauer K, Gumucio DL, Meisler MH. Expression of the human amylase genes: recent origin of a salivary amylase promoter from an actin pseudogene. Nucleic Acids Res. 1988;16:8261–76.

56. Hurst TP, Magiorkinis G. Activation of the innate immune response by endogenous retroviruses. J Gen Virol. 2015;96:1207–18. https://doi.org/10.1099/jgv.0.000017.

57. Pastuzyn ED, Day CE, Kearns RB, Kyrke-Smith M, Taibi AV, McCormick J, et al. The neuronal gene arc encodes a repurposed retrotransposon gag protein that mediates intercellular RNA transfer. Cell. 2018;173:275. https://doi.org/10.1016/j.cell.2018.03.024.

58. Karolchik D, Hinrichs AS, Furey TS, Roskin KM, Sugnet CW, Haussler D, et al. The UCSC table browser data retrieval tool. Nucleic Acids Res. 2004;32:D493–6. https://doi.org/10.1093/nar/gkh103.

59. Kent WJ, Sugnet CW, Furey TS, Roskin KM, Pringle TH, Zahler AM, et al. The human genome browser at UCSC. Genome Res. 2002;2002(12):996–1006. https://doi.org/10.1101/gr.229102.

60. Tamura K, Stecher G, Peterson D, Filipski A, Kumar S. MEGA6: molecular evolutionary genetics analysis version 6.0. Mol Biol Evol. 2013;30:2725–9. https://doi.org/10.1093/molbev/mst197.

61. Edgar RC. MUSCLE: multiple sequence alignment with high accuracy and high throughput. Nucleic Acids Res. 2004;32:1792–7. https://doi.org/10.1093/nar/gkh340.

62. Untergasser A, Cutcutache I, Koressaar T, Ye J, Faircloth BC, Remm M, et al. Primer3: new capabilities and interfaces. Nucleic Acids Res. 2012;40:e115. https://doi.org/10.1093/nar/gks596.

63. Soding J. Protein homology detection by HMM-HMM comparison. Bioinformatics. 2005;21:951–60. https://doi.org/10.1093/bioinformatics/bti125.

A CRISPR screen for factors regulating SAMHD1 degradation identifies IFITMs as potent inhibitors of lentiviral particle delivery

Ferdinand Roesch, Molly OhAinle and Michael Emerman[*] (iD)

Abstract

The InterFeron Induced TransMembrane (IFITM) proteins are interferon stimulated genes that restrict many viruses, including HIV-1. SAMHD1 is another restriction factor blocking replication of HIV-1 and other viruses. Some lentiviruses evolved Vpx/Vpr proteins to degrade SAMHD1. However, this viral antagonism can be perturbed by host mechanisms: a recent study showed that in interferon (IFN) treated THP1 cells, Vpx is unable to degrade SAMHD1. In the present work, we designed an Interferon Stimulated Genes (ISGs)-targeted CRISPR knockout screen in order to identify ISGs regulating this phenotype. We found that IFITM proteins contribute to the IFNα-mediated protection of SAMHD1 by blocking VSV-G-mediated entry of the lentiviral particles delivering Vpx. Consistent with this, IFNα treatment and IFITM expression had no effect when the A-MLV envelope was used for pseudotyping. Using an assay measuring viral entry, we show that IFNα and IFITMs directly block the delivery of Vpx into cells by inhibiting VSV-G viral fusion. Strikingly, the VSV-G envelope was significantly more sensitive to this IFNα entry block and to IFITMs than HIV-1's natural envelope. This highlights important differences between VSV-G pseudotyped and wild-type HIV-1, in particular relative to the pathways they use for viral entry, suggesting that HIV-1 may have evolved to escape restriction factors blocking entry.

Keywords: HIV-1, SAMHD1, Vpx, Pseudotypes, Interferon, IFITM, VSV-G, A-MLV, Viral entry

Background

Type I IFNs play a central role in activation of innate immunity by turning on a vast transcriptional program that results in enhanced expression of hundreds of Interferon Stimulated Genes (ISGs). Many of these ISGs encode proteins that have antiviral activity, inhibiting viruses at various steps of their life cycle including at the earliest stages of entry [1]. In particular, the InterFeron Induced TransMembrane (IFITM) proteins (IFITM1, IFITM2, and IFITM3) are ISGs localized at the cell surface and in endosomal compartments that restrict entry of many viruses, including HIV-1, VSV, Influenza A, some flaviviruses and alphaviruses [2–6].

After fusion, retroviruses release genomes and associated proteins into the cytoplasm during the uncoating process, ultimately resulting in the synthesis of reverse transcription products, formation of the preintegration complex, and nuclear import [7]. The accessory proteins Vpr and Vpx, which are encapsidated into budding virions through interaction with the p6 region of Gag [8], are also released from the incoming viral particles after fusion, in a process independent from uncoating of the viral core [9].

One of the functions of Vpx is to promote degradation of the host antiviral protein SAMHD1 [10, 11]. SAMHD1 is a dNTP triphosphohydrolase that depletes the cellular pools of dNTPs [12] in quiescent cells of the myeloid lineage and in resting CD4 + T cells [13], resulting in a block to reverse transcription [10, 11]. In some SIVs lacking Vpx, SAMHD1 antagonism is achieved by the related viral protein Vpr [14]. Vpx/Vpr proteins directly bind to

*Correspondence: memerman@fredhutch.org
Divisions of Human Biology and Basic Sciences, Fred Hutchinson Cancer Research Center, 1100 Fairview Ave N, Mailstop C2-023, Seattle, WA 98109, USA

SAMHD1 and recruit the DDB1/Cul4/DCAF1 ubiquitin ligase complex, resulting in proteasomal degradation of SAMHD1 [15, 16]. The recognition of SAMHD1 by Vpx/Vpr proteins is evolutionarily dynamic, with some viral proteins binding to the N-terminus of SAMHD1, and others to the C-terminus [17]. In addition to the evolution at the Vpx/SAMHD1 interface, the host has evolved other mechanisms to regulate SAMHD1. For instance, SAMHD1 enzymatic activity is controlled by cell cycle progression [18–20], and the host factor H11/HSPB8 has been reported to degrade Vpx, thus protecting SAMHD1 from degradation [21].

Dragin et al. [22] showed that interferon alpha (IFNα) treatment of THP1 cells prevents degradation of SAMHD1 following incubation with SIV_{MAC} virus-like particles containing Vpx (VLPs-Vpx). This observation suggests the existence of one or more proteins induced or activated by IFNα that directly or indirectly protect SAMHD1 from degradation. IFN treatment controls SAMHD1 enzymatic activity by phosphorylation [18], and reports have described induction of SAMHD1 expression in monocytes and some cell lines after IFNα treatment [23, 24] through mechanisms involving modulation of microRNAs and IRF3, respectively. However, none of these effects could explain how IFNα protects SAMHD1 from degradation by Vpx [22].

In the present work, we confirmed that treatment of THP1 cells with either interferon alpha (IFNα) or interferon gamma (IFNγ) indeed protects SAMHD1 from degradation by Vpx when Vpx is delivered to cells via VLPs that are pseudotyped with VSV-G. We designed a flow cytometry-based CRISPR knockout screen to identify ISGs involved in this phenotype and identified the InterFeron Induced TransMembrane (IFITM) proteins. Moreover, we show that IFNα protects SAMHD1 from degradation when Vpx-containing VLPs are pseudotyped with VSV-G for viral entry, but not when they are pseudotyped with the envelope from amphotropic murine leukemia virus (A-MLV), suggesting that the IFNα block occurs at the level of viral entry. By directly comparing the entry block imposed by IFNα and IFITMs on HIV-1 pseudotyped with different envelopes, we show that VSV-G is inhibited to a greater degree than HIV-1 wild-type envelope. This result suggests that HIV-1 may escape IFNα induced blocks to viral entry, potentially by using different cellular pathways for membrane fusion, as

suggested in a recent study [25]. Finally, our screen could also be used to identify factors blocking a variety of different viral envelopes, using SAMHD1 degradation as a proxy for cytoplasmic delivery of viral proteins.

Results

IFN treatment protects SAMHD1 from degradation by Vpx in THP1 cells

First, we confirmed the published observation that IFN treatment inhibited SAMHD1 degradation in THP1 cells [22]. SAMHD1 degradation in THP1 cells was achieved by overnight treatment with Virus-Like Particles (VLPs) that consist of the SIV_{MAC} Gag/Pol structural proteins and naturally package both Vpr and Vpx [26], with only Vpx being able to degrade SAMHD1 [14]. Vpx-containing VLPs (VLPs-Vpx) were pseudotyped with the Vesicular Stomatitis Virus glycoprotein (VSV-G), as has been done in previous studies [10, 12, 22, 27]. THP1 cells were treated with universal type I interferon alpha (IFNα), a recombinant human IFN alpha, or IFNγ for 24 h and transduced with VLPs-Vpx. We measured the endogenous levels of SAMHD1 using flow cytometry in order to monitor SAMHD1 degradation in a quantitative manner in cell populations. Over 99% of the cells expressed SAMHD1, and this proportion did not change with IFNα or IFNγ treatment (Fig. 1a, top row). Consistent with previously published data, SAMHD1 was degraded in the presence of VLPs-Vpx (Fig. 1a, bottom row) and high levels of SAMHD1 degradation can be achieved: it reached 50% in the dose response presented in Fig. 1b (black lines), and even higher levels if more VLPs-Vpx were used (not shown). However, in the presence of IFNα and IFNγ, SAMHD1 degradation was blocked, (Fig. 1a, bottom row), even at high doses of VLPs-Vpx (Fig. 1b, dashed lines). Averaged over three independent experiments, IFNα or IFNγ treatment blocked SAMHD1 degradation by fivefold (Fig. 1c). Therefore, we hypothesized the existence of one or several ISGs, induced by both IFNα and IFNγ, that protect SAMHD1 from degradation by Vpx-containing VLPs.

A CRISPR screen identifies IFITMs as factors blocking Vpx-mediated degradation of SAMHD1

IFNα could affect SAMHD1 degradation by Vpx by any of several mechanisms, such as blocking Vpx trafficking to the nucleus, post-translational modification of

(See figure on next page.)

Fig. 1 IFN treatment inhibits Vpx-mediated degradation of SAMHD1. THP1 cells were treated for 24 h with 1000 U/mL of IFNα, 1000 U/mL of IFNγ or left untreated. The indicated amount of VLPs-Vpx pseudotyped with VSV-G (as determined by RT activity) was added to cells for 16 h: cells were then collected and SAMHD1 degradation was measured by flow cytometry. **a** Representative flow cytometry pots. **b** Representative dose response experiment. THP1 were treated with the indicated amount of VLPs-Vpx. The percentage of cells in which SAMHD1 is degraded was determined as shown in **a**. **c** Combined data from three independent experiments, using a viral dose within linear range. *p < 0.05; **p < 0.01 (t test)

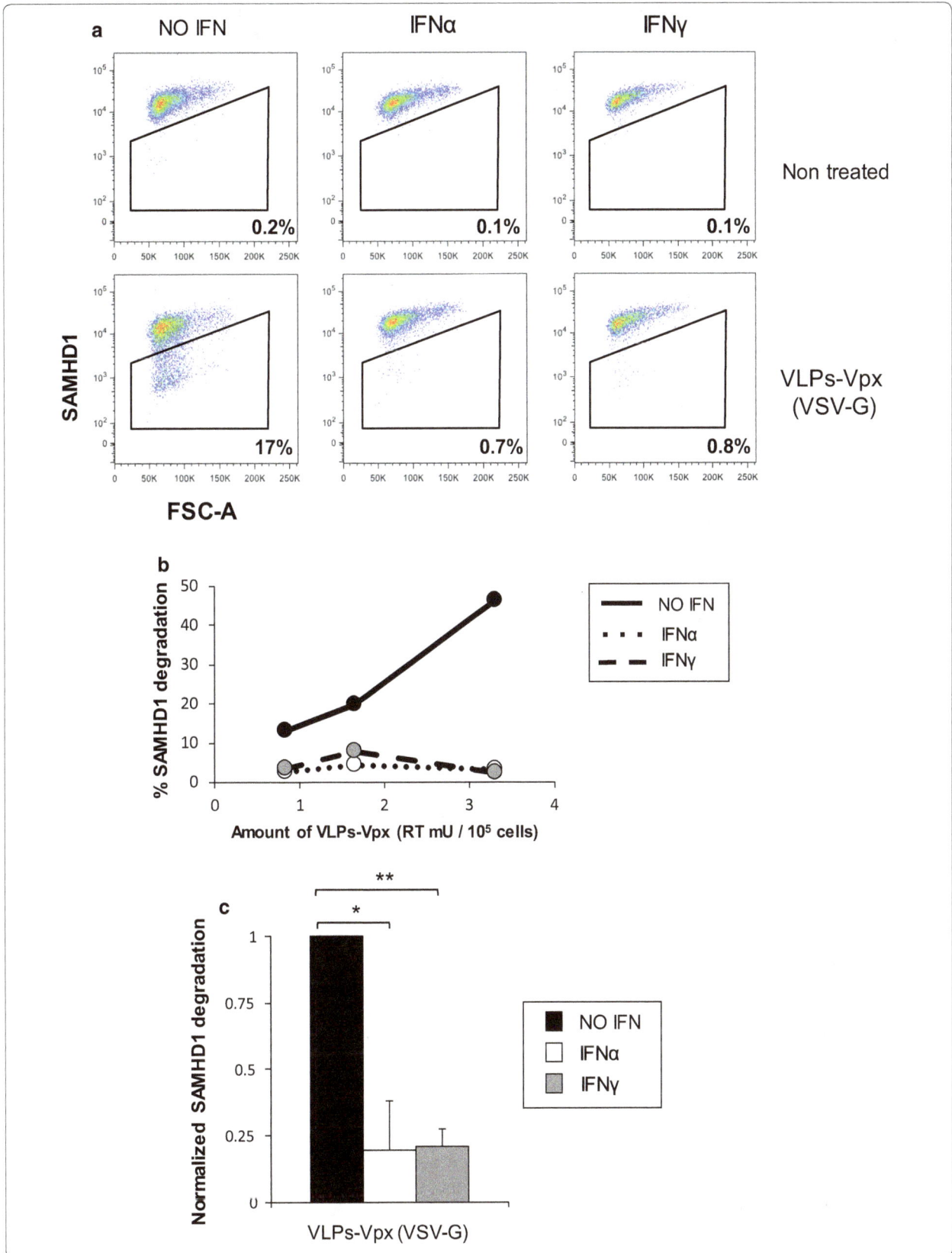

SAMHD1, interference with the degradation pathway through which Vpx targets SAMHD1, or, as described below, IFNα induction of genes affecting entry/fusion of the VLPs delivering Vpx. In order to identify the factor(s) responsible for this phenotype, we designed a CRISPR knockout screen taking advantage of the high-throughput qualities of both flow cytometry and next-generation sequencing technologies. We hypothesized that sgRNAs that target genes necessary for SAMHD1 protection from degradation would be enriched in the population of cells displaying low levels of SAMHD1. We first created a library of single-guide RNAs (sgRNAs) targeting 1906 human ISGs, with 8 different sgRNAs per gene and 200 non-targeting controls (NTCs) that do not target any loci in the human genome. We assembled sgRNAs into a lentiviral vector backbone that also encodes Cas9 and a puromycin resistance gene (OhAinle et al., manuscript in preparation). THP1 cells were transduced with this library, selected for puromycin resistance and cultured for 2 weeks to allow gene knockout to occur. The cells were treated with IFNα, and incubated with VSV-G pseudotyped VLPs-Vpx as described in Fig. 1. Endogenous SAMHD1 levels were measured and cells were sorted using flow cytometry.

The gating strategy for sorting a pure population of SAMHD1 negative cells is outlined in Fig. 2a. First, we sorted cells based on their morphology to remove dead cells, debris and cell doublets, which may skew subsequent analyses. Non-viable cells that cannot be identified solely by their morphology were eliminated by incubation with a viability dye, in which they appeared high in the DAPI channel. Finally, cells were sorted based on their SAMHD1 levels. As expected, only a small fraction of cells (about 7%) are SAMHD1 negative, which is consistent with data presented in Fig. 1 and with the hypothesis that only a very limited fraction of the CRISPR library will rescue SAMHD1 degradation. After sorting, we obtained 5×10^5 SAMHD1 negative cells and 3×10^6 SAMHD1 positive cells, which allows for a coverage of the library higher than 100X. The screen was performed with two technical replicates. After DNA extraction, sgRNA sequences in the different cell populations were amplified and deep-sequenced.

The frequency of each sgRNA within the SAMHD1 negative and positive populations was determined to calculate enrichment in the SAMHD1 negative population. sgRNAs enriched in the SAMHD1 negative fraction should target factors involved in IFN signaling, in SAMHD1 expression and stability, and may potentially target new ISGs protecting SAMHD1. In order to take into account results of all 8 sgRNAs targeting each gene in the library, we performed a gene-specific analysis with the MAGeCK tool that was developed for this purpose

[28]. This method assigns a score for each gene, factoring in the combined action of all sgRNAs, the enrichment of each sgRNA, and the biological replicate of the screen. Figure 2b shows the top 20 genes from screen ranked by their-log10 MAGeCK score on the X axis. As validation of our strategy, at the very top of this list is SAMHD1 itself since sgRNAs targeting this gene should result in low protein levels of SAMHD1 (Fig. 2b, blue square). Factors necessary for IFN signaling such as the IFN receptor IFNAR1, the signaling molecules STAT1 and STAT2, and the transcription factor IRF9 are among the top scoring hits from the screen (Fig. 2b, orange triangles), further validating our strategy.

After these positive controls, IFITM3 is one of the highest hits together with poorly characterized genes such as COMMD3, EIF3L and SLC35A2. Of note, IFITM1 is also present in our list of top hits, although with a lower MAGeCK score (Fig. 2b) and IFITM2 ranks 232, with a much lower gene score (Additional file 1: Table S1). It should be pointed out, however, that because of the extensive homology between IFITMs (up to 90% at the nucleotide level), the sgRNAs used in our screen cannot completely distinguish between the different homologs. In particular, one sgRNA for IFITM1, which was much more enriched than the others, displayed perfect homology with IFITM3 (not shown).

In order to explain the IFNα-induced protection of SAMHD1 phenotype, candidate hits should be significantly induced by IFNα treatment. Thus, we compared the gene scores from our screen to IFNα induction at the mRNA level in THP1 cells using a previously published dataset [29] (Fig. 2b, Y axis). While a number of our top hits, such as COMMD3, SLC35A2 and EIF3L, are reported to be poorly induced—if at all—at the transcriptional level by IFNα [29], IFITM proteins were highly induced by IFNα in THP1 cells [29], thus appearing to be the most likely candidate hits from this screen (Fig. 2b).

Knockout of IFITM2/3 explains most of the phenotype

To validate the results of our screen, we generated CRISPR knockout THP1 cells for specific IFITM proteins. Achieving knockout specificity for IFITMs is technically challenging, as previous studies have pointed out [25, 30], in particular for IFITM2 and IFITM3, which share 90% sequence identity at the nucleotide level. Therefore, we selected one sgRNA that specifically targets IFITM1 (12 and 13 nucleotide changes from IFITM2 and IFITM3, respectively) and one sgRNA that targets both IFITM2 and IFITM3 as it has perfect homology for both loci in THP1 cells, but differs by three nucleotides from IFITM1. A non-targeting control (NTC) sgRNA was included as a negative control. These sgRNAs were cloned into the

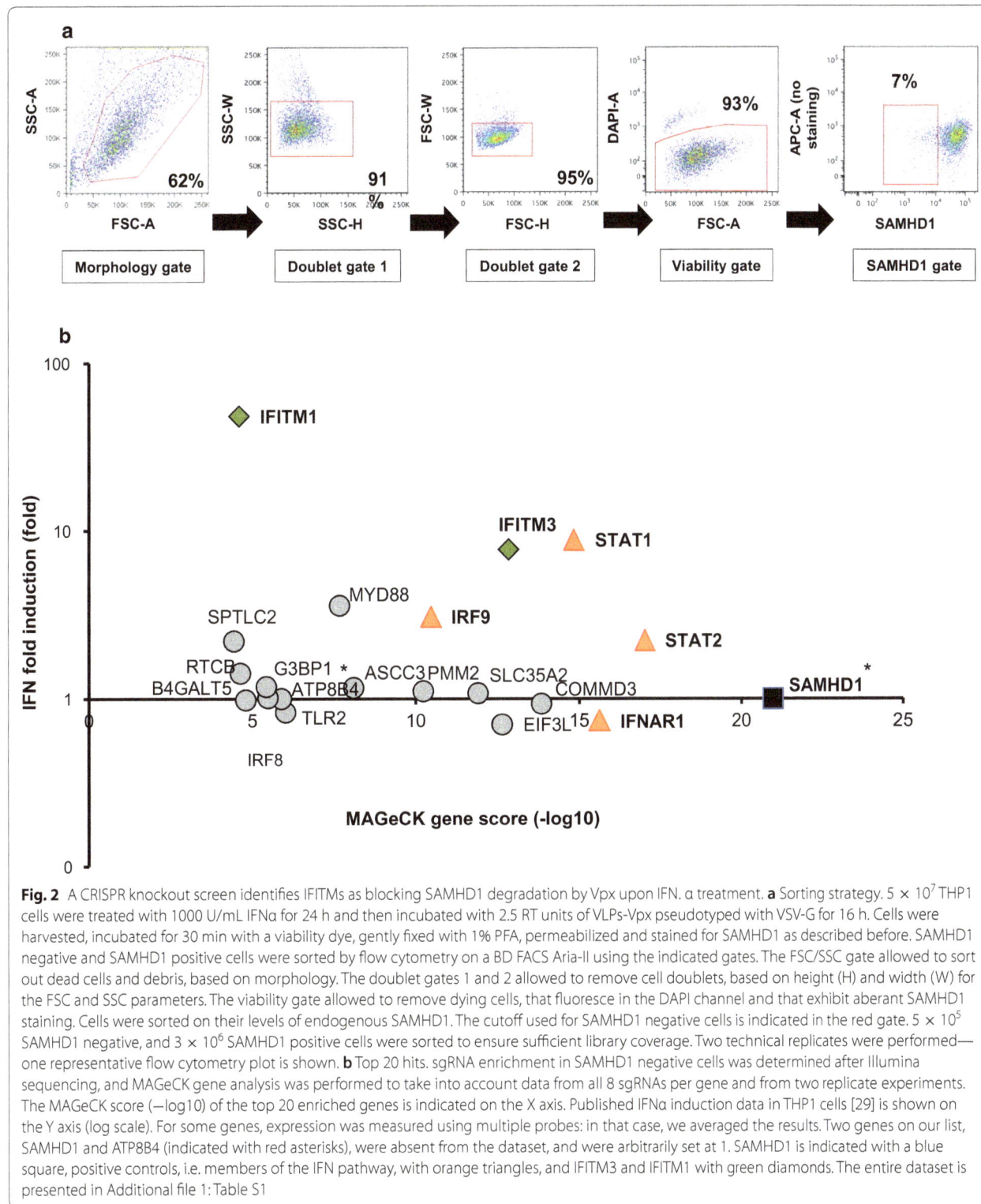

Fig. 2 A CRISPR knockout screen identifies IFITMs as blocking SAMHD1 degradation by Vpx upon IFN. α treatment. **a** Sorting strategy. 5×10^7 THP1 cells were treated with 1000 U/mL IFNα for 24 h and then incubated with 2.5 RT units of VLPs-Vpx pseudotyped with VSV-G for 16 h. Cells were harvested, incubated for 30 min with a viability dye, gently fixed with 1% PFA, permeabilized and stained for SAMHD1 as described before. SAMHD1 negative and SAMHD1 positive cells were sorted by flow cytometry on a BD FACS Aria-II using the indicated gates. The FSC/SSC gate allowed to sort out dead cells and debris, based on morphology. The doublet gates 1 and 2 allowed to remove cell doublets, based on height (H) and width (W) for the FSC and SSC parameters. The viability gate allowed to remove dying cells, that fluoresce in the DAPI channel and that exhibit aberrant SAMHD1 staining. Cells were sorted on their levels of endogenous SAMHD1. The cutoff used for SAMHD1 negative cells is indicated in the red gate. 5×10^5 SAMHD1 negative, and 3×10^6 SAMHD1 positive cells were sorted to ensure sufficient library coverage. Two technical replicates were performed— one representative flow cytometry plot is shown. **b** Top 20 hits. sgRNA enrichment in SAMHD1 negative cells was determined after Illumina sequencing, and MAGeCK gene analysis was performed to take into account data from all 8 sgRNAs per gene and from two replicate experiments. The MAGeCK score (—log10) of the top 20 enriched genes is indicated on the X axis. Published IFNα induction data in THP1 cells [29] is shown on the Y axis (log scale). For some genes, expression was measured using multiple probes: in that case, we averaged the results. Two genes on our list, SAMHD1 and ATP8B4 (indicated with red asterisks), were absent from the dataset, and were arbitrarily set at 1. SAMHD1 is indicated with a blue square, positive controls, i.e. members of the IFN pathway, with orange triangles, and IFITM3 and IFITM1 with green diamonds. The entire dataset is presented in Additional file 1: Table S1

Cas9-expressing lentiviral vector, and THP1 cells were transduced and selected by puromycin treatment. We first attempted to generate clonal knockout cell lines, but heterogeneity of the cell line, a known issue with THP1 cells [31], caused significant clone-to-clone variability and complicated interpretation of the results (not shown). Instead, we used pools of knockout cells, in which, after puromycin selection, levels of IFITM expression were greatly reduced, as measured by Western Blot (Fig. 3a). We observed that the IFITM1 sgRNA appeared to be specific, as it knocked-out almost entirely the expression of IFITM1 without significantly altering levels of IFITM2 and IFITM3. The sgRNA targeting IFITM2/3 led to low levels of expression of both IFITM3 and IFITM2, even in presence of IFNα, but left IFITM1 intact. Antibody specificity for IFITM2 vs IFITM3 is known to be difficult to achieve. Thus, to confirm our Western Blot results, we designed primers specific for the *ifitm2* and *ifitm3* loci (details in the Methods section), that were used for PCR amplification and sequencing of the CRISPR lesions present in THP1 knockout cells (Fig. 3b). Using TIDE analysis, a tool specifically designed to assess the percentage of cells edited by sgRNAs in heterogeneous populations [32], we determined that IFITM2/3 knockout cells are highly edited for *ifitm2* (71%) and *ifitm3* (78%), while NTC and IFITM1 knockout cells showed no editing at these loci. These results confirm that the sgRNA has specificity for both IFITM2 and IFITM3, as the IFITM2/3 knockout cells are edited at both the *ifitm2* and *ifitm3* loci, but not at the *ifitm1* locus.

To ask if IFITM knockout rescues SAMHD1 degradation, knockout cell lines were treated with IFNα and with Vpx, as described previously, and SAMHD1 degradation was measured. We observed that knockout of IFITM2/3, but not IFITM1, led to a significant rescue of SAMHD1 degradation in presence of IFNα. In the experiment presented in Fig. 3c, up to 34% of IFITM2/3 knockout cells (vs < 1% in NTC cells) had SAMHD1 degraded in the presence of IFNα. Averaged over three independent experiments, we observed that knocking out IFITM2/3 significantly rescued SAMHD1 degradation (Fig. 3d). These results suggest that IFITM3 and/or IFITM2, but not IFITM1, play a major role in inhibiting SAMHD1 degradation by VLPs-Vpx.

Since IFITM3 was the top ISG (apart from positive controls) enriched in our initial screen, we also generated a stable THP1 cell line over-expressing an HA-tagged version of IFITM3 (IFTIM3-HA), in which the levels of IFITM3 are within fivefold of those observed after IFNα treatment, as measured by Western Blot (Fig. 3e). We found that IFITM3-HA over-expression potently inhibited the ability of VSV-G pseudotyped VLPs-Vpx to degrade SAMHD1 in the absence of IFNα: averaged over 3 experiments, we observed a fourfold reduction in SAMHD1 degradation in IFITM3 expressing cells, compared to wild-type THP1 (Fig. 3f). The results of both knockout and over-expression experiments thus show that IFITM2/3 inhibit SAMHD1 degradation in THP1 cells.

IFNα protection of SAMHD1 is envelope-dependent and affects entry of Vpx bearing VLPs into cells

We hypothesized that IFITMs may act on SAMHD1 degradation by inhibiting VSV-G endosomal entry, as this envelope was used to pseudotype the Virus-Like Particles containing Vpx. Importantly, while IFITM3 restricts entry of VSV [6] and of lentiviral vectors pseudotyped with the VSV-G envelope [33], it has no effect on entry mediated by the Murine Leukemia Virus amphotropic envelope (A-MLV) [4]. Unlike VSV, MLV is thought to fuse mainly at the plasma membrane [34], although some reports suggest that it uses caveolae-mediated endocytosis [35, 36]. Thus, we compared VLPs-Vpx pseudotyped with VSV-G, which had been used in Fig. 1 and in previous studies [10, 12, 22, 27], with VLPs-Vpx pseudotyped with the Murine Leukemia Virus amphotropic envelope (A-MLV). We normalized the amounts of VLPs-Vpx used based on RT activity, and verified that the different VLPs packaged roughly similar levels of Vpx (Fig. 4a). When

---

(See figure on next page.)

Fig. 3 IFITMs block SAMHD1 degradation after treatment with VLPs-Vpx pseudotyped with VSV-G. **a** Knockout efficiency as measured by protein levels. THP1 were cells transduced with a lentivector coding for Cas9 and sgRNAs targeting either IFITM1 (IFITM1-KO, lanes 2 and 5) or IFITM2 and IFITM3 (IFITM2/3-KO, lanes 3 and 6) or encoding a non-targeting sgRNA (NTC, lanes 1 and 4). Cells were selected in puromycin for 2 weeks. Cells were treated for 24 h with 0 (lanes 1 through 3) or 1000 (lanes 4 through 6) U/mL IFNα and protein expression was measured by Western Blot. For IFNα treated cells, three times less lysate was loaded, in order to be able to visualize levels of IFITMs in the absence or presence of IFNα stimulation in the same exposure. Tubulin was used as a loading control. **b** Genomic DNA was extracted from THP1 NTC, IFITM1-KO or IFITM2/3-KO cells. The *ifitm2* and *ifitm3* loci were amplified using specific PCR primers with a 3' mismatch. For each cell type, we verified that the PCR was specific by Sanger sequencing. The sequences at the two loci were compared to the reference sequence using TIDE analysis and the percentage of editing was quantified. **c** Cells were treated for 24 h with 0 or 1000 U/mL IFNα and incubated with the indicated amount of VLPs-Vpx pseudotyped with VSV-G. SAMHD1 degradation was measured by flow cytometry 16 h after treatment. One dose response experiment is shown. **d** Combined data from three independent experiments, using a viral dose within linear range. Each symbol represents an experiment. *$p < 0.05$ (*t* test). **e** Overexpression of IFITM3 in THP1 cells was measured by Western Blot. Cells were lysed in NP40-DOC buffer and probed for IFITM3. Tubulin was used as a loading control. The band indicated with an asterisk corresponds to the HA tagged version of IFITM3. **f** SAMHD1 degradation assays. Cells were treated for 24 h with 0 or 1000 U/mL IFNα, then incubated with the indicated amount of VLPs-Vpx pseudotyped with VSV-G for 16 h and SAMHD1 degradation was measured by flow cytometry. Combined data from three independent experiments using a viral dose within linear range. *$p < 0.05$ (*t* test)

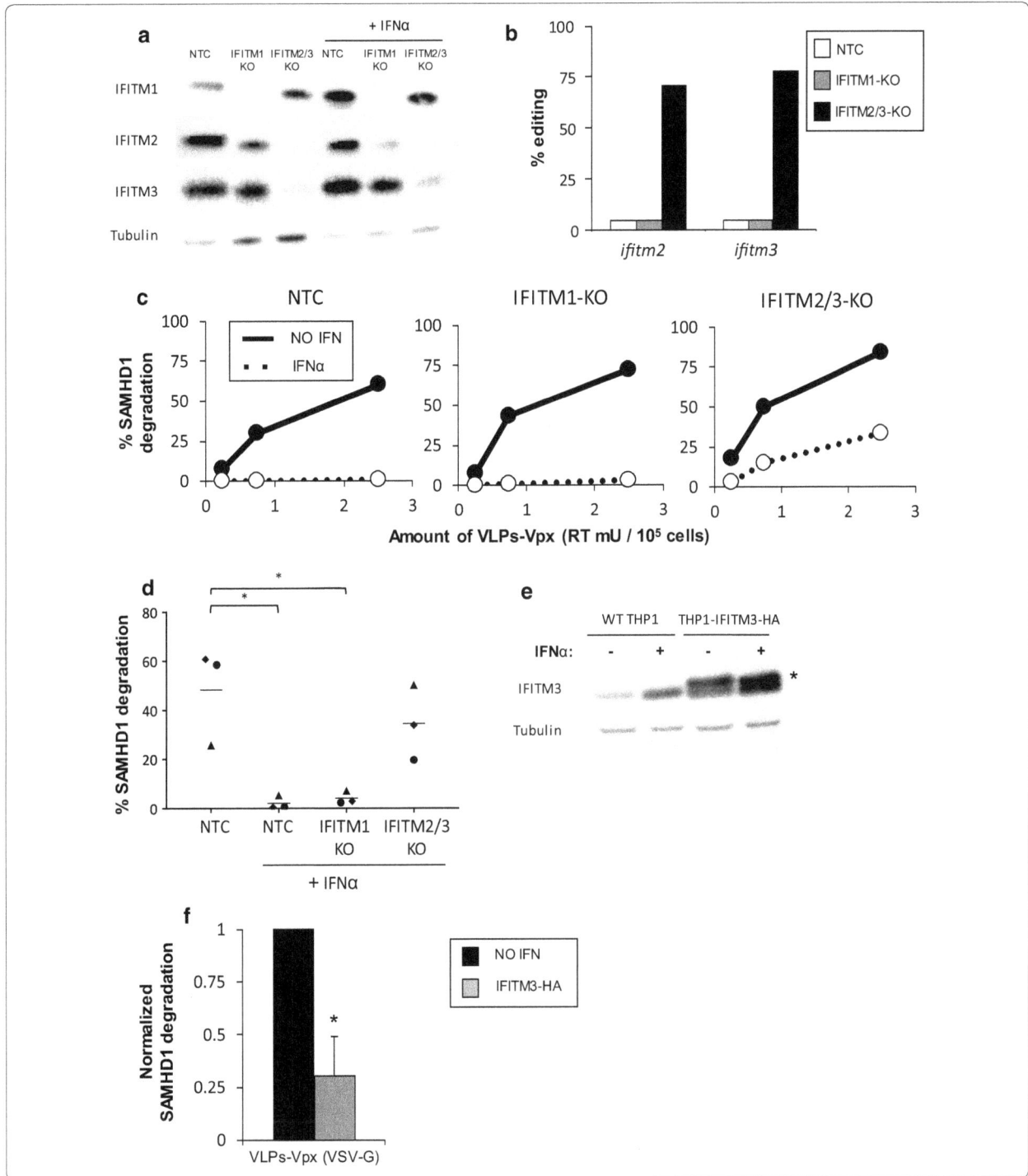

A-MLV was used instead of VSV-G, about 6 times more VLPs were required in order to achieve similar levels of SAMHD1 degradation, indicating that this envelope may be less fusogenic (Fig. 1b, ~ 1.5 RT mU of VLPs VSV-G lead to 20% degradation compared to 9 RT mU of VLPs A-MLV, Fig. 4b). Strikingly, we observed that while

A-MLV env-pseudotyped Vpx-containing particles were able to cause degradation of SAMHD1 in the absence of IFNα (Fig. 4b, black lines), IFNα treatment had no effect on Vpx-mediated SAMHD1 degradation (Fig. 4b, dashed line). Averaged over three independent experiments, we found that there is no significant difference in SAMHD1

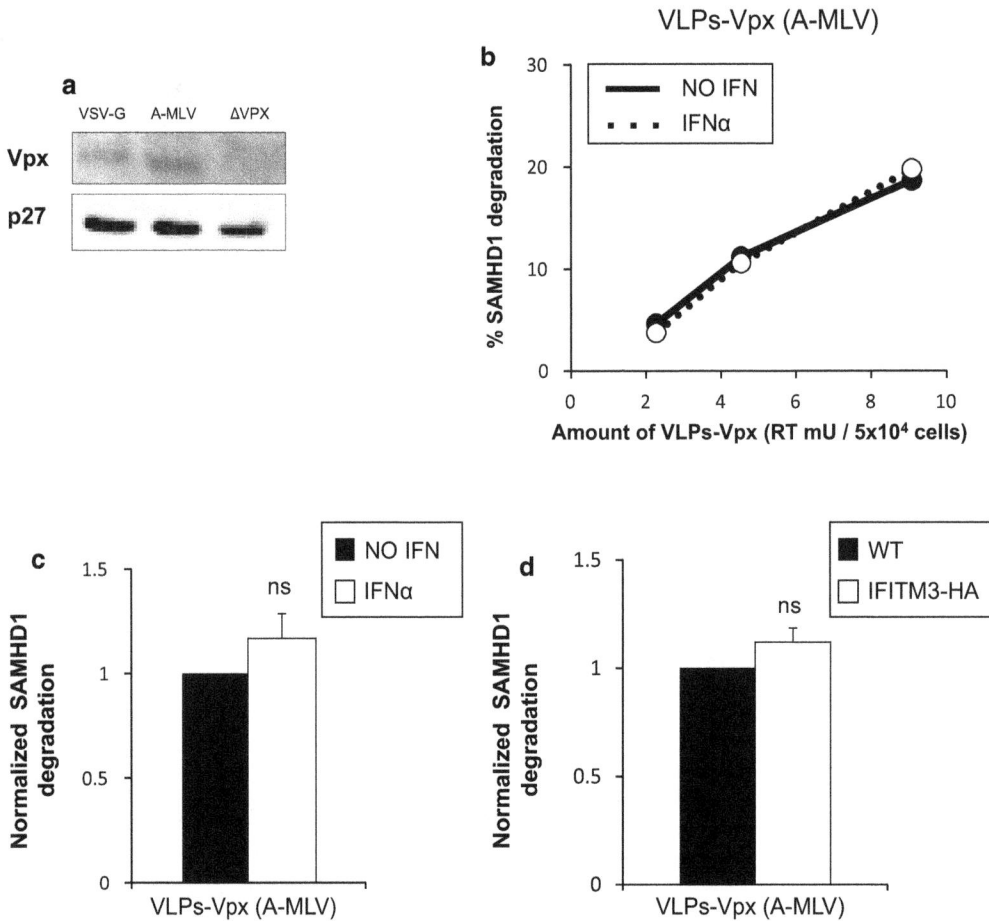

Fig. 4 IFN α does not block SAMHD1 degradation in THP1 cells when VLPs-Vpx are pseudotyped with A-MLV. **a** Levels of Vpx incorporation in VLPs pseudotyped with different envelopes. 250 RT mU of VLPs-Vpx pseudotyped with either VSV-G (left lane) or A-MLV (center lane) were loaded on a gel and levels of Vpx were probed by Western Blot. 250 RT mU of VLPs-Δvpx pseudotyped with VSV-G (rigth lane) were used as a negative control. 50 RT mU of the same VLPs preparations were loaded and probed for p27 as a loading control. **b** THP1 cells were treated for 24 h with 0 (solid lines) or 1000 (dotted lines) U/mL of IFNα, then with the indicated amount of VLPs–Vpx pseudotyped with A-MLV (as determined by RT activity). Cells were treated with the indicated amounts of VLPs-Vpx and SAMHD1 degradation was measured by flow cytometry 16 h later. One representative experiment is shown. **c** Combined data from three independent experiments for the effect of IFNα (white bar), using a viral dose within linear range. n = 3; *ns* non significant (*t* test). **d** Combined data from three independent experiments for the effect of IFITM3 overexpression (white bar), using a viral dose within linear range. n = 3; *ns* non significant (*t* test)

degradation by VLPs-Vpx particles pseudotyped with A-MLV (Fig. 4c), in contrast to VLPs-Vpx particles pseudotyped with VSV-G (Fig. 1c). IFITM3-HA over-expression also had no effect on SAMHD1 degradation when the A-MLV env was used (Fig. 4d), consistent with previous reports [4]. These results provide further evidence that, rather than directly acting on the SAMHD1/Vpx interface or on Vpx itself, IFNα likely acts at the earlier stage of Vpx delivery by VLPs.

In order to initiate degradation of SAMHD1, Vpx must be released from incoming virions, enter the nucleus [12] and engage the DCAF4/DDB1/Cul4a complex [15, 16]. Thus, monitoring SAMHD1 degradation is an indirect measure of the effects of IFNα and IFITMs on blocking release of viral components first into the cytoplasm. To show more directly that IFNα affects an early step of Vpx delivery into cells, we used the Vpr-β-lactamase (Vpr-BlaM) assay, which measures entry of viral cores into the cytoplasm specifically, without taking into account capture of viral particles in endosomes.

We produced HIVΔ*env* pseudotyped with VSV-G (HIVΔ*env*(VSV-G)) packaging Vpr-BlaM, and infected THP1 cells. Representative flow cytometry data and a dose response experiment are shown in Fig. 5a, b, respectively. IFITM3-HA over-expression signifi-cantly restricted VSV-G-mediated entry by about

(See figure on next page.)
Fig. 5 IFN α treatment and IFITMs directly block viral fusion. **a** THP1 wild-type or overexpressing IFITM3-HA were treated for 24 h with 0 or 1000 U/mL IFNα for 24 h, and then infected with the indicated amount of HIV-1Δenv(VSV-G) packaging the Vpr-β-lactamase fusion protein for 3 h. Cells were then incubated with the fluorescent CCF2-AM substrate for 2 h, fixed, and acquired by flow cytometry immediately. Representative flow cytometry plots are shown. **b** Representative dose response experiment. Solid black line: wild-type THP1 cells, dashed black line: wild-type THP1 treated with IFNα, grey dashed line: THP1 cells overexpressing IFITM3. **c** Combined data from three independent experiments, using a viral dose within linear range. **p < 0.01 (paired t test). **d** THP1 cells wild-type (in black) or knockout for IFITM2/3 (in grey) were treated with IFNα (dashed lines) or untreated (solid lines) and infected with the indicated amount or HIVΔenv(VSV-G). One representative dose response experiment is shown. **e** Combined data from four independent experiments, using a viral dose within linear range. Each symbol represents data from one experiment. **p < 0.01 (paired t test)

threefold (Fig. 5c), consistent with its effect on Vpx delivery (Fig. 3b). IFNα had an even stronger effect, inhibiting VSV-G entry by about eightfold. This result further demonstrates that IFNα treatment and IFITM3 expression are able to restrict entry of viral particles pseudotyped with VSV-G, excluding other indirect effects on Vpx or SAMHD1. Similar to our results using SAMHD1 degradation experiments (Fig. 3), knocking-out IFITM2/3 rescued VSV-G fusion in the presence of IFNα (Fig. 5d): the inhibition by IFNα decreased from roughly 30-fold to 1.5-fold when IFITM2/3 were knocked-out even though we used pools of cells where the knockout efficiency was around 75% (Fig. 3b). Averaged over four experiments, IFITM2/3 knockout significantly rescued entry of VSV-G pseudotyped particles into cells (Fig. 5e), demonstrating that IFITM2/3 indeed contribute to the IFNα entry block to VSV-G entry. Although we cannot exclude a role for other ISGs, we conclude that the main mechanism by which IFNα protects SAMHD1 from degradation is by inducing expression of IFITMs that block VSV-G-mediated entry of VLPs-Vpx.

IFNα and IFITMs impose a stronger block on VSV-G-pseudotyped viruses than on wild-type HIV-1

IFNα treatment, in part through the action of IFITMs, blocks entry of VSV-G pseudotyped viral particles. Because entry with the VSV-G envelope may differ from how HIV-1 enters cells we compared the magnitude of this block to the one imposed on HIV-1's own CXCR4-tropic envelope. Importantly, these two envelopes have different mechanisms for viral entry: while VSV-G-mediated entry occurs through pH-dependent fusion in the endosomes [37], productive entry of HIV-1 into its target cells likely happens by pH-independent fusion at the plasma membrane, although this remains controversial [38, 39]. Thus, we reasoned that the site of viral entry might dictate the sensitivity to IFNα and to IFITMs and affect lentiviruses bearing the HIV-1 or VSV-G envelopes differentially. To test this hypothesis, we directly compared the amount of IFNα block to HIV-1 that either contained its natural env or was pseudotyped with VSV-G in the entry assay described previously (Fig. 5).

Strikingly, while we observed stronger IFNα block on VSV-G-mediated entry than for HIV-1 env-mediated entry (24-fold vs 1.5-fold on average, respectively; Fig. 6a, b). Similarly, knockout of basal levels of IFITM2/3 (in absence of IFNα) had a significant impact on VSV-G-mediated entry, but much less on entry mediated by HIV-1 Env (fourfold vs 1.5-fold on average, Fig. 6c, d). In both cases, statistical analysis indicated that infection by VSV-G pseudotypes was significantly different than HIV-1 wt either in the presence of IFNα or in untreated cells lacking IFITM2 and IFITM3. These results suggest that VSV-G pseudotyping may expose the virus to a different subset of restriction factors that restrict viral fusion, including IFITMs, potentially by diverting HIV-1 from its natural entry pathway. These results are consistent with previous observations linking the route of HIV-1 entry and IFITM restriction [25].

To confirm that this difference in entry translates into different levels of infection in cell cultures, we performed single cycle infection assays. THP1 cells transduced with lentivectors encoding Non-Targeting Control (NTC) or IFITM2/3-targeting sgRNAs were infected with either HIV-1Δenv(VSV-G), which is only able to perform one cycle of infection, or with wild-type HIV-1. In order to ensure that the latter virus only performs one round of infection, the viral input was washed after 24 h and cells were treated with T-20, a peptide inhibiting membrane fusion of HIV-1 [40]. These experiments were performed in absence of IFNα with the rationale that other ISGs potently inhibiting HIV in THP1 cells, such as MxB could mask the effect of IFITMs [29]. Notably, IFITMs are significantly expressed at basal levels (Fig. 3a). Infection was monitored by measuring intracellular Gag levels 48 h post-infection. Consistent with our entry results, we observed that IFITM2/3 knockout greatly enhanced infection by HIV-1Δenv(VSV-G), but had a much less pronounced effect on wild-type HIV-1 infection (Fig. 6e, f). Taken together, these results suggest that basal levels of IFITM2 and IFITM3 expression inhibit VSV-G-mediated entry, but much less HIV-1 entry. Furthermore, we conclude that VSV-G-pseudotyping, although achieving higher rates of infection thanks to a higher envelope

a

THP1 WT	THP1 WT + IFNα	THP1 IFITM3 -HA	
0.2%	0.2%	0.2%	Non infected
22.8%	3.6%	10.0%	HIV-1Δ*env*(VSV-G)

CCF2-AM

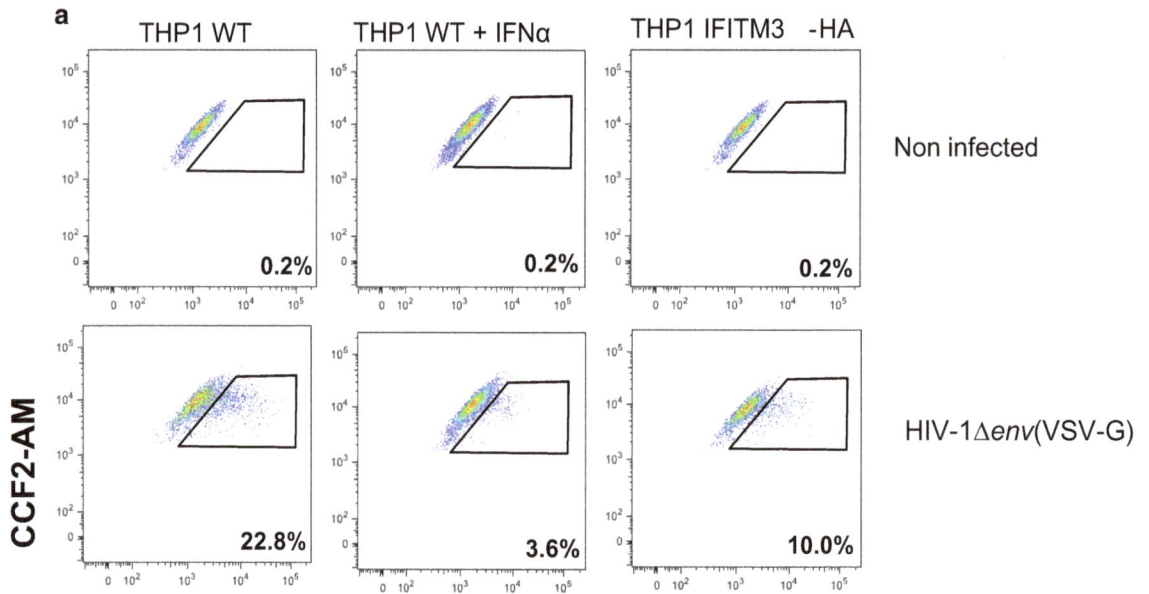

Cleaved CCF2-AM

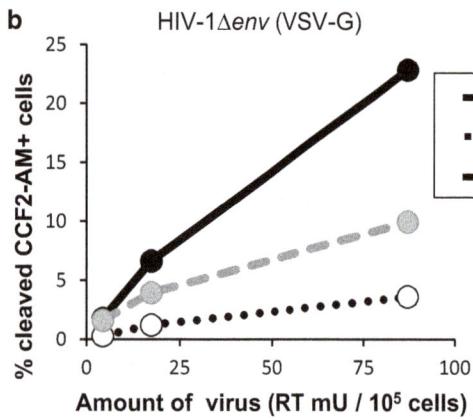

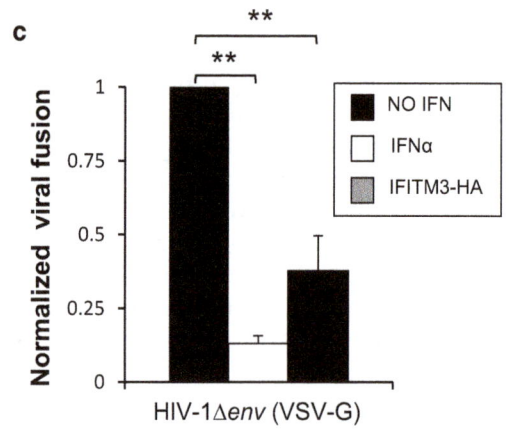

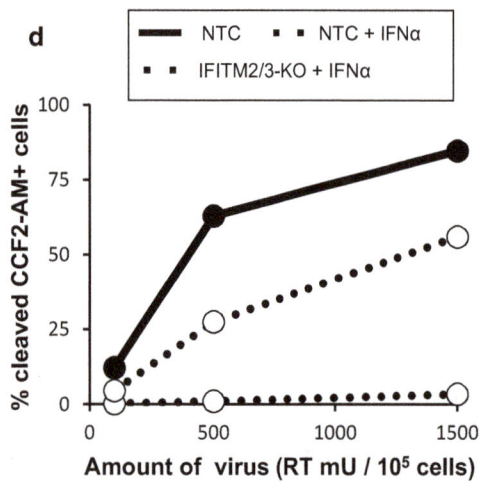

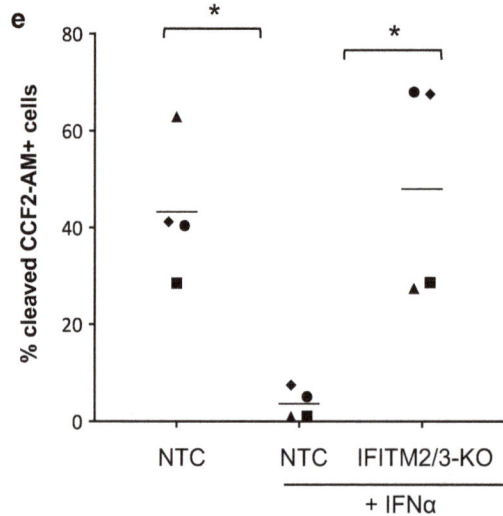

b

HIV-1Δ*env* (VSV-G)

% cleaved CCF2-AM+ cells

— NO IFN
···· IFNα
- - IFITM3-HA

Amount of virus (RT mU / 10^5 cells)

c

Normalized viral fusion

■ NO IFN
□ IFNα
▨ IFITM3-HA

HIV-1Δ*env* (VSV-G)

d

— NTC   · · NTC + IFNα
· · IFITM2/3-KO + IFNα

% cleaved CCF2-AM+ cells

Amount of virus (RT mU / 10^5 cells)

e

% cleaved CCF2-AM+ cells

NTC   NTC   IFITM2/3-KO
                        + IFNα

(See figure on next page.)
Fig. 6 VSV-G pseudotyping leads to stronger restriction by IFNα and IFITM2/3. **a, b** THP1 wild-type or overexpressing IFITM3-HA were treated for 24 h with 0 or 1000 U/mL IFNα for 24 h, and then infected with the indicated amounts of either HIV-1 WT (**a**, left panel) or HIV-1Δenv(VSV-G) (**a**, right panel) packaging the Vpr-β-lactamase fusion protein for 3 h. Cells were then incubated with the fluorescent CCF2-AM substrate for 2 h, fixed, and acquired by flow cytometry immediately. **a** Representative dose response experiment. **b** Combined data from four independent experiments, using a viral dose within linear range. Each symbol representing data from one experiment. *$p < 0.05$; **$p < 0.01$ (t test). **c, d** THP1 cells transduced with a Non-Targeting Control (NTC) sgRNA or with an sgRNA targeting both IFITM2 and IFITM3 (IFITM2/3) were infected, in the absence of IFNα, with HIV WT (**c**, left panel) or HIV-1Δenv(VSV-G) (**c**, right panel) packaging Vpr BlaM for 3 h. Viral entry was measured as in panel **a**. **c** One representative dose response experiment. **d** Combined data from four independent experiments, using a viral dose within linear range. Each symbol represents one experiment. *$p < 0.05$ (t test). **e, f** THP1 cells transduced with a non-targeting sgRNA (NTC) or with a sgRNA against IFITM2 and IFITM3 (IFITM2/3) were infected, in absence of IFNα, with HIV WT (**e**, left panel) or HIV-1Δenv(VSV-G) (**e**, right panel). After 24 h, viral input was washed, and cells were cultured in presence of 1 μM of the entry inhibitor T-20, to prevent subsequence rounds of infection. The percentage of Gag positive cells were measured by flow cytometry at 48 h p.i. E: One representative dose response experiment. **f** Combined data from four independent experiments, using a viral dose within linear range. Each symbol representing data from one experiment. Each symbol represents one experiment. *$p < 0.05$, **$p < 0.01$ (t test)

fusogenicity, changes the sensitivity of HIV-1 to an IFNα entry block by increasing sensitivity to IFITM-mediated restriction.

Discussion

A CRISPR screen for IFNα-induced factors that protect SAMHD1 from degradation

A flow cytometry-based CRISPR knockout screen approach identified IFITMs as being the most predominant ISGs underlying the protection of SAMHD1 from degradation after transduction with VSV-G-pseudotyped VLPs containing Vpx [22]. As the VSV-G used to pseudotype the VLPs delivering Vpx mediates entry into endosomes [37], where IFITMs (particularly IFITM3) are thought to act, our results argue that IFNα protects SAMHD1 from degradation by blocking viral entry of VLPs delivering Vpx into cells. The method described here that assays viral entry/fusion events by monitoring Vpx-mediated degradation of SAMHD1, could also be applied more generally to discover new genes affecting entry mediated by different envelope proteins.

IFITMs directly contribute to the effect of IFNα on SAMHD1 degradation by VLPs-Vpx

Because of high sequence homology, targeting IFITM3 without affecting levels of IFITM2 is challenging, as described in previous studies [25, 30]. Thus, we could not formally demonstrate if IFITM2 or IFITM3 act synergistically, or alone in this phenotype. Nonetheless, we did show that IFITM3-HA overexpression is sufficient to inhibit degradation of SAMHD1 by VLPs-Vpx (Fig. 3). Although one previous study observed only a minor effect of IFNα treatment on viral entry of VSV-G-pseudotyped lentivectors using the Vpr-BlaM assay [22], our eightfold IFNα block of VSV-G entry (Fig. 5), together with the fact that IFNα has no effect when an alternate delivery method was used (Fig. 4), strongly

supports the idea that IFITMs block delivery of Vpx into the cytoplasm of IFNα-treated cells. Therefore, the SAMHD1 protection phenotype described in the literature [22] can be explained by inhibition of Vpx delivery by IFITMs. Finally, other factors, such as COMMD3 or EIF3L also emerged as top hits from our screen (Fig. 2), and although they were minimally induced (if at all) by IFNα in THP1 cells, they may contribute to early events in VSV-G-mediated entry into cells.

VSV-G pseudotyping changes HIV-1 sensitivity to IFNα and IFITMs

In addition to blocking endosomal entry of VSV [6], IFITMs are also described to inhibit HIV-1 entry when expressed in target cells [41]. IFITM restriction in target cells may rely on a different mechanism than when IFITMs are expressed in producer cells. In addition to the role of IFITMs that are packaged into budding virions and restrict infection in target cells [33, 42, 43], IFITMs may, when expressed in target cells, also inhibit the hemifusion process [44, 45], and/or deregulate cholesterol homeostasis, resulting in reduced membrane fusion [46].

Changing the entry pathway used by HIV-1 by VSV-G pseudotyping directs membrane fusion to the endosomes instead of at the plasma membrane, and may influence HIV-1 sensitivity to ISGs, and to IFITMs in particular. Consistent with this idea, we observed that VSV-G pseudotypes are hyper sensitive to IFNα and IFITMs (Fig. 6). Moreover, the effect of IFITM3-HA on VSV-G-mediated entry did not completely recapitulate the magnitude of the IFNα block (Fig. 5), suggesting that other ISGs may play an additional role.

A recent report demonstrating that HIV-1 Transmitter/Founder strains are initially resistant to IFITM3, but become sensitive after viral escape from neutralizing antibodies [25]. Although it is important to note that the subcellular compartment in which HIV-1 fuses and enter

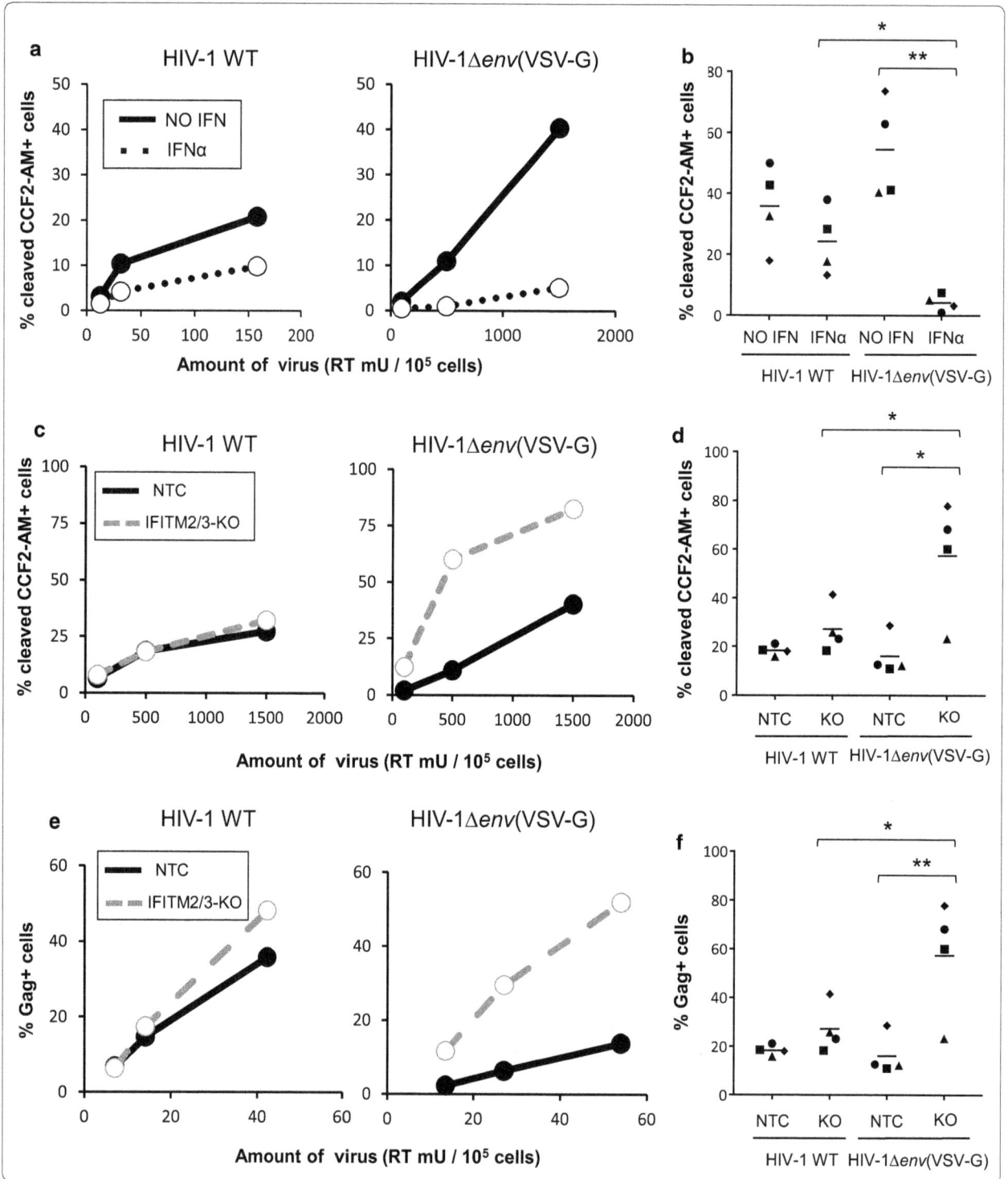

cells leading to productive infection remains controversial, and may depend on the cell type used [38, 39], one likely interpretation of our results is that in THP1 cells, HIV-1 fuses predominantly at the plasma membrane, rather than in endosomal vesicles where IFITM3 and other ISGs may act. VSV-G pseudotyping, by re-routing HIV-1 fusion to endosomes, may expose the virus to a different set of restriction factors. Our data suggest that HIV-1 strains that have evolved to fuse at the plasma membrane would avoid a potentially more restrictive environment imposed by IFITM2/3. The endosomal compartment may indeed represent a less productive route for HIV-1 entry, as has been suggested by a study in which a dominant negative variant of dynamin blocked endocytosis but had no effect on infection levels in T cells [47]. Importantly, VSV-G pseudotyping may not only affect viral entry, but also later steps in the viral life cycle, such as uncoating [48] or nuclear import and integration [49]. Thus, such considerations should be taken into account in studies that use VSV-G pseudotyping, as it may influence the antiviral factors that HIV-1 may be accessible to.

Conclusions

In this work, we used a CRISPR-Cas9 knockout flow cytometry screen to determine factor(s) are responsible for the block to SAMHD1 degradation in IFNα treated cells when Vpx is delivered via VSV-G pseudotyped viral particles. We identified IFITMs as the major factors involved in this phenomenon. Our results suggest that IFNα acts on Vpx delivery due to the effects of IFITMs on VSV-G-mediated entry/fusion rather than on the SAMHD1 degradation process itself. Indeed, we show that IFNα and IFITM2/3 have a much greater effect on entry of HIV-1 pseudotyped with VSV-G compared to HIV-1 bearing a CXCR4-tropic envelope. Thus, using VSV-G pseudotypes to study HIV restriction factors can be misleading because these pseudotypes may be exposed to antiviral factors that do not normally affect HIV-1. Finally, the CRISPR knockout screening approach we describe here could also be used to identify restriction factors specific for different viral envelopes using Vpx-mediated SAMHD1 degradation as an easy readout to screen for viral entry.

Material and methods
Cells, plasmids and viruses

THP1 cells were grown in RPMI 1640, supplemented with 10% Fetal Bovine Serum (FBS) and penicillin/streptomycin (100 µg/mL; Gibco #15140-122). HEK-293T cells were grown in Dulbecco modified Eagle medium (DMEM) supplemented with 10% FBS and penicillin/streptomycin. The SIV3+, SIV3Δvpx and Vpr-β-lactamase plasmids are kind gifts from Olivier Schwartz [10, 11, 27, 50]. The pHIV-dTomato plasmid was obtained through Addgene (#21374). The sgRNA library was synthesized in vitro (Twist Bioscience) and cloned in the lentiCRISPRv2 lentiviral backbone, and was a gift from Feng Zhang (Addgene plasmid # 52961). pMD2.G and psPAX2 were gifts from Didier Trono (Addgene plasmids #12259/12260). VLPs-Vpx were produced by transfecting HEK293T cells with SIV$_{MAC}$ Gag/Pol (SIV3+plasmid or SIV3Δvpx) and VSV-G (pMD2.G

plasmid) or A-MLV (A-MLV Env plasmid) at a 2.5: 1 ratio, and using 3 µL of TransIT LT1 (#MIR2305, Mirus) per µg of DNA. HIV-1 Vpr-β-lactamase viruses were produced by co-transfecting either HIV-1 proviral wild-type plasmid (pLAI) and Vpr-β-lactamase at a 3:1 ratio, or HIV-1Δenv (pLAIΔenv), VSV-G, and Vpr-β-lactamase at a 3:1:1 ratio. IFITM3-HA lentivector particles were made by co-transfecting the pHIV-dTomato-IFITM3-HA plasmid together with HIV-1 Gag/Pol (psPAX2 plasmid) and VSV-G at a 2:1.5:1 ratio. Lentiviral vector preparations containing the ISG library were made using the lentiC-RISPRv2_ISG library assembly together with psPAX2 and VSV-G at a 2:1.5:1 ratio. For all virus and VLP production, supernatants were harvested 48–72 h post transfection, clarified by centrifugation, passed through a 0.22 µm filter and concentrated by ultracentrifugation (90 min at 90,000 g). All transduction and infection experiments were carried out in presence of 20 µg/mL of DEAE-Dextran (Sigma; # D9885). The following reagents were obtained through the NIH AIDS Reagent Program, Division of AIDS, NIAID, NIH: T-20,(Enfuvirtide); SV-A-MLV-Env plasmid from Dr. Nathaniel Landau and Dr. Dan Littman [51].

SAMHD1 degradation assay

$5x10^4$ THP1 cells were plated in 96-well plates and treated with 1000 U/mL universal type I IFNα (#11200-2, PBL) or IFNγ (#11500-2, PBL) for 24 h. The next day the cells were treated with the indicated amount of VLPs-Vpx for 16 h. Cells were washed in PBS, and incubated for 15 min at room temperature with the Live/Dead Fixable Blue Dead Cell Stain Kit following instructions provided by the manufacturer (#L34962, ThermoFisher), then fixed in 4% formaldehyde solution (diluted in PBS from a 37% solution, Sigma #252549) for 5 min, and then permeabilized using PBS-Triton X-100 (Sigma, #X100) 0.5% for 15 min. Cells were then stained on ice for 30 min with anti-SAMHD1 antibody (clone I19-18, Millipore #MABF933,) diluted to 0.5 µg/mL in PBS 1% BSA, washed in PBS, and incubated on ice for 30 min with the Goat anti-mouse Alexa 488 secondary antibody (#A-11001, Thermo Fisher), diluted to 4 µg/mL in PBS 1% BSA. Flow cytometry data were acquired using a CANTO-II flow cytometer (BD).

Flow cytometry CRISPR screen

The screening experiment was performed with two technical replicates. $5x10^7$ THP1 cells were transduced with lentiviral vectors containing the lentiC-RISPRv2_ISG library. After 2 weeks of puromycin selection (0.5 µg/mL, #P8833, Sigma), cells were treated with 1000 U/mL of universal type I IFNα for 24 h and incubated with VLPs-Vpx for 16 h. Cells were washed in PBS and incubated for 30 min at room temperature with the Live/Dead Fixable Blue Dead Cell Stain Kit following instructions provided by the manufacturer. Cells were washed in PBS and fixed with 1% PFA for 15 min. The fixation process was stopped by addition of 0.2 M Glycine. Cells were washed in PBS, and permeabilized using PBS/Triton X100 0.5% for 15 min. Cells were washed with PBS, stained on ice for 60 min with anti-SAMHD1 antibody diluted at 0.5 µg/mL in PBS 1% BSA, washed in PBS, and incubated on ice for 45 min with the Goat anti-mouse Alexa 488 secondary antibody diluted to 4 µg/mL in PBS 1% BSA. Cells were washed and resuspended in sorting buffer (PBS 2% FBS, 25 mM Hepes, 5 mM EDTA) and filtered. 5×10^5 SAMHD1 negative and 3×10^6 SAMHD1 positive cells were then sorted using an ARIA-II flow cytometer (BD), in polypropylene tubes previously coated with PBS 4% BSA. Cells were pelleted and lysed in 300 µL of chromatin immunoprecipitation buffer (0.1% SDS, 10 mM EDTA, 20 mM EGTA, 300 mM NaCl, 10 mM Tris HCl pH 8.1). 3 µL of proteinase K (#19133, Qiagen) and 3 µL of RNAse A (10 µg/mL, #R4642-10MG, Sigma) were added to the lysates and cells were incubated at 65 °C for 16 h to reverse crosslinking of protein and DNA. DNA was extracted using phenol chloroform (#P2069-100 ML, Sigma), precipitated, washed in 70% ethanol, and resuspended in RNAse free water. sgRNAs were amplified from genomic DNA with a maximum of 2 µg of template DNA per reaction using the Herculase II Fusion DNA Polymerase kit (Agilent, #600679). A first PCR was carried out using the following primers: forward gagggcctatttcccatgattccttca and reverse ctgctgtccctgtaataaacccg. Round 1 PCR products were cleaned up using the QIAquick PCR purification kit (Qiagen, #28106) and used as a template for the round 2 PCR, that allows barcoding and addition of the sequencing adapters, using a common reverse primer caagcagaagacggcatacgagatgtgactggagttcagacgtgtgctcttccgatcttgccactttttcaagttgataacggact coupled with a unique barcoding forward primer for each sample, here: F1 aatgatacggcgaccaccgagatctacactctttccctacacgacgctcttccgatctatctcgcgtacgtcttgtggaaaggacgaaacaccg and F2 aatgatacggcgaccaccgagatctacactctttccctacacgacgctcttccgatctactacagtgtcttgtggaaaggacgaaacaccg. PCR products were cleaned up and size selected using the Agencourt Ampure XP beads kit (Beckman Coulter, # A63880), using a two-step purification with 1:1.2 and 1:1.5 DNA to beads ratios. Samples were quantified using the QUBIT dsDNA HS Assay Kit (Thermo Fisher Q32854), pooled at a 2 nM concentration and submitted for sequencing on one HiSeq2500 (Illumina) lane, using the Rapid Mode (60 cycles).

Statistical analysis

sgRNA enrichment was analyzed using the Bioconductor package edgeR [52] and gene-level analysis was performed using MAGeCK [28]. The IFNα induction data was generated using a dataset (GSE46599) published by Goujon et al. [29] and re-analyzed using the lumi [53] and limma [54] Bioconductor packages. When several probes were used for a single genes, fold induction values were averaged.

Reverse-transcriptase activity assay

Viral stocks were quantified using an RT activity assay described before [55]. Briefly, viral supernatants were lysed in 2X lysis buffer (0.25% Triton X-100, 50 mM KCl, 100 mM Tris HCl, glycerol 40%) in the presence of 4U RNAse inhibitor (Fermentas, #EO0382). qRT-PCR reactions were prepared following instructions from the Takyon Rox SYBR MasterMix dTTP Blue kit (Eurogentec, #UF-RSMT-B0101), with MS2 RNA used as a template (Roche, #10165948001) and the following primers: tcctgctcaacttcctgtcgag and cacaggtcaaacctcctaggaatg. qRT-PCR was performed using a ABI QuantStudio5 Real Time PCR machine. Reactions were performed in duplicates, and titers were calculated using a standard curve made with a virus stock of previously determined RT units.

Vpr-β-lactamase assays

Viral entry was assayed with a protocol adapted from Cavrois et al. [50]. Briefly, indicated amounts of virus containing the Vpr-β-lactamase fusion protein were used to infect 10^5 THP1 cells. After 3 h, cells were washed in cold CO_2-independent media (Invitrogen), without FBS, resuspended in CO_2-independent media supplemented with 10% FBS, and incubated with the CCF2-AM substrate following the instructions provided by the manufacturer (LiveBlazer FRET—B/G loading kit, #K1023, Invitrogen), in the presence of 1.8 mM Probenecid (#P8761-25G, Sigma), for 2 h at room temperature in the dark. Cells were washed three times in cold CO_2-independent media, then once in PBS, and finally fixed with 4% formaldehyde for 10 min. Fluorescence of the CCF2-AM substrate was immediately measured by flow cytometry on a Canto-II (BD) using the AmCyan and Pacific-Blue channels.

Generation of cell lines overexpressing IFITMs or with IFITM knockout

RNA was extracted from 10^6 THP1 cells using the Rneasy plus mini Kit (#74134, Qiagen). RT-PCR was performed to amplify IFITM3 cDNA and add a C-terminal HA-tag and restriction sites using the SuperScript® III One-Step RT-PCR System with Platinum Taq DNA Polymerase kit (#12574018, Invitrogen) and the following primers: gatctctagaatcgatatgaatcacactgtccaaacct and gatcggatccggtaccctaagcgtaatctggaacatcgtatgggtatccataggcctggaagatca. IFITM3-HA was then cloned into the pHIV-dTomato backbone using the XbaI/BamHI restriction sites, and clones were verified by sequencing. THP1 cells were spinoculated with lentivectors encoding IFITM3-HA, and overexpression was verified by monitoring dTomato levels. Cells were harvested and lysed in the NP40-DOC lysis buffer (NP40 1%, deoxycholate 0.2%, NaCl 120 mM, Tris 20 mM) and IFITM3 levels were also monitored by Western Blot analysis (#11714-1-AP, Proteintech; 1/1000). sgRNAs targeting IFITM1 or IFITM2/3 were cloned in the lentiCRISPRv2 backbone by BsmBI restriction of the backbone, annealing of sense and antisense oligos (5 min at 95 °C) and ligation. The following oligos were used (the 20 bp-gene targeting sequence in all caps): IFITM1 sense caccgCAGAGCCGAATACCAGTAAC and antisense aaacGTTACT GGTATTCGGCTCTGc; IFITM2/3 sense caccgGTGGATCACGGTGGACGTCG and antisense aaacCGACGTCCACCGTGATCCACc; NTC sense caccgACGGAGGCTAAGCGTCGCAA and antisense aaacTTGCGACGCTTAGCCTCCGTc. Lentiviral particles were produced as indicated before and used to transduce THP1 cells. After 1-2 weeks of puromycin selection (1 µg/mL, #P8833, Sigma), genomic DNA was extracted using the QuickExtract kit (Lucigen, QE09050) by resuspending cells in 100 µL of the solution, and by denaturing for 20 min at 60 °C and 20 min at 95 °C. The following primers, specific for each *ifitm* locus due to a mismatch at the 3' nucleotide, were used for locus specific amplification: IFITM2-F aagaggaaactgttgagaaaacgg, IFITM2-R cgtgtgaggataaagggctgatg, IFITM3-F accatcccagtaacccgaccg, IFITM3-R gctgatacaggactcggctcc. Amplicons were sequenced and the percentage of editing was quantified using TIDE analysis [32] (https://tide-calculator.nki.nl/). Knockout was also verified by Western Blot using NP40-DOC as the lysis buffer and antibodies specific for IFITM1 (#60074-1-Ig, Proteintech; 1/1000), IFITM2 (#66137-1-Ig, Proteintech; 1/1000), IFITM3 (#11714-1-AP, Proteintech; 1/1000).

Single cycle infection assays

10^5 cells were infected with HIV-1 WT or HIV-1Δ*env*(VSV-G) with the indicated amounts of virus. After 24 h, cells were washed in PBS and the T-20 entry inhibitor (NIH AIDS reagent program, #12732) was added at a 1 µM concentration to prevent subsequent rounds of infection. Intracellular Gag levels were measured by flow cytometry 36 h post infection using KC57-FITC (Beckman Coulter #664665).

Authors' contributions
FR designed and performed experiments, and analyzed results. MO helped perform experiments. ME helped design experiments and analyzed results. All authors wrote the manuscript and read and approved the final version.

Acknowledgements
We thank Olivier Schwartz for sharing reagents. We thank Loïc Dragin and Florence Margottin-Goguet for helpful discussion and Nicholas Chesarino and Amit Sharma for critical reading of the manuscript. We thank the Fred Hutch Flow Cytometry and Genomics Shared Resources. We thank Ryan Basom for help in data analysis.

Competing interests
The authors declare that they have no competing interests.

Funding
This work was supported by CCEH Pilot Grant P30 DK56465 to MO and R01 AI30927 and R01 GM11570 to ME. The funders had no role in study design, data collection and interpretation, or the decision to submit the work for publication.

References
1. Schoggins JW, Rice CM. Interferon-stimulated genes and their antiviral effector functions. Curr Opin Virol. 2011;1:519–25.
2. Bailey CC, Zhong G, Huang IC, Farzan M. IFITM-family proteins: the cell's first line of antiviral defense. Annu Rev Virol. 2014;1:261–83.
3. Weston S, Czieso S, White IJ, Smith SE, Wash RS, Diaz-Soria C, et al. Alphavirus restriction by IFITM proteins. Traffic. 2016;17:997–1013.
4. Brass AL, Huang IC, Benita Y, John SP, Krishnan MN, Feeley EM, et al. The IFITM proteins mediate cellular resistance to influenza A H1N1 virus, West Nile virus, and dengue virus. Cell. 2009;139:1243–54.
5. Narayana SK, Helbig KJ, McCartney EM, Eyre NS, Bull RA, Eltahla A, et al. The interferon-induced transmembrane proteins, IFITM1, IFITM2, and IFITM3 inhibit hepatitis C virus entry. J Biol Chem. 2015;290:25946–59.
6. Weidner JM, Jiang D, Pan XB, Chang J, Block TM, Guo JT. Interferon-induced cell membrane proteins, IFITM3 and tetherin, inhibit vesicular stomatitis virus infection via distinct mechanisms. J Virol. 2010;84:12646–57.
7. Ambrose Z, Aiken C. HIV-1 uncoating: connection to nuclear entry and regulation by host proteins. Virology. 2014.
8. Accola MA, Bukovsky AA, Jones MS, Gottlinger HG. A conserved dileucine-containing motif in p6(gag) governs the particle association of Vpx and Vpr of simian immunodeficiency viruses SIV(mac) and SIV(agm). J Virol. 1999;73:9992–9.
9. Jauregui P, Logue EC, Schultz ML, Fung S, Landau NR. Degradation of SAMHD1 by Vpx Is independent of uncoating. J Virol. 2015;89:5701–13.
10. Laguette N, Sobhian B, Casartelli N, Ringeard M, Chable-Bessia C, Segeral E, et al. SAMHD1 is the dendritic- and myeloid-cell-specific HIV-1 restriction factor counteracted by Vpx. Nature. 2011;474:654–7.
11. Hrecka K, Hao C, Gierszewska M, Swanson SK, Kesik-Brodacka M, Srivastava S, et al. Vpx relieves inhibition of HIV-1 infection of macrophages mediated by the SAMHD1 protein. Nature. 2011;474:658–61.
12. Lahouassa H, Daddacha W, Hofmann H, Ayinde D, Logue EC, Dragin L, et al. SAMHD1 restricts the replication of human immunodeficiency virus type 1 by depleting the intracellular pool of deoxynucleoside triphosphates. Nat Immunol. 2012;13:223–8.
13. Descours B, Cribier A, Chable-Bessia C, Ayinde D, Rice G, Crow Y, et al. SAMHD1 restricts HIV-1 reverse transcription in quiescent CD4(+) T-cells. Retrovirology. 2012;9:87.
14. Lim ES, Fregoso OI, McCoy CO, Matsen FA, Malik HS, Emerman M. The ability of primate lentiviruses to degrade the monocyte restriction factor SAMHD1 preceded the birth of the viral accessory protein Vpx. Cell Host Microbe. 2012;11:194–204.

15. Sharova N, Wu Y, Zhu X, Stranska R, Kaushik R, Sharkey M, et al. Primate lentiviral Vpx commandeers DDB1 to counteract a macrophage restriction. PLoS Pathog. 2008;4:e1000057.

16. Ahn J, Hao C, Yan J, DeLucia M, Mehrens J, Wang C, et al. HIV/simian immunodeficiency virus (SIV) accessory virulence factor Vpx loads the host cell restriction factor SAMHD1 onto the E3 ubiquitin ligase complex CRL4DCAF1. J Biol Chem. 2012;287:12550–8.

17. Fregoso OI, Ahn J, Wang C, Mehrens J, Skowronski J, Emerman M. Evolutionary toggling of Vpx/Vpr specificity results in divergent recognition of the restriction factor SAMHD1. PLoS Pathog. 2013;9:e1003496.

18. Cribier A, Descours B, Valadao AL, Laguette N, Benkirane M. Phosphorylation of SAMHD1 by cyclin A2/CDK1 regulates its restriction activity toward HIV-1. Cell Rep. 2013;3:1036–43.

19. Bonifati S, Daly MB, St Gelais C, Kim SH, Hollenbaugh JA, Shepard C, et al. SAMHD1 controls cell cycle status, apoptosis and HIV-1 infection in monocytic THP-1 cells. Virology. 2016;495:92–100.

20. Yan J, Hao C, DeLucia M, Swanson S, Florens L, Washburn MP, et al. CyclinA2-cyclin-dependent kinase regulates SAMHD1 protein phosphohydrolase domain. J Biol Chem. 2015;290:13279–92.

21. Kudoh A, Miyakawa K, Matsunaga S, Matsushima Y, Kosugi I, Kimura H, et al. H11/HSPB8 restricts HIV-2 Vpx to restore the anti-viral activity of SAMHD1. Front Microbiol. 2016;7:883.

22. Dragin L, Nguyen LA, Lahouassa H, Sourisce A, Kim B, Ramirez BC, et al. Interferon block to HIV-1 transduction in macrophages despite SAMHD1 degradation and high deoxynucleoside triphosphates supply. Retrovirology. 2013;10:30.

23. Riess M, Fuchs NV, Idica A, Hamdorf M, Flory E, Pedersen IM, et al. Interferons induce expression of SAMHD1 in monocytes through down-regulation of miR-181a and miR-30a. J Biol Chem. 2017;292:264–77.

24. Yang S, Zhan Y, Zhou Y, Jiang Y, Zheng X, Yu L, et al. Interferon regulatory factor 3 is a key regulation factor for inducing the expression of SAMHD1 in antiviral innate immunity. Sci Rep. 2016;6:29665.

25. Foster TL, Wilson H, Iyer SS, Coss K, Doores K, Smith S, et al. Resistance of transmitted founder HIV-1 to IFITM-mediated restriction. Cell Host Microbe. 2016;20:429–42.

26. Goujon C, Jarrosson-Wuilleme L, Bernaud J, Rigal D, Darlix JL, Cimarelli A. With a little help from a friend: increasing HIV transduction of monocyte-derived dendritic cells with virion-like particles of SIV(MAC). Gene Ther. 2006;13:991–4.

27. Berger G, Goujon C, Darlix JL, Cimarelli A. SIVMAC Vpx improves the transduction of dendritic cells with nonintegrative HIV-1-derived vectors. Gene Ther. 2009;16:159–63.

28. Li W, Xu H, Xiao T, Cong L, Love MI, Zhang F, et al. MAGeCK enables robust identification of essential genes from genome-scale CRISPR/Cas9 knock-out screens. Genome Biol. 2014;15:554.

29. Goujon C, Moncorge O, Bauby H, Doyle T, Ward CC, Schaller T, et al. Human MX2 is an interferon-induced post-entry inhibitor of HIV-1 infection. Nature. 2013;502:559–62.

30. Wu X, Dao Thi VL, Huang Y, Billerbeck E, Saha D, Hoffmann HH, et al. Intrinsic immunity shapes viral resistance of stem cells. Cell. 2017.

31. Aldo PB, Craveiro V, Guller S, Mor G. Effect of culture conditions on the phenotype of THP-1 monocyte cell line. Am J Reprod Immunol. 2013;70:80–6.

32. Brinkman EK, Chen T, Amendola M, van Steensel B. Easy quantitative assessment of genome editing by sequence trace decomposition. Nucleic Acids Res. 2014;42:e168.

33. Tartour K, Appourchaux R, Gaillard J, Nguyen XN, Durand S, Turpin J, et al. IFITM proteins are incorporated onto HIV-1 virion particles and negatively imprint their infectivity. Retrovirology. 2014;11:103.

34. McClure MO, Sommerfelt MA, Marsh M, Weiss RA. The pH independence of mammalian retrovirus infection. J Gen Virol. 1990;71(Pt 4):767–73.

35. Beer C, Andersen DS, Rojek A, Pedersen L. Caveola-dependent endocytic entry of amphotropic murine leukemia virus. J Virol. 2005;79:10776–87.

36. Katen LJ, Januszeski MM, Anderson WF, Hasenkrug KJ, Evans LH. Infectious entry by amphotropic as well as ecotropic murine leukemia viruses occurs through an endocytic pathway. J Virol. 2001;75:5018–26.

37. Sun X, Yau VK, Briggs BJ, Whittaker GR. Role of clathrin-mediated endocytosis during vesicular stomatitis virus entry into host cells. Virology. 2005;338:53–60.

38. Marin M, Melikyan GB. Can HIV-1 entry sites be deduced by comparing bulk endocytosis to functional readouts for viral fusion? J Virol. 2015;89:2985.

39. Herold N, Muller B, Krausslich HG. Reply to "Can HIV-1 entry sites be deduced by comparing bulk endocytosis to functional readouts for viral fusion?". J Virol. 2015;89:2986–7.

40. Kilby JM, Hopkins S, Venetta TM, DiMassimo B, Cloud GA, Lee JY, et al. Potent suppression of HIV-1 replication in humans by T-20, a peptide inhibitor of gp41-mediated virus entry. Nat Med. 1998;4:1302–7.

41. Lu J, Pan Q, Rong L, He W, Liu SL, Liang C. The IFITM proteins inhibit HIV-1 infection. J Virol. 2011;85:2126–37.

42. Compton AA, Bruel T, Porrot F, Mallet A, Sachse M, Euvrard M, et al. IFITM proteins incorporated into HIV-1 virions impair viral fusion and spread. Cell Host Microbe. 2014;16:736–47.

43. Yu J, Li M, Wilkins J, Ding S, Swartz TH, Esposito AM, et al. IFITM proteins restrict HIV-1 infection by antagonizing the envelope glycoprotein. Cell Rep. 2015;13:145–56.

44. Li K, Markosyan RM, Zheng YM, Golfetto O, Bungart B, Li M, et al. IFITM proteins restrict viral membrane hemifusion. PLoS Pathog. 2013;9:e1003124.

45. Desai TM, Marin M, Chin CR, Savidis G, Brass AL, Melikyan GB. IFITM3 restricts influenza A virus entry by blocking the formation of fusion pores following virus-endosome hemifusion. PLoS ONE. 2014;10:e1004048.

46. Amini-Bavil-Olyaee S, Choi YJ, Lee JH, Shi M, Huang IC, Farzan M, et al. The antiviral effector IFITM3 disrupts intracellular cholesterol homeostasis to block viral entry. Cell Host Microbe. 2013;13:452–64.

47. Herold N, Anders-Osswein M, Glass B, Eckhardt M, Muller B, Krausslich HG. HIV-1 entry in SupT1-R5, CEM-ss, and primary CD4+T cells occurs at the plasma membrane and does not require endocytosis. J Virol. 2014;88:13956–70.

48. Brun S, Solignat M, Gay B, Bernard E, Chaloin L, Fenard D, et al. VSV-G pseudotyping rescues HIV-1 CA mutations that impair core assembly or stability. Retrovirology. 2008;5:57.

49. Yu D, Wang W, Yoder A, Spear M, Wu Y. The HIV envelope but not VSV glycoprotein is capable of mediating HIV latent infection of resting CD4 T cells. PLoS Pathog. 2009;5:e1000633.

50. Cavrois M, De Noronha C, Greene WC. A sensitive and specific enzyme-based assay detecting HIV-1 virion fusion in primary T lymphocytes. Nat Biotechnol. 2002;20:1151–4.

51. Landau NR, Page KA, Littman DR. Pseudotyping with human T-cell leukemia virus type I broadens the human immunodeficiency virus host range. J Virol. 1991;65:162–9.

52. Robinson MD, McCarthy DJ, Smyth GK. edgeR: a Bioconductor package for differential expression analysis of digital gene expression data. Bioinformatics. 2010;26:139–40.

53. Du P, Kibbe WA, Lin SM. lumi: a pipeline for processing Illumina microarray. Bioinformatics. 2008;24:1547–8.

54. Wettenhall JM, Smyth GK. limmaGUI: a graphical user interface for linear modeling of microarray data. Bioinformatics. 2004;20:3705–6.

55. Vermeire J, Naessens E, Vanderstraeten H, Landi A, Iannucci V, Van Nuffel A, et al. Quantification of reverse transcriptase activity by real-time PCR as a fast and accurate method for titration of HIV, lenti- and retroviral vectors. PLoS ONE. 2012;7:e50859.

14

Measuring integrated HIV DNA ex vivo and in vitro provides insights about how reservoirs are formed and maintained

Marilia Rita Pinzone and Una O'Doherty[*]

Abstract

The identification of the most appropriate marker to measure reservoir size has been a great challenge for the HIV field. Quantitative viral outgrowth assay (QVOA), the reference standard to quantify the amount of replication-competent virus, has several limitations, as it is laborious, expensive, and unable to robustly reactivate every single integrated provirus. PCR-based assays have been developed as an easier, cheaper and less error-prone alternative to QVOA, but also have limitations. Historically, measuring integrated HIV DNA has provided insights about how reservoirs are formed and maintained. In the 1990s, measuring integrated HIV DNA was instrumental in understanding that a subset of resting CD4 T cells containing integrated HIV DNA were the major source of replication-competent virus. Follow-up studies have further characterized the phenotype of these cells containing integrated HIV DNA, as well as shown the correlation between the integration levels and clinical parameters, such as duration of infection, CD4 count and viral load. Integrated HIV DNA correlates with total HIV measures and with QVOA. The integration assay has several limitations. First, it largely overestimates the reservoir size, as both defective and replication-competent proviruses are detected. Since defective proviruses are the majority in patients on ART, it follows that the number of proviruses capable of reactivating and releasing new virions is significantly smaller than the number of integrated proviruses. Second, in patients on ART clonal expansion could theoretically lead to the preferential amplification of proviruses close to an *Alu* sequence though longitudinal studies have not captured this effect. Proviral sequencing combined with integration measures is probably the best estimate of reservoir size, but it is expensive, time-consuming and requires considerable bioinformatics expertise. All these reasons limit its use on a large scale. Herein, we review the utility of measuring HIV integration and suggest combining it with sequencing and total HIV measurements can provide insights that underlie reservoir maintenance.

Keywords: ART, HIV, Integrated HIV DNA, Proviral DNA, Reservoir, Sequencing

Background

The introduction of combination antiretroviral therapy (ART) has profoundly modified the history of human immunodeficiency virus (HIV) infection. The majority of patients on ART have undetectable viral loads and life expectancy close to the general population [1–3]. Unfortunately, ART is not curative, and in the majority of individuals HIV viral load promptly rebounds after ART cessation. This is due to the presence of long-lived viral reservoirs, containing replication-competent proviruses, which currently represent the barrier to any curative approach [4–6]. "Shock and kill" strategies rely on the activation and immune clearance of viral reservoirs. The evaluation of efficacy of such interventions requires the accurate measure of the individual viral reservoir.

Measuring HIV reservoirs has been challenging. Historically, quantitative viral outgrowth assay (QVOA) has been considered the reference standard to measure the fraction of the HIV reservoir that is replication-competent [7]. Polymerase chain reaction (PCR)-based assays, such as total and integrated HIV DNA, have represented a cheaper, less time-consuming and less error-prone

*Correspondence: unao@pennmedicine.upenn.edu
Department of Pathology and Laboratory Medicine, University of Pennsylvania, Philadelphia, PA, USA

approach to study the reservoir, but have their own short-comings [8, 9].

In this review, we summarize the technical and clinical strengths, as well as the weaknesses of measuring integrated HIV DNA. We also discuss the scenarios where, despite its limitations, integrated HIV DNA can still provide useful information, especially when combined with other techniques, such as proviral sequencing.

The challenge of measuring HIV reservoir size

Measuring integrated HIV DNA has been instrumental in increasing our understanding of HIV biology. In the 1990s, Siliciano's group published the first ground-breaking studies showing that resting CD4 T cells containing integrated HIV DNA were the main reservoir in patients on ART [10, 11]. The authors showed that replication-competent virus could be induced in vitro from resting CD4 T cells of patients with undetectable viremia by using QVOA. Initially, it was thought that latently infected cells form when HIV integrates in activated cells just before they return to a resting state [10–15]. However, additional studies demonstrated that resting CD4 T cells can be directly infected with HIV with delayed kinetics [16–25].

Historically, QVOA was extremely important because it captured a relevant attribute of the reservoir—that cells persisted without making any virus unless they were stimulated and then could produce virus. This was conceptually important because it explained why the reservoir was resistant to therapy. The assay relies on the purification of large numbers of resting CD4 T cells usually by negative selection, which are cultured in the presence of target cells to amplify released virions and activators to stimulate infected cells to release virions. QVOA requires a large amount of blood (~200 ml), or a leukapheresis product, in order to obtain the required number of resting CD4 T cells. QVOA is based on the limiting dilution method and the results are typically expressed as infectious units per million cells (IUPM) [7]. QVOA as currently performed is an underestimate of reservoir size as it is difficult to stimulate every replication-competent provirus. In fact, repeated stimulation of initially negative wells leads to reactivation of proviruses that were not induced in the previous round of stimulation [26]. This could be due to the stochastic nature of HIV reactivation [27]. Notably, repeated rounds of T cell stimulation can reactivate many of the latent proviruses that are resistant to expression. Proviral sequencing suggests the reservoir may be 6-fold larger than QVOA estimates [26]. Proviral sequencing studies have further called into question the value of QVOA as more intact proviruses were identified in effector memory (TEM) > transitional memory (TTM) > naive > central memory (TCM) T cells [28],

while QVOA suggested that TCM contained the largest fraction of replication-competent proviruses [29].

After ART interruption virological rebound always occurs even when the reservoir is extremely small, as shown by the Mississippi baby [30] and the Boston patients [31, 32]. "Undetectable" HIV in these publications indicates not detected in a large volume of blood (typically ~180 ml or ~20–50 million CD4s). These patients could now be described as having reservoirs below a certain detection limit, such as < 1 infectious unit per 50 million CD4s. QVOA is not appropriate to detect small changes in the size of the reservoir that may occur in pilot clinical trials because of its limited reproducibility, the large number of patient's cells, the expense, the technical expertise, and the significant labor required [33]. Considering these limitations, PCR-based methods were developed to provide upper limit estimates of HIV reservoirs, as an easier, cheaper and less error-prone tool that might compliment QVOA.

In the following paragraphs, we describe some scenarios where integrated HIV DNA provided unique insights about reservoir characterization, in settings where other assays could not be fully exploited because of the presence of unintegrated HIV DNA, ongoing replication (untreated infection, episodes of viremia on ART) or because of limited cell availability (studies on HIV persistence in cellular subsets).

Integrated HIV DNA in cellular subsets

In the last 20 years, the HIV field has progressively gained a better understanding of the cellular subsets contributing to the reservoir size. Ostrowski et al. [15] showed that memory CD4 T cells contain 16-fold more integrated HIV DNA than naive cells consistent with the idea that the memory CD4 T cells make up the largest portion of the HIV reservoir. However, the difference between memory and naive cells (defined as CD62L + CD45RA + cells) was much smaller in patients infected with C-X-C chemokine receptor type 4 (CXCR4) viruses. This could be explained by the near absence of C–C chemokine receptor type 5 (CCR5) and high levels of CXCR4 in naive cells. Similarly, Chomont et al. [34] showed that the pool of cells containing integrated HIV DNA is mostly represented by cells with a memory phenotype. Measurements of integration provided important evidence suggesting that naive T cells contribute to the reservoir, which were then confirmed in a small subset of patients by QVOA as well [15, 34, 35]. Given the long intermitotic half-life of naive T cells, this subset may prove to be a significant under-investigated barrier to cure and integration measurements remain the primary evidence of their contribution to the reservoir. Notably, this data should be evaluated in light of recent studies on

T memory stem cells (TSCM) [36–39], which are phenotypically similar to naive T cells, but can be distinguished by the expression of CD95 and interleukin 2 receptor subunit beta. Considering the long half-life of naive and TSCM, both cell subsets could be significant contributors to the reservoir.

Central memory (TCM, CD45RA-CCR7+CD27+) and transitional memory (TTM, CD45RA-CCR7-CD27+) CD4 T cells contain the majority of integrated HIV DNA, and could be responsible for reservoir maintenance/replenishment through several mechanisms, including antigen-driven and homeostatic proliferation. TCM were reported to be the main reservoir in immunological responders and individuals who started treatment early. On the other end of spectrum, in patients with low CD4 T cell counts the majority of HIV DNA was harboured by TTM. These cells have increased proliferative activity in comparison to TCM and may therefore contribute to the stability of the reservoir. The reservoir size was smaller in individuals with higher CD4 nadir, higher absolute CD4 counts and a CD4/CD8>1. Moreover, integrated HIV levels were significantly lower in patients who had started ART within the first year of infection [34].

Recent studies have provided an in-depth phenotypical analysis of cellular subsets that can be enriched for HIV DNA. Gosselin et al. [40] sorted blood memory cells according to the expression of CCR6, CCR4 and CXCR3 to differentiate the following subsets: T helper (Th)17 (CCR4 + CCR6+), Th2 (CCR4 + CCR6−), Th1Th17 (CXCR3 + CCR6+), and Th1 (CXCR3 + CCR6−). These subsets showed different susceptibility to HIV infection in vitro: in fact, cells with a Th17 and Th1Th17 profile appeared highly permissive to R5 and X4 HIV infection, whereas those with a Th2 profile were susceptible to X4 HIV replication only, and cells with a Th1 profile were relatively resistant to both R5 and X4 HIV replication. There was an enrichment for integrated HIV DNA in circulating CCR6 + T cells of HIV-infected subjects, both off and on ART, but a parallel depletion of these cells in comparison to uninfected controls, suggesting they may be preferentially infected and killed by HIV. Since the CCR6/C–C motif ligand-20 (CCL20) axis is important for mucosal homeostasis, more CCR6 + cells can potentially be recruited in tissues, such as the gut, the vagina and the brain, attracting additional susceptible cells at the sites of viral replication. The same group showed more recently that CCR6 + cells are enriched in the colon of individuals on ART in comparison to blood. Moreover, in both compartments CCR6 + cells harbour higher levels of total HIV DNA in comparison to CCR6- cells [41]. An enrichment for integrated DNA in CXCR3 + CCR6+ cells has been reported by others [42].

Immune checkpoint molecules are co-inhibitory receptors, physiologically involved in the containment of immune activation. Overexpression of several immune checkpoint molecules has been associated with T cell exhaustion and dysfunction. A recent study evaluated their association with HIV reservoir size [43]. In patients on stable ART, none of the markers alone was associated with integrated HIV DNA when adjusting for current CD4 count. However, the co-expression of Lymphocyte activation gene-3 (LAG-3), T cell Immunoglobulin and ITIM domain (TIGIT), and Programmed death-1 (PD-1) correlated with the frequency of cells harbouring integrated HIV DNA, after adjusting for nadir and current CD4 T cell count ($p = 0.038$). Memory CD4 T cells showed a gradual enrichment for integrated HIV DNA when expressing an increasing number of immune checkpoint molecules. Cells expressing the 3 markers were eightfold enriched for integrated HIV DNA in comparison to the whole CD4 population. The authors speculated that cells expressing these markers can be preferentially infected with HIV, or they may preferentially persist in comparison to the negative ones.

Dynamics of integrated HIV DNA in acute and chronic HIV infection

The first hint that treating patients early would be more effective at reducing reservoir size came from Strain et al. [44]. They showed that after one year of ART replication-competent HIV could not be detected by QVOA in any of the individuals starting ART during primary HIV infection (PHI) and in the majority of patients initiating therapy within 6 months after seroconversion.

Recent studies of the dynamics of integrated HIV DNA provide some clues to possible mechanisms behind restriction of reservoir size with early treatment including immune clearance. Both animal and human models have shown that HIV seeding occurs very early during HIV infection [45–47]. However, there is evidence that the earlier ART is started during acute infection the smaller the HIV reservoir is after virological suppression [48]. An in-depth study of acutely infected subjects in Thailand evaluated the dynamics of total, 2-Long Terminal Repeat (LTR) and integrated HIV DNA in untreated and treated acute HIV infection [49]. In untreated patients (Fiebig stage I/II (HIV RNA+, p24 ±, HIV IgM−)), integrated HIV DNA peaked at week 2 after enrollment, declined significantly between week 2 and week 6, and then gradually increased over time. By the end of the observation period (week 144), integration levels were significantly higher than at nadir ($p = 0.02$). Total HIV DNA did not capture this effect, likely because of the excess of unintegrated DNA: it increased rapidly, peaking at week 2, but did not change significantly afterwards in the untreated group. Treated individuals started ART immediately after enrollment (46% in Fiebig stage I/II). Integrated HIV DNA was 25-fold lower at week 2 and 100-fold lower at week 144 in comparison to untreated individuals. These findings have important clinical implications, since both total and integrated HIV DNA measures correlate with immune reconstitution, with immune activation and predict the time to viral rebound after ART interruption [50–53]. Thus, in certain settings integrated HIV DNA can be a correlate of reservoir size, despite the fact that it is an overestimate and has additional limitations discussed below.

Several studies have shown that initiating ART during acute infection is associated with a greater decline in the levels of integrated HIV DNA [54–56]. A limitation of these studies is their small size, but the consistent finding from all three groups that integrated HIV DNA was cleared more rapidly and effectively if patients were treated early makes these results more convincing. Murray et al. [56] showed the decline of integrated HIV DNA was biphasic and that the first phase of decay was significantly faster when patients were treated early after HIV infection with a half-life of 10 versus 43 days for the first phase of decay ($p = 0.04$) and then 63 versus 172 days. Meanwhile the rate of decay for total HIV was similar for both groups. Pinzone et al. showed that acutely infected individuals exhibited a significant drop in integrated HIV levels 12 months after ART initiation, while integration levels barely changed in patients treated during chronic infection [54], consistent with Koelsch et al. [55]. Moreover, Buzon et al. [57] found treating the earliest stages Fiebig III/IV resulted in a larger drop in integrated HIV DNA than treating in Fiebig V; uniquely, the decline in integrated HIV continued in those patients treated at the very earliest stages over several years. Pre-ART integration levels also correlated with viral load (r = 0.86) and negatively correlated with CD4/CD8 ratio (r = − 0.52), consistent with the idea that integrated HIV DNA can provide a surrogate marker for reservoir size [54] and consistent with [34, 56, 58]. These longitudinal studies highlight that integrated HIV DNA measures provide different and complementary information to total HIV DNA when an excess of unintegrated HIV DNA may exist.

Potential reasons for lower reservoirs when initiating ART early include (1) less escape from cytotoxic T lymphocyte (CTL) [59, 60], (2) more functional CTL during acute infection [59, 61, 62], (3) preferential protection of TCM [50, 63] and (4) increased susceptibility to ART. The latter possibility would seem likely if the fraction of HIV harbouring replication-competent proviruses is larger in acute infection. A limitation of these studies is the lack of information on the fraction of proviruses

that are replication-competent. If replication-competent proviruses plateau early after infection, then the reduction in integration levels observed in acute infection is likely to reflect the effectiveness of ART against replication-competent proviruses while in individuals with chronic infection the majority of proviruses are defective and only a small fraction of them will be cleared by antiretroviral drugs. If replication-competent proviruses continue to accrue at a constant rate, this would suggest that the immune system is more effective early after HIV infection. Bruner et al. [64] have recently provided the first attempt to characterize the proviral landscape by sequencing proviruses during acute infection. The authors showed that defective proviruses accumulate early in HIV infection, making up over 93% of the proviral pool, even when ART is started within the first 2–3 weeks from enrolment. Alternatively, it is possible that a significant fraction of the reservoir is expressed and potentially cleared even in individuals treated during chronic infection, but the clonal expansion of defective clones may mask a drop in reservoir size by DNA measures [65]. Sequencing proviruses at multiple time points could provide new insights on the dynamics of intact/defective proviruses over time.

Longitudinal studies show integrated HIV DNA increases over time

In the absence of ART, integrated HIV DNA accumulates over time after a brief decline that may be immune-mediated [49, 54]. Pinzone et al. [54] monitored longitudinally integrated HIV DNA in 6 individuals followed from acute to chronic infection (mean observation time 6 years), showing that integrated HIV DNA increased progressively over time (from 109 to 1941 copies/million peripheral blood mononuclear cells (PBMCs)). The authors compared the increase in reservoir size observed in chronic progressors (CPs) versus long-term nonprogressors (LTNPs). As expected [57, 66], they found that LTNPs have much lower integrated HIV DNA levels. However, in the absence of ART LTNPs experienced an increase in the levels of integrated HIV DNA over time (from 17 to 34 copies/million PBMCs over 5 years), consistent with evidence of ongoing replication [67–69]. Integration levels did not significantly change in ART controls. Among the chronic progressors, the rate of integration increase varied greatly; in fact, two patients showed some decline in integrated HIV DNA within the first 2 years of observation, followed by an increase in integration levels, suggesting that some transient immune control existed early during infection. The different accumulation rate observed in LTNPs and chronic individuals can be due to differences in CTL functions. However, loss of CTL function over time did not explain the increase in integrated HIV DNA in LTNP patients as CTL function did not decline over time. We speculate that reservoir expansion could be due to ongoing viral replication in sanctuary sites, such as the B-cell follicles, where CD8 T cells are functionally excluded [70–72]. The increase in integrated HIV DNA over time suggests that the true reservoir size increases over time [8, 32].

Structured Treatment Interruptions and integrated HIV DNA measures

Several studies have evaluated the changes in total HIV DNA levels after ART interruption [52, 53, 73, 74], but few have addressed changes in integrated HIV DNA [53, 75]. The VISCONTI cohort provides an example of enhanced frequency of functional cure for HIV, as a higher fraction of individuals who were started on ART within 2 months of infection were able to maintain undetectable viral loads for several years after ART withdrawal [50]. In the Spartac study and the ANRS 116 SALTO study, total HIV DNA levels were shown to be predictive of the timing of viral rebound in patients treated early after infection [52, 53]. Azzoni et al. showed in a small pilot study of patients on ART who received treatment intensification with pegylated interferon alpha-2a (IFN-α-2a) that integrated HIV DNA actually declined after treatment interruption in the subset of patients that maintained virologic control [51]. More data on the kinetics of integration levels coupled with proviral sequencing after STI would improve our understanding of reservoir expansion in this setting.

Integrated HIV DNA and reservoir clearance

Integrated HIV DNA can be an useful tool to assess CTL-mediated clearance of infected CD4 T cells [76]. Graf et al. measured the levels of integrated and 2-LTR intermediates in CD4 T cells from LTNPs that had been superinfected in vitro and cocultured with autologous CD8 T cells. They showed the preferential clearance of integrated over 2-LTR DNA in the presence of CTL. This was consistent with the hypothesis that Gag+ cells are preferentially cleared, since integrated HIV but not 2-LTR expresses Gag in an efficient manner under short-term coculture [77]. The authors also found that integrated HIV DNA inversely correlated with CTL capability to clear infected cells both in LTNPs and CPs. These findings again are consistent with the idea that CTL activity controls the expansion of HIV reservoirs and at least in the very early stages of infection immune clearance plays a role in limiting reservoir size.

Integration measures have helped capture the possible role of immune clearance in reservoir formation and maintenance. In fact, in the setting of untreated infection other assays, such as total HIV DNA or QVOA,

cannot be used to assess the dynamics of reservoir change over time. In the aforementioned study from the acute Thailand cohort [49] the drop in integrated HIV DNA between week 2 and 6 suggests clearance, possibly immune-mediated, of infected cells. Similarly, in the study from Buzon et al. [57] patients starting therapy in the earliest Fiebig stages did have smaller reservoirs. In [54], some chronic progressors did show an initial contraction of the reservoir during the acute phase of infection, followed by reservoir expansion, suggestive of initial immune control, which was then lost over time.

Integrated HIV DNA in studies using latency reversal agents (LRAs)

A few trials have evaluated the change in integrated HIV DNA levels after the administration of LRAs to disrupt latency, such as vorinostat [78], panobinostat [79], and romidepsin [80]. Interestingly, in none of these studies a significant change in integration levels was found at a cohort level. This could be due to the fact that only a minority of patients may respond to the intervention and the change in their reservoir size can be masked when looking at the average response in the cohort. Moreover, at an individual level, defective proviruses that contain no open reading frames (ORFs) would not be cleared by eradication strategies, and if such proviruses were prominent they would mask clearance in the population of intact proviruses. Since some studies only target one ORF (HIV Gag in the Vacc4x study) [80], only intact proviruses and proviruses expressing Gag would be expected to be cleared with this approach, resulting in only small changes in HIV integration (in most cases < twofold). Notably, one patient in Vacc4x study did show a reduction in integrated and total HIV DNA and QVOA, and may represent a responder [80]. Follow-up studies sequencing proviruses in this potential responder may clarify if the patient is a true responder. One potential advantage of measuring integrated HIV DNA is that the error of the assay is low and this makes it possible to identify a small reduction in individual responders by monitoring the patients longitudinally. While total HIV DNA measurements also have a small error, we speculate many therapeutic approaches, especially LRAs, have the potential to induce a round of reverse transcription (unpublished data). In this case, total HIV DNA might not capture a reduction in the size of the reservoir, which could be detected by integrated HIV DNA [81].

Combined use of HIV DNA intermediates to model the dynamics of reservoir over time

In some studies, mathematical modelling has provided important insights into how different HIV intermediates in resting and activated cells change over time on ART.

Murray et al. [58] analyzed longitudinally the dynamics of HIV intermediates in resting and activated cells of 8 patients with acute infection and 8 patients with chronic HIV starting an antiretroviral regimen containing raltegravir.

Before ART initiation, resting cells had the highest levels of 2-LTR and 2-LTR/integrated HIV DNA ratio. These observations are consistent with direct infection of resting cells in vivo [16–25], as supported by recent modelling [82]. 2-LTR would be expected to accumulate in resting cells as a consequence of the longer life span of resting cells as well as less efficient integration in resting cells [18, 19, 83].

Interestingly, after 1 year of ART, the levels of total, integrated and 2-LTR DNA were similar in resting and activated cells. This has important implications for eradication studies. At first blush, we would expect HIV DNA levels to quickly decline in activated cells after starting ART, if ongoing replication were stopped [84], as a result of several mechanisms, including cell death due to viral cytotoxicity. However, the persistence of HIV DNA in activated T cells suggest that cells may be converting from a resting to an activated phenotype and vice versa. This, in turn, suggests that activation of an HIV infected cells does not always result in cell death before the cell can return to a resting state. This, in turn, suggests the basic idea of "shock and kill" may be more difficult to achieve than initially thought since cell activation from latency may not result in cell death.

Integrated HIV DNA: technical aspects
Principles of the assay
HIV integration is measured using a nested real-time approach [85, 86]. The first step of PCR anchors a forward primer to the human *Alu* element and a reverse primer to the HIV genome. *Alu* is a repeat element in the human genome that occurs approximately every 3,000 base pairs. Only integrated HIV DNA is exponentially amplified by the first step, whereas unintegrated HIV DNA is linearly amplified by the HIV primer since only one strand can be copied. The second step is a real-time PCR approach within the HIV LTR. In order to adjust for the amount of unintegrated HIV DNA that can be linearly amplified, during the first step some wells contain only the HIV-specific primer. This controls for the background signal coming from unintegrated HIV and is used to define a threshold for a signal that represents a positive well for integration. *Alu*-HIV PCR is the most applied method to measure integrated HIV DNA. Less common methods include inverse PCR, linker ligation PCR and gel separation [10, 87, 88].

In the gel separation method, DNA samples are run on a gel to separate genomic high-molecular weight

DNA from episomal DNA. The genomic DNA recovered from the gel is then used to measure HIV DNA by PCR. Recently, Lada et al. used pulse-field gel electrophoresis combined with droplet digital PCR, and showed good correlation with *Alu*-HIV PCR (r = 0.7, $p = 0.023$), and efficient removal of unintegrated forms, but low yields from the gel (on average 21%) [87].

Choice of the PCR primers
Different labs measuring integrated HIV DNA use different HIV primers for the first amplification step. O'Doherty's lab uses a primer located in a conserved region of the Gag gene (primer SK431). Chomont's lab uses a primer annealing in the U3-R junction of the LTR [89]. The difference in primers used for the first step has important implications, as in the first case only proviruses containing an intact Gag region will be amplified, while with the second primer all the proviruses with an intact LTR will likely be amplified, including a larger number of massively deleted proviruses. One primer may have advantages over the other, depending on the specific experimental question that is being asked. For example, in studies evaluating reservoir clearance after priming for Gag CTL, the Gag primer may be preferred, as in that case integrated HIV decline may represent a surrogate of reservoir contraction. On the other hand, the *Alu*-LTR assay will capture all the integrated HIV DNA and therefore provides increased sensitivity over *Alu*-Gag. This could be an important advantage in the assessment of reservoir changes after therapeutic interventions (for instance bone marrow transplantation), when the levels of residual HIV DNA are expected to be extremely low and a very sensitive assay is required to detect any residual HIV.

Quality control for robust measurements
Consistency of amplification is affected by variations in master mixes, Taq polymerase, as well as variability between thermocyclers. Large volume PCR master mixtures minimize systematic variation. An integration standard can be included in all runs to test thermocycler conformity from run to run and to identify PCR inhibition (by adding the standard to patient samples) [9, 85]. Some laboratories utilize serial dilutions of cell lines (e.g. ACH-2) to create a standard curve to quantify integrated HIV DNA [89]. The ACH-2 cells are not entirely transcriptionally silent and contain variable numbers of HIV integrations (from 5 to 10 in our hands) [90]. Every lab should verify the number of proviruses per cell in a given lot of ACH-2 cells before using them as a standard in these assays. This is actually an advantage for the ACH-2 cells line, as it has sufficient diversity of integration sites to roughly capture the diversity of distances to *Alu*

present in acute infection and can be used to estimate integration frequency while other cell lines with 1–2 proviruses do not provide strong estimates.

For each infected cell, the distance between the integrated provirus and the nearest *Alu* element is variable. Therefore, each provirus will be amplified at different efficiency depending on its distance from the closest *Alu* [17]. This represents an important limitation of the assay, which is mitigated by repetitive sampling. Moreover, to reduce variability between runs as well as variability between different laboratories, our laboratory currently measures integrated HIV DNA using the Poisson distribution. This allows the quantification of integrated HIV DNA without using a standard curve. We target 30–80% of positive wells at two dilutions in a 96-well plate to obtain the most robust result, as error increases outside of this range. This implies that we need ~500 proviruses per patient to obtain a robust measure of the integration levels [unpublished data]. It follows that the number of cells required for the assay will largely vary depending on the individual integration levels. The chance that the well contains no integrated HIV DNA (negative reaction) or 1 or more proviruses (positive reaction) will follow the Poisson distribution. The number of copies of integrated HIV can be calculated from the frequency of positive wells by PCR without the need of a standard curve [91], though we do apply a correction factor as our assay detects ~10% of integrations [91] (20% of integrations are detected with recent improvements due to decreased gag background).

Measuring integrated HIV DNA robustly in LTNPs is challenging. It requires a large number of cells, as in some patients the integration level may be as low as 1–5 copies/million PBMCs, which can be a limitation if apheresis products are not available [66]. To increase the sensitivity of the assay, a large number of cells per well are needed, and this requires best-quality DNA in order to avoid PCR inhibition.

Some labs compensate for limited numbers of available cells by testing large numbers of patients [89]. However, a low number of repeats reduces the sensitivity of the assay, which implies that negative results should be interpreted carefully, as they may reflect the limited quantity of cells tested.

Measuring integrated HIV DNA: a summary of pros and cons
Strengths
On a technical level, integrated HIV DNA is relatively inexpensive, robust, and potentially high-throughput in comparison to QVOA. Total and integrated HIV DNA can be combined to capture ongoing replication. A full review of total HIV DNA as a measure of reservoir size

is provided in another chapter of this special issue [92]. In patients on long-term ART, integration levels are relatively similar to total HIV DNA and consistent with a relatively stable reservoir [34, 81]. Total and integrated HIV DNA provide different insights [93]. Total DNA showed a similar decline in acute and chronic infection with a sevenfold decline in the first year and a slower decline over the next few years from pre-ART levels [93]. In contrast, there was a tenfold decline of integrated HIV DNA levels in acute infection, whereas there was only a twofold decline in patients treated chronically [54].

Mexas et al. [81] showed the utility of combining total and integrated HIV DNA in clinical trials. In the presence of detectable viremia, the authors showed an increase in the ratio between total and integrated HIV. Moreover, they evaluated the change in reservoir size of patients on stable ART who received IFN-α-2a + ART for 5 weeks, followed by IFN-α-2a alone for 12 weeks. 45% of patients maintained a viral load < 400 copies/ml during ART interruption and were considered "responders". Treatment with IFN-α-2a led to an increase in total over integrated HIV DNA as well as an increase in viremia on ART and after ART interruption, suggesting that IFN-α-2a treatment induced ongoing replication. In responders, the administration of IFN-α-2a also led to a decrease in integrated but not total HIV DNA levels. This discrepancy between total and integrated HIV DNA could be due to the imbalance between the immune-mediated clearance of cells containing integrated HIV (reduction in integration levels) and de novo infection of new cells (increase in total DNA). These results suggest that the concomitant use of total and integrated HIV DNA can provide insights into the changes in reservoir size after therapeutic interventions.

Moreover, in some cases total HIV DNA cannot be used to measure reservoir size. In most patients off ART unintegrated HIV represents the most abundant form. In those cases, total HIV DNA measures would be largely driven by variable levels of linear and circular non-integrated forms. Therefore, integrated HIV DNA can represent a more appropriate tool to measure reservoir size in patients off ART.

Integrated HIV DNA is a robust assay, and can capture smaller changes than the QVOA assay. Integration levels correlated with QVOA in a comparative study of reservoir assays [33] (r = 0.7, p = 0.0008). In this study, QVOA did not correlate with total HIV DNA, probably because of data censoring; a few samples were negative for total HIV DNA by digital droplet PCR, thus reducing the strength of the correlation. Similarly, Mendoza et al. [94] reported that QVOA correlated with integrated HIV DNA in a cohort of LTNPs (r = 0.72, p = 0.03). More recently, similar findings were published by Kiselinova et al. [95] in a cohort of 25 long-term treated patients who started ART during chronic infection. The authors found that integrated HIV DNA correlated with total HIV DNA ($R^2 = 0.85$, $p < 0.001$) and QVOA ($R^2 = 0.44$, $p = 0.041$). Thus, while integration is an overestimate of reservoir size and while the number of defective proviruses vary between patients, in some settings measuring integrated HIV DNA can serve as a less error-prone surrogate of reservoir size.

Weaknesses: variable overestimate of reservoir size

Most of the integrated HIV DNA is not replication-competent, as it contains large deletions, mutations originating from viral reverse transcriptase or from innate host defense mechanisms (e.g. APOBEC3G). PCR-based methods overestimate reservoir size as the majority of proviruses are defective in individuals on ART [26, 96]. Those proviruses will not be distinguished from replication-competent ones using *Alu*-HIV assays. Table 1 provides three possible outcomes of eradication trials when using integrated HIV DNA to assess if a therapy is effective. In scenario 1, an intervention might be effective in reducing the "real" reservoir, but have no effect on defective proviruses such that integrated HIV DNA would remain unchanged. This might occur if clearance of the infected cells required virion release or if a strategy required high-level expression of Gag, which would require in turn expression of Tat and Rev; thus, these proviruses are generally largely intact and unlikely to be defective. In scenario 2, an intervention that targets only defective proviruses would decrease the levels of integrated HIV DNA, but this drop would not reflect a decrease in the size of the "true" reservoir. This might occur if replication-competent proviruses are more resistant to transcription or translation than defective ones. possibly due to the repressive nature of the site of integration. In scenario 3, a decline in integration would likely capture a reduction in reservoir size if an intervention targets both defective and replication-competent proviruses, though the reduction would not

likely capture the precise change in the true reservoir as defective and replication-competent proviruses are not expected to be targeted proportionally. This could occur if an immune therapy can clear both defective and replication-competent proviruses that are capable of expressing HIV proteins as was proposed to occur in [51, 81]. If transcription of replication-competent proviruses is not repressed more than transcription of defective proviruses, the immune response should be more effective at clearing replication-competent proviruses that defective ones, since replication-competent proviruses have 9 ORFs for the immune system to target. The previously mentioned IFN-α-2a trial suggested this third scenario could occur. Given that IFN-α-2a would likely increase immune clearance of all protein-expressing cells, it was likely that defective proviruses with intact ORFs as well as intact ones could both be cleared. Notably proviruses that contain no ORFs should not be cleared, though these represent a minority of proviruses [64, 97].

HIV integrates preferentially within regions of active transcription [98, 99]. *Alu* repeats are also more prominent in gene-rich regions. As described, the integration standard was designed to correct for the tendency of HIV to integrate closer to *Alu* sites. However, this correction did not account for clonally expanded integration sites. With time on ART clonal expansion occurs [100] and there appears to be selection with a tendency for clones that are near cell cycle genes. In fact, it has been shown that after several years on ART more than 40% of proviruses are located in the genome of cells that have undergone clonal expansion after HIV integration. Clonal expansion may result from selection of proviruses integrated HIV preferential selection into genes promoting cell growth, as recently shown by Maldarelli et al. [101]. These genes also tend to be close to *Alu* sites. As a consequence, proviruses that are closer to *Alu* sequences are likely to be preferentially expanded over time on ART. Thus, the presence of clonal expansion can result in apparently higher levels of integrated HIV DNA over time in comparison to total HIV DNA

Table 1 Possible outcomes of eradication trials when using integrated HIV DNA to assess the change in reservoir size

Possible outcome in eradication studies	How does the outcome affect reservoir measures?
1. Preferential reduction in intact proviruses	Integrated HV DNA is likely to be unchanged. Proviral sequencing would likely detect a reduction in the fraction of replication-competent proviruses which could be combined with integration measures to determine the absolute reduction in intact proviruses
2. Preferential reduction in defective proviruses	Integrated HIV DNA would decrease, without reflecting a contraction in the size of the "true" reservoir. Proviral sequencing would likely capture the change in the fraction of defective proviruses
3. Decrease in both intact and defective proviruses	If intact and defective proviruses are targeted differently, a decrease in integrated HIV DNA would occur, but would not likely be proportional to the decrease in the number of intact proviruses. Proviral sequencing combined with integration measures would likely capture the changes in the reservoir size and character

measures. Integration site analysis of patients with discrepant total and integration measurements may clarify why integration levels can appear to be slightly higher in some patients on ART. While clonal expansion is an appealing explanation for discrepancies between total and integrated HIV DNA, in our hands integrated and total HIV DNA are relatively constant over time on ART which is not consistent with this explanation. Regardless, the exact level is less important than the relative change for revealing reservoir expansion, contraction and ongoing replication.

There are some instances where knowing the exact level is important as well, for instance to estimate the total-body reservoir size. One scenario could be represented by STI after bone marrow transplantation, when the residual reservoir size is expected to be extremely low. In that case, the use of PCR assays, especially total HIV DNA, along with extensive sampling, likely represents the most sensitive tool to assess how much HIV persists in the body.

Solutions to the hurdles involve combining integration measures with proviral sequencing

Combining integration measures with proviral sequencing to identify intact proviruses may represent the best tool to estimate the size of the HIV reservoir, but the assay is expensive and labor-intensive, and requires considerable bioinformatics expertise, limiting its scalability in large cohorts. As more data accumulate on reservoir growth and decay, it may be possible to choose cohorts with similar reservoir size and sequence characteristics, in which case PCR measures of integration might be useful to identify responders to a therapy, but accurate measurement of reservoir reduction would likely involve sequencing as well.

Conclusions

Measuring HIV reservoirs robustly is still a challenge for the field. Every available marker has its own strengths and weaknesses. The choice of the most appropriate marker(s) depends on the experimental question that is being asked. Measuring integrated HIV DNA has increased our understanding of HIV dynamics but, as discussed, the assay has several limitations, which impose a careful use of this tool in clinical studies. Proviral sequencing combined with integration measurements will likely provide the closest estimate of reservoir size, and the most powerful tool to characterize and monitor the proviral landscape in HIV-infected individuals.

Abbreviations
ART: antiretroviral therapy; CXCR4: C-X-C chemokine receptor type 4; CCL20: C-C motif ligand 20; CCR5: C-C chemokine receptor type 5; CP: chronic progressor; CTL: cytotoxic T lymphocyte; CTLA-4: cytotoxic T-lymphocyte-associated protein-4; HIV: human immunodeficiency virus; IC: immune checkpoint molecule; IFN-α: interferon alpha; IUPM: infectious units per million cells; LAG-3: lymphocyte activation gene-3; LN: lymph node; LRA: latency reversal agent; LTNP: long-term nonprogressor; LTR: long terminal repeat; PBMC: peripheral blood mononuclear cell; PCR: polymerase chain reaction; PD-1: programmed death-1; PHI: primary HIV infection; ORF: open reading frame; STI: structured therapeutic interruption; TSCM: T memory stem cell; TCM: central memory T cell; TEM: effector memory T cell; Th: T helper; TIGIT: T cell Immunoglobulin and ITIM domain; TIM-3: T cell immunoglobulin-3; TTM: transitional memory T cell; QVOA: quantitative viral outgrowth assay.

Authors' contributions
Both authors read and approved the final manuscript.

Acknowledgements
We would like to acknowledge Daniel J. VanBelzen for his many insights into the measurement of HIV integration that have further enhanced our ability to apply this assay to appropriate clinical questions.

Competing interests
The authors declare they have no competing interests.

Funding
R01-AI-120011; R33-AI-104280; UM1-AI-126617.

References
1. Palella FJ Jr, Delaney KM, Moorman AC, Loveless MOFJ, Satten GA, Aschman DJHS. Declining morbidity and mortality among patients with advanced human immunodeficiency virus infection. HIV Outpatient Study Investigators. N Engl J Med. 1998;338:853–60.
2. Samji H, Cescon A, Hogg RS, Modur SP, Althoff KN, Buchacz K, et al. Closing the gap: increases in life expectancy among treated HIV-positive individuals in the United States and Canada. PLoS One. 2013;8(12):e81355. https://doi.org/10.1371/journal.pone.0081355.
3. Wada N, Jacobson LP, Cohen M, French A, Phair J, Munoz A. Cause-specific mortality among HIV-infected individuals, by CD4 + cell count at HAART initiation, compared with HIV-uninfected individuals. AIDS. 2014;28:257–65. https://doi.org/10.1097/QAD.0000000000000078.
4. Finzi D, Blankson J, Siliciano JD, Margolick JB, Chadwick K, Pierson T, et al. Latent infection of CD4 + T cells provides a mechanism for lifelong persistence of HIV-1, even in patients on effective combination therapy. Nat Med. 1999;5:512–7. https://doi.org/10.1038/8394.
5. Wong JK, Hezareh M, Günthard HF, Havlir DV, Ignacio CC, Spina CA, et al. Recovery of replication-competent HIV despite prolonged suppression of plasma viremia. Science. 1997;278:1291–5.
6. Siliciano JD, Kajdas J, Finzi D, Quinn TC, Chadwick K, Margolick JB, et al. Long-term follow-up studies confirm the stability of the latent reservoir for HIV-1 in resting CD4 + T cells. Nat Med. 2003;9:727–8.

7. Laird GM, Eisele EE, Rabi SA, Lai J, Chioma S, Blankson JN, et al. Rapid quantification of the latent reservoir for HIV-1 using a viral outgrowth assay. PLoS Pathog. 2013;9:e1003398. https://doi.org/10.1371/journal.ppat.1003398.

8. Avettand-Fènoë V, Hocqueloux L, Ghosn J, Cheret A, Frange P, Melard A, et al. Total HIV-1 DNA, a marker of viral reservoir dynamics with clinical implications. Clin Microbiol Rev. 2016;29:859–80.

9. Graf EH, O'Doherty U. Quantitation of integrated proviral DNA in viral reservoirs. Curr Opin HIV AIDS. 2013;8:100–5. https://doi.org/10.1097/COH.0b013e32835d8132.

10. Chun TW, Finzi D, Margolick J, Chadwick K, Schwartz D, Siliciano RF. In vivo fate of HIV-1-infected T cells: quantitative analysis of the transition to stable latency. Nat Med. 1995;1:1284–90.

11. Chun TW, Stuyver L, Mizell SB, Ehler LA, Mican JA, Baseler M, et al. Presence of an inducible HIV-1 latent reservoir during highly active antiretroviral therapy. Proc Natl Acad Sci USA. 1997;94:13193–7. https://doi.org/10.1073/pnas.94.24.13193.

12. Bukrinsky MI, Stanwick TL, Dempsey MP, Stevenson M. Quiescent T lymphocytes as an inducible virus reservoir in HIV-1 infection. Science. 1991;254:423–7. https://doi.org/10.1126/science.1925601.

13. Korin YD, Zack JA. Progression to the G1b phase of the cell cycle is required for completion of human immunodeficiency virus type 1 reverse transcription in T cells. J Virol. 1998;72:3161–8.

14. Stevenson M, Stanwick TL, Dempsey MP, Lamonica CA. HIV-1 replication is controlled at the level of T cell activation and proviral integration. EMBO J. 1990;9:1551–60. http://www.pubmedcentral.nih.gov/articlerender.fcgi?artid=551849&tool=pmcentrez&rendertype=abstract.

15. Ostrowski MA, Chun TW, Justement SJ, Motola I, Spinelli MA, Adelsberger J, et al. Both memory and CD45RA +/CD62L + naive CD4(+) T cells are infected in human immunodeficiency virus type 1-infected individuals. J Virol. 1999;73:6430–5.

16. Agosto LM, Yu JJ, Dai J, Kaletsky R, Monie D, O'Doherty U. HIV-1 integrates into resting CD4 + T cells even at low inoculums as demonstrated with an improved assay for HIV-1 integration. Virology. 2007;368(1):60–72.

17. Agosto LM, Yu JJ, Dai J, Kaletsky R, Monie D, O'Doherty U. HIV-1 integrates into resting CD4 + T cells even at low inoculums as demonstrated with an improved assay for HIV-1 integration. Virology. 2007;368:60–72.

18. Pace MJ, Graf EH, Agosto LM, Mexas AM, Male F, Brady T, et al. Directly infected resting CD4 + T cells can produce HIV gag without spreading infection in a model of HIV latency. PLoS Pathog. 2012;8:e1002818. https://doi.org/10.1371/journal.ppat.1002818.

19. Plesa G, Dai J, Baytop C, Riley JL, June CH, O'Doherty U. Addition of deoxynucleosides enhances human immunodeficiency virus type 1 integration and 2LTR formation in resting CD4 + T cells. J Virol. 2007;81:13938–42. https://doi.org/10.1128/JVI.01745-07.

20. Swiggard WJ, Baytop C, Yu JJ, Dai J, Li C, Schretzenmair R, et al. Human immunodeficiency virus type 1 can establish latent infection in resting CD4 + T cells in the absence of activating stimuli. J Virol. 2005;79:14179–88. https://doi.org/10.1128/JVI.79.22.14179-14188.2005.

21. Chavez L, Calvanese V, Verdin E. HIV latency is established directly and early in both resting and activated primary CD4 T cells. PLoS Pathog. 2015;11:e1004955. https://doi.org/10.1371/journal.ppat.1004955.

22. Vatakis DN, Bristol G, Wilkinson TA, Chow SA, Zack JA. Immediate activation fails to rescue efficient human immunodeficiency virus replication in quiescent CD4 + T cells. J Virol. 2007;81:3574–82. https://doi.org/10.1128/JVI.02569-06.

23. Saleh S, Solomon A, Wightman F, Xhilaga M, Cameron PU, Lewin SR. CCR7 ligands CCL19 and CCL21 increase permissiveness of resting memory CD4 + T cells to HIV-1 infection: a novel model of HIV-1 latency. Blood. 2007;110:4161–4.

24. Dahabieh MS, Ooms M, Simon V, Sadowski I. A doubly fluorescent HIV-1 reporter shows that the majority of integrated HIV-1 is latent shortly after infection. J Virol. 2013;87:4716–27. https://doi.org/10.1128/JVI.03478-12.

25. Lassen KG, Hebbeler AM, Bhattacharyya D, Lobritz MA, Greene WC. A flexible model of HIV-1 latency permitting evaluation of many primary CD4 T-cell reservoirs. PLoS One. 2012;7:e30176.

26. Ho Y-C, Shan L, Hosmane NN, Wang J, Laskey SB, Rosenbloom DIS, et al. Replication-competent noninduced proviruses in the latent reservoir increase barrier to HIV-1 cure. Cell. 2013;155:540–51. https://doi.org/10.1016/j.cell.2013.09.020.

27. Dar RD, Hosmane NN, Arkin MR, Siliciano RF, Weinberger LS. Screening for noise in gene expression identifies drug synergies. Science. 2014;344:1392–6. https://doi.org/10.1126/science.1250220.

28. Hiener B, Horsburgh BA, Eden J-S, Barton K, Schlub TE, Lee E, et al. Identification of genetically intact HIV-1 proviruses in specific CD4 + T cells from effectively treated participants. Cell Rep. 2017;21:813–22. https://doi.org/10.1016/j.celrep.2017.09.081.

29. Soriano-Sarabia N, Bateson RE, Dahl NP, Crooks AM, Kuruc JD, Margolis DM, et al. Quantitation of replication-competent HIV-1 in populations of resting CD4 + T cells. J Virol. 2014;88:14070–7. https://doi.org/10.1128/JVI.01900-14.

30. Persaud D, Gay H, Ziemniak C, Chen YH, Piatak M, Chun T-W, et al. Absence of detectable HIV-1 viremia after treatment cessation in an infant. N Engl J Med. 2013;369:1828–35. https://doi.org/10.1056/NEJMoa1302976.

31. Henrich TJ, Hu Z, Li JZ, Sciaranghella G, Busch MP, Keating SM, et al. Long-term reduction in peripheral blood HIV type 1 reservoirs following reduced-intensity conditioning allogeneic stem cell transplantation. J Infect Dis. 2013;207:1694–702.

32. Henrich TJ, Hanhauser E, Marty FM, Sirignano MN, Keating S, Lee TH, et al. Antiretroviral-free HIV-1 remission and viral rebound after allogeneic stem cell transplantation: report of 2 cases. Ann Intern Med. 2014;161:319–27.

33. Eriksson S, Graf EH, Dahl V, Strain MC, Yukl SA, Lysenko ES, et al. Comparative analysis of measures of viral reservoirs in HIV-1 eradication studies. PLoS Pathog. 2013;9:e1003174.

34. Chomont N, El-Far M, Ancuta P, Trautmann L, Procopio FA, Yassine-Diab B, et al. HIV reservoir size and persistence are driven by T cell survival and homeostatic proliferation. Nat Med. 2009;15:893–900. https://doi.org/10.1038/nm.1972.

35. Pierson T, Hoffman TL, Blankson J, Finzi D, Chadwick K, Margolick JB, et al. Characterization of chemokine receptor utilization of viruses in the latent reservoir for human immunodeficiency virus type 1. J Virol. 2000;74:7824–33. https://doi.org/10.1128/JVI.74.17.7824-7833.2000.

36. Tabler CO, Lucera MB, Haqqani AA, McDonald DJ, Migueles SA, Connors M, et al. CD4 + memory stem cells are infected by HIV-1 in a manner regulated in part by SAMHD1 expression. J Virol. 2014;88:4976–86. https://doi.org/10.1128/JVI.00324-14.

37. Buzon MJ, Sun H, Li C, Shaw A, Seiss K, Ouyang Z, et al. HIV-1 persistence in CD4 + T cells with stem cell-like properties. Nat Med. 2014;20:139–42. https://doi.org/10.1038/nm.3445.

38. Jaafoura S, de Herve MDG, Hernandez-Vargas EA, Hendel-Chavez H, Abdoh M, Mateo MC, et al. Progressive contraction of the latent HIV reservoir around a core of less-differentiated CD4+ memory T Cells. Nat Commun. 2014;5:5407. https://doi.org/10.1038/ncomms6407.

39. Chahroudi A, Silvestri G, Lichterfeld M. T memory stem cells and HIV: a long-term relationship. Curr HIV/AIDS Rep. 2015;12:33–40.

40. Gosselin A, Monteiro P, Chomont N, Diaz-Griffero F, Said EA, Fonseca S, et al. Peripheral blood CCR4 + CCR6 + and CXCR3 + CCR6 + CD4 + T cells are highly permissive to HIV-1 infection. J Immunol. 2010;184:1604–16. https://doi.org/10.4049/jimmunol.0903058.

41. Gosselin A, Wiche Salinas TR, Planas D, Wacleche VS, Zhang Y, Fromentin R, et al. HIV persists in CCR6 + CD4 + T cells from colon and blood during antiretroviral therapy. Aids. 2017;31:35–48. https://doi.org/10.1097/QAD.0000000000001309.

42. Khoury G, Anderson JL, Fromentin R, Hartogensis W, Smith MZ, Bacchetti P, et al. Persistence of integrated HIV DNA in CXCR3 + CCR6 + memory CD4 + T-cells in HIV-infected individuals on antiretroviral therapy. Aids. 2016. https://doi.org/10.1097/QAD.0000000000001029.

43. Fromentin R, Bakeman W, Lawani MB, Khoury G, Hartogensis W, DaFonseca S, et al. CD4 + t cells expressing PD-1, TIGIT and LAG-3 contribute to HIV persistence during ART. PLoS Pathog. 2016;12:e1005761. https://doi.org/10.1371/journal.ppat.1005761.

44. Strain MC, Little SJ, Daar ES, Havlir DV, Günthard HF, Lam RY, et al. Effect of treatment, during primary infection, on establishment and clearance of cellular reservoirs of HIV-1. J Infect Dis. 2005;191:1410–8. https://doi.org/10.1086/428777.

45. Chun TW, Engel D, Berrey MM, Shea T, Corey L, Fauci AS. Early establishment of a pool of latently infected, resting CD4(+) T cells during primary HIV-1 infection. Proc Natl Acad Sci USA. 1998;95:8869–73. https://doi.org/10.1073/pnas.95.15.8869.

46. Nishimura Y, Sadjadpour R, Mattapallil JJ, Igarashi T, Lee W, Buckler-White A, et al. High frequencies of resting CD4 + T cells containing integrated viral DNA are found in rhesus macaques during acute lentivirus infections. Proc Natl Acad Sci. 2009;106:8015–20. https://doi.org/10.1073/pnas.0903022106.

47. Whitney JB, Hill AL, Sanisetty S, Penaloza-MacMaster P, Liu J, Shetty M, et al. Rapid seeding of the viral reservoir prior to SIV viraemia in rhesus monkeys. Nature. 2014;512:74–7. https://doi.org/10.1038/nature13594.

48. Ananworanich J, Schuetz A, Vandergeeten C, Sereti I, de Souza M, Rerknimitr R, et al. Impact of multi-targeted Antiretroviral treatment on gut T cell depletion and HIV reservoir seeding during acute HIV infection. PLoS ONE. 2012;7:e33948. https://doi.org/10.1371/journal.pone.0033948.

49. Ananworanich J, Chomont N, Eller LA, Kroon E, Tovanabutra S, Bose M, et al. HIV DNA set point is rapidly established in acute HIV infection and dramatically reduced by early ART. EBioMedicine. 2016;11:68–72. https://doi.org/10.1016/j.ebiom.2016.07.024.

50. Sáez-Cirión A, Bacchus C, Hocqueloux L, Avettand-Fenoel V, Girault I, Lecuroux C, et al. Post-Treatment HIV-1 controllers with a long-term virological remission after the interruption of Early initiated antiretroviral therapy ANRS VISCONTI study. PLoS Pathog. 2013;9:e1003211.

51. Azzoni L, Foulkes AS, Papasavvas E, Mexas AM, Lynn KM, Mounzer K, et al. Pegylated interferon alfa-2a monotherapy results in suppression of HIV type 1 replication and decreased cell-associated HIV DNA integration. J Infect Dis. 2013;207:213–22.

52. Assoumou L, Weiss L, Piketty C, Burgard M, Melard A, Girard P-M, et al. A low HIV-DNA level in peripheral blood mononuclear cells at antiretroviral treatment interruption predicts a higher probability of maintaining viral control. Aids. 2015;29:2003–7. https://doi.org/10.1097/QAD.0000000000000734.

53. Williams JP, Hurst J, Stöhr W, Robinson N, Brown H, Fisher M, et al. HIV-1 DNA predicts disease progression and post-treatment virological control. Elife. 2014;3:e03821.

54. Pinzone MR, Graf E, Lynch L, McLaughlin B, Hecht FM, Connors M, et al. Monitoring integration over time supports a role for CTL and ongoing replication as determinants of reservoir size. J Virol. 2016. https://doi.org/10.1128/JVI.00242-16.

55. Koelsch KK, Boesecke C, McBride K, Gelgor L, Fahey P, Natarajan V, et al. Impact of treatment with raltegravir during primary or chronic HIV infection on RNA decay characteristics and the HIV viral reservoir. Aids. 2011;25:2069–78. https://doi.org/10.1097/QAD.0b013e32834b9658.

56. Murray JM, McBride K, Boesecke C, Bailey M, Amin J, Suzuki K, et al. Integrated HIV DNA accumulates prior to treatment while episomal HIV DNA records ongoing transmission afterwards. Aids. 2012;26:543–50.

57. Buzon MJ, Martin-Gayo E, Pereyra F, Ouyang Z, Sun H, Li JZ, et al. Long-term antiretroviral treatment initiated at primary HIV-1 infection affects the size, composition, and decay kinetics of the reservoir of HIV-1-infected CD4 T cells. J Virol. 2014;88:10056–65. https://doi.org/10.1128/JVI.01046-14.

58. Murray JM, Zaunders JJ, McBride KL, Xu Y, Bailey M, Suzuki K, et al. HIV DNA subspecies persist in both activated and resting memory CD4 + T cells during antiretroviral therapy. J Virol. 2014;88:3516–26. https://doi.org/10.1128/JVI.03331-13.

59. Radebe M, Gounder K, Mokgoro M, Ndhlovu ZM, Mncube Z, Mkhize L, et al. Broad and persistent gag-specific CD8 + T-cell responses are associated with viral control but rarely drive viral escape during primary HIV-1 infection. Aids. 2015;29:23–33. https://doi.org/10.1097/QAD.0000000000000508.

60. Deng K, Pertea M, Rongvaux A, Wang L, Durand CM, Ghiaur G, et al. Broad CTL response is required to clear latent HIV-1 due to dominance of escape mutations. Nature. 2015;517:381–5. https://doi.org/10.1038/nature14053.

61. Streeck H, Jolin JS, Qi Y, Yassine-Diab B, Johnson RC, Kwon DS, et al. Human immunodeficiency virus type 1-specific CD8 + T-cell responses during primary infection are major determinants of the viral set point and loss of CD4 + T cells. J Virol. 2009;83:7641–8. https://doi.org/10.1128/JVI.00182-09.

62. Trautmann L, Mbitikon-Kobo F-M, Goulet J-P, Peretz Y, Shi Y, Van Grevenynghe J, et al. Profound metabolic, functional, and cytolytic differences characterize HIV-specific CD8 T cells in primary and chronic HIV infection. Blood. 2012;120:3466–77. https://doi.org/10.1182/blood-2012-04-422550.

63. Descours B, Avettand-Fenoel V, Blanc C, Samri A, Mélard A, Supervie V, et al. Immune responses driven by protective human leukocyte antigen alleles from long-term nonprogressors are associated with low HIV reservoir in central memory CD4 T cells. Clin Infect Dis. 2012;54:1495–503.

64. Bruner KM, Murray AJ, Pollack RA, Soliman MG, Laskey SB, Capoferri AA, et al. Defective proviruses rapidly accumulate during acute HIV-1 infection. Nat Med. 2016;22:1043–9. https://doi.org/10.1038/nm.4156.

65. Estes JD, Kityo C, Ssali F, Swainson L, Nganou Makamdop K, Del Prete GQ, et al. Defining total-body AIDS-virus burden with implications for curative strategies. Nat Publ Gr. 2017. https://doi.org/10.1038/nm.4411.

66. Graf EH, Mexas AM, Yu JJ, Shaheen F, Liszewski MK, Di Mascio M, et al. Elite suppressors harbor low levels of integrated HIV DNA and high levels of 2-LTR circular HIV DNA compared to HIV + patients on and off HAART. PLoS Pathog. 2011;7:e1001300.

67. Mens H, Kearney M, Wiegand A, Shao W, Schønning K, Gerstoft J, et al. HIV-1 continues to replicate and evolve in patients with natural control of HIV infection. J Virol. 2010;84:12971–81. https://doi.org/10.1128/JVI.00387-10.

68. Julg B, Pereyra F, Buzón MJ, Piechocka-Trocha A, Clark MJ, Baker BM, et al. Infrequent recovery of HIV from but robust exogenous infection of activated CD4 + T cells in HIV elite controllers. Clin Infect Dis. 2010;51:233–8.

69. O'Connell KA, Brennan TP, Bailey JR, Ray SC, Siliciano RF, Blankson JN. Control of HIV-1 in elite suppressors despite ongoing replication and evolution in plasma virus. J Virol. 2010;84:7018–28. https://doi.org/10.1128/JVI.00548-10.

70. Connick E, Mattila T, Folkvord JM, Schlichtemeier R, Meditz AL, Ray MG, et al. CTL fail to accumulate at sites of HIV-1 replication in lymphoid tissue. J Immunol. 2007;178:6975–83. https://doi.org/10.4049/jimmunol.178.11.6975.

71. Fukazawa Y, Lum R, Okoye AA, Park H, Matsuda K, Bae JY, et al. B cell follicle sanctuary permits persistent productive simian immunodeficiency virus infection in elite controllers. Nat Med. 2015;21:132–9. https://doi.org/10.1038/nm.3781.

72. Connick E, Folkvord JM, Lind KT, Rakasz EG, Miles B, Wilson NA, et al. Compartmentalization of simian immunodeficiency virus replication within secondary lymphoid tissues of rhesus macaques is linked to disease stage and inversely related to localization of virus-specific CTL. J Immunol. 2014;193:5613–25. https://doi.org/10.4049/jimmunol.1401161.

73. Yerly S, Gunthard HF, Fagard C, Joos B, Perneger TV, Hirschel B, Perrin L. Proviral HIV-DNA predicts viral rebound and viral setpoint after structured treatment interruptions. Res Lett. 2004;18:1951–64.

74. Piketty C, Weis L, Assoumou L, Burgard M, Mélard A, Ragnaud JM, et al. ANRS 116 Salto Study Group. A high HIV DNA level in PBMCs at antiretroviral treatment interruption predicts a shorter time to treatment resumption, independently of the CD4 nadir. J Med Virol. 2010;82:1819–28.

75. Hurst J, Hoffmann M, Pace M, Williams JP, Thornhill J, Hamlyn E, et al. Immunological biomarkers predict HIV-1 viral rebound after treatment interruption. Nat Commun. 2015;6:8495. https://doi.org/10.1038/ncomms9495.

76. Graf EH, Pace MJ, Peterson BA, Lynch LJ, Chukwulebe SB, Mexas AM, et al. Gag-positive reservoir cells are susceptible to HIV-specific cytotoxic T lymphocyte mediated clearance in vitro and can be detected in vivo [corrected]. PLoS ONE. 2013;8:e71879. https://doi.org/10.1371/journal.pone.0071879.

77. Chan CN, Trinité B, Lee CS, Mahajan S, Anand A, Wodarz D, et al. HIV-1 latency and virus production from unintegrated genomes following direct infection of resting CD4 T cells. Retrovirology. 2016;13:1. https://doi.org/10.1186/s12977-015-0234-9.

78. Elliott JH, Wightman F, Solomon A, Ghneim K, Ahlers J, Cameron MJ, et al. Activation of HIV transcription with short-course vorinostat in HIV-infected patients on suppressive antiretroviral therapy. PLoS Pathog. 2014;10:1–19.

79. Rasmussen TA, Tolstrup M, Brinkmann CR, Olesen R, Erikstrup C, Solomon A, Winckelmann A, Palmer S, Dinarello C, Buzon M, Lichterfeld M, Lewin SR, Østergaard LSO. Panobinostat, a histone deacetylase inhibitor, for latent-virus reactivation in HIV-infected patients on suppressive antiretroviral therapy: a phase 1/2, single group, clinical trial. Lancet HIV. 2014;1:e13–21.

80. Leth S, Schleimann MH, Nissen SK, Højen JF, Olesen R, Graversen ME, Jørgensen S, Kjær AS, Denton PW, Mørk A, Sommerfelt MA, Krogsgaard K, Østergaard L, Rasmussen TA, Tolstrup MSO. Combined effect of Vacc-4x, recombinant human granulocyte macrophage colony-stimulating factor vaccination, and romidepsin on the HIV-1 reservoir (REDUC): a single-arm, phase 1B/2A trial. Lancet HIV. 2016;3:e463–72.

81. Mexas AM, Graf EH, Pace MJ, Yu JJ, Papasavvas E, Azzoni L, et al. Concurrent measures of total and integrated HIV DNA monitor reservoirs and ongoing replication in eradication trials. AIDS. 2012;26:2295–306. https://doi.org/10.1097/QAD.0b013e32835a5c2f.

82. Cardozo EF, Andrade A, Mellors JW, Kuritzkes DR, Perelson AS, Ribeiro RM. Treatment with integrase inhibitor suggests a new interpretation of HIV RNA decay curves that reveals a subset of cells with slow integration. PLoS Pathog. 2017;13:1–18.

83. Pace MJ, Graf EH, O'Doherty U. HIV 2-long terminal repeat circular DNA is stable in primary CD4 + T cells. Virology. 2013;441:18–21.

84. Andrade A, Guedj J, Rosenkranz SL, Lu D, Mellors J, Kuritzkes DR, et al. Early HIV RNA decay during raltegravir-containing regimens exhibits two distinct subphases (1a and 1b). AIDS. 2015;29:2419–26. https://doi.org/10.1097/QAD.0000000000000843.

85. Liszewski MK, Yu JJ, O'Doherty U. Detecting HIV-1 integration by repetitive-sampling Alu-gag PCR. Methods. 2009;47:254–60. https://doi.org/10.1016/j.ymeth.2009.01.002.

86. Yu JJ, Wu TL, Liszewski MK, Dai J, Swiggard WJ, Baytop C, et al. A more precise HIV integration assay designed to detect small differences finds lower levels of integrated DNA in HAART treated patients. Virology. 2008;379:78–86. https://doi.org/10.1016/j.virol.2008.05.030.

87. Lada, Steven M et al. Novel Assay to Measure Integrated HIV DNA in PBMC from ART-Suppressed Persons. CROI. 2017; Poster 300.

88. Kumar R, Vandegraaff N, Mundy L, Burrell CJ, Li P. Evaluation of PCR-based methods for the quantitation of integrated HIV-1 DNA. J Virol Methods. 2002;105:233–46.

89. Vandergeeten C, Fromentin R, Merlini E, Lawani MB, DaFonseca S, Bakeman W, et al. Cross-clade ultrasensitive PCR-based assays to measure HIV persistence in large-cohort studies. J Virol. 2014;88:12385–96. https://doi.org/10.1128/JVI.00609-14.

90. Symons J, Chopra A, Malatinkova E, Spiegelaere W De, Leary S, Cooper D, et al. HIV integration sites in latently infected cell lines: evidence of ongoing replication. Retrovirology. 2017;14:2.

91. De Spiegelaere W, Malatinkova E, Lynch L, Van Nieuwerburgh F, Messiaen P, O'Doherty U, et al. Quantification of integrated HIV DNA by repetitive-sampling Alu-HIV PCR on the basis of poisson statistics. Clin Chem. 2014;60:886–95. https://doi.org/10.1373/clinchem.2013.219378.

92. Rouzioux C, Avettand-Fenoel V. Total HIV-DNA: a global marker of HIV persistence. Retrovirology. 2018;15(1). **(In press).**

93. Besson GJ, Lalama CM, Bosch RJ, Gandhi RT, Bedison MA, Aga E, et al. HIV-1 DNA decay dynamics in blood during more than a decade of suppressive antiretroviral therapy. Clin Infect Dis. 2014;59:1312–21. https://doi.org/10.1093/cid/ciu585.

94. Mendoza D, Johnson SA, Peterson BA, Natarajan V, Salgado M, Robin L, et al. Comprehensive analysis of unique cases with extraordinary control over HIV replication comprehensive analysis of unique cases with extraordinary control over HIV replication. Blood. 2014;119:4645–55.

95. Kiselinova M, De Spiegelaere W, Buzon MJ, Malatinkova E, Lichterfeld M, Vandekerckhove L. Integrated and total HIV-1 DNA predict ex vivo viral outgrowth. PLoS Pathog. 2016;12:e1005472.

96. Bruner KM, Hosmane NN, Siliciano RF. Towards an HIV-1 cure: measuring the latent reservoir Katherine. Trends Microbiol. 2015;23:192–203.

97. Imamichi H, Dewar RL, Adelsberger JW, Rehm CA, O'Doherty U, Paxinos EE, et al. Defective HIV-1 proviruses produce novel protein-coding RNA species in HIV-infected patients on combination antiretroviral therapy. Proc Natl Acad Sci USA. 2016;113:201609057. https://doi.org/10.1073/pnas.1609057113.

98. Lewinski MK, Bisgrove D, Shinn P, Chen H, Hoffmann C, Hannenhalli S, et al. Genome-wide analysis of chromosomal features repressing human immunodeficiency virus transcription. J Virol. 2005;79:6610–9. https://doi.org/10.1128/JVI.79.11.6610-6619.2005.

99. Han Y, Lassen K, Monie D, Sedaghat AR, Shimoji S, Liu X, et al. Resting CD4 + T cells from human immunodeficiency virus type 1 (HIV-1)-infected individuals carry integrated HIV-1 genomes within actively transcribed host genes. J Virol. 2004;78:6122–33. https://doi.org/10.1128/JVI.78.12.6122-6133.2004.

100. Hughes S, Coffin J. What integration sites tell us about HIV persistence. Cell Host Microbe. 2016;19:588–98.

101. Maldarelli F, Wu X, Su L, Simonetti FR, Shao W, Hill S, et al. Specific HIV integration sites are linked to clonal expansion and persistence of infected cells. Science. 2014;345:2–7. https://doi.org/10.1126/science.1254194.

15

Myricetin antagonizes semen-derived enhancer of viral infection (SEVI) formation and influences its infection-enhancing activity

Ruxia Ren[1,2†], Shuwen Yin[1†], Baolong Lai[2], Lingzhen Ma[1], Jiayong Wen[1], Xuanxuan Zhang[1], Fangyuan Lai[1], Shuwen Liu[1*] and Lin Li[1*]

Abstract

Background: Semen is a critical vector for human immunodeficiency virus (HIV) sexual transmission and harbors seminal amyloid fibrils that can markedly enhance HIV infection. Semen-derived enhancer of viral infection (SEVI) is one of the best-characterized seminal amyloid fibrils. Due to their highly cationic properties, SEVI fibrils can capture HIV virions, increase viral attachment to target cells, and augment viral fusion. Some studies have reported that myricetin antagonizes amyloid β-protein (Aβ) formation; myricetin also displays strong anti-HIV activity in vitro.

Results: Here, we report that myricetin inhibits the formation of SEVI fibrils by binding to the amyloidogenic region of the SEVI precursor peptide (PAP248–286) and disrupting PAP248–286 oligomerization. In addition, myricetin was found to remodel preformed SEVI fibrils and to influence the activity of SEVI in promoting HIV-1 infection. Moreover, myricetin showed synergistic effects against HIV-1 infection in combination with other antiretroviral drugs in semen.

Conclusions: Incorporation of myricetin into a combination bifunctional microbicide with both anti-SEVI and anti-HIV activities is a highly promising approach to preventing sexual transmission of HIV.

Keywords: HIV, Myricetin, Amyloid fibrils, SEVI, Synergistic antiviral effects

Background

Since the first cases of acquired immune deficiency syndrome (AIDS) were reported in 1981, more than 70 million people have been infected by human immunodeficiency virus (HIV), and approximately 1 million die of the disease annually [1]. Currently, unprotected sex remains the major route of HIV transmission, accounting for more than 80% of new HIV infections worldwide [2].

It has been shown that semen functions as a critical carrier of virus during sexual transmission [3]. Notably, amyloid fibrils in semen are considered to be responsible for the reduced efficacy of antiretroviral therapies (cART)

in vivo because they facilitate virus attachment and internalization into cells [4]. A naturally occurring C-proximal proteolytic fragment of prostatic acid phosphatase (PAP) in semen, PAP248–286, has been reported to form aggregated amyloid fibrils (known as semen-derived enhancer of virus infection or SEVI) and to increase by several orders of magnitude the rate of HIV infection in vitro [5]. Because SEVI is highly cationic and the fibrils it forms are positively charged, it not only effectively captures HIV virions but also promotes viral attachment to target cells by neutralizing the inherent electrostatic repulsion between the negative charges on the surfaces of the virions and target cells [6]. Some other endogenous amyloid aggregates that increase HIV-1 infectivity, including the PAP N-proximal fragment (PAP85–120) and semenogelins (SEM1 and SEM2), have been identified in human semen [7, 8], which may explain the discrepancy between the low infectiousness of HIV in vitro and its observed efficient sexual transmission.

*Correspondence: liusw@smu.edu.cn; li75lin@126.com
†Ruxia Ren and Shuwen Yin contributed equally to this work
[1] Guangdong Provincial Key Laboratory of New Drug Screening, Guangzhou Key Laboratory of Drug Research for Emerging Virus Prevention and Treatment, School of Pharmaceutical Sciences, Southern Medical University, 1838 Guangzhou Avenue North, Guangzhou 510515, Guangdong, China
Full list of author information is available at the end of the article

As amyloid species that are naturally abundant in semen, including SEVI, play a critical role in the spread of HIV, they represent a particularly attractive target for the development of molecules that can reduce spread of the virus. Theoretically, eliminating seminal amyloid fibrils by antagonizing fibril formation or enhancing the degradation of mature endogenous fibrils can massively reduce any viral infection enhancement [9–11]. This strategy might be advantageous because it targets host factors rather than the virus itself.

It is well known that the aggregation of proteins into amyloid fibrils is associated with fatal diseases, including Alzheimer's disease, Parkinson's disease and diabetes, and many molecules that inhibit fibrillization in vitro have been reported. For instance, epigallocatechin-3-gallate (EGCG), the major catechin present in green tea, not only potently inhibits the amyloidogenesis of various polypeptides but is also able to disassemble a wide range of preformed amyloid fibrils [12, 13].

Myricetin, a common dietary flavonoid found in foods such as walnuts, onions, berries, herbs and red grapes, exerts a wide variety of biological and nutraceutical effects, including antioxidative, antiinflammatory, antidiabetic, antitumor and free radical-scavenging activities [14–16]. Moreover, myricetin shows activity against HIV-1 infection by inhibiting HIV-1 integrase [17, 18]. It is noteworthy that myricetin inhibits amyloid fibrillization by a variety of disease-associated amyloidogenic proteins, including amyloid β-protein (Aβ), tau protein, islet amyloid polypeptide and other amyloidogenic peptides [19–21]. As described above, SEVI is a possible drug target for preventing HIV sexual transmission due to its stable structure and high levels in semen [22]. The concentration of endogenous SEVI in pooled semen is approximately 35 µg/ml, which considerably exceeds the level (≥ 2 µg/ml) required to enhance infection [7, 23]. However, it is not known whether myricetin affects the formation of SEVI amyloid fibrils in semen. In the current study, we sought to elucidate the effects of myricetin on the formation of SEVI amyloid fibrils and on the enhancement of HIV-1 infection by SEVI. Strikingly, the results showed that myricetin influences the activity of SEVI in enhancing HIV-1 infection and that it exhibits synergistic effects in semen against HIV-1 infection when applied to cells in combination with other antiretroviral (ARV) agents. These findings will be helpful in the development of dual-function antiviral drugs or microbicides that possess both anti-HIV and anti-SEVI-enhancing activities.

Results

Myricetin inhibits the formation of SEVI fibrils and other seminal fibrils

Thioflavin T (ThT), a dye that is commonly used in the detection of amyloid fibrils, can intercalate into the β-sheet structure of amyloid fibrils, resulting in enhanced fluorescence and a characteristic redshift in the emission spectrum. Congo red, another amyloid-binding dye, exhibits apple-green birefringence under polarized light as well as increased fluorescence [7, 24]. To evaluate the effects of myricetin on the formation of SEVI fibrils by PAP248–286, we collected PAP248–286 aggregates formed in the presence or absence of various concentrations of myricetin at different time points and monitored them using both ThT fluorescence and Congo red staining assays. The results showed that myricetin antagonized the assembly of PAP248–286 monomers into SEVI fibrils in a dose-dependent manner. The addition of myricetin at 75 µg/ml increased the lag time of SEVI amyloid fibril formation by PAP248–286 to more than 48 h, as measured by ThT fluorescence (Fig. 1a), whereas the lag time of amyloid fibril formation by PAP248–286 in the absence of myricetin was less than 6 h. Congo red assays showed that the lag time of SEVI amyloid fibril formation in the presence of various concentrations of myricetin was extended to approximately 18 h (Fig. 1b). The morphology of SEVI fibrils in the presence and absence of myricetin was imaged by transmission electron microscopy (TEM). As shown in Fig. 1c, mature SEVI fibrils formed by PAP248–286 were identified after shaking for 24 h, whereas no amyloid fibrils were observed after adding 16 µg/ml of myricetin, even after shaking for 48 h.

Far-UV (190–260 nm) circular dichroism (CD) spectrum measurement is commonly used to detect the presence of the typical secondary β-sheet structure of fibrils; such fibrils display a spectrum with a minimum at approximately 218 nm. A characteristic β-sheet secondary structure undergoes higher-level association to form protein aggregates and mature fibrils. Thus, we further investigated the secondary structure of SEVI fibrils formed in the presence or absence of myricetin by measuring their CD spectra. As illustrated in Fig. 1e, the spectrum of PAP248–286 after agitation for 24 h displayed a single minimum at approximately 230 nm, indicating the presence of a typical β-sheet component. However, the spectrum of PAP248–286 after agitation for 24 h in the presence of 5 µg/ml myricetin (final concentration) indicated the presence of a characteristic random coil structure, suggesting that PAP248–286 did not adopt any ordered or stable conformation and indicating that β-sheet aggregation had not occurred.

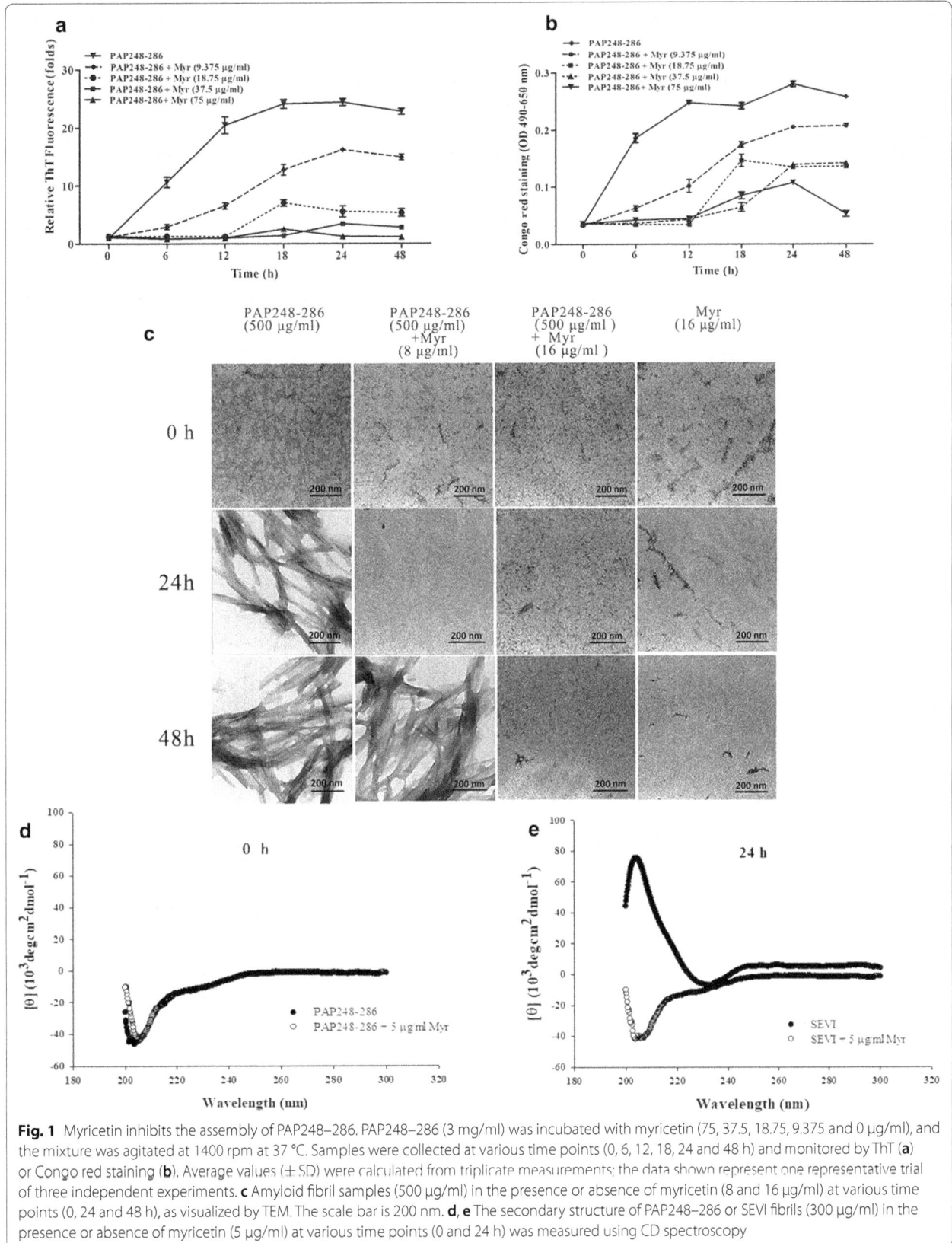

Fig. 1 Myricetin inhibits the assembly of PAP248–286. PAP248–286 (3 mg/ml) was incubated with myricetin (75, 37.5, 18.75, 9.375 and 0 μg/ml), and the mixture was agitated at 1400 rpm at 37 °C. Samples were collected at various time points (0, 6, 12, 18, 24 and 48 h) and monitored by ThT (**a**) or Congo red staining (**b**). Average values (±SD) were calculated from triplicate measurements; the data shown represent one representative trial of three independent experiments. **c** Amyloid fibril samples (500 μg/ml) in the presence or absence of myricetin (8 and 16 μg/ml) at various time points (0, 24 and 48 h), as visualized by TEM. The scale bar is 200 nm. **d**, **e** The secondary structure of PAP248–286 or SEVI fibrils (300 μg/ml) in the presence or absence of myricetin (5 μg/ml) at various time points (0 and 24 h) was measured using CD spectroscopy

Several studies have reported that the PAP248–286 monomer lacks the ability to promote HIV-1 infection [25]. To determine whether enhancement of HIV-1 infection by PAP248–286 is lost after the addition of myricetin, we characterized the HIV-1 infection-enhancing activity of PAP248–286 samples after agitation in the presence or absence of myricetin for various times (samples in Fig. 1a, b); the final concentrations of PAP and myricetin used in the cell-based HIV infection assay are only one-sixtieth of their initial concentrations. To eliminate the anti-HIV activity of myricetin itself, the above samples were first centrifuged at 12,000 rpm for 5 min to remove free myricetin. As shown in Fig. 2 and Additional

file 1: Figure S2, PAP248–286 that had been agitated for 6–48 h effectively enhanced HIV-1 infection by two HIV-1 clones in a time-dependent manner. However, the ability of PAP248–286 to enhance HIV-1 infection decreased after agitation in the presence of myricetin in a dose-dependent manner. The highest final concentration of myricetin tested (1.25 μg/ml) significantly neutralized SEVI-mediated enhancing activity by inhibiting the formation of SEVI fibrils (Fig. 2, Additional file 1: Figure S2). It is worth mentioning that inhibition of SEVI fibril formation was not observed after agitation of PAP248–286 in the presence of lower concentrations of myricetin for 24 h but was observed after agitation of PAP248–286 in

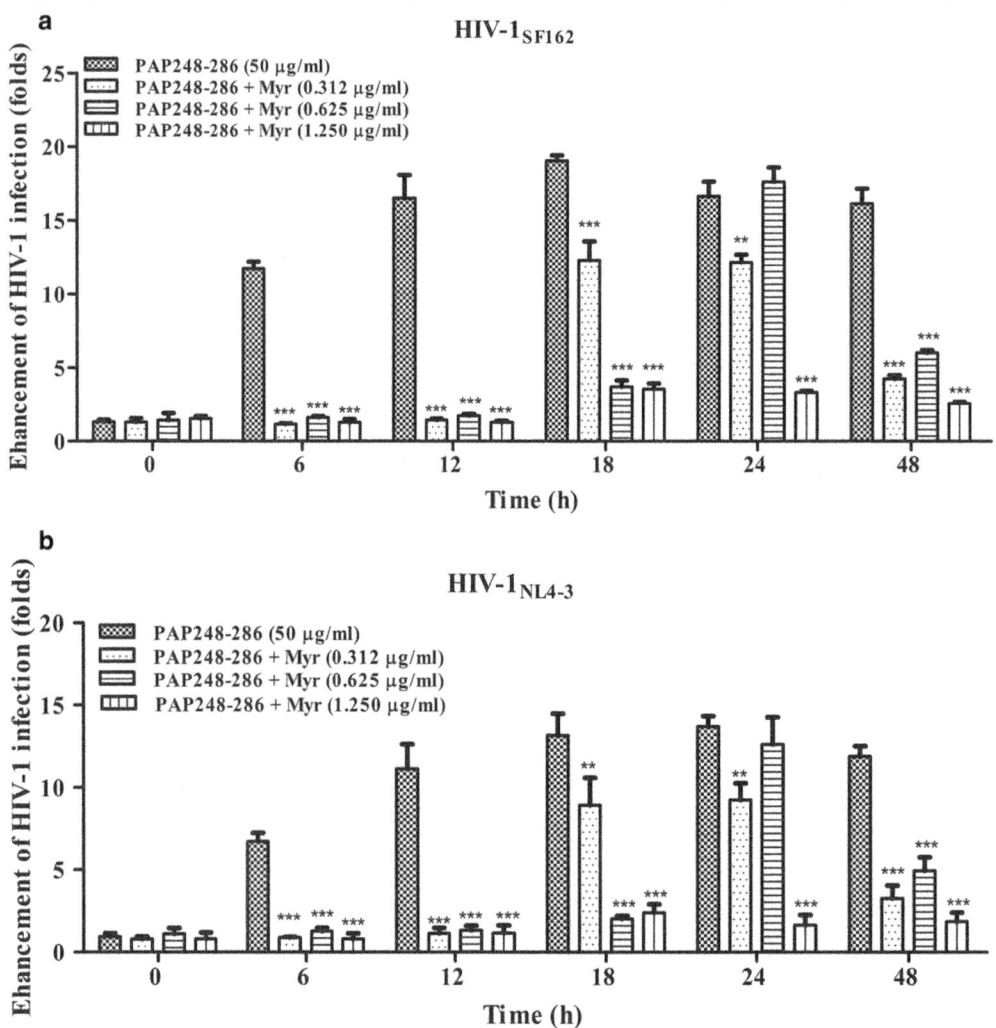

Fig. 2 Amyloid fibril samples display loss of enhancement of HIV-1 infection in the presence of myricetin. Mixed SEVI fibril samples prepared as described above in the presence or absence of myricetin were diluted to a final concentration of 50 μg/ml (PAP248–286). The samples were then incubated with HIV-1$_{SF162}$ (**a**) and HIV-1$_{NL4-3}$ (**b**) infectious clones. The mixtures were added to prepared TZM-b1 cells. Luciferase activities were measured at 72 h post-infection. The values shown represent the mean ± SD (n = 3). One-way ANOVA with Dunnett's post hoc multiple comparisons test was used to statistically analyze the differences between samples containing PAP248–286 alone and samples containing PAP248–286 and myricetin (*$p < 0.05$; **$p < 0.01$, ***$p < 0.001$)

the presence of the same concentrations of myricetin for 48 h (Fig. 2). The most likely reason for this is that the ability of myricetin to inhibit fibril formation may require long exposure times and full interaction. The results also indicated that myricetin may play a role in the degradation of mature SEVI fibrils. Taken together, these findings show that myricetin abrogates the formation of SEVI fibrils by PAP248–286, thereby influencing the activity of SEVI in enhancing HIV-1 infection.

The effects of myricetin on the formation of two other common seminal amyloid fibrils, SEM1 and SEM2, were also assessed. According to the results, myricetin also inhibited the formation of fibrils by both $SEM1_{86-107}$ and $SEM2_{86-107}$ in a dose-dependent manner (Additional file 1: Figure S1). The addition of myricetin at a concentration of 200 µg/ml completely blocked amyloid fibril formation, as measured by ThT fluorescence.

Myricetin shows binding affinity to functional regions of the PAP248–286 monomer

To clarify the molecular mechanism by which myricetin inhibits assembly of PAP248–286 into fibrils, we first analyzed potential interaction between myricetin and the PAP248–286 monomer by western blotting (WB). Myricetin is a negatively charged compound, whereas PAP248–286 is positively charged peptide. The inherent electrostatic repulsion that exists between two oppositely charged molecules might account for deposition of the PAP248–286 peptide via a change in isoelectric point. Using native acid gel electrophoresis, we observed a marked decrease in the level of PAP248–286 monomer in the supernatant after adding myricetin, a decrease that was dose dependent (Fig. 3a). The results indicate that myricetin binds to PAP248–286 monomers and forms insoluble aggregates via natural electrostatic interaction. The affinity between myricetin and the PAP248–286 monomer was further investigated using surface

plasmon resonance (SPR). As shown in Fig. 3b, myricetin bound to the PAP248–286 monomer with high affinity ($K_D = 3.02 \times 10^{-7}$ M). To confirm the specificity of this binding, an irrelevant peptide (N36) and an irrelevant flavonoid (phlorizin) were used as negative controls; N36 is a 36-mer synthetic peptide derived from the N-terminal heptad repeat region of the HIV gp41 envelope protein [26], and phlorizin is a natural phenol that is found in apple and pear tree leaves. Our results confirmed that myricetin does not bind to N36 and that phlorizin does not bind to the PAP248–286 monomer (Fig. 3c, d).

To further substantiate the interaction of myricetin with PAP248–286 at the atomic level, computational molecular docking was conducted to identify the potential amino acids involved in the binding of myricetin to PAP248–286 monomers. Our analysis, which was based on the 3D molecular structure of myricetin and the monocrystal PAP248–286 protein structure reported in Protein Data Bank (PDB; code No. 2L3H), showed that myricetin is able to bind to PAP248–286 and form hydrogen bonds via four potential residues: Leu258, Gln259, Met271 and Arg273. Myricetin is also able to bind to PAP248–286 via hydrophobic interactions with Val264 and Leu268 (Fig. 3e).

Some studies have reported that the central region of the SEVI precursor peptide PAP248–286, namely, PAP257–267, is an amyloidogenic region with high fibril-forming propensity [27]. Coincidentally, PAP268–271 plays a vital role in promoting SEVI fibrillation [27]. According to our computational molecular docking results, six potential residues of PAP248–286 are associated with myricetin binding (Fig. 3e). To replace PAP248–286, we synthesized a 15-amino acid PAP257–271 fragment that includes both of the amyloidogenic regions (PAP257–267 and PAP268–271) and all six of the amino acids (Leu258, Gln259, Val264, Leu268, Met271 and Arg273) shown to be important in the molecular

(See figure on next page.)
Fig. 3 Myricetin exhibits high-affinity binding to the functional region of the PAP248–286 monomer. **a** The electrostatic interaction of myricetin with PAP248–286. PAP248–286 (100 µg/ml) was incubated with serially diluted myricetin (12.5, 6.25, 3.13 and 1.56 µg/ml) at 37 °C for 30 min. The samples were then centrifuged at 5000 rpm for 15 min; the peptides remaining in the supernatant were electrophoresed through 10% acidic native polyacrylamide gels and detected by WB using a polyclonal antibody against PAP248–286. **b** Binding affinity of myricetin to PAP248–286. PAP248–286 (50 µg/ml) was immobilized on a sensor chip. Subsequently, twofold serial dilutions of recombinant myricetin were injected as the analyte. The affinity constant K_D is the ratio of the dissociation constant K_d to the association constant K_a ($K_D = K_d/K_a$). **c** Binding affinity of myricetin to an irrelevant N36 peptide (50 µg/ml). **d** Binding affinity of an irrelevant flavonoid (phlorizin) to PAP248–286 (50 µg/ml). **e** Presumed binding sites of myricetin to PAP248–286. According to the computational docking results, myricetin formed hydrogen bonds with Leu258, Gln259, Met271 and Arg273, and it bound to Val264 and Leu268 by hydrophobic interactions. **f** Amyloid fibril formation by wild-type PAP257–273 and six mutants. Wild-type and mutant peptides (3 mg/ml) were agitated at 1400 rpm at 37 °C for 40 h; the presence of fibrils was then monitored using ThT assays. **g** Myricetin inhibition of fibril formation by wild-type and mutants PAP257–273. Wild-type and mutants PAP257–273 were mixed with myricetin (200, 100, 50 and 25 µg/ml), and the mixtures were agitated at 1400 rpm at 37 °C. The samples were then collected and monitored using ThT assays. Percent inhibition was calculated from the following equation: (1-ThT fluorescence of fibrils with Myr/ThT fluorescence of fibrils without Myr) × 100. Average values (± SD) were calculated from triplicate measurements; the data shown represent one representative trial of three independent experiments

a

PAP248-286 (100 µg/ml)   +   +   +   +   +

Myr (µg/ml)   -   1.56   3.13   6.25   12.5

b

$K_D (Myr) = 3.02 \times 10^{-7}$ M

6.36 µg/ml Myr
3.18 µg/ml Myr
1.59 µg/ml Myr
0.80 µg/ml Myr
0.40 µg/ml Myr
0.20 µg/ml Myr

c

6.36 µg/ml Myr
3.18 µg/ml Myr
1.59 µg/ml Myr
0.80 µg/ml Myr
0.40 µg/ml Myr
0.20 µg/ml Myr

d

6.36 µg/ml Phlorizin
3.18 µg/ml Phlorizin
1.59 µg/ml Phlorizin
0.80 µg/ml Phlorizin
0.40 µg/ml Phlorizin
0.20 µg/ml Phlorizin

e

f

g

PAP257-273
PAP257-273 (L-258-A)
PAP257-273 (Q-259-A)
PAP257-273 (L-268-A)
PAP257-273 (R-273-A)

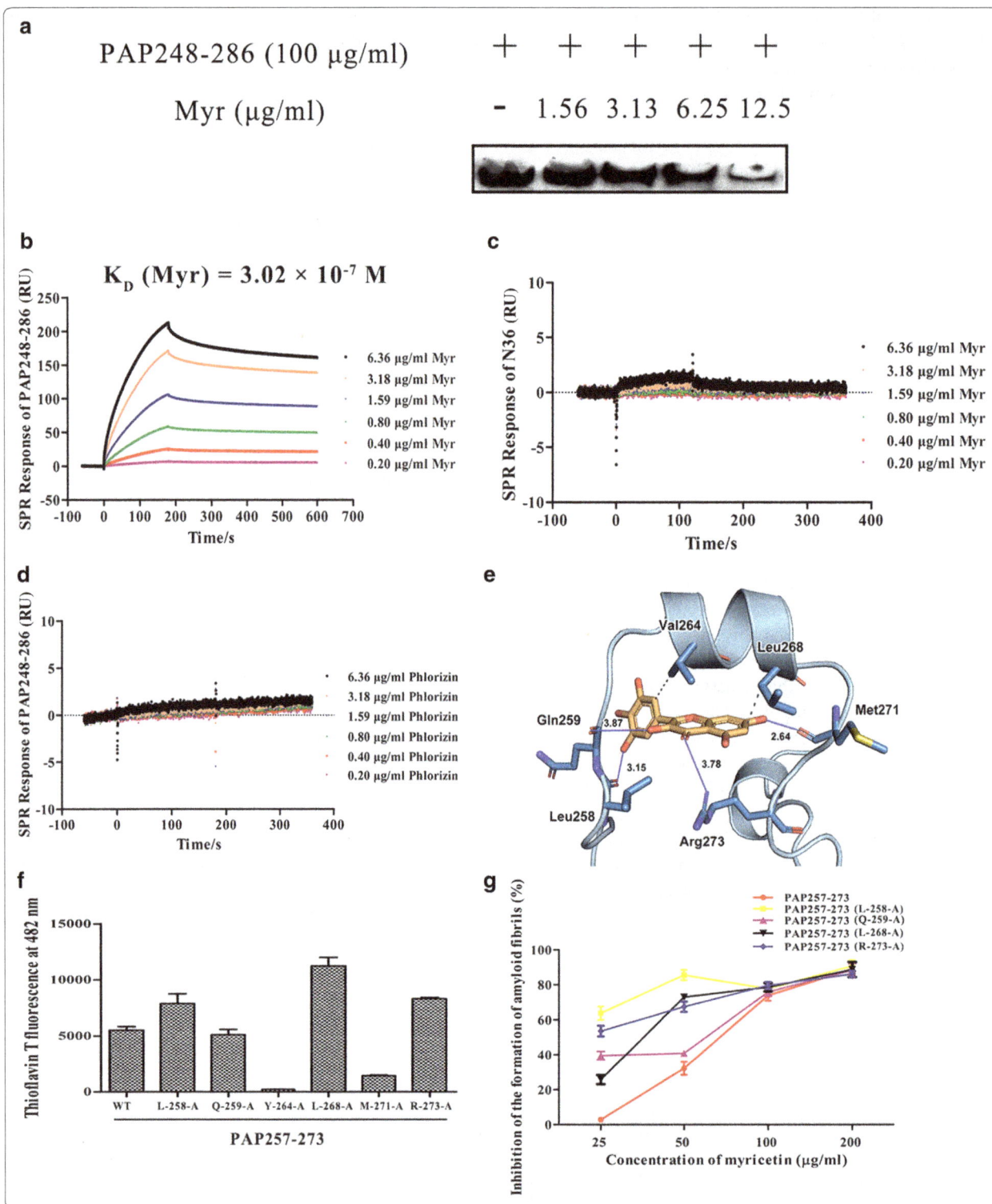

docking analysis. Importantly, due to its short length, the PAP257–271 peptide is simpler to synthesize on a large scale than is the SEVI peptide. In this study, we confirmed that the wild-type PAP257–273 fragment readily forms amyloid fibrils (Fig. 3f). To investigate whether the above-named six residues are essential for the formation of SEVI fibrils, we assessed the aggregation of PAP257–273 peptides containing site-directed mutations of these residues. As shown in Fig. 3f, four mutants of PAP257–273, i.e., Leu258A, Gln259A, Leu268A and Arg273A, exhibited fibril-forming propensity (Fig. 3f). Notably, PAP257–273 peptides with Val264A and Met271A mutations displayed attenuated aggregation during fibril formation, indicating that Val264 and Met271 of PAP248–286 might be critical for the assembly of PAP248–286 into fibrils. The inhibitory effects of myricetin on fibril formation by the four mutants of PAP257–273 were similar to or even stronger than their effects on wild-type PAP257–273, as measured by ThT assays (Fig. 3g).

Myricetin inhibits oligomerization of PAP248–286 monomers

Considerable evidence shows that the presence of low-n-order oligomers during the early stages of fibril formation indicates a lag phase in fibril assembly. It has been reported that myricetin inhibits Aβ aggregation by preventing amyloid β-protein oligomerization [28]. We therefore used photo-induced cross-linking of unmodified proteins (PICUP) to determine whether myricetin inhibits PAP248–286 monomer oligomerization and found that myricetin significantly inhibited oligomerization of PAP248–286 monomers in a dose-dependent manner (Fig. 4a). When 20 μg/ml of myricetin was mixed with 500 μg/ml of PAP248–286, oligomerization did not proceed to completion. In the presence of cross-linking agents, the PAP248–286 monomer, which was used as a positive control, predominantly existed as a mixture of oligomers on the order of 2–7. An irrelevant protein (glutathione S-transferase, GST) and an irrelevant flavonoid (phlorizin) were used as negative controls; GST normally exists as a mixture of homodimers and higher-order cross-linked species, thus providing an appropriate positive control for cross-linking chemistry. The results showed that phlorizin did not inhibit early oligomerization of PAP248–286 and that myricetin did not block oligomerization of GST (Fig. 4b, c).

Myricetin antagonizes assembly of SEVI seeded by preformed fibrils

It has been reported that the addition of a small amount of preformed SEVI fibrils as seeds to a suspension of soluble PAP248–286 monomers promotes fibril polymerization and eliminates the lag phase for assembly [23, 29]. In the present study, myricetin-mediated inhibition of SEVI aggregation seeded by preformed fibrils was determined by the ThT assay. In contrast to unseeded PAP248–286 solutions, PAP248–286 solutions seeded with preformed SEVI fibrils showed rapid assembly into fibrils (Fig. 4d). In addition to antagonizing unseeded PAP248–286 assembly (Fig. 1a, b), myricetin also completely obstructed SEVI-seeded fibrillization (Fig. 4d), indicating that myricetin antagonizes the growth and aggregation of SEVI fibrils after nucleation. ThT assay results were utilized to generate a dose–response curve for myricetin inhibition of PAP248–286 (2 mg/ml) seeded or not with 10% wt/wt mature SEVI fibrils agitated for 48 h (Fig. 4e, f), and we obtained a half maximal inhibitory concentration (IC_{50}) value of 41.51 μg/ml for myricetin inhibition of seeded PAP248–286 assembly compared to an IC_{50} value of 22.59 μg/ml for myricetin inhibition of spontaneous PAP248–286 assembly. Thus, higher concentrations of myricetin (200 μg/ml) were required to inhibit PAP248–286 assembly after the addition of SEVI seeds (Fig. 4d–f).

Myricetin remodels mature SEVI fibrils

ThT and Congo red assays were employed to determine whether myricetin can disassemble preformed fibrils, and the results showed that myricetin remodeled mature SEVI fibrils immediately in a dose-dependent but not in a time-dependent manner (Fig. 5a, b). Similar results showing that myricetin leads to a decrease in the β-sheet minimum of SEVI fibrils were obtained by CD, both immediately at 1 min and up to 48 h (Fig. 5c–e).

Myricetin influences the activity of SEVI in enhancing HIV-1 infection

The effects of myricetin on the SEVI-mediated enhancement of HIV-1 infection were assessed by fluorescence microscopy, flow cytometry and HIV-1 infection assays. CEMx174 5.25 M7 cells expressing a green fluorescent protein (GFP) reporter gene under the control of the HIV-1 promoter were chosen as target cells. Fluorescence microscopy images revealed faint background GFP$^+$ fluorescence expression in uninfected CEMx174 5.25 M7 cells and that SEVI fibril formation increased the fluorescence intensity of HIV-1-infected cells. However, myricetin notably decreased the fluorescence intensity of HIV-1-infected cells in the presence of SEVI fibrils (Fig. 6a). Subsequent flow cytometry assays further confirmed that myricetin reduced the number of cells infected by HIV-1 in the presence of SEVI fibrils (Fig. 6b). When SEVI fibrils were added to cells, the percentage of GFP$^+$ CEMx174 5.25 M7 cells was increased to 15.5%, whereas the initial percentage of GFP$^+$ cells of the control group in the absence of SEVI fibrils and HIV-1$_{SF162}$ was 2.37%. The percentage of GFP$^+$ cells of the HIV-1$_{SF162}$ group without SEVI fibrils was 2.57%, though the percentage of GFP$^+$ cells decreased to 1.97% upon incubation with myricetin (Fig. 6b). Similar to the HIV-1$_{SF162}$ control, the initial percentage of GFP$^+$ cells after incubation with HIV-1$_{SF162}$ and myricetin in the absence of SEVI fibrils was approximately 2.69%. To demonstrate

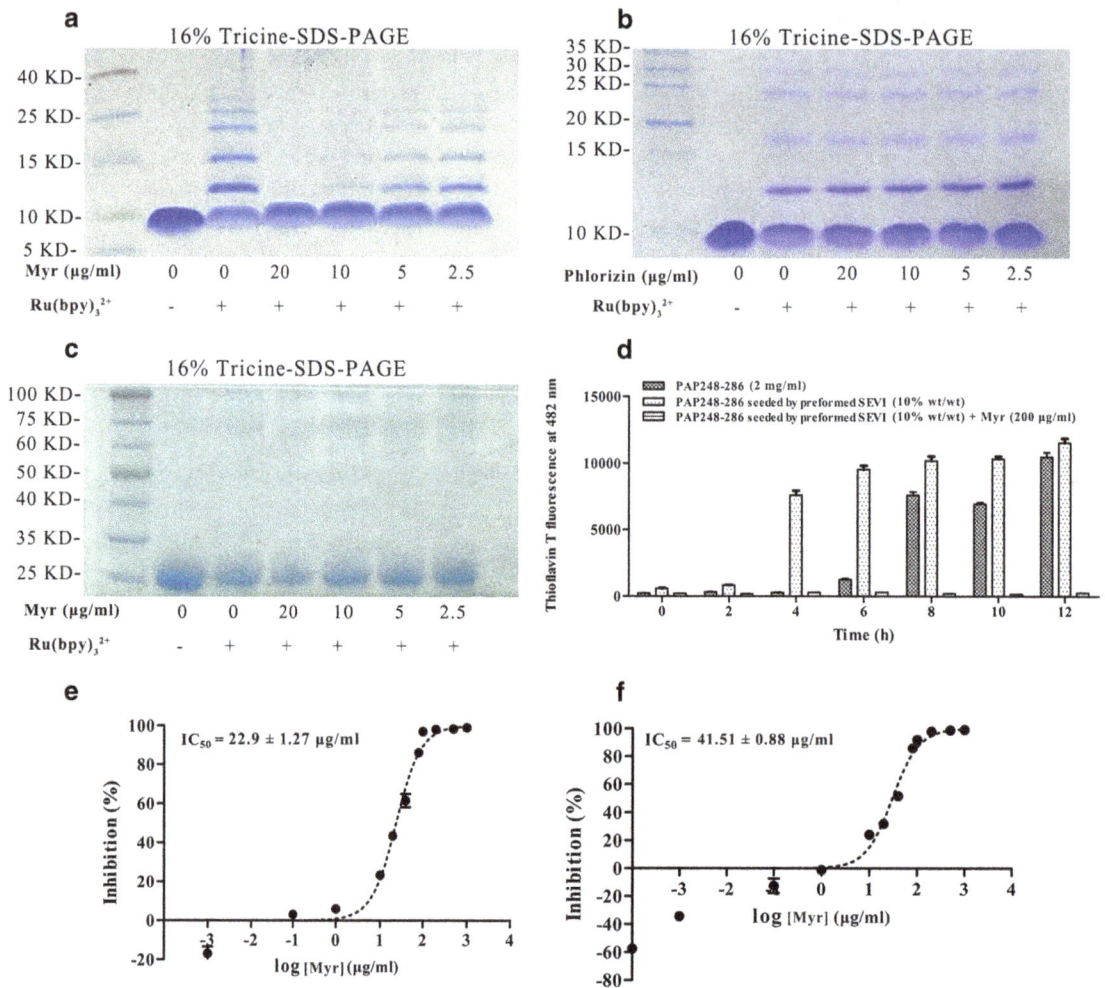

Fig. 4 Myricetin inhibits early oligomerization, fibril extension and degradation of PAP248–286. **a** The effects of myricetin on the oligomerization of PAP248–286, as assessed using 16% Tricine-SDS-PAGE and Coomassie blue staining. PAP248–286 monomer at 500 μg/ml with or without cross-linking served as the control. **b** The effects of an irrelevant flavonoid (phlorizin) on the oligomerization of PAP248–286. **c** The effects of myricetin on the oligomerization of GST. **d** The effects of myricetin on fibril extension by PAP248–286. Mature SEVI fibril seeds (1% wt/wt) were mixed with PAP248–286 peptide (2 mg/ml) in the presence or absence of myricetin (200 μg/ml), and the mixture was agitated at 1400 rpm at 37 °C. Aliquots were collected at various time points and assessed by ThT fluorescence. **e** Dose–response curve for myricetin inhibition of PAP248–286 (2 mg/ml) fibrillization after 48 h of agitation by ThT assay. **f** Dose–response curve for myricetin inhibition of PAP248–286 (2 mg/ml) fibrillization seeded by preformed SEVI fibrils (10% wt/wt) after 48 h of agitation by ThT assay. IC_{50} values were calculated. The values shown represent the mean ± SD (n = 3)

the reproducibility of the results, additional bar graph showing the averaged data of the percentages of GFP+ CEMx174 5.25 M7 cells from multiple experiments is presented in Fig. 6c.

To directly measure the effects of myricetin on SEVI-mediated enhancement of HIV-1 infection, we performed HIV-1 infection assays in the presence of SEVI fibrils. To eliminate the anti-HIV activity of myricetin itself as much as possible, we removed free myricetin by washing myricetin-treated SEVI samples one to five times with phosphate-buffered saline (PBS) followed by

centrifugation prior to the assays. In contrast to samples containing only SEVI fibrils, myricetin-treated SEVI fibrils after one wash resulted in significant attenuation in infectivity of CCR5-tropic HIV-1_{SF162} and CXCR4-tropic HIV-1_{NL4-3} infectious clones in a dose-dependent manner (Fig. 6e, f) [7]. Our results further showed that myricetin-mediated inhibition of SEVI-mediated enhancement of HIV infection was still observed after five washes (Additional file 1: Figure S3).

We further assessed the viability of on both CEMx174 5.25 M7 and TZM-bl cells after exposure to myricetin

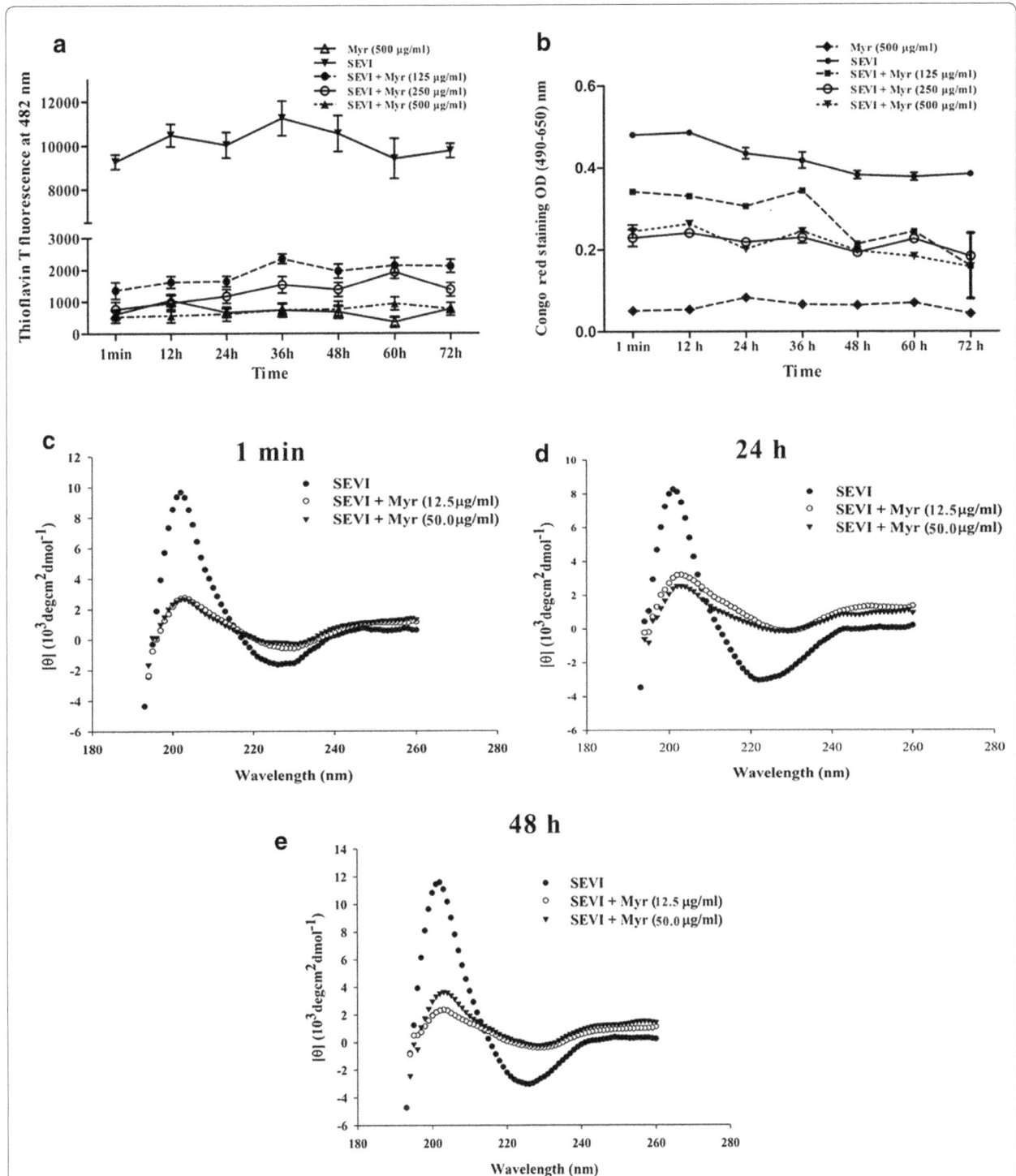

Fig. 5 Remodeling of fibrils was monitored using ThT (**a**) or Congo red (**b**) assays. Mature SEVI fibrils were incubated with various concentrations of myricetin (500, 250, 125 µg/ml) or PBS and agitated as described above for 72 h. Aliquots were removed at the indicated time points. **c–e** At various time points (1 min, 24 and 48 h), the samples collected in the above-described remodeling experiment were measured by CD. Average values (± SD) were calculated from triplicate measurements, the data shown represent one representative trial of three independent experiments

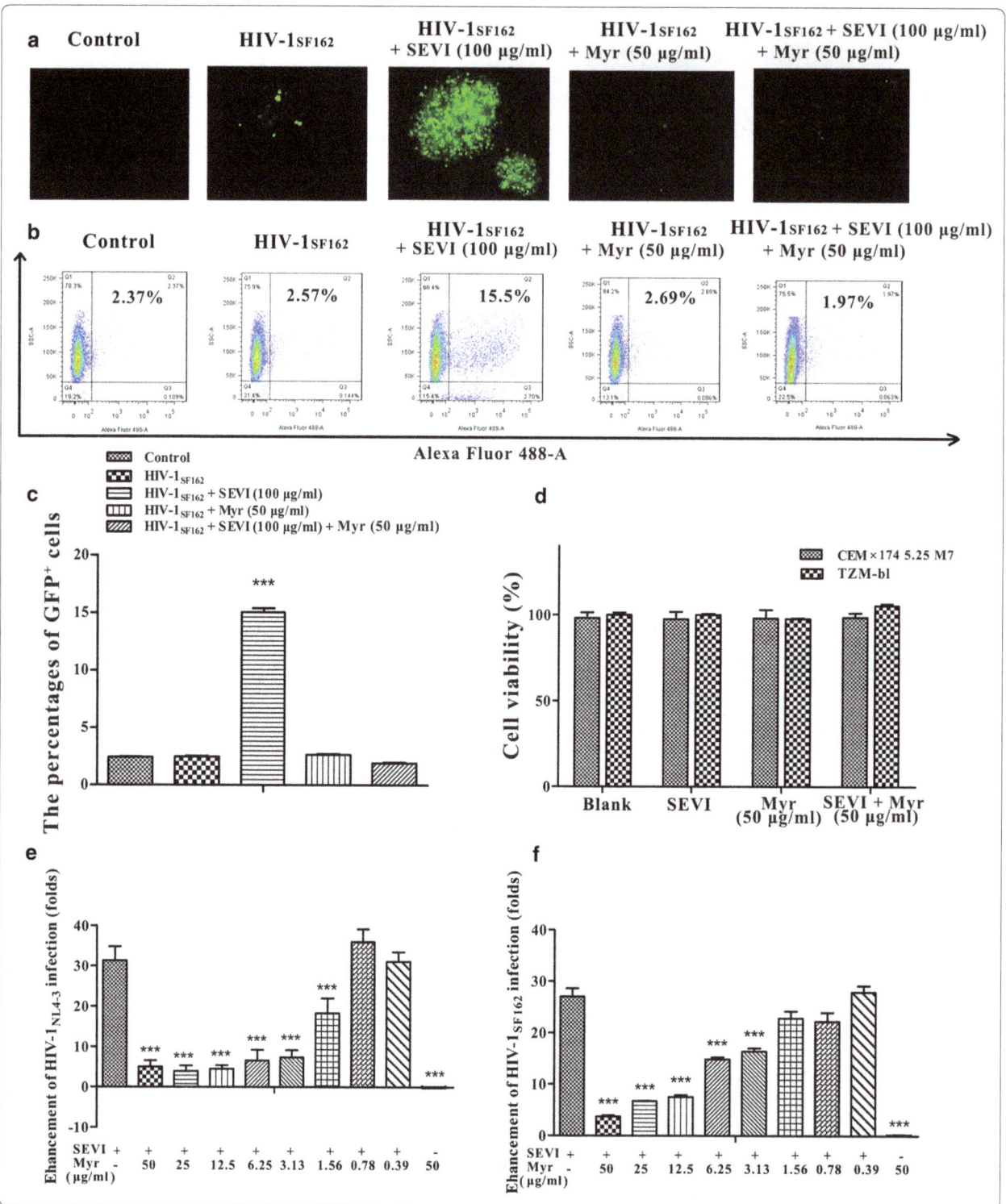

Fig. 6 Myricetin reduces the activity of SEVI in enhancing HIV-1 infection. CEMx174 5.25M7 cells infected by HIV-1 $_{SF162}$ in the presence or absence of SEVI (100 µg/ml) and myricetin (50 µg/ml) were imaged by fluorescence microscopy (**a**) and flow cytometric analysis (**b**). **c** The percentages of GFP$^+$ CEMx174 5.25 M7 cells from multiple experiments. **d** Cell viability assay of CEMx174 5.25 M7 and TZM-bl cells with or without SEVI (100 or 50 µg/ml) or/and myricetin (50 µg/ml). SEVI (50 µg/ml) was incubated with myricetin at various concentrations (50, 25, 12.5, 6.25, 3.13, 1.56, 0.78 and 0.39 µg/ml). The mixtures were centrifuged to remove soluble myricetin. The pellets were resuspended in the original volume of medium and mixed with CCR5-tropic HIV-1$_{SF162}$ (**e**) or CXCR4-tropic HIV-1$_{NL4-3}$ (**f**). The luciferase activities of the cultures were measured at 72 h post-infection. Average values (± SD) were calculated from triplicate measurements; the data shown represent one representative trial of three independent experiments. One-way ANOVA with Dunnett's post hoc multiple comparisons test was used to statistically analyze differences between samples containing SEVI alone and samples containing SEVI and myricetin ($^*p < 0.05$; $^{**}p < 0.01$, $^{***}p < 0.001$)

at the highest concentration in parallel with all infection assays under the exact same conditions. As shown in Fig. 6d, myricetin at 50 µg/ml exhibited no cytotoxicity toward CEMx174 5.25 M7 and TZM-b1 cells, with almost 100% cell viability being observed.

Interaction of SEVI with virions is affected by myricetin [30]

The effects of myricetin on the virus-binding ability of SEVI were examined using a virus pull-down assay. The results showed that SEVI fibrils alone bound to more than 51.6% of the input HIV-1 virions, including HIV-1$_{SF162}$ and HIV-1$_{NL4-3}$ infectious clones. Myricetin significantly abrogated the binding of all tested HIV-1 virions to SEVI fibrils in a dose-dependent manner (Fig. 7a–c), indicating that myricetin influences SEVI's activity in enhancing HIV-1 infection by preventing the formation of virion-amyloid complexes. The positive surface charge of SEVI fibrils facilitates virion attachment to target cells and enhances HIV infection by serving as a polycationic bridge [7]. Thus, we determined whether negatively charged myricetin attenuates the interaction of SEVI with HIV-1 virions by affecting the cationic properties of SEVI fibrils. Zeta potential is commonly employed to quantitate the magnitude of charge of materials; such charge is an important indicator of the stability and degree of electrostatic repulsion of colloidal dispersions [31, 32]. Myricetin significantly decreased the zeta potential of SEVI fibrils in a dose-dependent manner (Fig. 7d), indicating that it neutralized their surface positive charge.

Myricetin antagonizes the infection-enhancing properties of human semen

Multiple studies have reported that semen increases HIV-1 infection in vitro and that semen-mediated promotion of HIV-1 infection correlates with the levels of amyloidogenic fragments in semen. The combined effects of myricetin on fibril architecture and the formation of fibril–virion complexes led us to investigate whether myricetin possibly diminishes the infection-enhancing properties of the amyloid fibrils present in human semen. Figure 8a shows that after agitation in the absence of myricetin, seminal fluid (SE-F) samples displayed a slight increase in fluorescence intensity, indicating the formation of new seminal fibrils. Remarkably, myricetin slightly abrogated the new formation of seminal fibrils in SE-F. To determine whether myricetin depletes or affects semen of endogenous amyloids, we further measured the effects of myricetin using a sensitive TEM assay, the results of which showed weak inhibition of seminal fibril formation by myricetin at a final concentration of 40 µg/ml after agitation of 8 h (Fig. 8b). We further investigated whether myricetin affects the role of endogenous seminal fibrils in enriching virions. Based on fluorescence confocal microscopy, myricetin markedly inhibited the capture of HIV-1 virions by endogenous seminal fibrils (Fig. 8c). In our HIV-1 infection assay, semen was first incubated with myricetin for 1 h, and the sample was then centrifuged to remove the remaining free myricetin to avoid any direct activity against HIV. The treatment of cells with 2.5% SE-F in the absence of myricetin enhanced HIV-1 infection by 15- to 16-fold. In contrast, seminal fibrils alone promoted aggregation of virions and fibril–virion complex formation. However, the addition of myricetin decreased the enhancement of infection by SE-F in a dose-dependent manner, suggesting that myricetin antagonizes semen-mediated infection enhancement by HIV-1$_{SF162}$ (Fig. 8d) and HIV-1$_{NL4-3}$ (Fig. 8e).

Myricetin shows low cytotoxicity in vitro

The potential cytotoxic effects of myricetin on HIV target cells (TZM-bl and CEMx174 5.25 M7 cells) and reproductive tract epithelial cells (VK2/E6E7 and Ect/E6E7 cells) were assessed using MTT (3-[4,5-dimethyl-2-thiazolyl]-2,5-diphenyl-2H-tetrazolium bromide) or XTT [2,3-bis(2-methoxy-4-nitro-5-sulfophenyl)-5-(phenylamino)carbonyl-2H-tetrazolium hydroxide] and tris (2,2-bipyridyl)dichlororuthenium(II)(Ru(bpy)$_3^{2+}$) assays. Myricetin displayed low cytotoxicity in vitro toward all cell lines tested, with 50% cytotoxic concentration (CC$_{50}$) values ranging from 95.6 to 107.2 µg/ml (Fig. 9a–d). It should be noted that the final concentrations of myricetin used in these experiments were far below the CC$_{50}$ values. At a concentration of 50 µg/ml, myricetin displayed no obvious cytotoxicity toward

Fig. 7 Myricetin blocks the interaction of SEVI with HIV-1 virions. SEVI samples (200 µg/ml) were first incubated with graded concentrations of myricetin for 30 min. The samples were then centrifuged at 12,000 rpm for 5 min; the supernatant was removed, and the pellets were resuspended and mixed with HIV-1$_{SF162}$ (**a**) and HIV-1$_{NL4-3}$ (**b**). These mixtures were centrifuged, and the p24 antigens present in the pellet were evaluated using a p24-antigen ELISA. **c** The zeta potential of SEVI fibrils in the presence or absence of myricetin was measured using Zeta Nanosizer. Average values ($\pm$ SD) were calculated from triplicate measurements; the data shown represent one representative trial of three independent experiments. One-way ANOVA with Dunnett's post hoc multiple comparisons test was used to statistically analyze the differences between samples containing SEVI alone and samples containing SEVI and myricetin (*$p < 0.05$; **$p < 0.01$, ***$p < 0.001$)

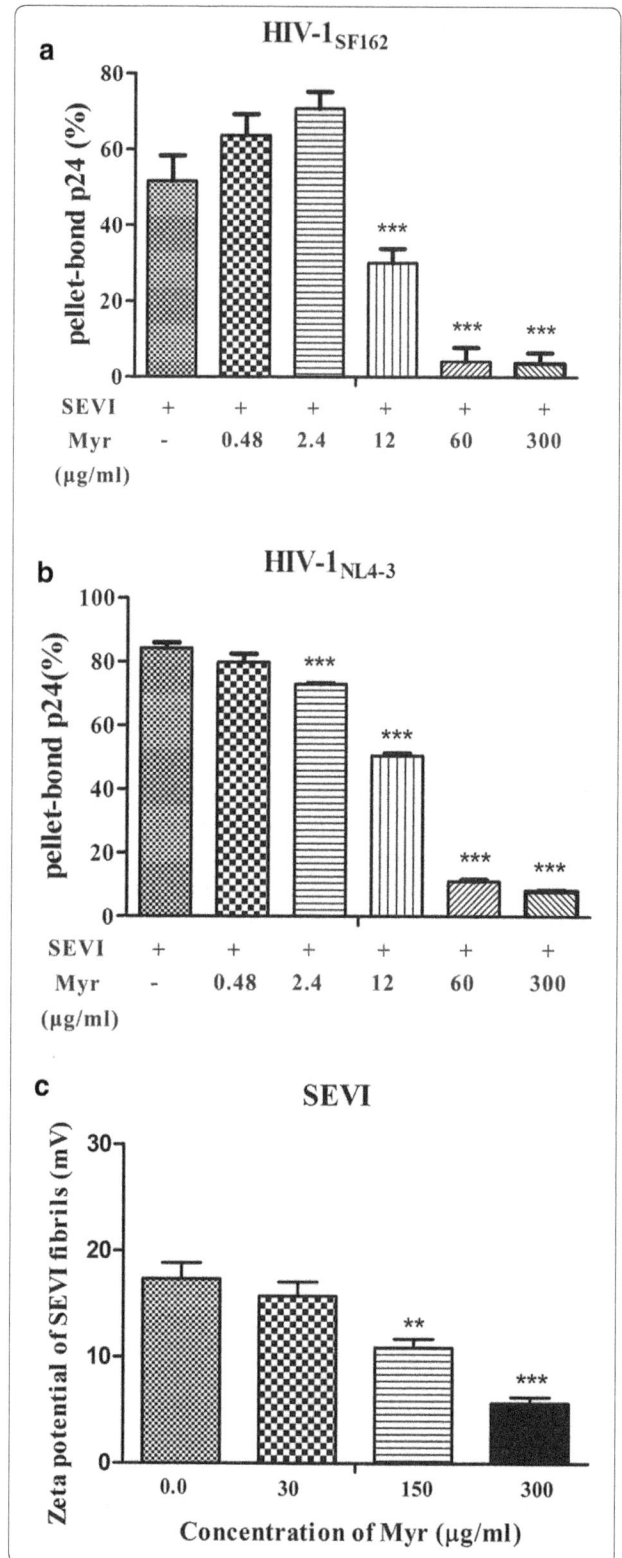

CEMx174 5.25 M7 or TZM-b1 cells (Fig. 6d). We also assessed direct inhibition of HIV-1$_{SF162}$ infection by myricetin alone and obtained an IC$_{50}$ of 1.952 µg/ml (Fig. 9e). The selectivity index (SI $=$ CC$_{50}$/IC$_{50}$) ranged from 49 to 55, indicating that myricetin might be safe for use in patients (Fig. 9f).

Combinations of myricetin and ARV drugs in 1% SE-F display synergistic effects against HIV-1 infection

In addition to binding to seminal amyloid fibrils, myricetin also appears to directly inhibit HIV-1 infection by targeting HIV integrase [18]. Accordingly, we determined the overall complementary effects of myricetin combined with various anti-retroviral (ARV) drugs on transmission of HIV-1 through semen, which is the most common route. The capacity of myricetin and ARV drugs alone or in combination to prevent infection of TZM-bl cells by 100 TCID$_{50}$ of HIV-1$_{SF162}$ in 1% SE-F was determined using luciferase assays. The ARV drugs used included an HIV entry inhibitor (maraviroc, MAR), nucleoside reverse transcriptase inhibitors (NRTIs) (zidovudine (AZT) and tenofovir (TNF)), non-nucleoside reverse transcriptase inhibitors (NNRTIs) (nevirapine (NVP) and efavirenz (EFV)) and an integrase inhibitor (raltegravir, RAL). The data in Table 1 show that combining myricetin with any of the above ARV drugs produced strong synergistic and complementary effects against infection by HIV-1$_{SF162}$ in 1% SE-F. The observed 50% competitive index (CI$_{50}$) values ranged from 0.051 to 0.450, and the IC$_{50}$ values of the individual drugs in each combination were reduced by approximately 2.91- to 154.87-fold. The synergistic effects of these combinations were also assessed intuitively, as shown in Fig. 10. The strongest

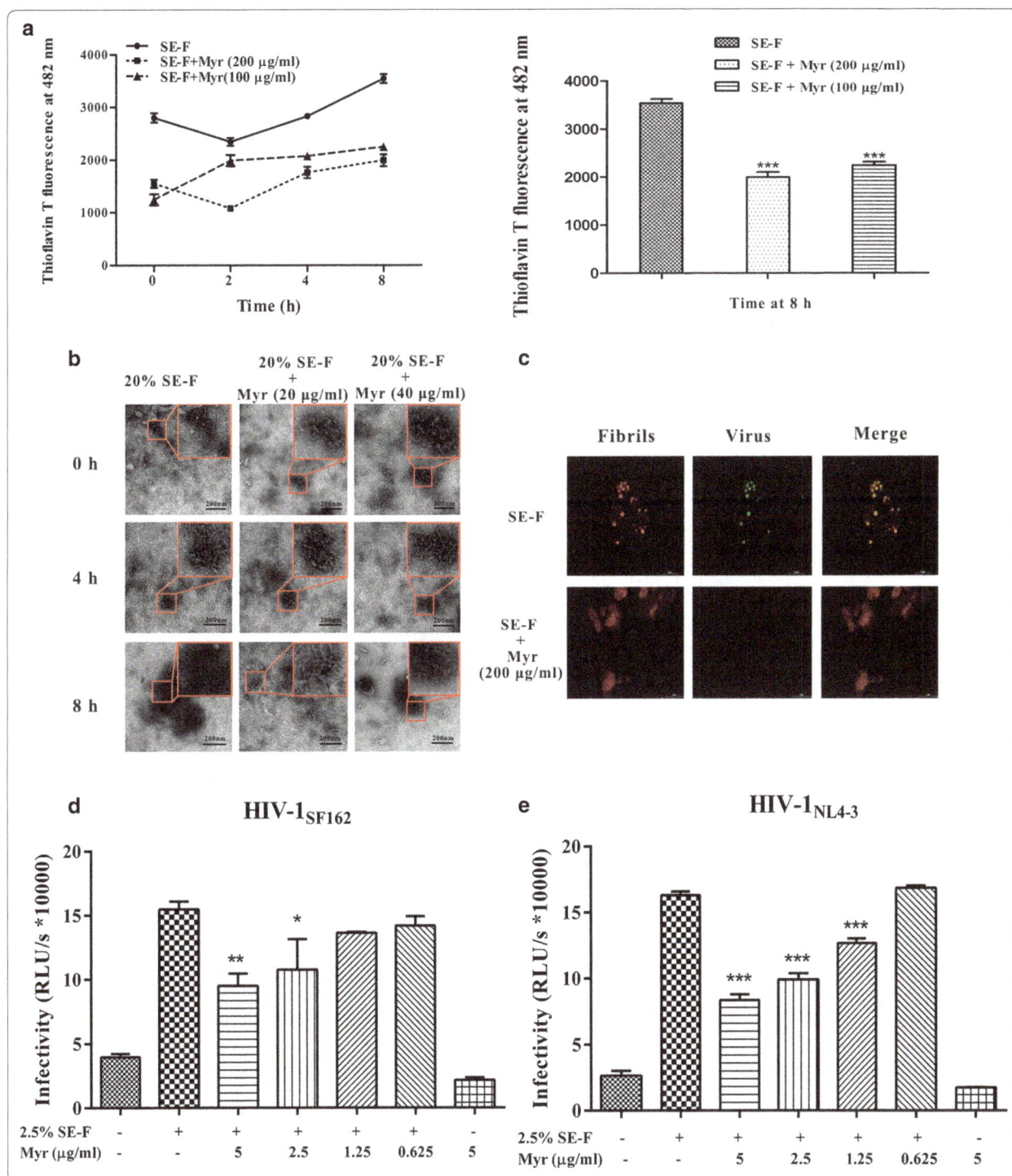

synergism was observed when myricetin was combined with the NRTI TNF: $CI_{50} = 0.051$, and dose reductions in the IC_{50} values of myricetin and TNF of approximately 24- and 107-fold, respectively, were observed (Table 1, Fig. 10). This combination is expected to exert synergistic antiviral effects and to help prevent the development of drug resistance during the prevention and treatment of HIV infection.

(See figure on previous page.)

Fig. 8 Myricetin antagonizes the infection-enhancing properties of human seminal fluid (SE-F). **a** Seminal amyloid fibril formation was antagonized by myricetin in a dose-dependent manner. SE-F samples containing myricetin (200, 100 or 0 µg/ml) were agitated at 1400 rpm at 37 °C for 8 h. Fibril integrity at the indicated time points (0, 4 and 8 h) was assessed using ThT fluorescence. **b** Seminal fibril samples (1:5 dilution) in the presence or absence of myricetin (20 and 40 µg/ml) at various time points (0, 4 and 8 h), as visualized by TEM. The scale bar is 200 nm. **c** Myricetin inhibited the assembly and attachment of HIV-1 virions to seminal fibrils by fluorescence confocal microscopy. The scale bar is 5 µm. The infection-enhancing properties of SE-F on HIV-1$_{SF162}$ (**d**) and HIV-1$_{NL4-3}$ (**e**) infection were attenuated by myricetin. SE-F samples were incubated with myricetin at various concentrations (200, 100, 50, 25 and 0 µg/ml) for 1 h. After centrifugation, the pellets were dissolved in fresh medium at a final dilution of 1:40 and incubated with various HIV-1 infectious clones. Luciferase activities were measured at 72 h post-infection. Average values ($\pm$ SD) were calculated from triplicate measurements; the data shown represent one representative trial of three independent experiments. One-way ANOVA with Dunnett's post hoc multiple comparisons test was used to statistically analyze differences between samples containing SE-F alone and samples containing SE-F and myricetin ($*p < 0.05$; $**p < 0.01$, $***p < 0.001$)

Discussion

There is evidence to support that human semen within the context of HIV-1 sexual transmission may have contributed to the failure of microbicides in previous clinical trials [33, 34]. Indeed, the antiviral efficacy of many candidate microbicides is greatly diminished in the presence of semen, and seminal amyloid fibrils have been found to be responsible for the semen-mediated enhancement of HIV infection [4, 9]. Due to their powerful positive charge, amyloid fibrils in semen can effectively capture virus and promote attachment to target cells by neutralizing the inherent electrostatic repulsion between the negative charges on the surfaces of HIV virions and target cells. Thus, a strategy of neutralizing the enhancing activity of seminal amyloid fibrils might be an attractive option for the development of ideal microbicides.

Several agents that block the enhancing activity of seminal amyloid fibrils in HIV infection have been reported. For example, based on its ability to abrogate SEVI-mediated enhancement of HIV-1 infection, the natural ingredient of green tea EGCG appears to be a promising supplement to antiretroviral microbicides [12, 13]. A component of EGCG, gallic acid, is able to directly abrogate the viral enhancement of seminal fibrils and might be able to prevent HIV infection via sexual transmission [35]. Unfortunately, EGCG has poor solubility and poor oral bioavailability and easily undergoes oxidation in vivo, complicating its use in clinical trials [36, 37]. Furthermore, EGCG was recently reported to promote the formation of toxic tau oligomers [38]. The small "molecular tweezer" CLR01 interacts with lysine and arginine residues on SEVI, leading to inhibition of the formation of infectivity-enhancing seminal amyloids and preformed fibril remodeling [29]. Of note, CLR01 interacts promiscuously and nonspecifically with the virus envelope; thus, it is also a broad-spectrum inhibitor of infection by enveloped viruses, including HIV-1, Herpes, Ebola and Zika [39]. The simplest and most logical explanation for the broad range of activity of CLR01 is that the inherent "stickiness" of

the molecule confers its promiscuous nature. However, the nonspecific binding of CLR01 to alkaline amino acids in the human body decreases the suitability of CLR01 as a therapy. Therefore, the development of effective, affordable and specific semen fibril antagonists is urgently needed.

The available literature verifies that myricetin possesses the potential to inhibit aggregation of the amyloid fibrils that play an important role in disease. In this work, we explored the potential impact of myricetin on the aggregation of seminal amyloid fibrils. First, myricetin at a concentration of 75 µg/ml was found to completely inhibit amyloidogenesis by peptide PAP248–286 in vitro (Fig. 1a, b); myricetin at a concentration of 200 or 40 µg/ml partially inhibited the formation of new amyloid fibrils in semen, as based on ThT and TEM assays (Fig. 8a, b). The ability of seminal fibrils to cause virion enrichment was inhibited by myricetin at a final concentration of 200 µg/ml (Fig. 8c). Second, myricetin was shown to be capable of blocking the enhancement of viral infection by abrogating interaction between SEVI and HIV-1 virions (Figs. 6, 7). It was clearly demonstrated that an SE-F sample agitated at 37 °C for 8 h significantly lost HIV-enhancing activity compared to the SE-F sample with no agitation [11, 40]. Correspondingly, the ability of semen to enhance HIV-1 infection after the addition of myricetin for 1 h incubation was decreased in a dose-dependent manner (Fig. 8d, e).

It is noteworthy that myricetin is known as a strong inhibitor of HIV reverse transcriptase and integrase, and it is possible that all of the inhibition described above is simply due to the known ability of myricetin to inhibit HIV infection, as opposed to its effects on SEVI. Indeed, we plan to compare the inhibitory activities of myricetin on HIV infection in the absence and presence of SEVI and semen. Regardless, one issue with such a comparison is that SEVI- or semen-mediated enhancement of HIV-1 infection occurs only at low infectivity [5], with myricetin completely preventing HIV infection, even very low concentrations. To avoid the direct activity of myricetin

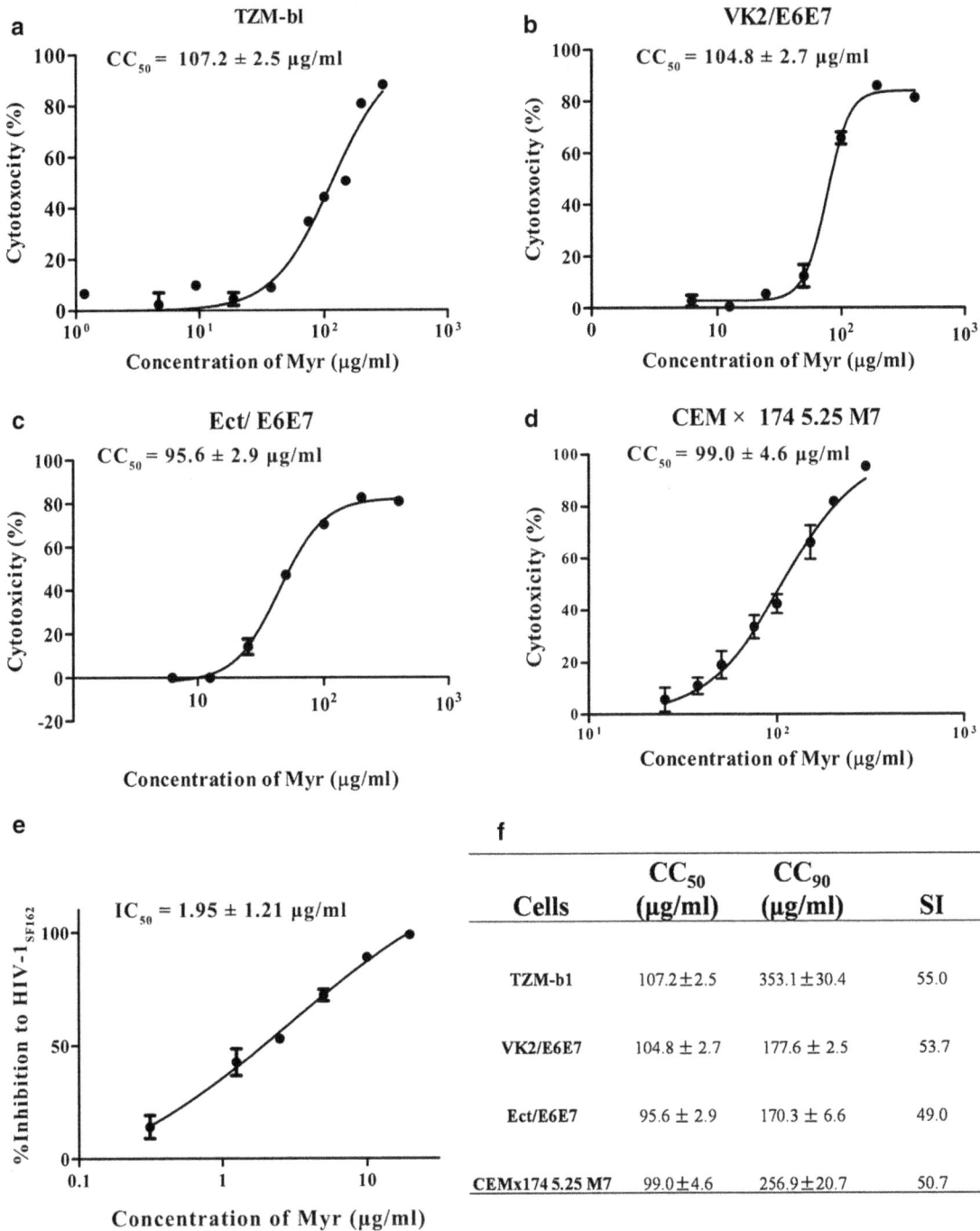

Fig. 9 Cytotoxicity of myricetin in vitro. **a** TZM-b1, **b** VK2/E6E7, **c** Ect/E6E7 and **d** CEMx174 5.25 M7 cells. The concentrations of myricetin for (**a**) and (**d**) were 300, 200, 150, 100, 75, 50, 37.5, and 25 μg/ml, for (**b**, **c**) were double dilution from 400 to 6.25 μg/ml. The MTT assay was used to evaluate adherent cells, and the XTT assay was used for cells in suspension. **e** %Inhibition of HIV-1$_{SF162}$ infection by myricetin alone without SEVI. The indicated concentrations of myricetin were incubated with the HIV-1$_{SF162}$ infectious clone for 30 min. The mixtures were then added to prepared TZM-b1 cells. Luciferase activities were measured at 72 h post-infection. Each sample was tested in triplicate, and the data are presented as the mean ± SD. **f** CC$_{50}$, CC$_{90}$ and SI values of myricetin against all tested cells. The assay was performed in triplicate; the data are presented as the mean ± SD

Table 1 Combination index (CI) and dose-reduction values for inhibition of HIV-1$_{SF162}$ infection determined by combining myricetin with ARVs in semen[a]

Drug combination, % inhibition	CI[b]	Mean value for[a]:					
		Myr			ARVs		
		Conc. (ng/ml)		Dose reduction	Conc. (ng/ml)		Dose reduction
Conc. (molar ratio)		Alone	Mixture		Alone	Mixture	
Myr:AZT (1571:1)							
50	0.331	600.52	105.97	5.67	0.37	0.06	6.17
90	0.145	16,962.76	1626.10	10.43	17.81	0.87	20.47
Myr:EFV (3142:1)							
50	0.450	2040.81	654.58	3.12	0.80	0.10	8.00
90	0.466	9407.22	2299.93	4.09	1.64	0.36	4.56
Myr:MAR (2095:1)							
50	0.275	1916.80	298.25	6.43	1.92	0.23	8.35
90	0.234	14,712.25	2335.84	6.30	24.03	1.80	13.35
Myr:RAL (3142:1)							
50	0.413	1613.13	372.91	4.33	0.46	0.08	5.75
90	0.514	7554.10	2592.53	2.91	3.37	0.58	5.81
Myr:TNF (62.8:1)							
50	0.051	1976.91	82.31	24.02	113.10	1.06	106.70
90	0.151	9440.37	1366.11	6.91	2721.14	17.57	154.87
Myr:NVP (628:1)							
50	0.262	2199.95	183.01	12.02	2.15	0.38	5.66
90	0.437	15,403.41	1709.88	9.01	11.02	3.59	3.07

[a] The data shown are the means of three independent assays performed in triplicate

[b] The CI value reflects the nature of the interaction between compounds

against HIV as much as possible, the mixture of SEVI/semen and myricetin was centrifuged at 12,000 rpm for 5 min to remove free myricetin from the samples. Thus, most of the inhibition caused by myricetin in our study is likely to have resulted from its effects on SEVI. Our findings indicate that myricetin is worth investigating as a possible candidate for the development of an ideal bifunctional microbicide with both anti-HIV and anti-SEVI activities.

According to native acid gel electrophoresis and SPR analyses, myricetin at 12.5 and 6.36 μg/ml was found to be able to bind to the PAP248–286 monomer (Fig. 3a, b). By using a computational molecular docking assay, we found that myricetin binds to specific amino acids in the PAP248–286 monomer, namely, Leu-258, Gln-259, Val-264, Leu-268, Met-271 and Arg-273, through salt bridges, hydrophobic interactions, and hydrogen bonds (Fig. 3e). Van der Waals forces may contribute to the interaction between myricetin and PAP248–286. Interestingly, the six residues identified as being involved in myricetin and PAP248–286 interaction are contained within the reported functional regions of PAP248–286. PAP257–267 is considered to be the central region of PAP248–286,

and this amyloidogenic region of the SEVI precursor peptide PAP248–286 has high fibril-forming propensity. Coincidentally, PAP268–271 has been reported to play an important role in promoting SEVI fibrillation [23]. Residues G260–N265 are thought to be involved in the initiation of fibrillation [40], and residues V262–H270 were shown to be the amyloidogenic region for SEVI fibrillation [41]. Therefore, one or several of the residues present at those six sites might be essential for the formation of SEVI fibrils [42]. The results of our study confirmed that wild-type PAP257–273, as well as PAP257–273 mutants containing Leu258A, Gln259A, Leu268A and Arg273A, readily formed amyloid fibrils (Fig. 3f). Notably, Val264A and Met271A mutations of PAP257–273 exhibited attenuated aggregation during fibril formation, indicating that the Val264 and Met271 residues of PAP248–286 may play a critical role in the assembly of PAP248–286 into fibrils. Myricetin clearly inhibited fibril formation by wild-type PAP257–273 and by four of the PAP257–273 mutants in a dose-dependent manner (Fig. 3g). These results suggest that inhibition of SEVI fibril formation by myricetin might be caused by the binding of myricetin to Val264 and Met271 of PAP248–286.

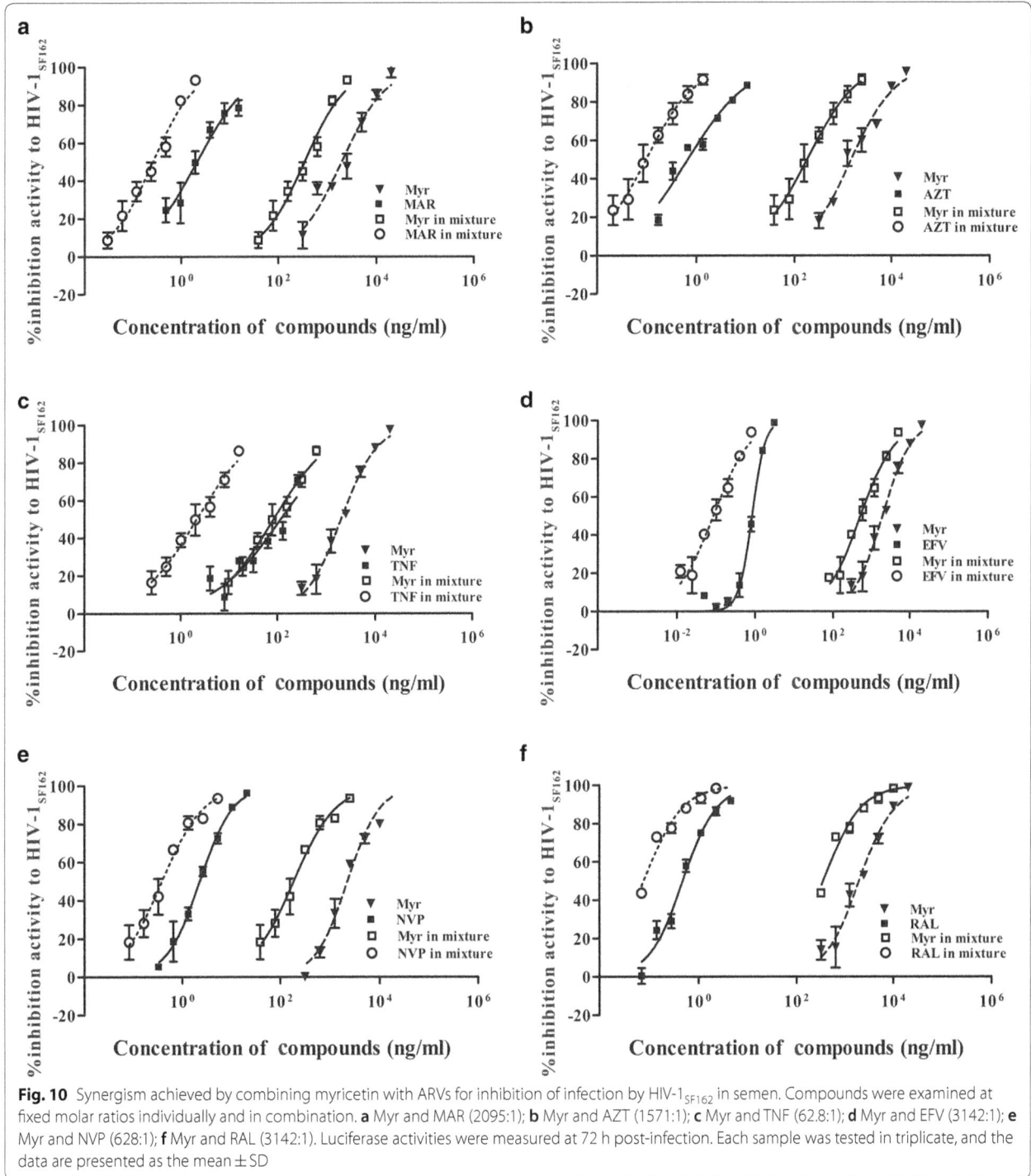

Fig. 10 Synergism achieved by combining myricetin with ARVs for inhibition of infection by HIV-1$_{SF162}$ in semen. Compounds were examined at fixed molar ratios individually and in combination. **a** Myr and MAR (2095:1); **b** Myr and AZT (1571:1); **c** Myr and TNF (62.8:1); **d** Myr and EFV (3142:1); **e** Myr and NVP (628:1); **f** Myr and RAL (3142:1). Luciferase activities were measured at 72 h post-infection. Each sample was tested in triplicate, and the data are presented as the mean ± SD

It is generally recognized that the formation of mature amyloid fibrils involves three stages: (i) monomers are first assembled into oligomers; (ii) fibrils evolve from protofibrils after nucleation; and (iii) the fibrils rapidly aggregate until equilibrium is reached [43]. Continuing investigations suggest that an oligomeric form of amyloid proteins plays a key role in disease causation and that low-n-order oligomers are especially important [28]. It would therefore be expected that the most efficacious therapeutic agents would be those that block the early assembly processes associated with amyloid protein oligomerization. Using a PICUP assay, we found that myricetin efficiently abrogated oligomerization of PAP248–286 in a dose-dependent manner (Fig. 4a). CD data also confirmed that myricetin at 5 μg/ml successfully inhibited the formation of β-sheet oligomers by PAP248–286 monomers (Fig. 1e).

Notably, myricetin decreased the zeta potential of SEVI in a dose-dependent manner (Fig. 7d). This might reflect a completely independent mechanism of inhibition of SEVI activity that is distinct from fibrillation inhibition. In general, the molecular electron-donating ability of a compound is determined by the highest occupied molecular orbital (HOMO) eigenvalue. Myricetin is a highly negatively charged compound with a HOMO eigenvalue of −5.7 eV [44]. The electrostatic interaction between myricetin and SEVI fibrils might cause myricetin to shield the surface cationic property of SEVI fibrils, leading to competitive inhibition of the binding of SEVI to the virus. In a similar manner, virus pull-down assays confirmed that myricetin inhibits the binding of HIV to SEVI fibrils in a dose-dependent manner (Fig. 7a–c). As shown in Additional file 1: Figure S4, myricetin did not affect the total amount of viral core protein p24, an observation that tends to exclude an antiviral effect of myricetin on the virus particles themselves. The observations are consistent with the idea that myricetin is an integrase inhibitor that affects the stage of viral growth but has no effect on the viral envelope.

Although anionic polymers are effective inhibitors of SEVI activity and HIV infection, they are not ideal candidates as anti-HIV vaginal microbicides because they are highly pro-inflammatory, disrupting the vaginal epithelial barrier [45]. One question that arises is does intravaginal application of anionic myricetin cause inflammation in female genital tract? There is a growing body of data indicating that myricetin displays strong anti-inflammatory activity in a variety of in vitro assays, as well as in both acute and chronic in vivo animal models, through regulation of multiple signaling pathways [15, 46, 47]. Therefore, myricetin with anti-inflammatory, anti-HIV and anti-SEVI activities might be developed as a promising microbicide to reduce the risk of HIV infection.

Previous studies have reported that fresh ejaculate contains semen fibrils; thus, assembly blockers might be inactive [10]. However, it is rare that agents exhibit the ability to degrade highly stable amyloid fibrils. Fortunately, we found that myricetin degraded SEVI fibrils in a dose-dependent manner, resulting in a lack of ability to seed the assembly of soluble PAP248–286 by SEVI (Fig. 5a, b). In addition, CD results showed that myricetin could immediately remodel SEVI into non-templating conformers (Fig. 5c). One of the advantages of using myricetin is that degradation occurs immediately,

whereas other reported remodeling inhibitors, including EGCG and CLR01, must be applied after several hours [12, 29]. Another advantage of using myricetin is its broad inhibition of the formation of seminal fibrils including SEVI, SEM1 and SEM2. Consequently, it is preferable to develop semen fibril antagonists that not only antagonize fibrillation but also remodel preformed fibrils. Future studies designed to determine the exact mechanism of action of myricetin with regard to the degradation of fibrils should be conducted.

It has previously been reported that brief exposure of HIV to semen reduced the antiviral efficacy of most microbicides [48]. Notably, myricetin is known to be an inhibitor of HIV-1 integrase, and we found that myricetin can partially weaken the semen-mediated enhancement of viral infection. Moreover, myricetin displays synergistic effects against HIV-1 infection in combination with other ARV agents in semen (Table 1; Fig. 10). As a key ingredient of various human foods and beverages, myricetin is relatively safe when used in patients. Our results also confirmed that myricetin has low cytotoxicity toward all tested cell lines in vitro, with CC_{50} values ranging from 95.6 to 107.2 μg/ml (Fig. 9). Therefore, it is likely that myricetin can be further developed into a candidate for inclusion in a combination microbicide to prevent HIV-1 sexual transmission.

Increasing evidence indicates that endogenous amyloids play natural and biological roles in the human body [49]. It was recently reported that semen amyloids may play a role in reproduction by participating in sperm selection and facilitating spermatozoal clearance [50]. Positively charged SEVI fibrils exert indirect antimicrobial activity by trapping microbial pathogens [51], though it remains unclear how inhibitors of amyloid formation or action may affect the antimicrobial and sperm-clearing natural role of amyloids in semen. To date, no studies have reported the side effects of semen fibril antagonists on the normal physiological function of amyloids. Before a semen fibril-targeted agent is clinically available, its potential effects on the normal physiological function of amyloids should be tested.

Conclusions

In this study, we found that myricetin interferes with various essential steps in the formation and remodeling of SEVI fibrils. Myricetin significantly inhibited all stages of SEVI formation, including early oligomerization and fiber extension, thereby blocking SEVI-mediated enhancement of HIV-1 infection. In addition, myricetin is capable of remodeling seminal amyloid fibrils and antagonizing semen-mediated enhancement of HIV-1 infection. Notably, myricetin displays synergistic effects against HIV-1 infection in semen when combined with other ARV agents and may work synergistically to reduce the rate of HIV transmission. It is likely that myricetin can be developed into a dual-functional microbicide candidate with both anti-HIV-1 and anti-SEVI-enhancing activities for use in preventing sexual transmission of HIV-1.

Methods

Cell lines, plasmids and reagents

TZM-bl, VK2/E6E7, Ect/E6E7 cells were obtained from the National Institutes of Health AIDS Research and Reference Reagent Program. HEK-293 T cells were purchased from American Type Culture Collection (ATCC) (Manassas, VA, USA). CEMx174 5.25M7 cells were kindly provided by Dr. C. Cheng-Mayer. Plasmids encoding CXCR4-tropic HIV-1$_{NL4-3}$ and CCR5-tropic HIV-1$_{SF162}$ infectious clones were kindly provided by Jan Münch of Ulm University (Ulm, Baden-Württemberg, Germany). The peptides PAP248–286, SEM1$_{86-107}$, SEM2$_{86-107}$ and N36 were synthesized by Scilight Biotechnology LLC (Beijing, China). Myricetin was purchased from Chengdu Must Biotechnology Co., Ltd. (Chengdu, China). ProteoStat Amyloid Plaque Detection Kits were purchased from Enzo Life Sciences (Plymouth Meeting, PA, USA). Thioflavin T (ThT), phlorizin, GST, Congo red, ammonium persulfate, DL-dithiothreitol (DTT), MTT, and XTT were purchased from Sigma (St. Louis, MO, USA). An anti-p24 monoclonal antibody (183-12H-5C), anti-HIV IgG, zidovudine (AZT), raltegravir (RAL) and maraviroc (MAR) were obtained from the National Institutes of Health AIDS Research and Reference Reagent Program. Tenofovir (TNF), nevirapine (NVP) and efavirenz (EFV) were purchased from Promega Biotech Co., Ltd. (Madison, WI, USA). Rabbit anti-PAP IgG was prepared, produced and purified by AbMax Biotechnology (Beijing, China).

Semen and seminal fluid samples

Pooled semen samples were obtained from 20 healthy donors at Nanfang Hospital (Guangzhou, China) after they had provided informed consent to participate in the study. Seminal fluid (SE-F) samples were collected by centrifugation of semen samples for 15 min at 10,000 rpm at 4 °C to remove spermatozoa and debris and were then stored at − 20 °C. The research protocols for this study were approved by the Ethical Committee of Nanfang Hospital of Southern Medical University and performed in accordance with relevant guidelines and regulations.

Formation of fibrils by PAP248–286, SEM1$_{86-107}$, SEM2$_{86-107}$ and formation of fibrils in semen

Solutions of the peptides PAP248–286, SEM1$_{86-107}$ and SEM2$_{86-107}$ (3 mg/ml) were agitated in the presence or absence of myricetin at the indicated concentrations (75, 37.5, 18.75 and 9.375 µg/ml for SEVI or 200, 100, 50 and 25 µg/ml for SEM1/2) for 48 h at 1400 rpm at 37 °C using an Eppendorf Thermomixer (Hamburg, Germany). At the indicated time points (0, 6, 12, 18, 24 and 48 h), aggregates were collected and stored at − 20 °C.

SE-F samples were collected and agitated at 1400 rpm at 37 °C in the presence or absence of myricetin at the indicated concentrations (200 and 100 µg/ml) for 8 h. At the indicated time points (0, 2, 4 and 8 h), aggregates were collected and stored at − 20 °C.

Remodeling of SEVI fibrils

SEVI fibrils (3 mg/ml) were agitated in the presence of myricetin (500, 250, 125 and 0 µg/ml) for 3 days at 37 °C at 1400 rpm. At various time points (1 min, 12, 24, 36, 48, 60 and 72 h), the sample mixtures were tested in ThT, Congo red and CD assays. Myricetin alone (500 µg/ml) was used as a negative control.

ThT fluorescence assay

Ten microliters of sample prepared as described above was mixed with 195 µl of ThT working solution (50 µM). The fluorescence of the mixture was measured using an RF-5301 PC spectrofluorophotometer (Shimadzu) at an excitation wavelength of 440 nm and an emission wavelength of 482 nm [23, 52].

Congo red staining assay

Five microliters of sample were mixed with 200 µl of Congo red reagent obtained from a Congo red kit for 2 min at room temperature (RT). The samples were then centrifuged at 12,000 rpm for 5 min, and the red-colored fiber precipitate was dissolved in 50 µl of dimethyl sulfoxide (DMSO). The absorbance of the solution at 490 nm was recorded using an enzyme-linked immunosorbent assay (ELISA) reader (Tecan, Research Triangle Park, NC, USA) [23, 52].

TEM

Suspensions of the collected samples (the final concentration of PAP248–286 was 500 µg/ml, and the final dilution of SE-F was 1:5) were deposited onto glow-discharged, carbon-coated grids for 2 min. The grids were then negatively stained with 2% phosphotungstic acid for an additional 2 min. The morphology of SEVI or seminal fibrils in the presence and absence of myricetin (16, 8 µg/ml for SEVI or 40, 20 µg/ml for semen) was visualized using an H-7650 TEM (Hitachi Limited, Tokyo, Japan). Myricetin (16 µg/ml) was used as a negative control.

CD

The secondary β-sheet structure of SEVI fibrils (the final concentration of PAP248–286 in the sample was 300 μg/ml) in the presence and absence of myricetin (5 μg/ml of the formation or 50, 12.5 μg/ml of the remodeling) was determined by CD spectroscopy in the "far-UV" spectral region (198–260 nm) using a Jasco 715 spectropolarimeter equipped with a thermostat-controlled cell housing and cells with a 1-mm path length (Jasco Inc., Japan). Each CD spectrum was collected three times [53].

HIV-1 infection assay

Enhancement of SEVI fibrils and SE-F samples in the presence and absence of myricetin was measured using HIV-1 infection assays as previously described [30, 54]. First, SE-F samples were collected as described above. Next, the SE-F samples were incubated with myricetin at various concentrations (200, 100, 50, 25 and 0 μg/ml) for 1 h at 37 °C; SEVI fibrils (50 μg/ml) were first incubated with graded concentrations of myricetin (50, 25, 12.5, 6.25, 3.13, 1.56, 0.78, 0.39 and 0 μg/ml) for 30 min. To eliminate the anti-HIV activity of myricetin itself as much as possible, the SEVI or SE-F and myricetin mixtures were centrifuged at 12,000 rpm for 5 min to remove free myricetin. The pellets of SE-F samples were dissolved in fresh medium at a final dilution of 1:40. Thus, the final concentrations of myricetin in 2.5% SE-F were 5, 2.5, 1.25, 0.625 and 0 μg/ml. The pellets of SE-F and SEVI fibrils in fresh medium were then incubated with CXCR4-tropic HIV-1$_{NL4-3}$ and CCR5-tropic HIV-1$_{SF162}$ infectious clones at RT for 10 min. Subsequently, 100 μl of the fibril–virus mixture was added to TZM-bl cells, which were cultured at 37 °C for 3 h, after which the culture supernatant was replaced with fresh medium. At 3 days post-infection, the cells were collected, washed and lysed with lysing reagent, and the luciferase activity was measured using a luciferase assay kit (Promega, Corp., Madison, WI, USA). HIV and myricetin were used as negative controls. The viability of TZM-bl cells with or without SEVI fibrils was detected in parallel with all infection assays under the exact same conditions.

The direct anti-HIV activity of myricetin on HIV-1$_{SF162}$ infection was detected. First, 1×10^5/ml TZM-bl cells were seeded in 96-well plates at 37 °C overnight, and 100 TCID$_{50}$ HIV-1 virus was incubated with myricetin (20, 10, 5, 2.5, 1.25, 0.625, 0.3125 and 0 μg/ml) at graded concentrations at 37 °C for 30 min. The mixture was then added to cells and further incubated for 72 h. The cells were collected, washed and lysed with the lysing reagent included in a luciferase assay kit. IC$_{50}$ values were calculated using CalcuSyn software [55], kindly provided by T. C. Chou (Sloan-Kettering Cancer Center, New York, NY).

Cytotoxicity assay in vitro

The cytotoxicity of myricetin toward TZM-bl, VK2/E6E7 and Ect/E6E7 cells was evaluated using MTT assays, and the cytotoxicity of myricetin toward CEMx174 5.25 M7 cells was evaluated using an XTT assay. Briefly, approximately 90% confluent cells were plated in 96-well plates at 1×10^5/ml, and the plates were incubated at 37 °C overnight. Different concentrations of myricetin were added, and the cells were incubated for an additional 48 h at 37 °C. For the MTT assays, the culture supernatant was discarded, and 100 μl of 0.5 mg/ml MTT solution was added to the cells. After incubating the cells for an additional 4 h, the cell-free supernatant was removed, and the formazan crystals formed were dissolved in 150 μl of DMSO. The absorbance of the resulting solution at 570 or 450 nm was measured using an ELISA reader. For the XTT assay, 50 μl of XTT solution (1 mg/ml) containing 0.02 μM phenazine methosulfate (PMS) was added. After 4 h, the absorbance at 450 nm was measured using an ELISA reader. CC$_{50}$ was calculated using CalcuSyn software.

Fluorescence microscopy and flow cytometry assays

Lymphoid CEMx174 5.25M7 cells that had been stably transduced with a long terminal repeat (LTR)-luciferase and LTR-green fluorescent protein cassette were used as target cells [5]. SEVI (100 μg/ml) was incubated with myricetin (50 μg/ml) at 37 °C for 30 min; the samples were then centrifuged at 12,000 rpm for 5 min to remove free myricetin. The resulting pellets were dissolved in fresh medium and mixed with an equal volume of HIV-1$_{SF162}$ for 5 min at RT. The mixture was then added to CEMx174 5.25M7 cells, which were cultured at 37 °C for 48 h. The fluorescence intensity of the resulting cell suspensions was observed by fluorescence microscopy (Nikon, Japan). The cells were washed, resuspended and analyzed by flow cytometry (BD FACSCanto TM^{II}). HIV and myricetin were used as negative controls. The viability of CEMx174 5.25M7 cells with or without SEVI fibrils was detected in parallel with all infection assays under the exact same conditions.

Seeding function of preformed SEVI

Preformed SEVI seeds (200 μg/ml) were added to 2 mg/ml PAP248–286 peptide solution in the presence or absence of myricetin (500, 200, 100, 80, 40, 20, 10 and 1 μg/ml), and the mixture was agitated at 1400 rpm at 37 °C. At the indicated time points (0, 2, 4, 6, 8, 10, and 12 h), samples were collected and subjected to ThT fluorescence assays as described above [29]. The IC$_{50}$ values of myricetin for the formation of PAP248–286 with or without SEVI seeds at 48 h time points were calculated using CalcuSyn software.

Virus pull-down assays

SEVI fibrils (200 µg/ml) were incubated with myricetin at various concentrations (300, 60, 12, 2.4, 0.48 and 0 µg/ml) at 37 °C for 30 min. The mixture was then challenged with 100 ng/ml HIV-1 virions (HIV-1$_{NL4-3}$ and HIV-1$_{SF162}$) for an additional 30 min. The samples were centrifuged at 12,000 rpm for 5 min, and the supernatants were removed. p24 antigens present in the pellets were detected by ELISA as previously described [56]. Total p24 antigens of the mixtures with myricetin at various concentrations and 100 ng/ml HIV-1 virions (HIV-1$_{NL4-3}$ and HIV-1$_{SF162}$) without SEVI fibrils were detected in parallel using virus pull-down assays under the exact same conditions.

Confocal microscopy

eGFP-labeled HIV-1 virions (R5-tropic) were produced by transfecting HEK-293T cells with proviral DNA expression plasmids and eGFP-Vpr plasmids by polyethylenimine (PEI) transfection. Semen samples were stained with a Proteostat dye contained in ProteoStat Amyloid Plaque Detection Kit at RT [10]. After staining, the fibril samples were incubated 1:1 with eGFP-labeled HIV-1 virions (100 ng/ml p24) with or without myricetin (200 µg/ml) at 37 °C for 3 h. The samples were then centrifuged at 5000 rpm for 3 min and imaged using a laser scanning Nikon A1 confocal microscope (Nikon, Japan). Proteostat and eGFP were excited using a 561 nm and a 488 nm laser line, respectively, and the emissions were collected using appropriate beam splitters.

Zeta potential

SEVI (200 µg/ml) was incubated in the presence or absence of myricetin at various concentrations (300, 150 and 30 µg/ml) for 30 min at RT. The samples were then centrifuged at 12,000 rpm for 5 min to remove free myricetin. The resulting pellets were resuspended in 1 mM KCl buffer, and the surface zeta potential of the resuspended samples was measured using a Zeta Nanosizer (Malvern Instruments, UK) [29].

WB assay

PAP248–286 monomers (100 µg/ml) were incubated with serially diluted myricetin (12.5, 6.25, 3.13 and 1.56 µg/ml) at 37 °C for 30 min, and the samples were centrifuged at 5000 rpm for 15 min. The PAP248–286 peptides remaining in the supernatant were analyzed by electrophoresis through 10% polyacrylamide continuous native gels as previously described [52]. The gels were subjected to WB

analysis to specifically identify the remaining PAP248–286 peptides using rabbit anti-PAP IgG.

Photo-induced cross-linking of unmodified proteins (PICUP)

Samples were chemically cross-linked using PICUP as previously reported [28]. First, PAP248–286 monomer (500 µg/ml) was incubated with various concentrations of myricetin (20, 10, 5 and 2.5 µg/ml) at 37 °C for 30 min. Next, 1 µl of 40 mM tris(2,2-bipyridyl) dichlororuthenium(II)(Ru(bpy)$_3^{2+}$) and 1 µl of 800 mM ammonium persulfate were added to 18 µl of the mixed sample. The mixture was then exposed to visible light for 5 s, and the cross-linking reaction was terminated by the addition of 2 µl of 5 M DTT. Non-cross-linked PAP248–286 monomer served as a negative control. The samples were separated by 10–20% gradient tricine sodium dodecyl sulfate-polyacrylamide gel electrophoresis (SDS-PAGE), and Coomassie blue staining was used to determine the frequency distribution of monomers and oligomers of PAP248–286. An irrelevant protein (GST) and an irrelevant flavonoid (phlorizin) were used as negative controls.

Computational docking analysis

The binding of PAP248–286 (RCSB Protein Data Bank (PDB) No. 2L3H) to myricetin was analyzed using the extensible molecular visualization UCSF Chimera program of AutoDock software [42, 57]. High-quality atomic charges for computer simulations of organic molecules in polar media can be generated by a novel charge model called AM1-BCC [58]. Hydrogen atoms were added using the Dock Prep module. The protein–ligand interaction online analysis tool Protein–Ligand Interaction Profiler [59] was applied, and images were generated by PyMOL software [31].

SPR analysis

The affinity of myricetin binding to PAP248–286 was measured using the BIAcore T100 system (GE Healthcare, Sweden) as previously described [60]. After PAP248–286 (50 µg/ml) was attached to the surface of a CM5 sensor chip as a cross-linker, myricetin (6.36, 3.18, 1.59, 0.80, 0.40 and 0.20 µg/ml) was injected at a flow rate of 20 µl/min, with a contact time of 2 min and a dissociation time of 2.5 min. The running buffer was water. The chip platform was regenerated with 10 mM HEPES, 150 mM NaCl, and 0.01% vol/vol Tween 20 (pH 7.4) and washed with the running buffer. A binding affinity (K_D) value was calculated using BIAcore software. An irrelevant peptide (N36) and an irrelevant flavonoid (phlorizin) were used as negative controls.

Combination treatment in SE-F

The inhibitory activity of myricetin and other ARV drugs and combinations on infection by HIV-1$_{SF162}$ infectious clones was determined as previously described [30, 31, 61]. Briefly, HIV-1$_{SF162}$ at 100 TCID$_{50}$ (50% tissue culture infective dose) was incubated in the presence or absence of various concentrations of myricetin, ARV drugs or combinations thereof in SE-F at 37 °C for 30 min. SE-F was diluted to 1:100 to prevent cytotoxicity, which slightly enhanced HIV infection. The mixture of myricetin, ARV drugs or combinations in 1% SE-F was added to TZM-bl cells, and the cells were incubated for 3 h at 37 °C; the medium was then replaced with fresh medium. Compounds were examined at fixed molar ratios in combination according to their individual IC$_{50}$ values. At 72 h post-infection, the luciferase activity of the cell cultures was measured as described above. The effective concentrations resulting in 50 and 90% inhibition (EC$_{50}$ and EC$_{90}$) were calculated using CalcuSyn software. The data were analyzed for cooperative effects using the Chou-Talalay method. Combination index (CI) values were calculated using the CalcuSyn program. The CI value reflects the nature of the interaction between compounds. CI values of $< 1, = 1$ and > 1 indicate synergy, additivity and antagonism, respectively. In detail, CI < 0.10 indicates very strong synergism, 0.10–0.30 indicates strong synergism, 0.30–0.70 indicates synergism, 0.70–0.85 indicates moderate synergism, and 0.85–0.90 indicates slight synergism. Dose reductions were calculated as the ratio of the EC$_{50}$ values of the compounds when used alone and when used in combination.

Statistical analysis

Statistical analysis of the experimental data was performed using a one-way analysis of variance (ANOVA) test in GraphPad Prism 5.0 (San Diego, CA, USA). A p value of < 0.05 was regarded as statistically significant; the probability level is indicated by single or multiple asterisks (*) (*$p < 0.05$; **$p < 0.01$; ***$p < 0.001$). All values represent the mean $\pm$ SD (standard deviation) of at least three measurements.

Additional file

Additional file 1: Figure S1. Myricetin inhibits other seminal amyloid fibril formation, as shown by ThT assays. (**a**) SEM186-107; (**b**) SEM286-107. Peptide (3 mg/ml) was incubated with myricetin (200, 100, 50 and 10 µg/ml) and agitated at 1,400 rpm at 37 °C. Then samples were collected and monitored by ThT. Average values ($\pm$ SD) were calculated from triplicate measurements, and the data represent one representative trial of three independent experiment. **Figure S2**. Amyloid fibril samples display loss of enhancement of HIV-1 infection in the presence of myricetin. The raw luciferase activities of mixed SEVI fibril samples prepared in the presence or absence of myricetin with HIV-1$_{SF162}$ (**a**) and HIV-1$_{NL4-3}$ (**b**) infectious clones. The values shown here represent the mean $\pm$ SD (n = 3). One-way

ANOVA with Dunnett's post hoc multiple comparisons test was used to statistically analyze the differences between samples containing PAP248-286 alone and samples containing PAP248-286 and myricetin (*$p < 0.05$; **$p < 0.01$, ***$p < 0.001$). **Figure S3**. SEVI (50 µg/ml) was incubated with myricetin at various concentrations (50, 25, 12.5, 6.25, 3.13, 1.56, 0.78 and 0.39 µg/ml). The mixtures were washed one to five times with PBS buffer and centrifuged to remove soluble myricetin. The pellets were resuspended in the original volume of medium and mixed with CCR5-tropic HIV-1$_{SF162}$ (**a**) or CXCR4-tropic HIV-1$_{NL4-3}$ (**b**). The luciferase activities of the cultures were measured at 72 h post-infection. Average values ($\pm$ SD) were calculated from triplicate measurements; the data shown here represent one representative trial of three independent experiments. One-way ANOVA with Dunnett's post hoc multiple comparisons test was used to statistically analyze the differences between samples containing SEVI alone and samples containing SEVI and myricetin (*$p < 0.05$; **$p < 0.01$, ***$p < 0.001$). **Figure S4**. The total p24 antigens of the mixtures of myricetin at various concentrations and 100 ng/ml HIV-1 virions without SEVI fibrils were detected in parallel with virus pull-down assays under the exact same conditions. (**a**) HIV-1$_{SF162}$ and (**b**) HIV-1$_{NL4-3}$. Average values ($\pm$ SD) were calculated from triplicate measurements, and the data represent one representative trial of three independent experiment.

Authors' contributions

LL and SL conceived the idea and designed the research. RR, SY, BL, LM, JW, XZ and FL performed the research. RR, LM, SL and LL analyzed the data and wrote the manuscript. All authors read and approved the final manuscript.

Author details

[1] Guangdong Provincial Key Laboratory of New Drug Screening, Guangzhou Key Laboratory of Drug Research for Emerging Virus Prevention and Treatment, School of Pharmaceutical Sciences, Southern Medical University, 1838 Guangzhou Avenue North, Guangzhou 510515, Guangdong, China. [2] Department of Pharmacy, The Seventh Affiliated Hospital of Sun Yat-sen University, Shenzhen 518107, China.

Acknowledgements

We thank Dr. Shibo Jiang of Fudan University, China for providing technical help. We thank Chunyan Wang of Nanfang Hospital of Southern Medical University, China, for the kind gift of human semen samples. This study was supported by the National Natural Science Foundation of China (8167348T to Lin Li).

Competing interests

The authors declare that they have no competing interests.

References

1. Lu L, Yu F, Cai L, Debnath AK, Jiang S. Development of small-molecule HIV entry inhibitors specifically targeting gp120 or gp41. Curr Top Med Chem. 2016;16:1074–90.

2. UNAIDS. Global AIDS Update 2017; http://aidsinfo.unaids.org/. UNAIDS. Core Epidemiology Slides; June 2017.

3. Sabatte J, Remes Lenicov F, Cabrini M, Rodriguez Rodrigues C, Ostrowski M, Ceballos A, Amigorena S, Geffner J. The role of semen in sexual transmission of HIV: beyond a carrier for virus particles. Microbes Infect. 2011;13:977–82.

4. Zirafi O, Kim KA, Roan NR, Kluge SF, Muller JA, Jiang S, Mayer B, Greene WC, Kirchhoff F, Munch J. Semen enhances HIV infectivity and impairs the antiviral efficacy of microbicides. Sci Transl Med. 2014;6:262ra157.

5. Munch J, Rucker E, Standker L, Adermann K, Goffinet C, Schindler M, Wildum S, Chinnadurai R, Rajan D, Specht A, et al. Semen-derived amyloid fibrils drastically enhance HIV infection. Cell. 2007;131:1059–71.

6. Roan NR, Münch J, Arhel N, Mothes W, Neidleman J, Kobayashi A, Smith-McCune K, Kirchhoff F, Greene WC. The cationic properties of SEVI underlie its ability to enhance human immunodeficiency virus infection. J Virol. 2009;83:73–80.

7. Arnold F, Schnell J, Zirafi O, Sturzel C, Meier C, Weil T, Standker L, Forssmann WG, Roan NR, Greene WC, et al. Naturally occurring fragments from two distinct regions of the prostatic acid phosphatase form amyloidogenic enhancers of HIV infection. J Virol. 2012;86:1244–9.

8. Roan NR, Muller JA, Liu H, Chu S, Arnold F, Sturzel CM, Walther P, Dong M, Witkowska HE, Kirchhoff F, et al. Peptides released by physiological cleavage of semen coagulum proteins form amyloids that enhance HIV infection. Cell Host Microbe. 2011;10:541–50.

9. Castellano LM, Shorter J. The surprising role of amyloid fibrils in HIV infection. Biology (Basel). 2012;1:58–80.

10. Usmani SM, Zirafi O, Muller JA, Sandi-Monroy NL, Yadav JK, Meier C, Weil T, Roan NR, Greene WC, Walther P, et al. Direct visualization of HIV-enhancing endogenous amyloid fibrils in human semen. Nat Commun. 2014;5:3508.

11. Roan NR, Liu H, Usmani SM, Neidleman J, Muller JA, Avila-Herrera A, Gawanbacht A, Zirafi O, Chu S, Dong M, et al. Liquefaction of semen generates and later degrades a conserved semenogelin peptide that enhances HIV infection. J Virol. 2014;88:7221–34.

12. Hauber I, Hohenberg H, Holstermann B, Hunstein W, Hauber J. The main green tea polyphenol epigallocatechin-3-gallate counteracts semen-mediated enhancement of HIV infection. Proc Natl Acad Sci USA. 2009;106:9033–8.

13. Castellano LM, Hammond RM, Holmes VM, Weissman D, Shorter J. Epigallocatechin-3-gallate rapidly remodels PAP85-1, SEM1 (45–107), and SEM2 (49–107) seminal amyloid fibrils. Biol Open. 2015;4:1206–12.

14. Devi KP, Rajavel T, Habtemariam S, Nabavi SF, Nabavi SM. Molecular mechanisms underlying anticancer effects of myricetin. Life Sci. 2015;142:19–25.

15. Semwal DK, Semwal RB, Combrinck S, Viljoen A. Myricetin: a dietary molecule with diverse biological activities. Nutrients. 2016;8:90.

16. Shih YW, Wu PF, Lee YC, Shi MD, Chiang TA. Myricetin suppresses invasion and migration of human lung adenocarcinoma A549 cells: possible mediation by blocking the ERK signaling pathway. J Agric Food Chem. 2009;57:3490–9.

17. Pasetto S, Pardi V, Murata RM. Anti-HIV-1 activity of flavonoid myricetin on HIV-1 infection in a dual-chamber in vitro model. PLoS ONE. 2014;9:e115323.

18. Chaniad P, Wattanapiromsakul C, Pianwanit S, Tewtrakul S. Anti-HIV-1 integrase compounds from Dioscorea bulbifera and molecular docking study. Pharm Biol. 2016;54:1077–85.

19. Hirohata M, Hasegawa K, Tsutsumi-Yasuhara S, Ohhashi Y, Ookoshi T, Ono K, Yamada M, Naiki H. The anti-amyloidogenic effect is exerted against Alzheimer's beta-amyloid fibrils in vitro by preferential and reversible binding of flavonoids to the amyloid fibril structure. Biochemistry. 2007;46:2488–99.

20. Zelus C, Fox A, Calciano A, Faridian BS, Nogaj LA, Moffet DA. Myricetin inhibits islet amyloid polypeptide (IAPP) aggregation and rescues living mammalian cells from IAPP toxicity. Open Biochem J. 2012;6:66–70.

21. He J, Wang Y, Chang AK, Xu L, Wang N, Chong X, Li I I, Zhang B, Jones GW, Song Y. Myricetin prevents fibrillogenesis of hen egg white lysozyme. J Agric Food Chem. 2014;62:9442–9.

22. Duan JM, Qiu JY, Tan SY, Liu SW, Li L. Semen-derived enhancer of viral infection—a key factor in sexual transmission of HIV. Bing Du Xue Bao. 2012;28:84–8.

23. Chen J, Ren R, Yu F, Wang C, Zhang X, Li W, Tan S, Jiang S, Liu S, Li L. A degraded fragment of HIV-1 Gp120 in rat hepatocytes forms fibrils and enhances HIV-1 infection. Biophys J. 2017;113:1425–39.

24. Frid P, Anisimov SV, Popovic N. Congo red and protein aggregation in neurodegenerative diseases. Brain Res Rev. 2007;53:135–60.

25. Olsen JS, DiMaio JTM, Doran TM, Brown C, Nilsson BL, Dewhurst S. Seminal plasma accelerates semen-derived enhancer of viral infection (SEVI) fibril formation by the prostatic acid phosphatase (PAP248–286) peptide. J Biol Chem. 2012;287(15):11842–9.

26. Le Y, Jiang S, Hu J, Gong W, Su S, Dunlop NM, Shen W, Li B, Ming Wang J. N36, a synthetic N-terminal heptad repeat domain of the HIV-1 envelope protein gp41, is an activator of human phagocytes. Clin Immunol. 2000;96(3):236–42.

27. Elias AK, Scanlon D, Musgrave IF, Carver JA. SEVI, the semen enhancer of HIV infection along with fragments from its central region, form amyloid fibrils that are toxic to neuronal cells. Biochim Biophys Acta. 2014;1844:1591–8.

28. Ono K, Li L, Takamura Y, Yoshiike Y, Zhu L, Han F, Mao X, Ikeda T, Takasaki J, Nishijo H, et al. Phenolic compounds prevent amyloid beta-protein oligomerization and synaptic dysfunction by site-specific binding. J Biol Chem. 2012;287:14631–43.

29. Lump E, Castellano LM, Meier C, Seeliger J, Erwin N, Sperlich B, Sturzel CM, Usmani S, Hammond RM, von Einem J, et al. A molecular tweezer antagonizes seminal amyloids and HIV infection. Elife. 2015;18:4.

30. Xun T, Li W, Chen J, Yu F, Xu W, Wang Q, Yu R, Li X, Zhou X, Lu L, et al. ADS-J1 inhibits semen-derived amyloid fibril formation and blocks fibril-mediated enhancement of HIV-1 infection. Antimicrob Agents Chemother. 2015;59:5123–34.

31. Osipovitch M, Lambrecht M, Baker C, Madha S, Mills JL, Craig PA. Automated protein motif generation in the structure-based protein function prediction tool. ProMOL. 2015;16:101–11.

32. Li L, Tan S, Lu H, Lu L, Yang J, Jin H, Liu S, Jiang S. Combinations of 3-hydroxyphthalic anhydride-modified ovalbumin with antiretroviral drug-based microbicide candidates display synergistic and complementary effects against HIV-1 infection. J Acquir Immune Defic Syndr. 2011;56:384–92.

33. Solomon MM, Lama JR, Glidden DV, Mulligan K, McMahan V, Liu AY, Guanira JV, Veloso VG, Mayer KH, Chariyalertsak S, et al. Changes in renal function associated with oral emtricitabine/tenofovir disoproxil fumarate use for HIV pre-exposure prophylaxis. Aids. 2014;28:851–9.

34. Karim SS, Kashuba AD, Werner L, Karim QA. Drug concentrations after topical and oral antiretroviral pre-exposure prophylaxis: implications for HIV prevention in women. Lancet. 2011;378:279–81.

35. LoRicco JG, Xu CS, Neidleman J, Bergkvist M, Greene WC, Roan NR, Makhatadze GI. Gallic acid is an antagonist of semen amyloid fibrils that enhance HIV-1 infection. J Biol Chem. 2016;291:14045–55.

36. Landis-Piwowar K, Chen D, Foldes R, Chan TH, Dou QP. Novel epigallocatechin gallate analogs as potential anticancer agents: a patent review (2009–present). Expert Opin Ther Pat. 2013;23:189–202.

37. Chen Z, Zhu QY, Tsang D, Huang Y. Degradation of green tea catechins in tea drinks. J Agric Food Chem. 2001;49:477–82.

38. Sinha S, Du Z, Maiti P, Klärner FG, Schrader T, Wang C, Bitan G. Comparison of three amyloid assembly inhibitors: the sugar scyllo-inositol, the polyphenol epigallocatechin gallate, and the molecular tweezer CLR01. ACS Chem Neurosci. 2012;3:451–8.

39. Röcker AE, Müller JA, Dietzel E, Harms M, Krüger F, Heid C, Sowislok A, Riber CF, Kupke A, Lippold S, von Einem J, et al. The molecular tweezer CLR01 inhibits Ebola and Zika virus infection. Antiviral Res. 2018;152:26–35.

40. Kim KA, Yolamanova M, Zirafi O, Roan NR, Staendker L, Forssmann WG, Burgener A, Dejucq-Rainsford N, Hahn BH, Shaw GM, et al. Semen-mediated enhancement of HIV infection is donor-dependent and correlates with the levels of SEVI. Retrovirology. 2010;7:55.

41. Sievers SA, Karanicolas J, Chang HW, Zhao A, Jiang L, Zirafi O, Stevens JT, Munch J, Baker D, Eisenberg D. Structure-based design of non-natural amino-acid inhibitors of amyloid fibril formation. Nature. 2011;475:96–100.

42. Nanga RP, Brender JR, Vivekanandan S, Popovych N, Ramamoorthy A. NMR structure in a membrane environment reveals putative amyloidogenic regions of the SEVI precursor peptide PAP(248–286). J Am Chem Soc. 2009;131:17972–9.

43. Straub JE, Thirumalai D. Toward a molecular theory of early and late events in monomer to amyloid fibril formation. Annu Rev Phys Chem. 2011;62:437–63.

44. Sadasivam K, Kumaresan R. Antioxidant behavior of mearnsetin and myricetin flavonoid compounds–a DFT study. Spectrochim Acta A Mol Biomol Spectrosc. 2011;79:282–93.

45. Roberts L, Liebenberg L, Barnabas S, Passmore JA. Vaginal microbicides to prevent human immunodeficiency virus infection in women: perspectives on the female genital tract, sexual maturity and mucosal inflammation. Best Pract Res Clin Obstet Gynaecol. 2012;26(4):441–9.

46. Ross JA, Kasum CM. Dietary flavonoids: bioavailability, metabolic effects, and safety. Annu Rev Nutr. 2002;22:19–34.

47. Rahimifard M, Maqbool F, Moeini-Nodeh S, Niaz K, Abdollahi M, Braidy N, Nabavi SM, Nabavi SF. Targeting the TLR4 signaling pathway by polyphenols: a novel therapeutic strategy for neuroinflammation. Ageing Res Rev. 2017;36:11–9.

48. Vuorinen H, Maatta K, Torronen R. Content of the flavonols myricetin, quercetin, and kaempferol in finnish berry wines. J Agric Food Chem. 2000;48:2675–80.

49. Myers C, Muthusubramanian A, Sutton RB, Wylie BJ, Cornwall G. Functional amyloids in reproduction. Biomolecules. 2017. https://doi.org/10.3390/biom7030046.

50. Roan NR, Sandi-Monroy N, Kohgadai N, Usmani SM, Hamil KG, Neidleman J, Montano M, Ständker L, Röcker A, Cavrois M, et al. Semen amyloids participate in spermatozoa selection and clearance. Elife. 2017. https://doi.org/10.7554/eLife.24888.

51. Easterhoff D, Ontiveros F, Brooks LR, Kim Y, Ross B, Silva JN, Olsen JS, Feng C, Hardy DJ, Dunman P. Semen-derived enhancer of viral infection (SEVI) binds bacteria, enhances bacterial phagocytosis by macrophages, and can protect against vaginal infection by a sexually transmitted bacterial pathogen. Antimicrob Agents Chemother. 2013;57:2443–50.

52. Tan S, Lu L, Li L, Liu J, Oksov Y, Lu H, Jiang S, Liu S. Polyanionic candidate microbicides accelerate the formation of semen-derived amyloid fibrils to enhance HIV-1 infection. PLoS ONE. 2013;8:e59777.

53. Ye Z, French KC, Popova LA, Lednev IK, Lopez MM, Makhatadze GI. Mechanism of fibril formation by a 39-residue peptide (PAPf39) from human prostatic acidic phosphatase. Biochemistry. 2009;48:11582–91.

54. Chen J, Ren R, Tan S, Zhang W, Zhang X, Yu F, Xun T, Jiang S, Liu S, Li L. A peptide derived from the HIV-1 gp120 coreceptor-binding region promotes formation of PAP248–286 amyloid fibrils to enhance HIV-1 infection. PLoS ONE. 2015;10:e0144522.

55. Chang TT, Chou TC. Rational approach to the clinical protocol design for drug combinations: a review. Acta Paediatr Taiwan. 2000;41:294–302.

56. Tan S, Li L, Lu L, Pan C, Lu H, Oksov Y, Tang X, Jiang S, Liu S. Peptides derived from HIV-1 gp120 co-receptor binding domain form amyloid fibrils and enhance HIV-1 infection. FEBS Lett. 2014;588:1515–22.

57. Pettersen EF, Goddard TD, Huang CC, Couch GS, Greenblatt DM, Meng EC, Ferrin TE. UCSF Chimera—a visualization system for exploratory research and analysis. J Comput Chem. 2004;25:1605–12.

58. Jakalian A, Jack DB, Bayly CI. Fast, efficient generation of high-quality atomic charges. AM1-BCC model: II. Parameterization and validation. J Comput Chem. 2002;23:1623–41.

59. Salentin S, Schreiber S, Haupt VJ, Adasme MF, Schroeder M. PLIP: fully automated protein–ligand interaction profiler. Nucleic Acids Res. 2015;43:W443–7.

60. Li R, Liu T, Liu M, Chen F, Liu S. Anti-influenza A virus activity of dendrobine and its mechanism of action. J Agric Food Chem. 2017;65:3665–74.

61. Jiang S, Lu H, Liu S, Zhao Q, He Y, Debnath AK. N-substituted pyrrole derivatives as novel human immunodeficiency virus type 1 entry inhibitors that interfere with the gp41 six-helix bundle formation and block virus fusion. Antimicrob Agents Chemother. 2004;48:4349–59.

Assessment of the gorilla gut virome in association with natural simian immunodeficiency virus infection

Mirela D'arc[1,2], Carolina Furtado[1], Juliana D. Siqueira[1], Héctor N. Seuánez[1,2], Ahidjo Ayouba[3], Martine Peeters[3] and Marcelo A. Soares[1,2*] (iD)

Abstract

Background: Simian immunodeficiency viruses (SIVs) of chimpanzees and gorillas from Central Africa crossed the species barrier at least four times giving rise to human immunodeficiency virus type 1 (HIV-1) groups M, N, O and P. The paradigm of non-pathogenic lentiviral infections has been challenged by observations of naturally infected chimpanzees with SIVcpz associated with a negative impact on their life span and reproduction, CD4[+] T-lymphocyte loss and lymphoid tissue destruction. With the advent and dissemination of new generation sequencing technologies, novel promising markers of immune deficiency have been explored in human and nonhuman primate species, showing changes in the microbiome (dysbiosis) that might be associated with pathogenic conditions. The aim of the present study was to identify and compare enteric viromes of SIVgor-infected and uninfected gorillas using noninvasive sampling and ultradeep sequencing, and to assess the association of virome composition with potential SIVgor pathogenesis in their natural hosts.

Results: We analyzed both RNA and DNA virus libraries of 23 fecal samples from 11 SIVgor-infected (two samples from one animal) and 11 uninfected western lowland gorillas from Campo-Ma'an National Park (CP), in southwestern Cameroon. Three bacteriophage families (Siphoviridae, Myoviridae and Podoviridae) represented 67.5 and 68% of the total annotated reads in SIVgor-infected and uninfected individuals, respectively. Conversely, mammalian viral families, such as Herpesviridae and Reoviridae, previously associated with gut- and several mammalian diseases were significantly more abundant ($p < 0.003$) in the SIVgor-infected group. In the present study, we analyzed, for the first time, the enteric virome of gorillas and their association with SIVgor status. This also provided the first evidence of association of specific mammalian viral families and SIVgor in a putative dysbiosis context.

Conclusions: Our results suggested that viromes might be potentially used as markers of lentiviral disease progression in wild gorilla populations. The diverse mammalian viral families, herein described in SIVgor-infected gorillas, may play a pivotal role in a disease progression still unclear in these animals but already well characterized in pathogenic lentiviral infections in other organisms. Larger sample sets should be further explored to reduce intrinsic sampling variation.

Keywords: Gorilla, SIVgor, Pathogenesis, Virome, Dysbiosis

Background

The human immunodeficiency virus (HIV) types 1 and 2 have arisen from multiple zoonotic transmissions of simian immunodeficiency viruses (SIVs) circulating in African non-human primates (NHP) to humans. SIVs from chimpanzees and gorillas from Central Africa crossed the species barrier at least four times giving rise to HIV-1 groups M, N, O, and P [1, 2]. Likewise, at least nine independent transmissions between sooty mangabeys from West Africa and humans have already been described, originating the different HIV-2 groups found in humans [3–5].

*Correspondence: masoares@biologia.ufrj.br
[1] Instituto Nacional de Câncer (INCA), Rio de Janeiro, Brazil
Full list of author information is available at the end of the article

Although SIVs have been referred to as immunodeficiency viruses, the clinical manifestations in SIV-infected hosts were not reported during the first decades when natural infections were initially described in the wild and in naturally infected animals, captive sooty mangabeys and African green monkeys kept in zoos or primate centers. SIV lineages have already been documented in more than 40 species of African NHP [6]. Despite high SIV viral loads, individuals of these species have been initially reported as effective controllers of disease progression [7–9]. However, following the experimental or accidental SIV infections of Asian macaques (that are not natural reservoirs of lentiviruses), these latter primates developed an AIDS-like disease that was very similar to the human condition [10, 11].

The paradigm of non-pathogenic lentiviral infections has been recently challenged by observations of wild chimpanzees (*P. t. schweinfurthii*) in Gombe, Tanzania, in which infection by their natural SIV strain (SIVcpz*Pts*) was associated with a negative impact on their life span and reproduction [12, 13]. Moreover, retrospective analysis of conserved tissues from dead SIVcpz*Pts*-infected animals showed signs of immune deficiency similar to those found in AIDS-affected humans [13]. In addition, SIVcpz infection has also been associated with CD4$^+$ T lymphocyte loss and lymphoid tissue destruction (alike HIV infection), leading to premature death in a naturally infected chimpanzee in a sanctuary in Cameroon [14]. Altogether, these findings underscored the need for further studies of wild NHP populations, particularly among apes, because of their highly endangered status and the potential impact of SIV infection on their survival and eventual population decline [1, 7, 15]. However, the study of these wild populations is particularly difficult and can only be carried out by noninvasive sampling.

With the advent and dissemination of next generation sequencing (NGS) technologies, novel and promising markers of immune deficiency have been explored in humans and NHP species, notably changes in the microbiome (dysbiosis) potentially associated with pathogenic conditions. In humans, HIV infection is markedly associated with expansion of enteric adenoviruses and significant loss of enteric bacterial diversity and richness, clearly involved in disease progression [16]. Similar evidence of microbiome instability was found in naturally infected chimpanzees in Gombe [17]. To present, there is no available data on the pathogenicity of SIV in gorillas. Moeller et al. [18] examining 186 fecal samples of wild gorillas from Cameroon, did not find association between SIV status and specific patterns of the gut bacteriome. Nevertheless, as gorillas are infected with SIVgor through cross-species transmission of SIVcpz from chimpanzees,

it is plausible that SIVgor might negatively impact the health of gorillas in the wild [2].

By combining noninvasive sampling and NGS approaches, Handley et al. [19] reported the expansion of the enteric virome associated with disease progression in an AIDS-like context in rhesus macaques, but not with the nonpathogenic SIV infection of African green monkeys. These findings showed that pathogenic SIV infection was associated with an enteropathy that contributed to the AIDS-like disease progression seen in macaques [19]. In this report, we used a similar strategy for identifying enteric virome disturbances as dysbiosis markers in wild gorillas to understand the potential impact of SIVgor infection in their natural hosts. We identified and compared enteric viromes of SIVgor-infected and uninfected gorillas using noninvasive sampling and NGS to assess the relationship of their viromes with potential SIVgor pathogenesis. Here we present the first virome description of SIVgor-infected and uninfected gorillas, identifying viral family profiles in each studied group. Furthermore, we herein provide the first evidence of association of specific mammalian virus families (such as Adenoviridae, Herpesviridae and Reoviridae) with presence of SIVgor in a putative dysbiosis context in wild animals.

Methods

Sample collection

Twenty-three fecal samples from 22 wild western lowland gorillas (*Gorilla gorilla gorilla*) were studied. Samples were collected between May 2008 and February 2014 in Campo Ma'an National Park (CP), Cameroon, in a long-term follow-up project of gorilla communities in this region, where we previously reported 29% of SIVgor-infected animals in some groups [20, 21]. These samples, from 11 SIVgor-infected and 11 uninfected individuals, had been previously analyzed with serological and/ or molecular tools for confirming or excluding SIVgor infection [2, 20–22] (Table 1). Animals were individualized with microsatellite analysis as previously described [1, 21]. SIVgor viral load (VL) was measured with a previously reported real-time RT-qPCR assay capable of quantifying all HIV-1 groups and a wide diversity of SIVcpz and SIVgor strains [23]. The fecal samples selected for the study also included being the most fresh (the shortest elapsed time from deposition to collection), having a good amount of material and also covered a wide range of VL (including the highest VL ever measured in an infected gorilla). VL estimates of SIVgor ranged from 20 to 31,497 copies per mL (cp/mL) (Table 1). Two sequential samples were collected within a time interval of approximately 1 year from a single gorilla (CPg-ID074),

Table 1 Description of noninvasive samples used in this study

Lab code	ID[a]	Collection date (dd/mm/yyyy)	Estimated freshness (h)	SIV-specific RT-PCR[b]	SIVgor VL (cp/mL)[c]	SIV serology	GPS coordinates
CP3376	CPg-ID046	12/05/2008	11	NA	NA	NEG	2.334617°N 10.191633°W
CP3385	CPg-ID059	12/05/2008	11	NA	NA	NEG	2.334617°N 10.191633°W
CP3403	CPg-ID030	12/05/2008	ND	gp41/polmini	45	POS	2.334444°N 10.183889°W
CP3409	CPg-ID031	12/05/2008	10	NEG	20	POS	2.33055°N 10.201833°W
CP3453	CPg-ID090	12/10/2008	22	NA	NA	NEG	2.34425°N 10.229833°W
CP3469	CPg-ID034	12/10/2008	ND	gp41	4.217	POS	2.341389°N 10.211389°W
CP5781	CPg-ID066	27/04/2010	14	gp41	1.095	POS	2.325°N 10.1781°W
CP5819	CPg-ID017	30/04/2010	6	NA	NA	NEG	2.32865°N 10.168633°W
CP6535	CPg-ID142	17/03/2011	8	NA	NEG	NEG	2.34647°N 10.28754°W
CP7880	CPg-ID086	27/01/2012	12	NA	NEG	NEG	2.34329°N 10.18654°W
CP7885	CPg-ID004	27/01/2012	12	gp41	655	POS	2.34329°N 10.18654°W
CP7890	CPg-ID005	27/01/2012	12	gp41	2.346	POS	2.34329°N 10.18654°W
CP8084	CPg-ID006	23/04/2012	24	gp41	1.242	POS	2.32763°N 10.18388°W
CP8789	CPg-ID074[d]	12/11/2012	12	gp41/gp120 (V1–V4)	31.497	POS	2.34434°N 10.25066°W
CP8797	CPg-ID021	12/11/2012	12	NA	NEG	NEG	2.34434°N 10.25066°W
CP8804	CPg-ID114	12/11/2012	8	NA	NEG	NEG	2.34362°N 10.25137°W
CP9667	CPg-ID041	13/07/2013	14	gp41/polmini	2.460	POS	2.32650°N 10.20193°W
CP9679	CPg-ID035	13/07/2013	6	polmini	700	POS	2.32650°N 10.20193°W
CP9683	CPg-ID108	13/07/2013	6	NA	NA	NEG	2.32650°N 10.20193°W
CP9686	CPg-ID102	13/07/2013	6	NA	NA	NEG	2.32650°N 10.20193°W
CP9725	CPg-ID074[d]	27/10/2013	12	gp41/gp120/ polmini	4.924	POS	2.31423°N 10.19226°W
CP9852	CPg-ID122	19/02/2014	2	NA	NA	NEG	2.31021°N 10.24563°W
CP9854	CPg-ID047	19/02/2014	6	NEG	980	POS	2.31021°N 10.24563°W

ND not done, *NA* not applicable, *POS* positive, *NEG* negative

[a] Samples individualized (ID) by microsatellite analysis [2, 20, 21]

[b] SIV-specific RT-PCR using primers CPZ-gp41 (~ 450 bp), polmini (280 bp) and gp120 V1–V4 (~ 1000 bp), as previously described [1, 21, 22, 24]

[c] Viral Load (VL), as previously described [23]

[d] Samples of the same individual

one sample (CP8789) in 2012, with an estimated VL of 31,497 cp/mL, and another (CP9725) in 2013, with a VL of 4924 cp/mL.

Library preparation, quantification and NGS

The NucliSens Magnetic Extraction kit (BioMerieux, Craponne, France) and QIAamp Stool DNA Miniprep Kit (QIAGEN, Courtaboeuf, France) were used to extract nucleic acids (total nucleic acids or DNA, respectively) as previously described [20, 21]. Total nucleic acids were initially treated with the TURBO DNA-free™ kit (Life Technologies, CA, USA) and purified using the RNeasy® MinElute® Cleanup kit (QIAGEN), following the manufacturers' instructions. For removal of ribosomal RNA (from plant, bacteria and mammalian host) prior to RNA library preparation, total purified RNA was subjected to the ScriptSeq™ Complete Gold Kit: Epidemiology (Epicentre, Wisconsin, USA). The MinElute PCR Purification Kit (QIAGEN) and the Agencourt AMPure XP System: PCR Purification kit (Beckman Coulter, CA, USA) were used to purify PCR-amplified products whenever requested by the ScriptSeq™ kit protocol. DNA libraries were constructed using the Nextera® DNA Sample Preparation kit (Illumina®, CA, USA), following the manufacturer's instructions. For all RNA and DNA library preparations, an average of 2 µg and of 50 ng of purified nucleic acid were used for each sample library, respectively. Quality control and absolute quantification of libraries were carried out in the ECO™ system (Eco Real-Time PCR System, Illumina®) using the KAPA Library Quantification kit (KAPA Biosystems, MA, USA), according to the manufacturers' specifications. Libraries were diluted to a final concentration of 12 pM and NGS by synthesis was carried out in an Illumina® HiSeq 2500 platform (2 × 100 paired-end runs). Sequencing data files are available in the SRA database under

BioProject accession PRJNA419744 (BioSample accesion: SAMN08143625—SAMN0814362547).

Bioinformatics and statistical analyses

Quality analysis of the generated sequencing reads was conducted with FastQC (Babraham Bioinformatics, Cambridge, UK) and reads with good quality (Phred score > 30 and ≥ 90 bp) were selected with Sickle-Master [25]. Reads were submitted to a BLASTX search [26] onto the GenBank nonredundant viral protein database, with a minimal e-value cutoff of $1e^{-5}$, and reads assigned to viruses were kept for further analysis. Virus taxonomic assignment was carried out using the Lowest-Common Ancestor (LCA) algorithm in MEGAN v. 6.3.5, built 4 (April 2016). The following LCA parameters were used: Min Score 50; Max Expected 1×10^{-5}; Top Percent 10; Min Support Percent 75; Min Support 5; Min Complexity 0.3. Sequences without any significant hit were designated as unassigned. The MEGAN's square-root normalization protocol enabled intra- and intergroup comparisons. We compared the virus taxa distribution between SIVgor-infected (POS) and uninfected (NEG) animals. For this and onward analyses, annotated reads of the two samples from the same SIVgor-infected animal (CPg-ID074) were pooled and averaged. Assigned sequence counts per taxa were exported for subsequent statistical analysis using GraphPad Prism v.7. Fisher's exact test with Bonferroni correction was used for multiple comparisons. Data were presented as heatmaps with outlier data points removed whenever specified. All graphs were generated using Microsoft Excel® for Mac and R Studio v. 0.99.902. Results were considered statistically significant when p values were < 0.01.

Results

Viral diversity in enteric samples of western lowland gorillas

To assess the diversity of the enteric virome of wild gorillas, RNA and DNA libraries of 23 fecal samples from 11 SIVgor-infected and 11 uninfected western lowland gorillas were sequenced. We recovered 473,357,985 high-quality reads (mean = 20,580,781.96/sample, ranging from 4386,718 to 94,513,993) for all RNA libraries and 559,920,656 reads (mean = 24,344,376.35/sample, ranging from 2511,994 to 125,855,508) for all DNA libraries. After applying MEGAN square-root normalization, a reduction in read counts to 132,138.5 reads (mean = 6006.3/sample, ranging from 2575 to 14,064) was achieved for RNA libraries and to 150,539 reads (mean = 6842.7/sample, ranging from 2409 to 23,131) for DNA libraries. BLASTX analysis showed that approximately 24 and 29% of normalized reads could be annotated for identifying virus families using a viral database for RNA and DNA libraries, respectively (Fig. 1).

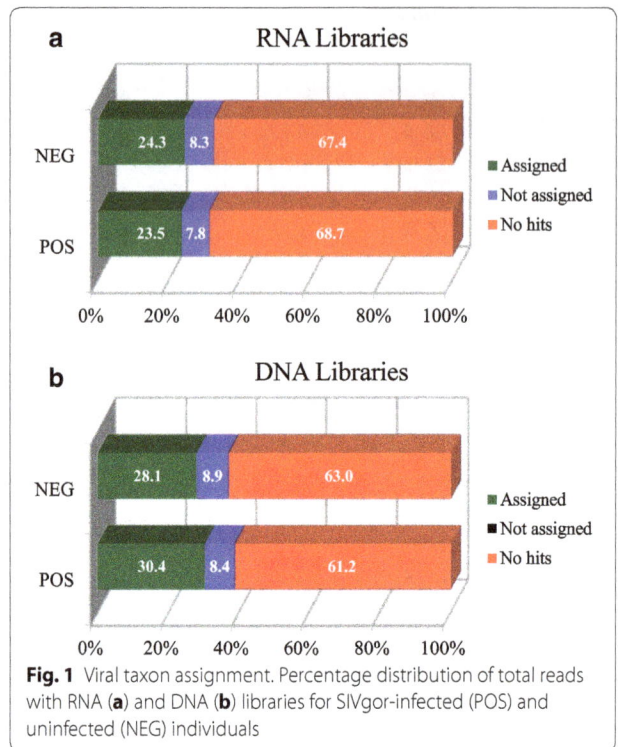

Fig. 1 Viral taxon assignment. Percentage distribution of total reads with RNA (**a**) and DNA (**b**) libraries for SIVgor-infected (POS) and uninfected (NEG) individuals

The Siphoviridae bacteriophage family was more frequent in SIVgor-infected individuals (32.7 vs 23.4% in uninfected individuals), while two other bacteriophage families were more frequent in uninfected individuals, Myoviridae (31.7 vs 25.8% in infected individuals) and Podoviridae (12.9 vs 9.0% in infected individuals). Altogether, these three viral families accounted for 67.5 and 68% of the total annotated reads in SIVgor-infected and uninfected individuals, respectively (Table 2). The majority of the other viral families showed frequencies below 1% of total reads. Viral family profiles diverged significantly between the two samples collected from a single individual (CPg-ID074; data not shown), a finding that precluded further analysis.

Association of gorilla virome profiles with SIVgor status

We compared the virome of the SIVgor-infected and uninfected gorillas and investigated the potential association of SIV status with virome profiles. As some viral families were represented in only one or two individuals of each group, outlier data were excluded from analysis to avoid spurious associations. In the SIVgor-infected group, 22 viral families were identified, with three taxa (Alloherpesviridae, Polydnaviridae and Reoviridae) exclusively represented in this group. Conversely, 21 viral families were identified among the uninfected gorillas, with two exclusive taxa (Microviridae and Tymoviridae). Despite the restrictive criteria of excluding outliers, we found a distinct profile

Table 2 Total number of annotated reads of viral families in SIVgor-infected (POS) and uninfected (NEG) individuals

Family	POS (%)	NEG (%)
Siphoviridae	12,433.5 (32.66)	8818 (23.39)
Myoviridae	9821 (25.80)	11,939 (31.66)
Podoviridae	3439 (9.03)	4859 (12.89)
Mimiviridae	2464.5 (6.47)	2536 (6.73)
Phycodnaviridae	2452.5 (6.44)	2455 (6.51)
Unclassified dsDNA phages	1266 (3.33)	1405 (3.73)
Unclassified phages	2477.5 (6.51)	2146 (5.69)
Unclassified dsDNA viruses	821 (2.16)	847 (2.25)
Unclassified Caudovirales	491.5 (1.29)	487 (1.29)
Herpesviridae	401.5 (1.06)	356 (0.94)
Others[a]	2006 (5.27)	1857 (4.93)
Total	38,074 (100)	37,705 (100)

[a] Other viral families with abundance frequency below 1% of annotated reads: Adenoviridae; Alloherpesviridae; Alphaflexiviridae; Ascoviridae; Asfarviridae; Baculoviridae; Betaflexiviridae; Bicaudaviridae; Bromoviridae; Caulimoviridae; Circoviridae; Closteroviridae; Dicistroviridae; Hytrosaviridae; Inoviridae; Iridoviridae; Leviviridae; Marseilleviridae; Mesoniviridae; Microviridae; Nudiviridae; Parvoviridae; Picobirnaviridae; Polydnaviridae; Potyviridae; Poxviridae; Reoviridae; Retroviridae; Rhabdoviridae; Rudiviridae; Streptococcaceae Virus; Tectiviridae; Tymoviridae; Unclassified ssDNA Viruses; Unclassified ssRNA Negative-strand Viruses; Unclassified ssRNA Positive-strand Viruses; Unclassified Viruses; and Virgaviridae

Table 3 Comparison of viral family abundance between SIVgor-infected (POS) and uninfected (NEG) individuals after outlier exclusion

Virus Family	POS (%)	NEG (%)	p value[a]
Alloherpesviridae	15 (0.07)	0 (0.00)	*0.0024*
Baculoviridae	32 (0.15)	50 (0.20)	0.9976
Herpesviridae	257 (1.19)	198 (0.79)	*0.0024*
Inoviridae	45 (0.21)	18 (0.07)	*0.0024*
Iridoviridae	39 (0.18)	15 (0.06)	0.2105
Marseilleviridae	53 (0.25)	66 (0.26)	1
Microviridae	0 (0.00)	22 (0.09)	*0.0024*
Mimiviridae	1838 (8.52)	2036 (8.15)	0.981
Myoviridae	6577 (30.47)	8645 (34.62)	*0.0024*
Nudiviridae	108 (0.50)	112 (0.45)	1
Parvoviridae	76 (0.35)	96 (0.38)	1
Phycodnaviridae	1759 (8.15)	1811 (7.25)	*0.0072*
Picobirnaviridae	35 (0.16)	64 (0.26)	0.5608
Podoviridae	1725 (7.99)	2322 (9.30)	*0.0024*
Polydnaviridae	2 (0.01)	0 (0.00)	0.9969
Poxviridae	19 (0.09)	44 (0.18)	0.235
Reoviridae	23 (0.11)	0 (0.00)	*0.0024*
Retroviridae	251 (1.16)	262 (1.05)	0.9989
Rhabdoviridae	2 (0.01)	32 (0.13)	*0.0024*
Siphoviridae	5666 (26.25)	5764 (23.08)	*0.0024*
Tymoviridae	0 (0.00)	65 (0.26)	*0.0024*
Unclassified Caudovirales	264 (1.22)	261 (1.05)	0.8284
Unclassified dsDNA Phages	831 (3.85)	1005 (4.02)	1
Unclassified dsDNA Viruses	575 (2.66)	603 (2.41)	0.8993
Unclassified Phages	1389 (6.44)	1479 (5.92)	*0.0024*
Total	21,582 (100)	24,970 (100)	

[a] p values were estimated with Fisher's Exact Test with Bonferroni correction (significant values are shown in italic)

for the SIVgor-infected group, with two significantly more abundant mammalian viral families (Herpesviridae and Reoviridae; p < 0.003; Table 3). The uninfected group also showed a distinct virome profile, with one significantly more abundant mammalian viral family (Rhabdoviridae; p < 0.003; Table 3). Unsupervised clustering analysis with the virome profiles of all 22 individuals revealed that some viral families served as putative proxies for SIVgor infection status, like Reoviridae and Alloherpesviridae in the SIVgor-infected group, and Tymoviridae, Microviridae and Rhabdoviridae in the uninfected group (Fig. 2).

Detection of disease-associated viruses in SIVgor-infected gorillas

A specific assessment of mammalian viral families previously associated with intestinal disease in their hosts was conducted in the studied specimens. Adenoviridae reads were found only in two SIVgor-infected gorillas. The association of this specific family with prolonged infections was characterized in CPg-ID004 (VL of 655 cp/mL) and CPg-ID047 (VL of 980 cp/mL) individuals, known to be SIVgor-infected since 2007 and 2011, respectively [20, 21]. Mammalian viral families that have been associated with gut and other diseases in humans [27–44] were also significantly more abundant in the SIVgor-infected group (p < 0.003), like Herpesviridae and Reoviridae, while only the Rhabdoviridae was more abundantly recovered in the uninfected group (p < 0.003).

Discussion

Studies on natural history of lentiviral infections in apes have been mostly limited to captive or semi-free ape communities due to the restrictions of working in the wild and to the endangered status of these species. However, noninvasive techniques developed during the last 30 years allowed for the study of prevalence, diversity and impact of SIV infection in several wild primate populations [6]. These advances prompted us to assess novel dysbiosis markers in previously studied wild gorilla communities, using fecal samples collected in CP.

In this study, 24 and 29% of normalized reads from RNA and DNA libraries, respectively, were annotated using a virus database. These rates were in agreement with similar reports on the complexity of virome annotation [31] and the finding of a large proportion of reads frequently found in the "No Hit" category in fecal samples [28]. These drawbacks may persist even when

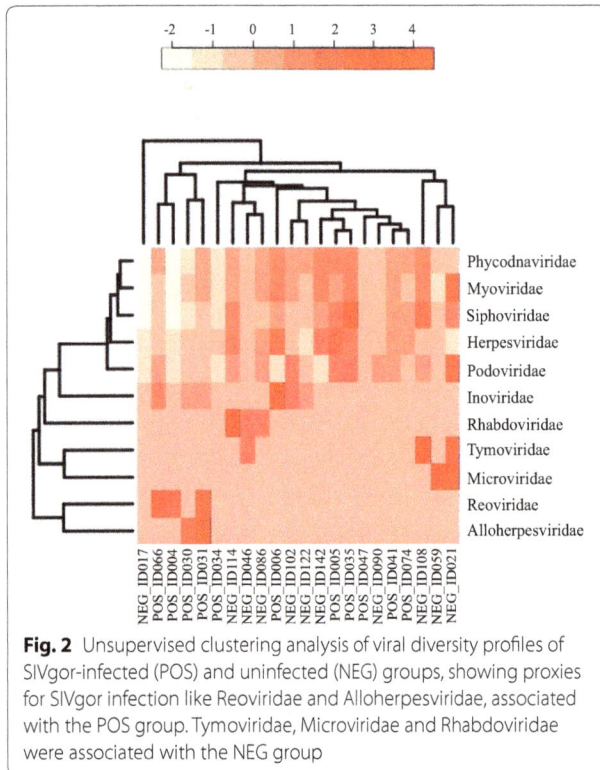

Fig. 2 Unsupervised clustering analysis of viral diversity profiles of SIVgor-infected (POS) and uninfected (NEG) groups, showing proxies for SIVgor infection like Reoviridae and Alloherpesviridae, associated with the POS group. Tymoviridae, Microviridae and Rhabdoviridae were associated with the NEG group

pretreatment for reducing bacterial or general eukaryotic material is carried out, because a substantial amount of non-viral sequences can still be found in fecal samples. It is also important to consider that a substantial proportion of the fecal virome is related to dietary components and associated viruses, like plant viruses [19, 45, 46]. In our study, a large number of annotated reads was related to non-mammalian viruses, mostly bacteriophages and plant viruses. Currently, the convergence of bacterial communities of sympatric individuals living off the same diet has been well established [19, 45, 47]. Moreover, the bacteriophage community, intrinsically linked with the bacteriome, can be an indicator of the general stability of the gut microbiome in a disease context. Mammalian viruses, on the other hand, might be important markers of disease progression despite their low frequency found during annotation.

In this study, we analyzed for the first time the enteric virome of gorillas in association with SIVgor status. This also provided the first evidence of association of specific mammalian viral families with SIVgor infection in a putative dysbiosis context. This was the case of SIV-infected rhesus macaques that presented unsuspected adenovirus infection associated with intestinal disease and enteric epithelial pathology, as well as enteric parvoviruses and advanced AIDS [19]. In the gorillas herein studied, adenoviruses were only recovered from SIVgor-infected

individuals, while parvoviruses were differently represented in samples with higher VL ($\geq$ 1000 copies/mL) than with lower VL (< 1000 copies/mL) (data not shown), suggesting that parvovirus infection might vary according to VL. The picobirnaviruses recovered in this study also showed to be more frequent in animals with higher VL than with lower VL, while reoviruses were significantly more abundant in SIVgor-infected animals than in their uninfected counterparts. Infection by picobirnaviruses and reoviruses has been associated with gastrointestinal complications in advanced HIV infections [29, 30, 41, 43]. Herpesviruses were also significantly more abundant in SIVgor-infected gorillas; these viruses have already been described in AIDS patients [36–40, 42] indicating persistent infections. These findings strongly suggest that SIVgor infection might be associated with dysbiosis, although further studies will be required for validation.

Epidemiological surveys showed that SIVgor as well as SIVcpz are less prevalent and considerably less evenly distributed among wild ape communities than the non-pathogenic SIVs in sooty mangabeys and African green monkeys [6]. These distribution disparities raise the possibility that apes may not be the natural reservoirs of these viruses, and that might be subjected to pathogenic conditions similar to those in other non-natural lentiviral hosts like humans and rhesus macaques [15, 19, 48, 49]. Currently SIVcpz, like HIV-1, is known to cause significant morbidity and mortality in infected chimpanzee communities [12, 13, 50], in association to compositional changes of the bacteriome rather than the virome, with disease progression with known (or suspected) immunodeficiency in late stages [51]. A similar study in wild gorillas failed to show association between SIVgor status and the bacteriome [52], while data on their virome has been, to present, wanting.

This study is underpinned by important limitations. In the great apes, it is well known that the gut microbiome community and abundance profiles are shaped by individual and external factors, like sex, age, time elapsed since fecal deposition, and dietary habits related with the rain or dry seasons of CP. With respect to sex, samples of SIVgor-infected and uninfected females showed larger numbers of reads of families of bacterial, amoebal, algal, invertebrate, and vertebrate viruses, both in SIVgor-infected and uninfected groups (not shown). In view of the small number of individuals within each group, this sex bias was not considered in further analyses. Moreover, our samples did not allow us to identify any age-related virome variation, since age estimation through noninvasive material is a very difficult, maybe unfeasible task.

Campo Ma'an is located in the southwest coast of Cameroon, a region with coastal equatorial climate where a heavy rain season (from August to November) is followed by a long dry season (from December to March), a short rain season (from April to May) and a short dry season (June and July). These alternate seasons might impose drastic diet changes resulting from different feeding strategies which, in turn, might be reflected in the fecal virome. Because we did not use seasonality as a factor for sample selection, both SIV-infected and uninfected groups had samples from dry and wet seasons, and such analysis was not considered in the present study, but deserves further assessment.

Despite the restrictive criteria herein adopted to minimize viral misidentification, the small number of studied individuals may produce imprecise estimates of microbiome profiles. Finally, the computational pipeline developed by us was characterized by a simple sequence of algorithms for identifying viral families without further characterization of full-length viral sequences or discovering novel viruses. On the other hand, the stringency for removing unreliable reads, despite hindering virus discovery, allowed robust description of the virome composition of SIVgor-infected and uninfected gorillas. However, higher number of samples will be necessary for reducing intrinsic sampling variation.

Conclusions

We herein describe, for the first time, the virome of wild gorillas, although these preliminary observations were carried out in a small number of individuals. This study suggests that the virome of SIVgor-infected individuals might differ from the one present in uninfected animals, in contrast to what has been reported for the bacteriome in this species [18]. The microbiome of SIVgor-infected animals must be further explored to validate present findings and to confirm whether virome dysbiosis might be consistent with the characteristic disease profile observed in SIVcpz-infected chimpanzees [17], the more classic pathogenic SIVmac infection in rhesus macaques, and HIV-1 infection in humans. The diverse mammalian viral families, herein described for the first time in SIVgor-infected gorillas, may play a pivotal role in a disease progression that still remains unclear in these animals but is already well characterized in pathogenic lentiviral infections. Our results suggest that viromes might be considered as markers of lentiviral disease progression in wild gorilla populations and should be further explored on a larger sample set.

Authors' contributions
MD, MP and MAS conceived the study. MP and AA collected and provided the gorilla samples. MD processed the gorilla fecal samples for the NGS assays. MD, CF and AA carried out the construction and quantification of the RNA and DNA libraries, and ran the samples on the Illumina® HiSeq 2500 platform. MD and JS performed the data analyses. HNS, MP and MAS provided reagents and infrastructure for the conduction of the study. MD, AA, MP, HNS and MAS

wrote the manuscript. All authors read and approved the final version of the manuscript.

Author details
[1] Instituto Nacional de Câncer (INCA), Rio de Janeiro, Brazil. [2] Universidade Federal do Rio de Janeiro (UFRJ), Rio de Janeiro, Brazil. [3] UMI233/INSERM1175 Institut de Recherche pour le Développement (IRD), University of Montpellier, Montpellier, France.

Acknowledgements
We wish to thank lab personnel form the Institut de Recherche pour le Développement—IRD (Montpellier, France) and Institut Bouisson Bertrand—IBB (France), mainly Dr. Eric Delaporte (Head of the Laboratory UMI233/INSERM1175 and Head of the IBB) for providing infrastructure for the conduction of the study and Amandine Esteban (technician of the laboratory UMI233/INSERM1175) for sample processing.

Competing interests
The authors declare that they have no competing interests.

Funding
This work was supported by grants from the Rio de Janeiro State Science Foundation (FAPERJ) E26/170.026/2008 and the Brazilian Research Council (CNPq) 573806/2008-0, both funded by the Brazilian National Institute of Science and Technology (INCT) for Cancer Control to H. N. S and M. A. S., the Graduate Program in Genetics (PGGEN) of Universidade Federal do Rio de Janeiro (UFRJ) Grant #1629742 to M. D., the National Institute of Health (RO1 AI 50529) and the Agence Nationale de Recherches sur le SIDA (ANRS 12125/12182/12325) to M. P. and A. A.

References
1. Keele BF, Van Heuverswyn F, Li Y, Bailes E, Takehisa J, Santiago ML, et al. Chimpanzee reservoirs of pandemic and nonpandemic HIV-1. Science. 2006;313:523–6.
2. D'arc M, Ayouba A, Esteban A, Learn GH, Boué V, Liegeois F, et al. Origin of the HIV-1 group O epidemic in western lowland gorillas. Proc Natl Acad Sci. 2015;112:E1343–52.
3. Santiago ML, Range F, Keele BF, Li Y, Bailes E, Bibollet-Ruche F, et al. Simian immunodeficiency virus infection in free-ranging sooty mangabeys (*Cercocebus atys atys*) from the Taï Forest, Côte d'Ivoire: implications for the origin of epidemic human immunodeficiency virus type 2. J Virol. 2005;79:12515–27.
4. Sharp PM, Bailes E, Chaudhuri RR, Rodenburg CM, Santiago MO, Hahn BH. The origins of acquired immune deficiency syndrome viruses: where and when? Philos Trans R Soc Lond B Biol Sci. 2001;356:867–76.
5. Ayouba A, Akoua-Koffi C, Calvignac-Spencer S, Esteban A, Locatelli S, Li H, et al. Evidence for continuing cross-species transmission of SIVsmm to humans: characterization of a new HIV-2 lineage in rural Côte d'Ivoire. AIDS. 2013;27:2488–91.
6. Peeters M, D'Arc M, Delaporte E. The origin and diversity of human retroviruses. AIDS Rev. 2014;16:23–34.
7. Paiardini M, Pandrea I, Apetrei C, Silvestri G. Lessons learned from the natural hosts of HIV-related viruses. Annu Rev Med. 2009;60:485–95.
8. Silvestri G. Naturally SIV-infected sooty mangabeys: are we closer to understanding why they do not develop AIDS? J Med Primatol. 2005;34:243–52.
9. Silvestri G. Immunity in natural SIV infections. J Int Med. 2009;265:97–109.

10. Daniel MD, Letvin NL, King NW, Kannagi M, Sehgal PK, Hunt RD, et al. Isolation of T-cell tropic HTLV-III-like retrovirus from macaques. Science. 1985;228:1201–4.

11. Kanki PJ, McLane MF, King NW, Letvin NL, Hunt RD, Sehgal P, et al. Serologic identification and characterization of a macaque T-lymphotropic retrovirus closely related to HTLV-III. Science. 1985;228:1199–201.

12. Keele BF, Jones JH, Terio KA, Estes JD, Rudicell RS, Wilson ML, et al. Increased mortality and AIDS-like immunopathology in wild chimpanzees infected with SIVcpz. Nature. 2009;460:515–9.

13. Rudicell RS, Holland Jones J, Wroblewski EE, Learn GH, Li Y, Robertson JD, et al. Impact of simian immunodeficiency virus infection on chimpanzee population dynamics. PLoS Pathog. 2010;6:e1001116.

14. Etienne L, Nerrienet E, LeBreton M, Bibila GT, Foupouapouognigni Y, Rousset D, et al. Characterization of a new simian immunodeficiency virus strain in a naturally infected *Pan troglodytes troglodytes* chimpanzee with AIDS related symptoms. Retrovirology. 2011;8:4.

15. Sharp PM, Hahn BH. Origins of HIV and the AIDS pandemic. Cold Spring Harb Perspect Med. 2011;1:a006841.

16. Monaco CL, Gootenberg DB, Zhao G, Handley SA, Ghebremichael MS, Lim ES, et al. Altered virome and bacterial microbiome in human immunodeficiency virus-associated acquired immunodeficiency syndrome. Cell Host Microbe. 2016;19:311–22.

17. Moeller AH, Shilts M, Li Y, Rudicell RS, Lonsdorf EV, Pusey AE, et al. SIV-induced instability of the chimpanzee gut microbiome. Cell Host Microbe. 2013;14:340–5.

18. Moeller AH, Peeters M, Ayouba A, Ngole EM, Esteban A, Hahn BH, et al. Stability of the gorilla microbiome despite simian immunodeficiency virus infection. Mol Ecol. 2015;24:690–7.

19. Handley SA, Thackray LB, Zhao G, Presti R, Miller AD, Droit L, et al. Pathogenic simian immunodeficiency virus infection is associated with expansion of the enteric virome. Cell. 2012;151:253–66.

20. Etienne L, Locatelli S, Ayouba A, Esteban A, Butel C, Liegeois F, et al. Noninvasive follow-up of simian immunodeficiency virus infection in wild-living nonhabituated western lowland gorillas in Cameroon. J Virol. 2012;86:9760–72.

21. Neel C, Etienne L, Li Y, Takehisa J, Rudicell RS, Bass IN, et al. Molecular epidemiology of simian immunodeficiency virus infection in wild-living gorillas. J Virol. 2010;84:1464–76.

22. Van Heuverswyn F, Li Y, Neel C, Bailes E, Keele BF, Liu W, et al. Human immunodeficiency viruses: SIV infection in wild gorillas. Nature. 2006;444:164.

23. Etienne L, Eymard-Duvernay S, Aghokeng A, Butel C, Monleau M, Peeters M. Single real-time reverse transcription-PCR assay for detection and quantification of genetically diverse HIV-1, SIVcpz, and SIVgor strains. J Clin Microbiol. 2013;51:787–98.

24. Takehisa J, Kraus MH, Ayouba A, Bailes E, Van Heuverswyn F, Decker JM, et al. Origin and biology of simian immunodeficiency virus in wild-living western gorillas. J Virol. 2009;83:1635–48.

25. Joshi N, Sickle FJ.: A sliding-window, adaptive, quality-based trimming tool for FastQ files. https://github.com/najoshi/sickle (2011). Accessed 15 Jan 2015.

26. Altschul SF, Gish W, Miller W, Myers EW, Lipman DJ. Basic local alignment search tool. J Mol Biol. 1990;215:403–10.

27. Brenchley JM, Price DA, Schacker TW, Asher TE, Silvestri G, Rao S, et al. Microbial translocation is a cause of systemic immune activation in chronic HIV infection. Nat Med. 2006;12:1365–71.

28. Cotten M, Oude Munnink B, Canuti M, Deijs M, Watson SJ, Kellam P, et al. Full genome virus detection in fecal samples using sensitive nucleic acid preparation, deep sequencing, and a novel iterative sequence classification algorithm. PLoS ONE. 2014;2:e93269.

29. Cunningham AL, Grohman GS, Harkness J, Law C, Marriott D, Tindall B, et al. Gastrointestinal viral infections in homosexual men who were symptomatic and seropositive for human immunodeficiency virus. J Infect Dis. 1988;158:386–91.

30. Gilger MA, Matson DO, Conner ME, Rosenblatt HM, Finegold MJ, Estes MK. Extraintestinal rotavirus infections in children with immunodeficiency. J Pediatr. 1992;120:912–7.

31. Handley SA. The virome: a missing component of biological interaction networks in health and disease. Genome Med. 2016;8:32.

32. Li SK, Leung RKK, Guo HX, Wei JF, Wang JH, Kwong KT, et al. Detection and identification of plasma bacterial and viral elements in HIV/AIDS patients in comparison to healthy adults. Clin Microbiol Infect. 2012;18:1126–33.

33. Marchetti G, Tincati C, Silvestri G. Microbial translocation in the pathogenesis of HIV infection and AIDS. Clin Microbiol Rev. 2013;26:2–18.

34. Minot S, Bryson A, Chehoud C, Wu GD, Lewis JD, Bushman FD. Rapid evolution of the human gut virome. Proc Natl Acad Sci USA. 2013;110:12450–5.

35. Naeger DM, Martin JN, Sinclair E, Hunt PW, Bangsberg DR, Hecht F, et al. Cytomegalovirus-specific T cells persist at very high levels during long-term antiretroviral treatment of HIV disease. PLoS ONE. 2010;29(5):e8886.

36. Sandler NG, Douek DC. Microbial translocation in HIV infection: causes, consequences and treatment opportunities. Nat Rev Microbiol. 2012;10:655–66.

37. Springer KL, Weinberg A. Cytomegalovirus infection in the era of HAART: fewer reactivations and more immunity. J Antimicrob Chemother. 2004;54:582–6.

38. Williams B, Landay A, Presti RM. Microbiome alterations in HIV infection a review. Cell Microbiol. 2016;18:645–51.

39. Zou S, Caler L, Colombini-Hatch S, Glynn S, Srinivas P. Research on the human virome: where are we and what is next. Microbiome. 2016;24(4):32.

40. Chang Y, Cesarman E, Pessin MS, Lee F, Culpepper J, Knowles DM, et al. Identification of herpesvirus-like DNA sequences in AIDS-associated Kaposi's sarcoma. Science. 1994;266:1865–9.

41. Giordano MO, Martinez LC, Rinaldi D, Gúinard S, Naretto E, Casero R, et al. Detection of picobirnavirus in HIV-infected patients with diarrhea in Argentina. J Acquir Immune Defic Syndr Hum Retrovirol. 1998;18:380–3.

42. González GG, Pujol FH, Liprandi F, Deibis L, Ludert JE. Prevalence of enteric viruses in human immunodeficiency virus seropositive patients in Venezuela. J Med Virol. 1998;55:288–92.

43. Raini SK, Nyangao J, Kombich J, Sang C, Gikonyo J, Ongus JR, et al. Human rotavirus group a serotypes causing gastroenteritis in children less than 5 years and HIV-infected adults in Viwandani slum, Nairobi. Ethiop J Health Sci. 2015;25:39–46.

44. Stevens SJC, Blank BSN, Smits PHM, Meenhorst PL, Middeldorp JM. High Epstein–Barr virus (EBV) DNA loads in HIV-infected patients: correlation with antiretroviral therapy and quantitative EBV serology. AIDS. 2002;16:993–1001.

45. Minot S, Sinha R, Chen J, Li H, Keilbaugh SA, Wu GD, et al. The human gut virome: inter-individual variation and dynamic response to diet. Genome Res. 2011;21:1616–25.

46. Zhang T, Breitbart M, Lee WH, Run J-Q, Wei CL, Soh SWL, et al. RNA viral community in human feces: prevalence of plant pathogenic viruses. PLoS Biol. 2006;4:e3.

47. Moeller AH, Peeters M, Ndjango JB, Li Y, Hahn BH, Ochman H. Sympatric chimpanzees and gorillas harbor convergent gut microbial communities. Genome Res. 2013;23:1715–20.

48. Hazenberg MD, Otto SA, van Benthem BHB, Roos MTL, Coutinho RA, Lange JMA, et al. Persistent immune activation in HIV-1 infection is associated with progression to AIDS. AIDS. 2003;17:1881–8.

49. Brenchley JM, Silvestri G, Douek DC. Nonprogressive and progressive primate immunodeficiency lentivirus infections. Immunity. 2010;32:737–42.

50. Terio KA, Kinsel MJ, Raphael J, Mlengeya T, Lipende I, Kirchhoff CA, et al. Pathologic lesions in chimpanzees (*Pan trogylodytes schweinfurthii*) from Gombe National Park, Tanzania, 2004–2010. J Zoo Wildl Med. 2011;42:597–607.

51. Barbian HJ, Li Y, Ramirez M, Klase Z, Lipende I, Mjungu D, et al. Destabilization of the gut microbiome marks the end-stage of simian immunodeficiency virus infection in wild chimpanzees. Am J Primatol. 2015. https://doi.org/10.1002/ajp.22515.

52. Moeller AH, Peeters M, Ayouba A, Ngole EM, Esteban A, Hahn BH, et al. Stability of the gorilla microbiome despite simian immunodeficiency virus infection. Mol Ecol. 2015;24:690–7.

Permissions

All chapters in this book were first published in RETROVIROLOGY, by BioMed Central; hereby published with permission under the Creative Commons Attribution License or equivalent. Every chapter published in this book has been scrutinized by our experts. Their significance has been extensively debated. The topics covered herein carry significant findings which will fuel the growth of the discipline. They may even be implemented as practical applications or may be referred to as a beginning point for another development.

The contributors of this book come from diverse backgrounds, making this book a truly international effort. This book will bring forth new frontiers with its revolutionizing research information and detailed analysis of the nascent developments around the world.

We would like to thank all the contributing authors for lending their expertise to make the book truly unique. They have played a crucial role in the development of this book. Without their invaluable contributions this book wouldn't have been possible. They have made vital efforts to compile up to date information on the varied aspects of this subject to make this book a valuable addition to the collection of many professionals and students.

This book was conceptualized with the vision of imparting up-to-date information and advanced data in this field. To ensure the same, a matchless editorial board was set up. Every individual on the board went through rigorous rounds of assessment to prove their worth. After which they invested a large part of their time researching and compiling the most relevant data for our readers.

The editorial board has been involved in producing this book since its inception. They have spent rigorous hours researching and exploring the diverse topics which have resulted in the successful publishing of this book. They have passed on their knowledge of decades through this book. To expedite this challenging task, the publisher supported the team at every step. A small team of assistant editors was also appointed to further simplify the editing procedure and attain best results for the readers.

Apart from the editorial board, the designing team has also invested a significant amount of their time in understanding the subject and creating the most relevant covers. They scrutinized every image to scout for the most suitable representation of the subject and create an appropriate cover for the book.

The publishing team has been an ardent support to the editorial, designing and production team. Their endless efforts to recruit the best for this project, has resulted in the accomplishment of this book. They are a veteran in the field of academics and their pool of knowledge is as vast as their experience in printing. Their expertise and guidance has proved useful at every step. Their uncompromising quality standards have made this book an exceptional effort. Their encouragement from time to time has been an inspiration for everyone.

The publisher and the editorial board hope that this book will prove to be a valuable piece of knowledge for researchers, students, practitioners and scholars across the globe.

List of Contributors

Eric Mauro
Fundamental Microbiology and Pathogenicity Laboratory, UMR 5234 CNRS-University of Bordeaux, SFR TransBioMed, 146 rue Léo Saignat, Bordeaux Cedex, France
International Associated Laboratory (LIA) of Microbiology and Immunology, CNRS, University de Bordeaux/ Heinrich Pette Institute-Leibniz Institute for Experimental Virology, Bordeaux, France

Xavier Robert
MMSB-Institute of the Biology and Chemistry of Proteins, UMR 5086 CNRS-Lyon 1 University, Lyon, France

Csaba Miskey and Zoltán Ivics
Division of Medical Biotechnology, Paul Ehrlich Institute, Langen, Germany

Stéphane Chaignepain
UMR CNRS 5248 CBMN (Chimie Biologie des Membranes et Nanoobjets), Université de Bordeaux, 33076 Bordeaux, France

Daniel R. Henriquez
Virology Program, ICBM, Faculty of Medicine, University of Chile, Santiago of Chile, Chile

Marc Ruff
Département de Biologie Structurale Intégrative, UDS, U596 INSERM, UMR7104 CNRS, IGBMC (Institut de Génétique et de Biologie Moléculaire et Cellulaire), Illkirch, France
Viral DNA Integration and Chromatin Dynamics Network (DyNAVir), Bordeaux, France

Matthew S. Parsons and Amy W. Chung
Department of Microbiology and Immunology, The University of Melbourne, at the Peter Doherty Institute for Infection and Immunity, Victoria, Australia

Stephen J. Kent
Department of Microbiology and Immunology, The University of Melbourne, at the Peter Doherty Institute for Infection and Immunity, Victoria, Australia

ARC Centre of Excellence in Convergent Bio-Nano Science and Technology, The University of Melbourne, Victoria, Australia
Melbourne Sexual Health Centre, Alfred Hospital, Monash University Central Clinical School, Victoria, Australia

Quang N. Nguyen, Jonathon E. Himes, Qifeng Han, Amit Kumar, Riley Mangan, Nathan I. Nicely, Guanhua Xie, Nathan Vandergrift and Xiaoying Shen
Duke Human Vaccine Institute, Duke University School of Medicine, Durham, NC, USA

Sallie R. Permar
Duke Human Vaccine Institute, Duke University School of Medicine, Durham, NC, USA
Department of Molecular Genetics and Microbiology, Duke University School of Medicine, Durham, NC, USA
Department of Pediatrics, Duke University School of Medicine, Durham, NC, USA.
Department of Immunology, Duke University School of Medicine, Durham, NC, USA

David R. Martinez
Duke Human Vaccine Institute, Duke University School of Medicine, Durham, NC, USA
Department of Molecular Genetics and Microbiology, Duke University School of Medicine, Durham, NC, USA

R.Whitney Edwards and Justin Pollara
Duke Human Vaccine Institute, Duke University School of Medicine, Durham, NC, USA
Department of Surgery, Duke University School of Medicine, Durham, NC, USA

Georges Khoury, Michelle Y. Lee, Jonathan Jacobson, Leigh Harty and Damian F. J. Purcell
Department of Microbiology and Immunology, The Peter Doherty Institute for Infection and Immunity, University of Melbourne, Melbourne, Australia

Talia M. Mota
Department of Microbiology and Immunology, The Peter Doherty Institute for Infection and Immunity, University of Melbourne, Melbourne, Australia

The Peter Doherty Institute for Infection and Immunity, Royal Melbourne Hospital, University of Melbourne, Melbourne, Australia

Carolin Tumpach and Jenny L. Anderson
The Peter Doherty Institute for Infection and Immunity, Royal Melbourne Hospital, University of Melbourne, Melbourne, Australia

Sharon R. Lewin
The Peter Doherty Institute for Infection and Immunity, Royal Melbourne Hospital, University of Melbourne, Melbourne, Australia
Department of Infectious Diseases, Alfred Health and Monash University, Melbourne, Australia

Shuang Li
School of Life Sciences, Peking University, Beijing, China

Hayato Murakoshi, Chengcheng Zou, Nozomi Kuse, Tomohiro Akahoshi, Takayuki Chikata and Masafumi Takiguchi
Center for AIDS Research, Kumamoto University, 2-2-1 Honjo, Chuo-ku, Kumamoto 860-0811, Japan
International Research Center of Medical Sciences, Kumamoto University, Kumamoto, Japan

Hiroyuki Gatanaga and Shinichi Oka
Center for AIDS Research, Kumamoto University, 2-2-1 Honjo, Chuo-ku, Kumamoto 860-0811, Japan
AIDS Clinical Center, National Center for Global Health and Medicine, Tokyo, Japan

Tomáš Hanke
International Research Center of Medical Sciences, Kumamoto University, Kumamoto, Japan
The Jenner Institute, University of Oxford, Old Road Campus Research Building, Roosevelt Drive, Oxford, UK

Jacqui Brener, Nora Lavandier,Chrissy Bolton, Reena Dsouza and Philip J. R. Goulder
Department of Paediatrics, University of Oxford, Oxford, UK

Astrid Gall
Department of Veterinary Medicine, University of Cambridge, Cambridge, UK

Paul Kellam
Wellcome Trust Sanger Institute, Wellcome Trust Genome Campus, Hinxton, Cambridge, UK

Division of Infection and Immunity, University College London, Gower Street, London, UK

Philippa C. Matthews and Jacob Hurst
Nuffield Department of Medicine, University of Oxford, Oxford, UK

Todd Allen and Rebecca Batorsky
Ragon Institute of MGH, MIT and Harvard, Boston, MA, USA

Fabian Chen
Department of Sexual Health, Royal Berkshire Hospital, Reading, UK

Anne Edwards
Department of GU Medicine, The Churchill Hospital, Oxford University NHS Foundation Trust, Oxford, UK

Oliver G. Pybus
Department of Zoology, University of Oxford, Oxford, UK

Neal N. Padte, Jian Yu, Yaoxing Huang and David D. Ho
Aaron Diamond AIDS Research Center, The Rockefeller University, 455 First Avenue, New York, NY 10016, USA

Defang Zhou, Jingwen Xue, Shuhai He, Xusheng Du, Jing Zhou, Chengui Li, Libo Huang and Ziqiang Cheng
College of Veterinary Medicine, Shandong Agricultural University, Tai'an 271018, China

Venugopal Nair and Yongxiu Yao
The Pirbright Institute & UK-China Centre of Excellence on Avian Disease Research, Pirbright, Ash Road, Guildford, Surrey GU24 0NF,UK

Maureen Oliveira, Ruxandra-Ilinca Ibanescu and Kaitlin Anstett
McGill University AIDS Centre, Lady Davis Institute for Medical Research, Jewish General Hospital, 3755 Côte Ste-Catherine Road, Montreal, QC H3T 1E2, Canada

Thibault Mésplède
McGill University AIDS Centre, Lady Davis Institute for Medical Research, Jewish General Hospital, 3755 Côte Ste-Catherine Road, Montreal, QC H3T 1E2, Canada

Department of Microbiology and Immunology, McGill University, Montreal, QC, Canada

Bluma G. Brenner
McGill University AIDS Centre, Lady Davis Institute for Medical Research, Jewish General Hospital, 3755 Côte Ste-Catherine Road, Montreal, QC H3T 1E2, Canada
Department of Microbiology and Immunology, McGill University, Montreal, QC, Canada
Faculty of Medicine (Surgery, Experimental Medicine, Infectious Disease), McGill University, Montreal, QC, Canada

Jean-Pierre Routy
Faculty of Medicine (Surgery, Experimental Medicine, Infectious Disease), McGill University, Montreal, QC, Canada

Marjorie A. Robbins
BC Children's Hospital Research Institute, Vancouver, BC, Canada

Francois Venter and Helen Rees
Wits Reproductive Health and HIV Institute, Faculty of Health Sciences, University of the Witwatersrand, Hillbrow Health Precinct, 22 Esselen Street, Hillbrow, Johannesburg 2001, South Africa

Robyn Eakle
Wits Reproductive Health and HIV Institute, Faculty of Health Sciences, University of the Witwatersrand, Hillbrow Health Precinct, 22 Esselen Street, Hillbrow, Johannesburg 2001, South Africa
Faculty of Public Health and Policy,London School of Hygiene and Tropical Medicine, London, United Kingdom

Emily N. Pawlak, Brennan S. Dirk, Rajesh Abraham Jacob, Aaron L. Johnson and Jimmy D. Dikeakos
Department of Microbiology and Immunology, Schulich School of Medicine and Dentistry, University of Western Ontario, Dental Sciences Building, Room 3007J, London, ON N6A 5C1, Canada

Zachary H. Williams and John M. Coffin
Department of Molecular Biology and Microbiology, Tufts University School of Medicine, Boston, MA, USA

Meagan Montesion
Department of Molecular Biology and Microbiology, Tufts University School of Medicine, Boston, MA, USA
Present Address: Foundation Medicine, Inc., Cambridge, MA, USA

Ravi P. Subramanian
Department of Molecular Biology and Microbiology, Tufts University School of Medicine, Boston, MA, USA
Present Address: Excerpta Medica, New York, NY,USA

Charlotte Kuperwasser
Department of Developmental, Chemical, and Molecular Biology, Tufts University School of Medicine, Boston, MA, USA
Raymond and Beverly Sackler Convergence Laboratory, Tufts University School of Medicine, Boston, MA, USA

Ferdinand Roesch, Molly OhAinle and Michael Emer
Divisions of Human Biology and Basic Sciences, Fred Hutchinson Cancer Research Center, 1100 Fairview Ave N, Mailstop C2-023, Seattle, WA 98109, USA

Marilia Rita Pinzone and Una O'Doherty
Department of Pathology and Laboratory Medicine, University of Pennsylvania, Philadelphia, PA, USA

Shuwen Yin, Lingzhen Ma, Jiayong Wen, Xuanxuan Zhang, Fangyuan Lai, Shuwen Liu and Lin Li
Guangdong Provincial Key Laboratory of New Drug Screening, Guangzhou Key Laboratory of Drug Research for Emerging Virus Prevention and Treatment, School of Pharmaceutical Sciences, Southern Medical University, 1838 Guangzhou Avenue North, Guangzhou 510515, Guangdong, China

Ruxia Ren
Guangdong Provincial Key Laboratory of New Drug Screening, Guangzhou Key Laboratory of Drug Research for Emerging Virus Prevention and Treatment, School of Pharmaceutical Sciences, Southern Medical University, 1838 Guangzhou Avenue North, Guangzhou 510515, Guangdong, China

Department of Pharmacy, The Seventh Affiliated Hospital of Sun Yat-sen University, Shenzhen 518107, China

Baolong Lai
Department of Pharmacy, The Seventh Affiliated Hospital of Sun Yat-sen University, Shenzhen 518107, China

Carolina Furtado and Juliana D. Siqueira
Instituto Nacional de Câncer (INCA), Rio de Janeiro, Brazil

Ahidjo Ayouba and Martine Peeters
UMI233/INSERM1175 Institut de Recherche pour le Développement (IRD), University of Montpellier, Montpellier, France

Mirela D'arc, Héctor N. Seuánez and Marcelo A. Soares
Instituto Nacional de Câncer (INCA), Rio de Janeiro, Brazil
Universidade Federal do Rio de Janeiro (UFRJ), Rio de Janeiro, Brazil

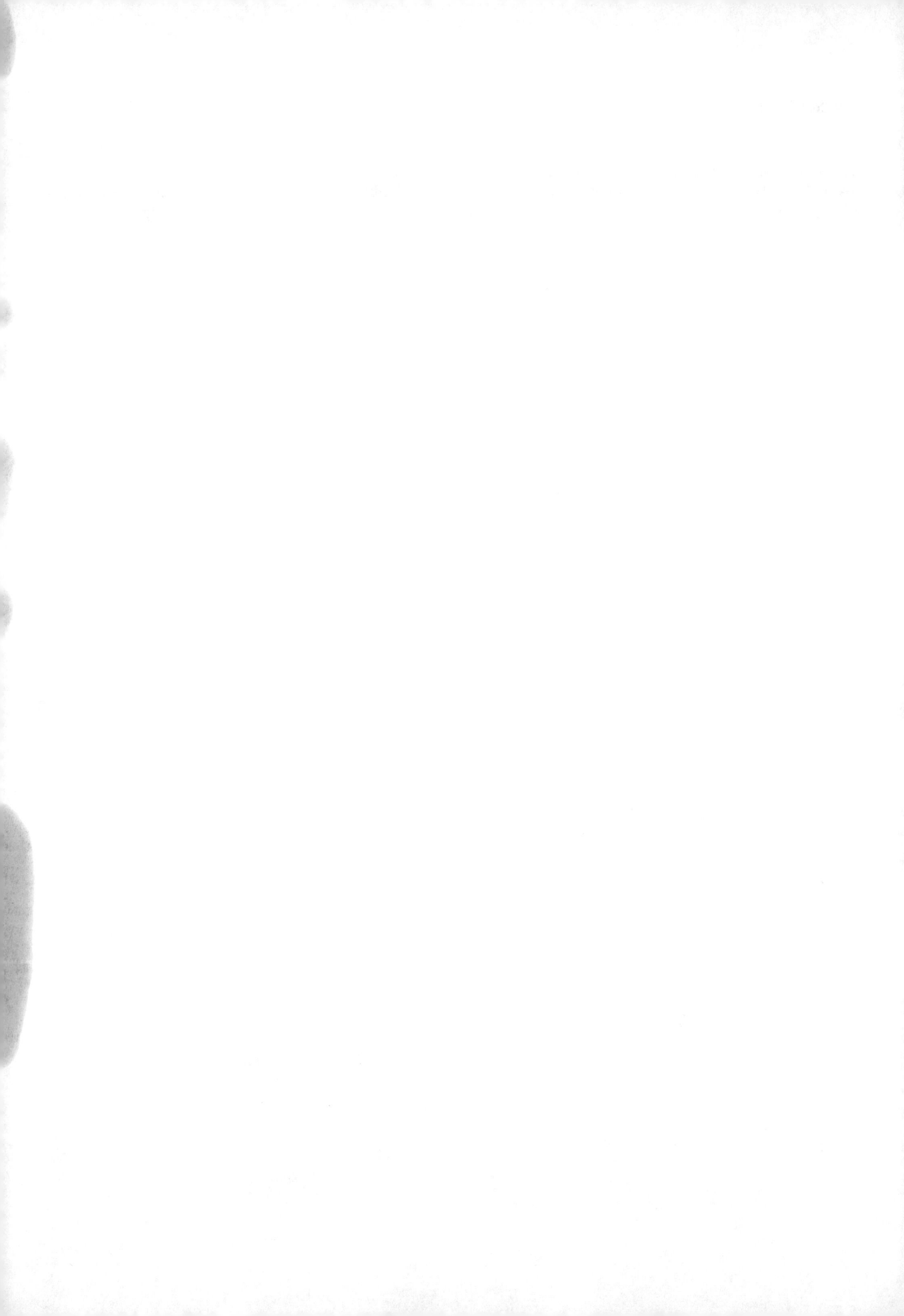

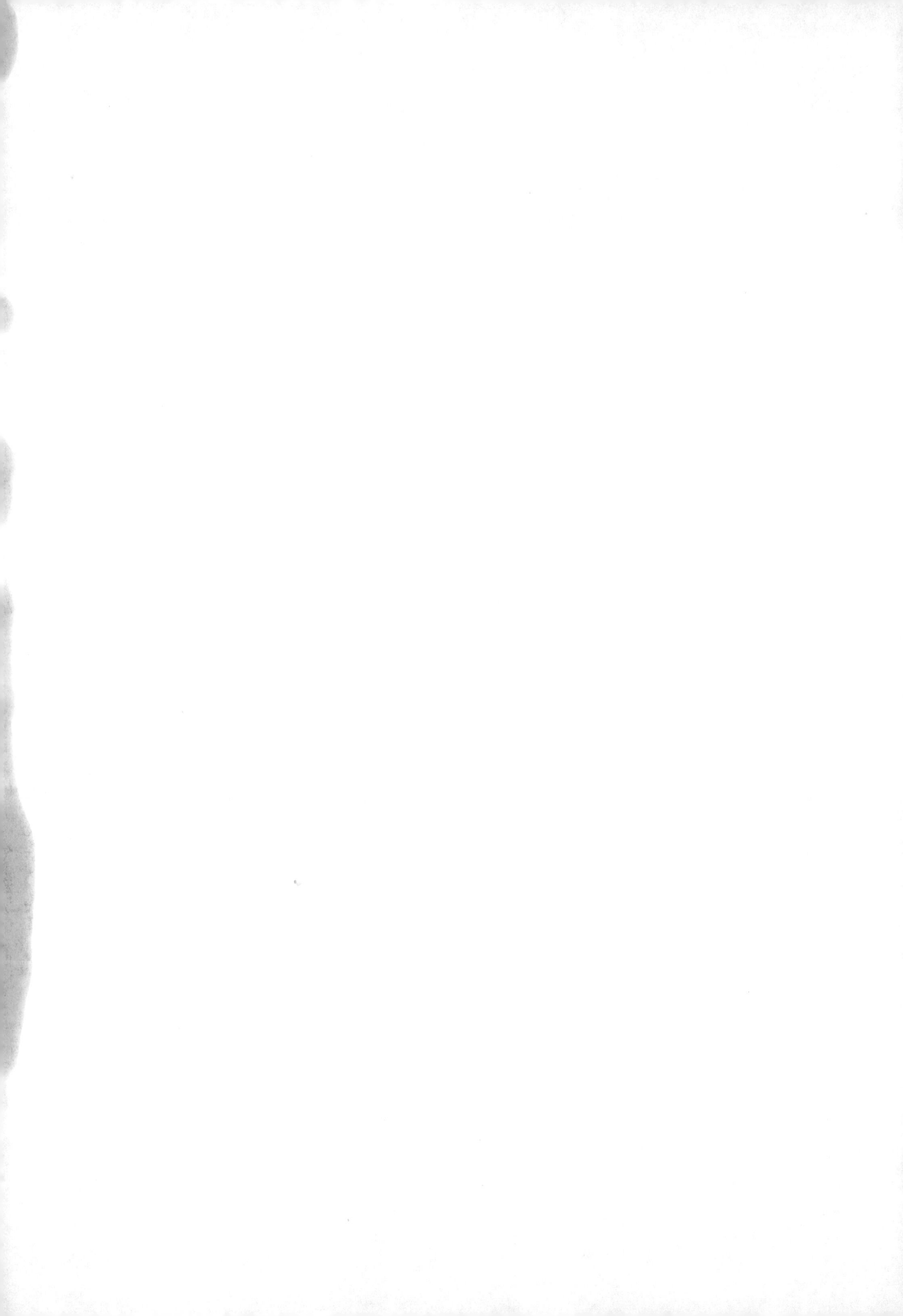

www.ingramcontent.com/pod-product-compliance
Lightning Source LLC
Chambersburg PA
CBHW061257190326
41458CB00011B/3694